Molecular Biology Intelligence Unit

MHC Ligands and Peptide Motifs

Hans-Georg Rammensee
Jutta Bachmann
Stefan Stevanović
University of Tübingen
Tübingen, Germany

Springer-Verlag
Berlin Heidelberg GmbH

LANDES BIOSCIENCE
Austin, Texas
U.S.A.

Molecular Biology Intelligence Unit

MHC Ligands and Peptide Motifs

LANDES BIOSCIENCE
Austin, Texas, U.S.A.

Springer

International ISBN 978-3-662-22164-8

While the authors, editors and publisher believe that drug selection and dosage and the specifications and usage of equipment and devices, as set forth in this book, are in accord with current recommendations and practice at the time of publication, they make no warranty, expressed or implied, with respect to material described in this book. In view of the ongoing research, equipment development, changes in governmental regulations and the rapid accumulation of information relating to the biomedical sciences, the reader is urged to carefully review and evaluate the information provided herein.

Library of Congress Cataloging-in-Publication Data

Rammensee, Hans-Georg, 1953- .
MHC ligands and peptide motifs / Hans-Georg Rammensee, Jutta Bachmann, Stefan Stevanović
p. cm. — (Molecular biology intelligence unit)
Includes bibliographical references and index.
ISBN 978-3-662-22164-8 ISBN 978-3-662-22162-4 (eBook)
DOI 10.1007/978-3-662-22162-4
1. Major histocompatibility complex. I. Bachmann, Jutta, 1961- . II. Stevanović, Stefan, 1959- . III. Title. IV. Series.
[DNLM: 1. Major Histocompatibility Complex--physiology. WO 680 R174m 1997]
QR184.315.R35 1997
616.07'9—dc21
DNLM/DLC
for Library of Congress 97-18997
CIP

Publisher's Note

Landes Bioscience produces books in six Intelligence Unit series: *Medical, Molecular Biology, Neuroscience, Tissue Engineering, Biotechnology* and *Environmental*. The authors of our books are acknowledged leaders in their fields. Topics are unique; almost without exception, no similar books exist on these topics.

Our goal is to publish books in important and rapidly changing areas of bioscience for sophisticated researchers and clinicians. To achieve this goal, we have accelerated our publishing program to conform to the fast pace at which information grows in bioscience. Most of our books are published within 90 to 120 days of receipt of the manuscript. We would like to thank our readers for their continuing interest and welcome any comments or suggestions they may have for future books.

Shyamali Ghosh
Publications Director
Landes Bioscience

CONTENTS

PREFACE

This book is not a textbook on a subdiscipline of immunology. It is an attempt to combine a wealth of information on the peptides associated with MHC molecules, a wealth that has been accumulated since 1990 in an astonishing speed, much to the amazement of the authors who witnessed the excitement around the discovery of the first few of these peptides. This book has been written and put together for all those somehow practically or theoretically involved with MHC-associated peptides—immunologists dealing with antigen-specific T-cell responses involved in the defense against viruses, bacteria, parasites, and malignancies, or with T cell responses causing autoimmune disease and allergy, as well as in the development of T cells, that is, positive and negative selection and T cell activation. Working with related problems ourselves, we felt the need for a handy source of information containing not only MHC peptide motifs, MHC ligands and T cell epitopes, but also the amino acid sequences of MHC molecules, in order to consider the structural basis for MHC motifs, that is, the nature of the pockets. Thus, this book is for our own use in the first place; since the number of people dealing with MHC-associated peptides must be rather high (we get quite a number of information requests) we thought that this book should be useful and of interest to all those people.

The core of this book is the collection of motifs, ligands, and T cell epitopes, and the relation of motifs to pocket composition. The meaning of this information in the context of the immune response is also addressed, i.e., the events before ligand and MHC get together, and the reaction of T cells against the final MHC/peptide complex. These parts, unfortunately, had to be kept somewhat superficial in order to stay within the size limit.

In collecting the data covered, we tried to be as accurate and as comprehensive as possible. Given the vast amount of data to be screened, however, we are afraid that some MHC ligands or even motifs have been omitted inadvertently. We apologize in advance for this and also for any errors that were overlooked in spite of very thorough cross-checking. The T cell epitopes included should be looked at as a representative selection rather than as a complete collection. Especially for class II-restricted T cell epitopes, but also for HIV-epitopes, we found it difficult to extract and judge for relevance all the peptide sequences reported to be recognized by T cells. The T cell epitopes that are covered, as well as some additional aspects, are influenced by our personal bias, e.g., MHC I-related items are usually given slightly more attention than those connected with class II.

We gratefully acknowledge the impact and help of many individuals who made this work possible: Jan Klein, to whom we owe our familiarity with MHC; Kirsten Falk and Olaf Rötzschke, who started the work on acid extraction of MHC-associated peptides in this laboratory and the many other coworkers who have continued in this field; Günther Jung and his colleagues, who shared their expertise in peptide chemistry with us; Niels Emmerich and Thomas Seitz, who extracted the new MHC motifs, ligands and T cell epitopes from the literature, and organized the new information; Thomas Friede, who checked part of the class II listings; Tilman Dumrese, who collected the minor H epitopes; Lynne Yakes, who translated passages into English and carried out all the secretarial work with the help of Petra Fellhauer; Patricia Hrstić for checking the many tables; Hansjörg Schild, Tobias Dick, and Christian Münz for their comments on Chapter 5 and for contributing illustrations; all the remaining members of our group who contributed knowledge and ideas in continuous discussion; Werner Mayer for critically reading chapter 2; John Trowsdale and R. Duncan Campbell for contributing an excellent figure on MHC gene organization; Steven Marsh for the preprint of the 'Nomenclature for factors of the HLA system, 1996'; all the editors and authors who allowed the reproduction of materials and who shared unpublished information, preprints, and reprints with us. In addition to these individuals, we would like to thank the organizations supporting our practical and theoretical work: Max Planck Institute for Biology, Tübingen; German Cancer Research Center, Heidelberg; University of Tübingen; Deutsche Forschungsgemeinschaft; Bundesministerium für Bildung, Wissenschaft, Forschung und Technologie; and Hoffman-La Roche.

Finally, we hope that our efforts in collecting, weighing, and organizing data related to MHC function will be useful for the advance of our understanding of the immune system, and for progress in prevention and treatment of infectious, autoimmune and malignant diseases.

Tübingen, March 1997

Hans-Georg Rammensee
Jutta Bachmann
Stefan Stevanović

CHAPTER 1

History and Overview

HISTORY

The traits of *MHC* genes have been noticed as early as in the beginning of the 20th century: a tumor grafted from a mouse to a genetically different mouse was rejected, whereas a tumor transplanted to a mouse of the same strain was not rejected. Thus, the tumor was not rejected on account of tumor-specific antigens but rather because of genetic differences between the mouse strains involved.[1] It was not until 1936, however, that what is now known as the MHC was discovered by Peter Gorer, then in London.[2] He had produced a rabbit-anti-mouse serum for the sake of blood group studies. The reactivity of this serum, called Nr. II, showed a striking correlation with tumor rejection: a tumor of the mouse strain A was rejected by C57 mice and in a certain proportion of (A x C57)F_1 x C57 backcross mice. All mice not reactive with the serum rejected the tumor. On the other hand, those mice rejecting the tumor developed antibodies with the same reactivity as rabbit serum Nr. II. Thus, it appeared that what caused tumor rejection was a blood-group like antigen shared by normal and tumor cells.[2] Since this antigen was originally discovered because of its recognition by rabbit anti-mouse serum Nr. II and because it resulted in tumor rejection, it was called histocompatibility antigen 2 or H-2—not immediately, however, but about 10 years later by George Snell and Gorer.[1]

George Snell then went on and started to isolate this and other histocompatibility genes in the form of congenic strains. For this project, he replaced tumor transplantations by skin grafting. This had two advantages: the rejection process was easier to follow and, more importantly, those mice not rejecting did survive and could be used for further breeding.

It turned out that the different mouse strains harbored a large number of such *H* genes; the latter could be grouped, however, into those causing fast rejection of skin grafts (within 20 days) and those taking many weeks or months. Those *H* genes with the strong effect were called major *H* genes, as opposed to the others, the minor *H* genes.[3,4,5] When it was found later that the major *H* genes of the mouse were all located within a cluster on chromosome 17, they were called the 'H-2 complex' and the corresponding gene groups in other species (the next was the chicken) were called major histocompatibility complexes.

After Snell had received his Nobel Prize for his contribution to MHC genetics, he visited Jan Klein in Tübingen and I, Hans-Georg Rammensee, was therefore fortunate enough to meet him in person and to discuss my studies on minor *H* genes in wild mice with him.[6]

While the mouse MHC was discovered by a combination of transplantation studies (histogenetics) and serological methods, the human MHC was discovered entirely by

MHC Ligands and Peptide Motifs, by Hans-Georg Rammensee, Jutta Bachmann, Stefan Stevanović.

antibodies (reviewed in ref. 1). In 1952, Jean Dausset in Paris found that some blood transfusion recipients produced antibodies able to agglutinate donor leukocytes.[7] Rose Payne at Stanford extended these studies and in 1958 discovered that mothers produced antibodies against the paternal leukocyte antigens expressed by their children. The same observation was made independently by Jon van Rood in Leiden, who wrote a most impressive PhD thesis about this discovery and the extensive serological studies it made possible. I am fortunate enough to be in possession of a signed copy of this, "perhaps the most famous thesis ever written."[1] Like the other workers of that time, van Rood had to struggle with extensive checkerboard tables indicating which antibody lot had reacted with which leukocyte sample. It took a while and several International Histocompatibility Workshops until the conclusion was reached that all these leukocyte reactive antibodies that Dausset, Payne and van Rood worked on were the counterparts of the mouse H-2 antigen, and thus, the human MHC molecules. Likewise, it took a number of years until the name of the human MHC was fixed to be HLA—for human leukocyte antigen.

In the mid-sixties the word 'complex' in the term MHC was seen to have been given righteously: no other genetic system in man or mouse appeared to be more polymorphic. At the same time, nothing was known about the physiological function of MHC molecules; their involvement in allograft rejection could possibly not be their natural function. Two major conceptual achievements between 1965 and 1975 shed some light on MHC function and indicated that MHC molecules have something to do with normal immune responses. When Hugh McDevitt immunized mice with synthetic polypeptides produced by Michael Sela, some strains produced antibodies to certain polypeptides but not others, and other strains reacted with different patterns.[8] Thus, the reactivity against a given (simple) antigen was genetically controlled—as also found by B. Benacerraf; genes involved were called Immune response (*Ir*) genes.[9] Using mice, H.O. McDevitt discovered that these genes correlated strongly with the H-2 haplotype.[10] Thus, MHC genes were likely to have something to do with the regulation of the immune response. The next major achievement was the discovery of MHC restriction by Zinkernagel and Doherty, then in Canberra, Australia. They studied the cellular immune response of several mouse strains against Lymphocytotropic choriomeningitis virus (LCMV). Target cells infected with LCMV were only killed if they shared MHC genes with the responder CTL. Thus, the CTL had 'dual specificity'; they not only recognized virus antigens on the infected cells but also depended somehow on MHC molecules expressed on the infected cell.[11] A similar but less clear conclusion had been drawn earlier upon the interaction between T (helper) and B cells by Berenice Kindred (then at the University of Konstanz) and Donald Shreffler: "Therefore the H-2 complex must play an active role in an enduring cooperation between bone marrow-derived (B) cells and thymus-derived (T) cells" (original citation see ref. 12). I was fortunate to have known Berenice personally; she was at the Max-Planck-Institut für Biologie in Tübingen for the last 5 years of her life (1980 to 1985), and I owe a good deal of immunological knowledge to her, as well as fruitful advice as to which laboratory I should choose for a postdoctoral fellowship.

Thus, in the mid-seventies it was known that both types of T cells—helpers and killers—recognized their antigen somehow together with MHC molecules. To recognize this, new cell culture techniques, such as the mixed lymphocyte reaction and the ^{51}Cr release assay pioneered by Mishell and Dutton[13] and Brunner and Cerrottini,[14] respectively, were instrumental. Using both techniques as in vitro correlates for allorejection, the MHC products were classified into two categories, one more efficiently stimulating CTL, the other more efficiently stimulating T cell proliferation in MLR. In 1979, Jan Klein introduced the now familiar terms MHC class I and class II for the two categories,[15] which, as we now know, differ in their function. Class II molecules are responsible for the Kindred/Shreffler phenomenon, whereas the Doherty/Zinkernagel observation is based on the function of class I molecules.

The few years after the discovery of MHC restriction were characterized by intense speculation on the nature of the molecular interaction between MHC, the antigen and the then elusive T cell receptor. Two issues were heatedly debated. One was the nature of the T cell receptor. Two hypotheses were popularly used to account for MHC-restriction: one, called the dual receptor hypothesis, postulated the existence of two different T cell receptors, one for the MHC molecule, the other for the antigen. The other, called the altered self hypothesis, assumed only one receptor with low affinity for self MHC; if the self MHC molecule is 'altered' somehow by foreign antigen, the receptor gains high affinity for the complex. These discussions were both complicated as well as inspired by Michael Bevan's discovery of positive selection of T cells by thymic tissue.[16] The other issue of debate was the nature of antigen-MHC interaction. One school believed in determinant selection (that is, MHC molecules somehow bind antigen directly, possibly as fragments).[17,18] This view was opposed by the assumption that MHC and antigen do not bind each other directly, or at least not specifically but rather are somehow connected via the T cell receptor.

All this was in the absence of any information on the T cell receptor or on the structure of MHC molecules. It was a great relief, therefore, when T cell receptors could be precipitated with monoclonal antibodies and the first T cell receptor genes (for the TCR β chain) were cloned and sequenced by Mark Davis and Tak Mak and their respective colleagues.[19,20]

A further step in the unraveling of MHC function was the discovery of the fragmentary nature of the antigen recognized by T cells together with MHC. Class II restricted T cells recognize fragments of antigen, whereby the fragmented antigen produced by macrophages can be replaced by a protease digest of the protein antigen, even if the antigen-presenting cells are fixed and not able to process antigen any more.[21,22] For class II-presented antigens, this came not as a surprise, at least to most researchers, since handling or 'processing' of antigens by macrophages was a familiar aspect.[23] A surprise, however, was the demonstration by Alan Townsend that class I-restricted antigens, as required by virus-specific CTL, are also fragments of the entire protein antigen[24] that can be replaced by exogenously added synthetic peptides.[25]

Sequence determination,[26] protein isolation[27,28] and finally crystallization and X-ray crystallography[29] allowed for the emergence of the view of the trimolecular complex between MHC molecule, antigenic peptide and T cell receptor as it is familiar to us now. However, the nature of the peptide in the MHC was still elusive. In 1989,[30] and even later, the peptide was still viewed as being in an α-helical conformation. Elution and sequence determination of individual and pooled MHC I ligands in 1990/91[31-33] identified the primary structure of such peptides as nonamers and produced the first peptide motifs. Finally, crystals with single peptide ligands[34,35] showed the extended conformation of the peptides, the detailed molecular interaction between peptide and MHC, and explained the allele-specific peptide motifs detected by peptide sequencing. With a few years delay, the corresponding information on MHC II molecules was obtained. The first identification of naturally processed class II ligands was published in 1991 by A. Rudensky et al from Charles Janeway's laboratory,[36] followed soon after by several other reports.[37-39] Allele-specific class II motifs were not evident immediately because class II-associated peptides are not uniform in length and not in a uniform frame, in contrast to class I ligands. Alignments of individual ligands did not help much to produce motifs. However, peptide-binding assays gave the first hints of anchors,[40] and binding assays using peptide libraries,[41,42] as well as pool sequencing of natural ligand mixtures,[39] gave indications about class II motifs that were placed on a molecular basis and explanation when a complex of a class II molecule, DR1, with an individual peptide ligand was crystallized and its structure determined by the Wiley laboratory.[43,44]

As of today, we know of a large number of better motifs and ligands and, thanks to the crystal structures, we have a good idea how the peptides interact with the MHC binding groove. The wealth of information on MHC associated peptides is the focus of this book.

OVERVIEW

The Transfer of Information by MHC Molecules

The function of MHC molecules is to transfer information about the current stock of proteins within a cell to the cell surface. This enables the immune system to survey the cell's general condition, allowing it, if necessary, to react. How the immune system then reacts depends on the circumstances and can range from the killing of a virus-infected cell by a cytotoxic T lymphocyte to the activation of a B cell by a helper T lymphocyte.

In order to comprehend the immune system, especially if one's interest lies in manipulating it in some way, a precise understanding of the function of the MHC is absolutely necessary. At the present time, the targeted activation of T cells that can destroy tumors, along with the targeted inhibition of autoreactive T cells, would seem to be within our grasp. In addition, we should also consider the function of the MHC in the design and development of new vaccines.

Terms

MHC stands for major histocompatibility complex and the designation can only be fully comprehended against its historical background. The first most obvious characteristic of MHC gene products was their tissue compatibility: skin or a tumor that is transplanted from one mouse to another is rejected if the donating and the receiving mice have a different MHC. Today, we would call MHC molecules 'antigen presenters' or 'peptide announcers' because we are acquainted with their physiological function. MHC is merely a generic term for categorizing the respective genes or molecules of all species. Furthermore, the MHC of every species has its own name, such as H-2 for the mouse MHC, B for the domestic fowl, and HLA (Human Leukocyte Antigen) for the human MHC. The designations for the remaining species have been applied somewhat more systematically; we have BoLA for cattle, for example, or RhLA for the rhesus monkey.

There are two classes of MHC molecules that differ in both structure and function, and therefore will be dealt with separately at a later point. The class I MHC molecules are expressed on most mammalian cells, whereas class II molecules are found only on very few cell types, most important of which are B cells, macrophages, dendritic cells and the thymic epithelium.

Genes and the Primary Structure

An MHC molecule of class I, or MHC class I molecule for short, consists of a heavy chain of approximately 350 amino acids (AA) with three sections that are similar to immunoglobulin domains and a transmembrane region, as well as a noncovalently bound light chain of 112 AA that comprises one domain only. In humans, the genes for the heavy chains in the MHC region are located on the short arm of chromosome 6. The gene for the light chain, which is also known as β2-microglobulin, is on chromosome 15. In addition to the 'classical' *MHC class I* genes *HLA-B*, *-C* and *-A* (Fig. 1.1), whose function has already been characterized, humans possess a whole series of class I genes such as *HLA-E*, *-F* and *-G*, the functions of which still have not been described in any detail.

MHC class II molecules consist of two chains of approximately equal size (250 AA), α and β, both of which contain two immunoglobulin-like domains and a transmembrane region. All *MHC* class *II* genes are found within the *MHC* region on chromosome 6; *DRA*, *DQA* and *DPA* code for the α chains, *DRB1*, *DQB* and *DPB* for the corresponding β chains (Fig. 1.1).

One prominent characteristic of the *MHC* genes is their enormous polymorphism (see Chapter 2). There are, for example, over 180 *HLA-B* alleles and over 190 *HLA-DRB* alleles in the population that not only differ to a great extent in their sequences, but also in their function as peptide receptors. The number of known *HLA* alleles for each locus is presented in Figure 1.1. Along with the *MHC* genes, there are also several other genes in the *MHC* region whose products play a role in the function of the MHC, in particular that of loading it with information in the form of peptides. These are the peptide transporter, TAP; the proteasome subunits LMP2 and LMP7; and the chaperones DMA and DMB. The remaining genes that are found in the *MHC* region (e.g., those for enzymes) have nothing to do with the function of the MHC.

Structure of the MHC

The two domains, α1 and α2, in the MHC class I heavy chain that are furthest away from the membrane form a peptide-binding groove (Fig. 1.2) that tightly holds a peptide normally comprising 9 amino acids in place in the final MHC class I molecule by means of its noncovalent binding ability. N and C termini of these peptides are fixed in the ends of the groove and several side chains fill complementary pockets in the class I groove. The organization and specificity of the pockets differ among the various allelic products (see Chapter 3). Further side chains can be reached on the surface of the complex.

In the case of class II molecules, a similar peptide-binding groove is formed by the α1 and β1 domains furthest away from the membrane in both chains (Fig. 1.2). The binding capabilities exert their effects chiefly between the backbone of the peptide and the peptide-binding groove along a section of 9 amino acids in a peptide of variable length. The N and C termini of the peptides are not fixed in the groove; side chains located in certain defined positions in the 9-amino acid stretch in the groove interact in a similar way with complementary pockets, as is the case with class I (see Chapter 3).

Loading of MHC Class I Molecules

The function of an MHC class I molecule is to acquire a selection of peptides that result from protein degradation in the cytosol and lumen of the endoplasmic reticulum (ER) and to transport them to the surface of the cell. Loading of the class I MHC molecule takes place after renewed synthesis in the ER. In a sense, the peptide is actually part of the final molecule that thus consists of three noncovalently bound parts: the heavy chain, β2-microglobulin and the peptide.

The path leading to development of the peptides is also termed antigen processing (see also Chapter 4b), although in most cases the MHC class I ligands are not antigens. The path resulting in the appearance of class I ligands is not yet understood in detail but it basically takes the following course (Fig. 1.3). A protein in the cytosol is degraded by the proteasome into peptides. Both the 26S proteasome that cleaves ubiquitinated proteins and the 20S proteasome are involved in degradation. The natural substrate type for the 20S proteasome has not yet been precisely determined; it could either be denatured protein or protein fragments produced by different proteases, including the 26S proteasome. The elucidation of the structure of a bacterial proteasome (from the archebacterium *Thermoplasma acidophilum*) revealed it to be barrel-shaped and to consist of 28 subunits arranged into four sets of seven rings, one on top of the other. The two inner sets of rings were found to be made up of β-subunits and the two outer sets of rings of α-subunits. The proteolytically active centers, which are novel threonine protease sites, are located next to the β-subunits, although only three of the seven centers are active in the eukaryotic proteasome with a chymo-trypsin, trypsin and peptidyl-glutamyl-peptide hydrolytic specificity. The distance between each of the seven active centers located in the β-ring is 28Å in the *Thermoplasma* proteasome, giving an extended peptide length of approximately nine AA. One can thus view the series of octamers to dodecamers produced by this proteasome as products of a double cleavage. As far as the eukaryotic proteasome is concerned, in which the position of the three different active centers has not yet been published, single cleavage is carried out by the normal 20S proteasome.

Three of the constitutive β-subunits are replaced by LMP2, LMP7 and MECL1 upon interferon-γ (IFNγ) induction, for example during a viral infection of the cell. Furthermore, IFNγ induces the PA28 regulator (a complex of rings made up of three α and three β subunits) to bind to the rings of the 20S proteasome that consist of α-subunits. The 20S proteasome/PA28 complex then cuts peptides with a length of 9-11 AA from the longer stretches of peptides by double cleavage; these have exactly the right length for MHC class I transport.[46] The dominant class I ligands, which as such have a large number of copies per cell, are presumably produced directly by this method (e.g., SYFPEITHI from the tyrosine kinase JAK1), whereas other ligands have to be shortened by exopeptidase after leaving the proteasome (e.g., YPHFMPTNL from the pp89 protein of the mouse cytomegalovirus). The peptides that come from the proteasome are transported into the ER by the peptide transporter TAP (transporter associated with antigen processing), a heterodimer comprising the subunits TAP-1 and TAP-2 coded in the MHC region.

It is not known how peptides reach the TAP from the proteasome; it is possible that chaperones such as Hsc70 play a role in this process. The TAP transports in an ATP-dependent way preferentially chosen peptides with a length of 7-13 AA; again, this is the length that conforms to the class I ligands. Apart from this, the human TAP is only selective to a very minor degree. Peptides with proline at position 2, for example, are only transported poorly. In contrast, the mouse transporter is selective for peptides with a hydrophobic C-terminus. If a peptide reaches the luminal TAP end, its fate depends on several factors. Many class I molecules, such as HLA-A2, for example, bind to TAP via the adapter molecule tapasin.[47] If the newly arriving peptide fits into the groove of such an MHC molecule it binds to it and the fully loaded MHC molecule is subsequently liberated from its helper molecules and brought to the cell surface in the usual way. A newly synthesized MHC class I molecule must go through several stages before it can bind peptide: to begin with, the chaperone calnexin assists in folding the newly-synthesized heavy chain. After β2-microglobulin is bound to this new heavy chain, the heterodimer associates with calreticulin; this complex is then the one that finally binds to the TAP by means of tapasin.

If by any chance the peptide that arrives via the TAP does not immediately fit the TAP-bound MHC molecule, or if the MHC molecule is unable to bind to TAP, as is the case with a number of HLA-B molecules, what happens next is not known. It probably binds to protein disulfide isomerase representing the dominant acceptor for TAP-translocated peptides.[48] It might also bind to gp96[49,50] which is also able to accept peptides but with a lower affinity.[51] From these molecules, it may be transferred to a newly synthesized MHC class I molecule that is still associated with calreticulin or prior to this it may even be shortened by exopeptidase.[52] Of the peptides that arrive via the TAP in the ER, 95% probably do not fit the peptide specificity of the MHC molecules available; these have to be disposed of by some means. They may be handed over to exporters such as SEC61 by the luminal peptide acceptors and be carried by these into the cytosol to be degraded, as is the case with misfolded proteins; they may even be degraded immediately in the ER.[53,54] Along the lines described here, part of the peptides produced by the protein turnover will always be removed, placed onto class I molecules, and transported to the cell surface. Selection of the relevant peptides depends more or less on the peptide specificity of the MHC molecules.

Peptide Specificity of MHC Class I Molecules

Of the 83 HLA-A, 186 HLA-B and 46 HLA-C allelic products, every single one has its own individual peptide specificity that is defined primarily by the position and specificity of the pockets that accommodate the side chains of the anchoring amino acids and secondarily by interactions and non-anchoring amino acid residues of the peptides. The allelic dependence of MHC peptide specificity is easy to understand in the light of the fact that not only the pockets but also those remaining parts of the groove that come into contact with the peptide are strongly affected by MHC polymorphism. Table 1.1 lists MHC ligands showing the anchoring amino acids in bold print in order to emphasize the peptide specificity or the peptide motifs of individual MHC molecules. Information on the allelic specificity of the motifs (including preferences and abhorrences beyond the anchor, as already mentioned) enable the prediction of MHC ligands and thus also T cell epitopes. The central part of this book deals with this subject (see Chapter 4).

T Cell Response (MHC Class I Molecules)

A normal cell presents approximately 10^4 different peptides on its 10^5 to 10^6 MHC class I molecules; the individual numbers of peptides range between 1 and over 10,000. All of these peptides originate from normal cell proteins and the immune system (or more precisely, the relevant class I restricted L subpopulation of $CD8^+$ T cells) is tolerant of these peptides, whether as a result of negative selection during T cell differentiation in the thymus or by peripheral mechanisms of tolerance. If new peptides join the 10^4 self peptides already present, for example, after a virus infection of the cell, these can be recognized by $CD8^+$ T cells as foreign. However, there are further prerequisites for the primary activation of virus-specific T cells beyond those centered around the appearance of new peptides, namely antigen presentation on dendritic cells in combination with soluble 'stress' mediators. In such a case, the heterodimer consisting of α- and β-chains in the T cell receptor binds to the MHC:peptide complex. The signal transfer to the T cell takes place by means of the CD3 molecules that belong to the T cell receptor complex but in addition, costimulatory acceptor molecules such as CD28 on the T cell must be occupied on the antigen-presenting cell by binding to costimulator molecules such as B7. The border between self and foreign is not clearly defined during T-cell recognition. T cells, for example, can be stimulated to react against self peptides that are present on normal cells in only small numbers. Several tumor-destroying $CD8^+$ T cells are actually targeted against normal self peptides that are expressed at a higher density in tumors than in normal tissue. (One example is tyrosinase in melanomas: YMNGTMSQV is recognized on HLA-A1.) Further targets of tumor-destroying CTL possibly include oncogene products, mutations in normal proteins, tumor-suppressing gene products, tissue-specific proteins and aberrantly expressed proteins.

'MHC class I-restricted T cells' is the designation for T cells that recognize peptide on MHC class I. They are not only important for combating virus-infected and malignant cells, but also for removing cells that are infested by parasites or infected by certain bacteria (see Chapter 5).

Loading of MHC Class II Molecules

The class II α and β chains that are newly synthesized in the ER first associate with a multipurpose molecule similar to a chaperone, the membrane-inserted so-called invariant chain (Ii), to form nonamers; complexes of three αβ dimers and three invariant chains are thus assembled (see also Chapter 4). As the Ii chain is able to close the MHC class II groove with its middle section, it is impossible for peptides in the ER, such as those of the class I loading pathway, to enter the groove. One additional function of the invariant chain is to direct the class II molecules into a special lysosome-like vesicle that is termed MHC class II-loading compartment, MIIC. It is here that loading of the peptides takes place. First of all, the invariant chain is proteolytically degraded by cathepsin S,[55] leaving short peptides called CLIPs (for class II-associated invariant chain peptide) that stay for the time being in the MHC groove and block it (Fig. 1.4). To exchange CLIPs for 'proper' peptides (that is, prospective MHC class II ligands), one further accessory molecule is required, HLA-DM. HLA-DM is again one of the antigen-processing accessory molecules that are coded in the MHC region, and comprise the heterodimer DMA/DMB. DM exchanges CLIPs for peptides emerging from lysosomal proteolysis. The exact mechanism of this exchange has yet to be elucidated. DM exhibits strong homology to MHC class II molecules and it was therefore originally believed to possess a peptide-binding groove that enabled it to absorb the CLIPs from the MHC class II groove, thereby liberating it. DM-associated peptides have, however, not yet been discovered. The 'proper' peptide ligands that were exchanged for CLIPs are produced by a whole series of lysosomal proteases, such as cathepsin D, that function in acidic pH. It is very likely that exopeptidases such as aminopeptidase N (CD13) are involved in the production. This conclusion is drawn from the appearance of Pro in position 2 of the class II ligands that has often been observed. The exact location within the cells during peptide production for MHC class II loading has still to be determined: Do proteolysis and loading take place in the same compartment? If not, how do peptides enter the loading compartment, by fusion of vesicles or by some form of transporter mechanism? The peptides that are sent into the class II loading pathway nevertheless usually arise from vesicle-associated proteins; they are either membrane-bound proteins or proteins that have entered the vesicle by means of phagocytosis, endocytosis, or pinocytosis. The fully loaded MHC class II molecules, comprising α and β chains and the peptide, are finally transported to the cell surface. If loaded MHC class II molecules reach an acidic vesicle again, for example during the process of phagocytosis, the bound peptides can be released and exchanged for others, because the MHC class II peptide association becomes labile in acidic environments.

Peptide Specificity of MHC Class II Molecules

Here again, the pockets and the regions of the MHC molecule that otherwise interact with the bound peptide are most particularly affected by MHC polymorphism. Of the nine amino acids in a typical class II ligand (consisting altogether of 12-25 amino acids), between three and four are anchored in the pockets. Specificity and spacing of the pockets define primarily the peptide specificity of every allelic product. As in the case of class I, the nonanchoring amino acids play a secondary but still significant role. The pocket specificity ranges from extremely high for the acidic amino acid residues Asp or Glu to very degenerative for all amino acids with the exception of the basic amino acids (see Chapter 3). A number of class II ligand examples are listed in Table 1.1 in order to illustrate the allele-specific peptide motifs of class II molecules; chapter 4 contains detailed lists of ligands and motifs. As several closely related class II alleles that are associated to a varying degree with autoimmune diseases differ in their peptide specificity, one could conclude that the variance in presented peptides is in some way connected with such diseases (see Chapter 5).

T Cell Response (MHC Class II Molecules)

The T cells that are associated with MHC class II molecules belong to the subpopulation of $CD4^+$ T cells. If such a T cell recognizes a foreign MHC class II presented peptide on a professional antigen-presenting cell (a macrophage or dendritic cell) and if a 'stress' signal is also present, the T cell is activated to produce cytokines such as IL-2, IL-4 and IFNγ. The spectrum of produced cytokines depends on the background of the T cell as well as the respective level of cytokines that are already available. The $CD4^+$ T cells can be divided into two subgroups according to the arrays of cytokines that they produce: T helper 1 (Th_1) cells with the leading cytokine IFNγ and Th_2 cells with the leading cytokine IL-4, although there are certain overlaps and exceptions. Th_1 cells are inflammatory and can bring about the destruction of extracellular parasites such as *Leishmania* by activating effector cells that are nonspecific for antigen. In addition, Th_1 cells are involved in B cell regulation. Th_2 cells are considered primarily as regulators of humoral immunity because they activate mainly B cells.

After a B cell has bound its antigen by means of its membrane-bound antigen receptors (immunoglobulin with its respective signal transduction molecules), it brings it to the degradation vesicle by receptor-induced endocytosis. The peptides produced by the antigen are loaded onto MHC class II molecules and can then be recognized by $CD4^+$ T cells on the cell surface. By doing so, B cells, and the T cells that regulate them, recognize different parts of the same antigen. The immunoglobulin, for example, may recognize the glycosyl residue of a glycoprotein, whereas the class II molecules, and as such the T cell, recognize a peptide from the protein section (see also Chapter 5).

If a $CD4^+$ T cell, which normally has already been activated by macrophages or dendritic cells, has bound the MHC class II peptide complex of an antigen-presenting B cell, activation of the B cell occurs by cell-cell contact and above all by cytokines: IL-4, for example, incites B cells to produce IgG1 and IgE; Th_2 cells are therefore also responsible for IgE-associated allergies. IL-5 drives IgA and INFγ IgG2a production.

Crosstalk

The main routes for peptide loading of MHC class I and class II molecules thus differ to a great extent. However, there are overlaps between the two that may have far-reaching consequences: even peptides from exogenous antigens can be bound to class I molecules after phagocytosis by macrophages or after being taken up in dendritic cells (see also Chapter 4b). This can take place both by infiltration of the exogenous antigen into the normal MHC class I pathway and by a different loading process in an endocytic vessel. MHC class I loading is particularly efficient when carried out with exogenous antigen that has been aggregated, for example by heat treatment or by binding to particles. Class I loading by exogenous antigen could be important for therapeutic use in developing new vaccines because in this process the activation of $CD8^+$ T cells is possible even without a vaccine that is capable of initiating infection. Of particular interest is the ability of one of the luminal ER peptide acceptor molecules, gp96, to transfer antigen to other cells along the MHC class I pathway. On the other hand, MHC class II molecules can be loaded with peptides from cytosolic proteins, whereby the loading takes place independently of the TAP. The protein, or a peptide derived from it, must therefore enter one of the vesicles by a different route.

CONCLUSION

The physiological function of MHC molecules is well established but even so, there is still a great deal to be learned about it. This includes the precise cleavage specificity of the proteases that are involved in antigen processing, such as proteasome and the cathepsins, as well as their regulation. In addition, we still know too little about the fate of the peptides and the steps that lead up to them. On the other hand, knowledge of the allelic specificity of MHC peptides can be applied to finding methods of manipulating the immune response against infection, malignant diseases and transplants, as well as in autoimmune diseases and other immunopathological cases (see also Chapter 5).

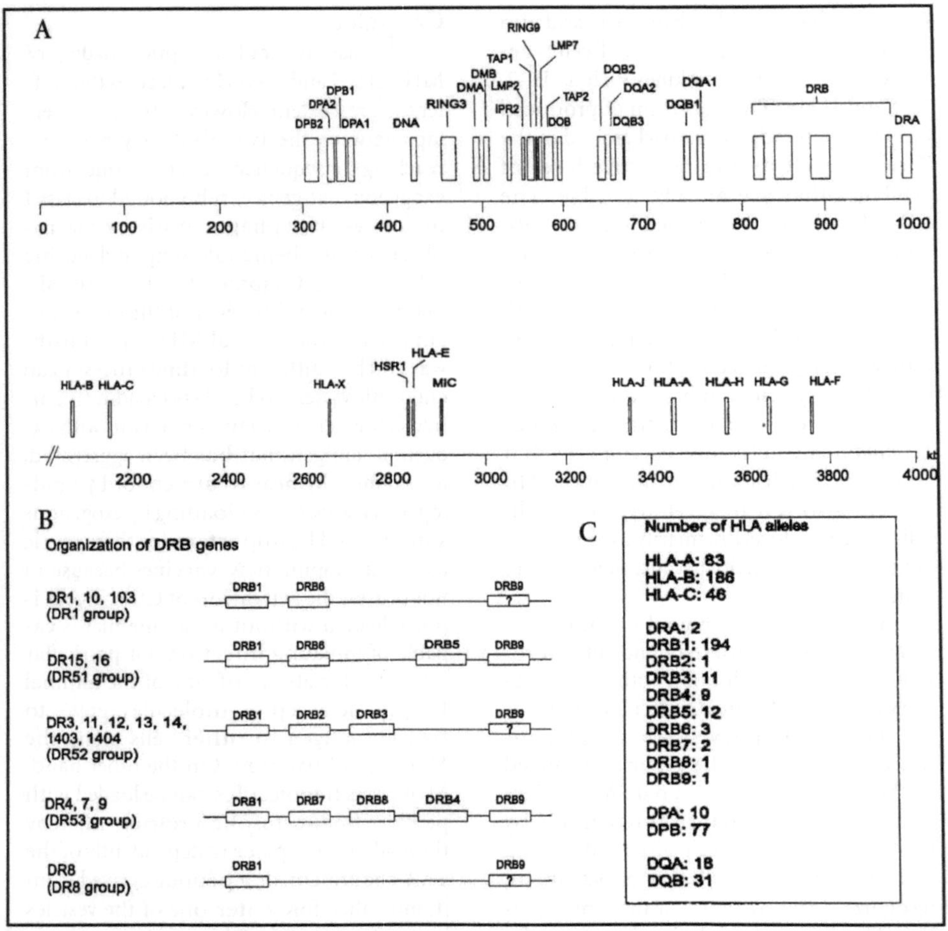

Fig. 1.1. A: Schematic map of the human MHC, B: *DRB* gene organization, C: number of alleles. The map has been modified from Campbell and Trowsdale, Immunol Today 1993;14:349-52. See ref. 45.

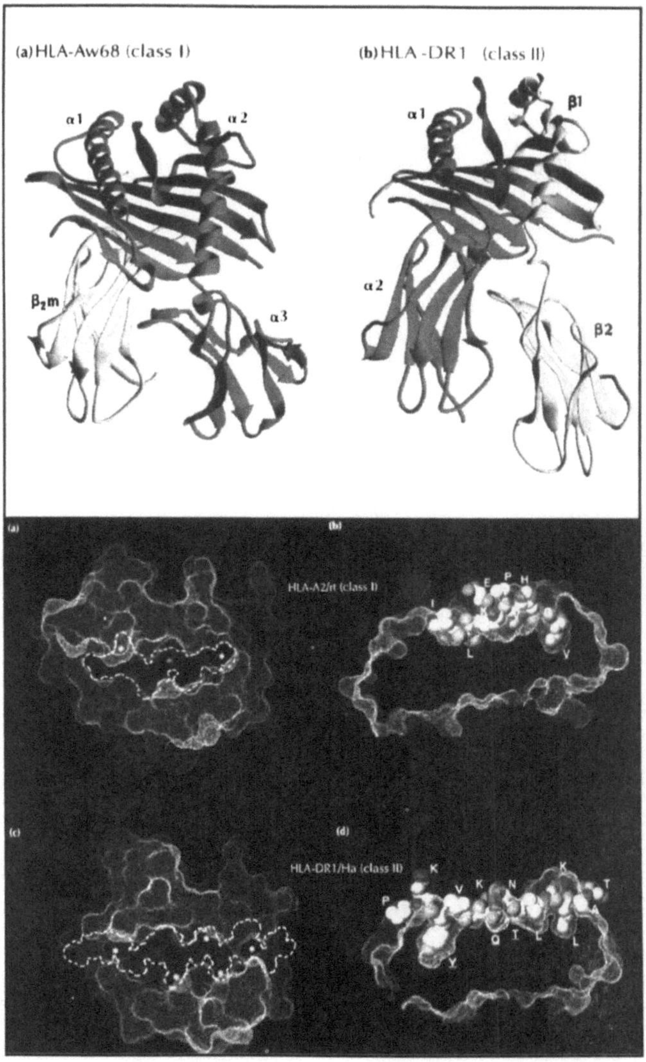

Fig. 1.2. MHC crystal structure. Top: Ribbon diagrams of HLA class I (HLA-Aw68) and class II (HLA-DR1) molecules.
Bottom: View of the peptide-binding groove of class I (HLA-A2) and class II (HLA-DR1) molecules
Left: Top view, with the peptide removed.
Right: Cross-section, bound peptide in colour. The peptide within the A2 molecule is ILKEPVHGH from the reverse transcriptase of HIV-1. L and V are anchors. The peptide within the HLA-DR1 molecule is PKYVKQNTLKLAT from Influenza hemagglutinin; Y, Q, T, and L are anchors. Reprinted with permission from: Stern LJ, Wiley DC. Structure 1994; 2:245-251 ©1994 Current Biology Limited.

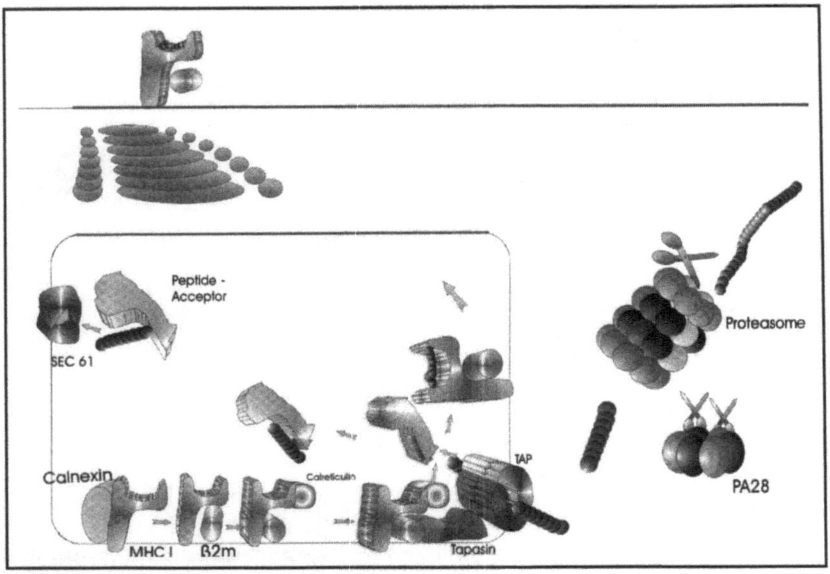

Fig. 1.3. Hypothetical and rather simplified overview of the interactions during peptide loading of MHC I: protein degradation in the cytosol, MHC assembly in the ER. Reprinted with permission from: Rammensee HG. Biospektrum 1997; 1:35-40 ©1997 Spektrum Akademischer Verlag.

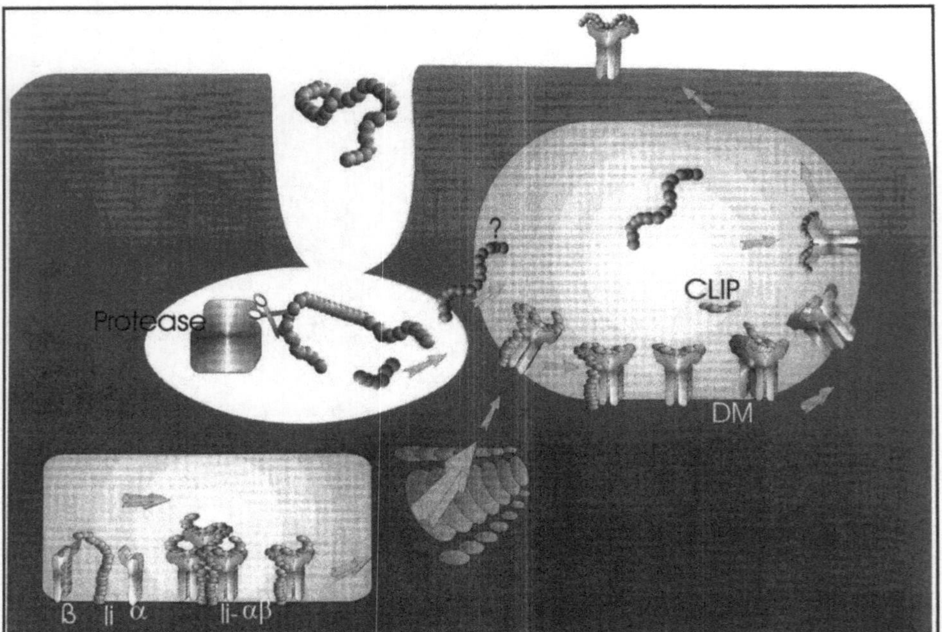

Fig. 1.4. Schematic representation of peptide loading of MHC class II molecules: Complex formation of α and β chains with the invariant chain to nonamers in the ER; the nonamers are later shown only as trimers. Removal of Ii, binding of peptide within the MHC class II loading compartment is shown. It has not yet been determined whether the proteolysis of the peptide donor (antigen) takes place in a separate compartment. Reprinted with permission from: Rammensee HG. Biospektrum 1997; 1:35-40 © 1997 Spektrum Akademischer Verlag.

Table 1.1 Examples for typical MHC associated peptides

a) MHC-I

MHC Molecule	Relative Peptide Position 1	2	3	4	5	6	7	8	9		Protein Source
HLA-A*0101	A	T	**D**	F	K	F	A	M	**Y**		Cyclin protein
	M	I	**E**	P	R	T	L	Q	**Y**		Ribosomal protein S16
	S	T	**D**	H	I	P	I	L	**Y**		Fructose-6-amino transferase
	S	S	**E**	Q	T	F	M	Y	**Y**		Ornithine decarboxylase
	E	A	**D**	P	T	G	H	S	**Y**		MAGE-1
	E	V	**D**	P	I	G	H	L	**Y**		MAGE-3
	C	T	**E**	L	K	L	S	D	**Y**		Influenza-nucleoprotein
HLA-A*0201	G	**I**	L	G	F	V	F	T	**L**		Influenza-matrix protein
	S	**L**	L	P	A	I	V	E	**L**		Protein phosphatase 2A
	Y	**L**	L	P	A	I	V	H	**I**		RNA-helicase
	Y	**M**	D	G	T	M	S	Q	**V**		Tyrosinase
	I	**L**	K	E	P	V	H	G	**V**		HIV-reverse transcriptase
HLA-B*2705	G	**R**	L	T	K	H	T	K	**F**		Ribosomal protein L
	T	**R**	Y	P	I	L	A	G	**H**		Cytochrome P450
	R	**R**	S	K	E	I	T	V	**R**		RNA-helicase
	S	**R**	Y	W	A	I	R	T	**R**		Influenza-nucleoprotein
	R	**R**	Y	P	D	A	V	Y	**L**		Measles F-protein
	R	**R**	I	Y	D	L	I	E	**L**		EBNA-6
	G	**R**	A	F	V	T	I	G	**K**		HIV-1 gp120
H-2K^d	S	**Y**	F	P	E	I	T	H	**I**		Tyrosine kinase JAK1
	T	**Y**	Q	R	T	R	A	L	**V**		Influenza-nucleoprotein
	G	**Y**	K	D	G	N	E	Y	**I**		Lysteriolysine O
	S	**Y**	I	P	S	A	E	K	**I**		*Plasmodium berghei* CSP
	K	**Y**	L	K	K	I	K	N	S	L	*P. falciparum* CSP

b) MHC-II

MHC Molecule		Relative Peptide Position 1	2	3	4	5	6	7	8	9		Protein Source
HLA-DRB1*0101	PK	**Y**	V	K	**Q**	N	**T**	L	K	**L**	AT	Influenza-hemagglutinin
	LAT	**W**	T	I	**Q**	G	**A**	A	N	**A**	LSGDVW	Transferrin receptor
	STPE	**F**	T	I	**L**	N	**T**	F	H	**I**	PSFTI	Apolipoprotein B
	LDHK	**F**	D	L	**M**	Y	**A**	K	R	**A**	FVHWY	Tubulin α1-chain
HLA-DRB1*0301	ISNQ	**L**	T	L	**D**	S	**N**	T	K	**Y**	FHKLN	Apolipoprotein B
	VDT	**F**	L	E	**D**	V	**K**	N	L	**Y**	HSEA	α1-antitrypsin
	KPRA	**I**	V	V	**D**	P	**V**	H	G	**F**	MY	LDL-receptor
	GPPKLD	**I**	R	K	**E**	E	**K**	Q	I	**M**	IDIFH	IFNγ-receptor
	GDVV	**A**	V	V	**D**	I	**K**	E	K	**G**	KDKWIELK	Lolium pollen protein
HLA-DRB1*0402	IKI	**I**	S	K	**I**	E	**N**	**H**	E	**G**	VR	Pyruvate kinase
	FGR	**I**	G	R	**L**	V	**T**	**R**	A	**A**	FN	GAPDH
	CNE	**I**	I	N	**W**	L	**D**	**K**	N	**Q**		Hsc 70
	QDF	**L**	T	K	**H**	A	**S**	**H**	T	**G**	SWIG	IgE Fc-receptor
	LNSK	**I**	A	F	**K**	I	**V**	**S**	Q	**E**	PA	Desmoglein 3

b) MHC-II (con't)

MHC Molecule	Relative Peptide Position											Protein Source
HLA-DRB1*0404	TPDF	**I**	V	P	**L**	T	**D**	**L**	R	**I**	PS	Apolipoprotein
	IKILN	**I**	F	G	**V**	I	**K**	**G**	F	**V**	E	Transferrin receptor
	AQGALAN	**I**	A	V	**D**	K	**A**	**N**	L	**E**	IMT	DR α-chain
	GSHS	**M**	R	Y	**F**	H	**T**	**A**	M	**S**	RPGRGE	HLA-B60
	MGQKDSY	**V**	G	D	**E**	A	**Q**	**S**	K	**R**		Actin
HLA-DRB1*0405	FRE	**F**	K	L	**S**	K	V	**W**	R	**D**	QH	Transferrin receptor
	KPPQ	**Y**	I	A	**V**	H	V	**V**	P	**D**	Q	MIF
	THY	**Y**	A	V	**A**	V	V	**K**	K	**D**	TDFK	Transferrin
	YLL	**Y**	Y	T	**E**	F	T	**P**	T	**E**	KD	β_2-microglobulin
	VADK	**I**	Q	L	**I**	N	**N**	**M**	L	**D**		Phosphoglycerate kinase

References

1. Klein J. Natural History of the Major Histocompatibility Complex. New York: J. Wiley & Sons; 1986.
2. Gorer PA. The genetic and antigenic basis of tumor transplantation. J Pathol Bacteriol 1937; 44:691-7.
3. Graff RJ, Snell GD. Histocompatibility genes of mice. 8. The alleles of the H-1 locus. Transplantation 1968; 6:598-617.
4. Counce S, Smith P, Barth R et al. Strong and weak histocompatibility gene differences in mice and their role in the rejection of homografts of tumors and skin. Ann Surg 1956; 144:198-204.
5. Graff RJ, Polinsky SL, Snell GD. Histocompatibility genes of mice. Transplantation 1971; 11:56-62.
6. Rammensee HG, Klein J. Polymorphism of minor histocompatibility genes in wild mice. Immunogenetics 1983; 17:637-47.
7. Dausset J. The challenge of the early days of human histocompatibility. Immunogenetics 1980; 10:1-5.
8. McDevitt HO, Sela M. Genetic control of the antibody response. I. Demonstration of determinant-specific differences in response to synthetic polypeptide antigens in two strains of inbred mice. J Exp Med 1965; 122:517-31.
9. Green I, Paul WE, Benacerraf B. Genetic control of immunological responsiveness in guinea pigs to 2,4-dinitrophenyl conjugates of poly-L-arginine, protamine, and poly-L-ornithine. Proc Natl Acad Sci USA 1969; 64:1095-102.
10. McDevitt HO, Chinitz A. Genetic control of the antibody response: relationship between immune response and histocompatibility (H-2) type. Science 1969; 163:1207-8.
11. Zinkernagel RM, Doherty PC. Restriction of in vitro T cell-mediated cytotoxicity in lymphocytic choriomeningitis within a syngeneic or semiallogeneic system. Nature 1974; 248:701-2.
12. Kindred B, Shreffler DC. H-2 dependence of co-operation between T and B cells in vivo. J Immunol 1972; 109:940-3.
13. Mishell RI, Dutton RW. Immunization of normal mouse spleen cell suspensions in vitro. Science 1966; 153:1004-6.
14. Brunner KT, Mauel J, Cerottini JC et al. Quantitative assay of the lytic action of immune lymphoid cells on 51-Cr-labelled allogeneic target cells in vitro; inhibition by isoantibody and by drugs. Immunology 1968; 14:181-96.
15. Klein J. The major histocompatibility complex of the mouse. Science 1979; 203:516-21.
16. Bevan MJ. In a radiation chimaera, host H-2 antigens determine immune responsiveness of donor cytotoxic cells. Nature 1977; 269:417-8.
17. Nagy Z, Klein J. Macrophage or T cell—that is the question. Immunol Today 1981; 2:228-229.
18. Shevach E. Is determinant selection dead? Immunol Today 1982; 3:31-34
19. Hedrick SM, Cohen DI, Nielsen EA et al. Isolation of cDNA clones encoding T cell-specific membrane-associated proteins. Nature 1984; 308:149-53.
20. Yanagi Y, Yoshikai Y, Leggett K et al. A human T cell-specific cDNA clone encodes a protein having extensive homology to immunoglobulin chains. Nature 1984; 308:145-9.

21. Shimonkevitz R, Kappler J, Marrack P et al. Antigen recognition by H-2-restricted T cells. I. Cell-free antigen processing. J Exp Med 1983; 158:303-16.
22. Allen PM, Strydom DJ, Unanue ER. Processing of lysozyme by macrophages: identification of the determinant recognized by two T-cell hybridomas. Proc Natl Acad Sci U S A 1984; 81:2489-93.
23. Unanue ER. Cooperation between mononuclear phagocytes and lymphocytes in immunity. N Engl J Med 1980; 303: 977-85.
24. Townsend AR, Gotch FM, Davey J. Cytotoxic T cells recognize fragments of the influenza nucleoprotein. Cell 1985; 42: 457-67.
25. Townsend AR, Rothbard J, Gotch FM et al. The epitopes of influenza nucleoprotein recognized by cytotoxic T lymphocytes can be defined with short synthetic peptides. Cell 1986; 44:959-68.
26. Steinmetz M, Frelinger JG, Fisher D et al. Three cDNA clones encoding mouse transplantation antigens: homology to immunoglobulin genes. Cell 1981; 24: 125-34.
27. Orr HT, López de Castro JA, Lancet D et al. Complete amino acid sequence of a papain-solubilized human histocompatibility antigen, HLA-B7. 2. Sequence determination and search for homologies. Biochemistry 1979; 18:5711-20.
28. Henning R, Milner RJ, Reske K et al. Subunit structure, cell surface orientation, and partial amino-acid sequences of murine histocompatibility antigens. Proc Natl Acad Sci U S A 1976; 73:118-22.
29. Bjorkman PJ, Saper MA, Samraoui B et al. Structure of the human class I histocompatibility antigen, HLA-A2. Nature 1987; 329:506-12.
30. Bjorkman PJ, Davis MM. Model for the interaction of T-cell receptors with peptide/MHC complexes. Cold Spring Harbor Symp Quant Biol 1989; 54:365-74.
31. Rötzschke O, Falk K, Wallny HJ et al. Characterization of naturally occurring minor histocompatibility peptides including H-4 and H-Y. Science 1990; 249:283-7.
32. Rötzschke O, Falk K, Deres K et al. Isolation and analysis of naturally processed viral peptides as recognized by cytotoxic T cells. Nature 1990; 348:252-4.
33. Falk K, Rötzschke O, Stevanović S et al. Allele-specific motifs revealed by sequencing of self-peptides eluted from MHC molecules. Nature 1991; 351:290-6.
34. Madden DR, Gorga JC, Strominger JL et al. The structure of HLA-B27 reveals nonamer self-peptides bound in an extended conformation. Nature 1991; 353: 321-5.
35. Fremont DH, Matsumura M, Stura EA et al. Crystal structures of two viral peptides in complex with murine MHC class I H-2Kb [see comments]. Science 1992; 257:919-27.
36. Rudensky AY, Preston Hurlburt P, Hong SC et al. Sequence analysis of peptides bound to MHC class II molecules. Nature 1991; 353:622-7.
37. Hunt DF, Michel H, Dickinson TA et al. Peptides presented to the immune system by the murine class II major histocompatibility complex molecule I-Ad. Science 1992; 256:1817-20.
38. Chicz RM, Urban RG, Gorga JC et al. Specificity and promiscuity among naturally processed peptides bound to HLA-DR alleles. J Exp Med 1993; 178:27-47.
39. Falk K, Rötzschke O, Stevanović S et al. Pool sequencing of natural HLA-DR, DQ, and DP ligands reveals detailed peptide motifs, constraints of processing, and general rules. Immunogenetics 1994; 39:230-42.
40. Jardetzky TS, Gorga JC, Busch R et al. Peptide binding to HLA-DR1: a peptide with most residues substituted to alanine retains MHC binding. EMBO J 1990; 9:1797-803.
41. Hammer J, Valsasnini P, Tolba K et al. Promiscuous and allele-specific anchors in HLA-DR-binding peptides. Cell 1993; 74:197-203.
42. Hammer J, Takacs B, Sinigaglia F. Identification of a motif for HLA-DR1 binding peptides using M13 display libraries. J Exp Med 1992; 176:1007-13.
43. Brown JH, Jardetzky TS, Gorga JC et al. Three-dimensional structure of the human class II histocompatibility antigen HLA-DR1. Nature 1993; 364:33-9.
44. Stern LJ, Brown JH, Jardetzky TS et al.

Crystal structure of the human class II MHC protein HLA-DR1 complexed with an influenza virus peptide. Nature 1994; 368:215-21.
45. Campbell RD, Trowsdale J. Map of the human MHC. Immunol Today 1993; 14:349-52.
46. Dick TP, Ruppert T, Groettrup M et al. Coordinated dual cleavages induced by the proteasome regulator P28 lead to dominant MHC ligands. Cell 1996; 86:253-62.
47. Sadasivan B, Lehner PJ, Ortmann B et al. Roles for calreticulin and a novel glycoprotein, tapasin, in the interaction of MHC class I molecules with TAP. Immunity 1996; 5:103-114
48. Lammert E, Stevanović S, Brunner J et al. Protein disulfide isomerase is the dominant acceptor for peptides translocated into the endoplasmic reticulum. [In Press] Eur J Immunol.
49. Arnold D, Faath S, Rammensee HG et al. Cross-priming of minor histocompatibility antigen-specific cytotoxic T cells upon immunization with the heat shock protein gp96. J Exp Med 1995; 182:885-9.
50. Suto R, Srivastava PK. A mechanism for the specific immunogenicity of heat shock protein-chaperoned peptides. Science 1995; 269:1585-8.
51. Lammert E, Arnold D, Nijenhuis M et al. The endoplasmic reticulum-resident stress protein gp96 binds peptides translocated by TAP. Eur J Immunol 1997; 27:923-927.
52. Hughes EA, Ortmann B, Surman M et al. The protease inhibitor, N-acetyl-L-leucyl-L-leucyl-leucyl-L-norleucinal, decreases the pool of major histocompatibility complex class I-binding peptides and inhibits peptide trimming in the endoplasmic reticulum. J Exp Med 1996; 183:1569-78.
53. Schekman R. Polypeptide Translocation: A Pretty Picture Is Worth a Thousand Words. Cell 1996; 87:593-5.
54. Wiertz EJ, Jones TR, Sun L et al. The human cytomegalovirus US11 gene product dislocates MHC class I heavy chains from the endoplasmic reticulum to the cytosol. Cell 1996; 84:769-79.
55. Riese RJ, Wolf PR, Bromme D et al. Essential role for cathepsin S in MHC class II-associated invariant chain processing and peptide loading. Immunity 1996; 4:357-66.

CHAPTER 2

The *MHC* Genes

INTRODUCTION

The major histocompatibility complex (*MHC*) is a region of highly polymorphic genes whose products are expressed on a variety of cells. Due to the history of discoveries, human MHC molecules are also designated as human leukocyte antigens (HLA) based on their recognition with alloantisera on human leukocytes. The *MHC* genes are functionally, structurally and evolutionary related to each other. The two major gene families, class *I* and class *II*, encode two different types of MHC molecules, which are functionally specialized in displaying antigenic peptides either to $CD8^+$ (MHC class I) or to $CD4^+$ (MHC class II) T-lymphocytes. This dichotomy of antigen presentation reflects an attractive logic, in that the almost ubiquitous expression of MHC class I molecules corresponds to the need to eliminate cells of any lineage harbouring intracellular pathogens, a task performed by $CD8^+$ cytotoxic T cells (CTL). This is in contrast to the restricted distribution of MHC class II molecules to certain antigen-presenting cell types (APC).

A major characteristic of the *MHC* is its extensive polymorphism. It has, with very few exceptions, been conserved in evolution and is believed to be the result of the role *MHC* gene products play in immune recognition. The HLA antigens, e.g., form the most polymorphic antigen system in humans which is related to its cardinal role in the defence of vertebrates against parasites and other pathogens and also to its contribution to autoimmune diseases.[1-3]

GENOMIC ORGANIZATION OF THE HUMAN *MHC*

The human *MHC* (*HLA*) genes map to a 3.800 kb DNA stretch on the p21.3 band on the short arm of chromosome 6.[4] In mice the *MHC* (*H2*) genes are located on chromosome 17. A recent map of the human *MHC* (*HLA*) is shown in Figure 2.1.[5] The class *I* loci map to the telomeric end of the short arm of chromosome 6 with *HLA-A* being the most telomeric locus. The *HLA* class *I* region spans approximately 1.800 kb.[6,5] The *HLA* class *II* region spans at least 800 kb and consists of three main subregions, *DP*, *DQ* and *DR*, arranged in that order in the direction from the centromere to the telomere.[7,1]

Intercalated between the class *I* loci on the telomeric side and the class *II* loci on the centromeric side of the *HLA* complex is an island of unrelated chromatin (UC) which is inhabited by loci encoding complement proteins such as Factor B, C2 and C4, and the

MHC Ligands and Peptide Motifs, by Hans-Georg Rammensee, Jutta Bachmann, Stefan Stevanović.

cytochrome P-450 enzyme steroid 21-hydroxylase(CYP21).[8-10] This region is sometimes also referred to as "class *III* region" and spans approximately 1.100 kb of DNA. All three regions harbor, however, many other loci with functions not involved in the immune system, most of which are found in the UC.

Nomenclature

Owing to the increasing number of genes and alleles which are found in the *MHC* region, the nomenclature of the genes and their products are constantly under revision.[11-15] As many alleles and genes are mentioned throughout the book we felt the necessity to devote a short paragraph to the nomenclature.

The *MHC* has been given different names in different species, e.g., *HLA* in humans, *H2* in the mouse, *RT1* in the rat, *ChLA* in the chimpanzee, *RhLA* in the Rhesus macaque, *BoLA* in domestic cattle, *B* in domestic fowl, etc., where "LA" stands for leukocyte or lymphocyte antigen. Except for *HLA*, the use of common names, however, fails in many cases to identify the species, genus or the family in an appropriate way. Therefore, new designations were proposed without, however, changing well-established designations such as *HLA* and *H2*.[16] In accordance with internationally accepted genetic nomenclature, the locus is indicated first, followed by the identification number of the allele, separated from the designation of the locus by an asterisk. There was a need to make the species designations more specific, i.e., instead of the old *MHC* designations which only denoted the common species name, the proposed new designations take account of the genus' (the first two letters) and the species' (third and fourth letter) scientific names. Therefore, for example, *ChLA* became *Patr* (for *Pan troglodytes*) and the macaque *MHC* (*RhLA*) has been further differentiated into *Mamu* (*Macaca mulatta*), *Mane* (*Macaca nemestrina*) or *Mafa* (*Macaca fascicularis*) to name just a few examples. Further examples for the proposed alterations of *MHC* allele designations can be found in Klein et al.[16] The designation of the complex is then followed by a dash and the locus symbol, *A*, *B*, *C*, etc. For example *HLA-A2* is designated *HLA-A*02* and the to date known 21 subtypes *HLA-A*0201* to *HLA-A*0221* (Table 2.1). The *HLA* class *II* genes are indicated by the subregion of localization (*DR*, *DQ*, *DP*) and whether they encode the α (e.g., *DRA*) or β (e.g., *DRB*) sequences. Table 2.1, 2.2 and 2.3 list the to date known *HLA-A*, *-B*, and *-C* alleles, Table 2.4, 2.5 and 2.6, the *DR*, *DQ* and *DP* alleles. If done correctly, gene names should be printed in italics, and molecule names in plain text. Since frequently a definition like MHC or HLA-A2 could mean both, gene and molecule, we felt unable to strictly follow this rule in this book. Another complication of nomenclature rules is the use of lowercase letters (except for the initial) for mouse genes, but capitals for human genes. The tables include sequences recognized by the WHO Nomenclature Committee until 1996.[15,17] Where possible, *HLA* specificity, accession numbers and selected references are also given.

HLA CLASS I REGION

Classical HLA Class I Loci

HLA class I antigens are heterodimeric membrane-bound glycoproteins made up of a heavy chain of 45 kD, which is noncovalently associated with beta-2 microglobulin (β2m). The two chains of the class I molecule associate in the endoplasmic reticulum (ER) and are subsequently transported to the cell surface.[498] The heavy chain consists of 340 amino acids and has three membrane-external domains (α1, α2, α3) of approximately 90 amino acids each. The transmembrane region consists of 25-30 hydrophobic amino acids, and the intracytoplasmic portion of another 25-30 amino acids.

The classical (Ia) molecules (HLA-A, -B, and -C) play a central role in T cell recognition by binding and displaying peptides for recognition by $CD8^+$ T cells. The *HLA-A*, *-B*, and *-C* genes are highly polymorphic, with the majority of polymorphic differences located in the peptide-binding regions (PBR) within the α1 and α2 domains (Figs. 2.2, 2.3, 2.4). In codons encoding amino acid residues of this region, nonsynonymous nucleotide substitutions dominate over synonymous ones. This seems to be the result of strong selection acting on the PBR for recognition of continously changing pathogens.[500-505] The substitution of even a few amino acids can be sufficient to alter serological and T cell recognition.[506] The polymorphism, diversity and function of the MHC molecules is interrelated. It has, with a very few exceptions, been conserved in evolution. The high polymorphism observed in *MHC* alleles in humans and other primates (or vertebrates altogether) makes it possible to generate effective immune responses against a wide variety of foreign antigens. Exposure to pathogens over an evolutionary timescale can select for expression of particular *MHC* alleles. This is indicated by the strong association of the *HLA-B53* allele with recovery from a potentially lethal form of malaria; this allele is very common in individuals from West Africa where malaria is endemic.[507-509]

Class *I* and also class *II* alleles often differ in up to 10% of their nucleotide sequences.[505] The frequency of individual alleles in a population varies according to the ethnic group or population studied. HLA-A2 is for example found in 45% of the European Caucasoid population, but in African blacks the frequency is only 20%.[1]

HLA-B has the greatest number of alleles (186) and gene diversity is concentrated at positions that directly influence peptide binding. About twice as many alleles exist for the *HLA-B* locus compared with *HLA-A* (83) and only a few *HLA-C* alleles (46) (Fig. 2.5)[17]. Furthermore, multiple amino acid differences are found between alleles, but alleles at the same locus are more similar to one another than to alleles of another locus. This phenomenon has also been observed in interspecific sequence comparisons, e.g., between humans and nonhuman primates: alleles of one locus are more similar between species than the alleles of two different loci within a single species. This phenomenon led to the trans-species hypothesis of evolution.[510]

HLA-C molecules differ in positions mainly found peripheral to the peptide binding site.[506] This may suggest that HLA-C proteins are not widely used. They have, however, been shown to be a factor in natural killer (NK) cells.[511] In the mouse class *I* cluster an analogous situation is present, since the *H2-K* and *H2-D* loci display a higher degree of polymorphism than the *H2-L* locus.[1] A selection of mouse class *I* alleles is found in Figure 2.20.

The organization of class *I* genes in different species studied so far is rather similar. They consist of eight exons, and the exon-intron organization reflects the domain structure of the molecule. The first exon usually contains the 5' untranslated (UT) sequence as well as the signal sequence. Then follow separate exons for each of the external domains, α1, α2 and α3. The fifth exon codes for the transmembrane region and exons 6-8 for the cytoplasmic domain and the 3' UT region (Fig. 2.6). Fine differences are observed between the different class *I* loci: *HLA-B* locus molecules have no coding sequences on exon 8 while *HLA-A* and *-B* genes possess three more nucleotides in exon 5 compared to *HLA-C*. Some evidence exists for the occurence of differential splicing in class *I* genes.[1,512]

Nonclassical HLA Class I Loci

There can be a large number of nonclassical (*Ib*) *MHC* class *I* genes (> 50 in mouse). Some class *Ib* genes appear to be under a different regulatory control from the classical *MHC* class *I* genes. Many of them are pseudogenes, with a restricted range of tissue expression.[514-516] Many have yet to be characterized functionally. In humans, they comprise *HLA-E, -X, -F, -G, -H,* and *-J* which are less polymorphic than the classical class *I* genes. *HLA-E* is located between the *HLA-B* and *-C* loci, *HLA-F, -G,* and *-H* are sited telomeric to *HLA-A*, separated from *HLA-A* by a recombination distance of 8.0 cM.[517,518] HLA-E, -F and -G products are expressed in the association with β2m.[519] HLA-F and -G may play an important role during development, *HLA-E* is highly transcribed in most tissues, and two differentially-regulated transcripts can be detected.[519-523] These genes are the human homologs of the mouse *Qa/Tl* genes. One of the mouse molecules, H2-M3, can even present peptides with N-formylated aminotermini.

On the sequence level there is a strong homology between the class Ib molecules and Ia antigens. The nucleotide sequences of *HLA-G, -E* and *-F* contain so-called frameshift mutations, different positions of termination codons and splicing defects in exon 6, which leads to a shorter cytoplasmic domain. *HLA-H* is expressed intracellularly; it misses a cysteine in the α3 domain and is not associated with β2m. All nonclassical *MHC* class *I* genes, however, exhibit little polymorphism and follow a different expression pattern than the classical ones.

MHC Related Loci

Other genes, such as the recently discovered *MICA* and *MICB* genes, the *MOG* and *B-T* gene also map to the *MHC* class *I* region (Fig. 2.1). The *MIC* family (MIC: MHC class I chain-related) is located about 40 kb centromeric to the *HLA-B* locus. Within this family, the closely related *MICA* and *MICB* genes encode transcripts of 1382 and 2376 bp, respectively.[520,524-526] These MIC molecules are encoded by unusually long genes of 11722 bp (*MICA*) or 12930 bp (*MICB*). The genomic organization of the two genes is distinct from other class *I* genes in that a large intron of 8840 bp (*MICA*) or 7352 bp (*MICB*) separates the first two exons, and a single sixth exon of 308 bp (*MICA*) or 1338 bp (*MICB*) encodes both the cytoplasmic tail and 3'UT sequence. Their promotors contain elements similar to the heat-shock consensus sequence.[520,527,528]

The *MOG* (myelin-oligodendrocyte glycoprotein) gene and the related *B-T* (butyrophilin) gene were originally identified in the mouse *M* region and were mapped to the distal end of the *MHC* class *Ib* region.[529-532] The human *MOG* gene lies 60 kb telomeric to *HLA-F* in a head-to-head orientation, whereas the mouse *Mog* gene lies 25 kb telomeric to *H2-M5* in a tail-to-tail orientation.[529] The gene contains nine exons and eight introns, the latter containing numerous repetitive DNA elements, including 14 *Alu* sequences within three introns. It spans about 17 kb and undergoes alternative splicing to produce six different transcripts, one of which involves a previously unknown exon.[529,533] Both these genes are related to the chicken *B-G* genes, a set of polymorphic loci located close to the chicken *MHC* genes.[534-537] It may be a factor in *MHC*-linked susceptibility to the demyelating autoimmune condition multiple sclerosis.[531] It is an intrinsic membrane molecule with two transmembrane domains and a member of the Ig superfamily.

MHC Class I Unrelated Loci

Many unrelated loci are peppered throughout the class *I* region and the function of most of them still remains to be determined. GNL1, or HSR1, is a member of GTP (guanine) binding proteins. The *GNL1* gene shows a high degree of homology with its mouse counterpart.[538] It is located less than 2 kb centromeric to *HLA-F* in the same transcriptional orientation (Fig. 2.1).

The gene encoding the octamer-binding transcription factor (OTF3) was mapped within or close to the human MHC class I region to 6p22-p21.3.[539,540] The homologous mouse gene, *Otf-3*, is located on mouse chromosome 17 between the *Q* and *T* regions of the *MHC*. Transcription factors containing the POU-homeo domain have been shown to be important regulators of tissue-specific gene expression in lymphoid and pituitary differentiation and in early mammalian development.

Other genes mapping to the *MHC* class *I* region comprise *ZNF173*, an acid finger protein that contains cysteine- and histidine-rich domains similar to those characteristic for metal-dependent DNA-binding proteins, and several *CAT* genes of varying or to date unknown functions.[541-544] An excellent overview of presently known *HLA* genes has recently been published by Campbell and Trowsdale.[5]

Regulation of MHC Class I Expression

The expression of class I and class II MHC molecules is controlled by the embryonic development, by the degree of cellular differentiation and the level of cell activation, as well as by exogenous immune and inflammatory stimuli. Inflammatory mediators such as interferons, lymphokines and cytokines increase MHC class I expression the transformation of epithelial cells by viruses (e.g., Adenovirus 12) leads to decreased levels of class I expression. In addition to the transcriptional regulation of MHC expression post-translational maturation is required for cell surface expression of functional proteins.[545]

On the molecular level the expression is regulated by the simultaneous interactions of cis- and trans-acting factors and the promotor sequences of the *MHC* genes.[546-550]

The 5' end of a eukaryotic gene usually contains regulatory elements such as promoter sequences (*TATA* box, *CCAAT* box) and enhancer elements. Figure 2.6 shows the genomic organization of an *HLA* α gene with a more detailed presentation of the regulatory elements involved in class *I* gene transcription. The constitutive expression of class *I* genes is governed by the class *I* regulatory elements (*CRE*/enhancer *A*) and its binding factors.[546-548] The *CRE* (cyclic AMP response element) is located at position -203 to -160, and the IFN consensus/response sequences (*ICS/IRS*) are juxtaposed at position -167 to -137. The existence of more than one CRE-binding protein suggests that the *CRE* motif could serve multiple regulatory functions.[551] These two sequences are the major cis-elements controlling *MHC* class *I* promoter activation. The α site with its core sequence TGACGC is located at positions -107 to -121 in the enhancer *B* region and enhances the transcription in a tissue-specific manner.[552] The *CRE*/enhancer *A* region acts as positive (in cells that are induced to differentiate) or negative (in undifferentiated cells) regulatory element, depending on the differentiation status of the cell.[553,554]

The developmental regulation is influenced by many cis-/trans-acting factors, such as:

1) Factors which bind to a negative regulatory element (*NRE*, located in the 5' part of the *ICS*) involving the enhancer *A/ICS* sequences.[554]
2) Enhancer/silencer elements outside the immediate 5' flanking region of *MHC* class *I* genes.[555,556]
3) H2RIIBP (H2 region II binding protein or RXRβ), a member of the nuclear hormone receptor family, binds to the 5' region of the *CRE* that activates transcription of class *I* genes in response to retinoic acid.[557-559]
4) IFNα, -β, -γ act as transcription activators by inducing transacting nuclear factors (IRF) to bind the consensus IFN sequence (*ICS/IRS*) in the class *I* gene promotors.[560,561]

Also IFNγ promotes synthesis of genes that enhance assembly of class I molecules, such as TAP and LMP.[562-564] IFNs do not only upregulate MHC class I expression in cells that constitutively express these antigens but can also induce expression in cells that do not normally express them.[565]

HLA CLASS II REGION

The class II molecules are heterodimeric membrane-bound glycoproteins which consist of an heavy chain of 35 kD and a light chain of 28 kD with the two chains being noncovalently associated. Both chains have two membrane-external domains of approximately 90 amino acids, and a transmembrane region and cytoplasmic domain of about 40 amino acids. There are three separate isotypes of the class *II* or *HLA-D* region, namely *DR*, *DP* and *DQ*. These molecules are encoded by genes located in distinct subregions and exhibit different degrees of polymorphisms, with *HLA-DR* being more polymorphic than *DP* and *DQ* (Fig. 2.7). Each subregion contains characteristic *A* and *B* genes. Their products assemble to give rise to the class II heterodimer.

The entire *HLA-D* region spans approximately 10^6 bp, the *DP* subregion is located at the centromeric end, *DR* at the telomeric, and *DQ* in between.[7,566,567] The gene structure of both *A* and *B* genes shows the typical correspondence between functional domains and intron-exon structure as already described for the class *I* genes but exhibit a larger variability in their organization. In mammals, the α chain encoding genes generally have five exons and the β chains (with the exception of *DQB* which has five), six (Fig. 2.8 and 2.9).[1,233,416,568] The basic plan is, however, similar to that of the class *I* genes: the first exon contains the 5'UT region and signal sequence, which is followed by two exons for each of the extracellular domains (α1, α2, β1, β2). Only in cichlid fishes is this pattern is broken in the class *IIB* genes: the third exon is split by an additional 97 bp intron (in *Auha-DXB*).[569] Otherwise all fish class *II* genes have one exon less than their mammalian counterparts. Certain genes, such as *DQA2*, do not follow the above mentioned pattern: they have connecting peptide, transmembrane, and cytoplasmic sequences on the same exon as part of the 3'UT sequence. Others, again, use a separate exon for the 3'UT region or for part of the cytoplasmic domain and the 3'UT region.[570,1] Mammalian class *II* genes tend to contain large introns, the length of which accounts for a main difference—on the molecular level—between the species studied so far.

DR Subregion

The *DR* subregion varies in length from 60 kb to about 260 kb. Within the *DR* subregion there is one *DRA* and several *DRB* genes. The *DRA* gene can hardly be called polymorphic, actually there is only one amino acid substitution (leucine for valine) at position 217 (Fig. 2.10).[231,233] On the other hand, the *DRB* genes are extremely polymorphic, not only is there variation in the number of *DRB* loci within the subregion, but also in the number of loci which are expressed and in the number of alleles at each individual locus. All *DR* haplotypes contain one *DRA* gene. In those *DR* haplotypes in which there are more than two *DRB* genes, only two *DRB* genes are expressed on the cell surface; the other are pseudogenes. To date, 194 alleles have been identified at the *DRB1* locus and 32 at the second expressed locus (*DRB3, DRB4,* or *DRB5*). There are five major groups of haplotypes, *DR2, DR1, DR52, DR8* and *DR53*, each characterized by a particular organization of its *DRB* genes. The *DRB1* gene is expressed in all haplotypes, the second expressed *DRB* locus differs according to the haplotype. The variation of organization of the *DRB* loci in different haplotypes is illustrated in Figure 2.11.

To date, nine *DRB* loci have been described, *DRB1, DRB3, DRB4,* and *DRB5* are functional genes, *DRB2, DRB6, DRB7, DRB8,* and *DRB9* are pseudogenes. Table 2.4 lists the presently recognized *DRB* alleles. The comparison of the allelic *DRB* sequences shows that the substitutions are mainly located within the peptide binding groove (Fig. 2.12).

DQ Subregion

The *DQ* subregion contains two pairs of *DQA* and *DQB* genes which are present in all haplotypes studied. In contrast to the *DR* subregion, both the *A* and *B* genes are polymorphic. The *DQA1* and *B1* genes are expressed and render well-characterized protein products, the *DQA2* and *B2* genes (formerly *DX* genes) are transcribed though no protein product from these loci has been found. As in the *DRB* genes, the allelic polymorphism resides predominantly within the membrane-distal α1 and β1 domains of the molecules (Fig. 2.13 and Fig. 2.14). They do, however, not have the same discrete regions of allelic hypervariablity as found in the *DRB* genes.[242] At the time of writing 18 *DQA* and 31 *DQB* alleles were recognized as such by the WHO Nomenclature Committee.[17]

DP Subregion

There are two sets of *HLA-DP* genes within the subregion which are—contrary to other class *II* genes—oriented in tail-to-tail fashion and span 75 kb (Fig. 2.1). However, only the *DPA1* and *DPB1* genes are expressed as a product. The *DPA2* and *DPB2* genes are nonfunctional pseudogenes: they possess several deleterious mutations in the coding sequences. In the case of *DPB2*, one nucleotide deletion in exon 3 leads to a frameshift mutation and therefore to 4 premature termination codons, and in the case of *DPA2* there are several frameshift mutations due to deletions in exon 2, 4 and 5. The deletion in exon 2 leads to a premature transcription stop in exon 3; a frame-shift mutation in exon 5 leads to the transcription of a longer α-chain.[573,574] A major characteristic of the *DP* subregion is the numerous insertions: a ribosomal pseudogene of the L32 family is integrated in intron 1 of the *HLA-DPB1* gene, *Alu* elements have also been found in introns of *DP* genes,[441,457,575] as well as a *Kpn*-repetitive element and a sequence similar to *IgCε*.[443] To date, 10 *DPA* and 77 *DPB* alleles have been recognized (Fig. 2.7 and Table 2.4) and their allelic differences are outlined in Figures 2.15 and 2.16.[17]

HLA-DO and *HLA-DN*

The *HLA-DOB* gene's sequence shows approximately 70% identity with known *DRB*, *DQB* and *DPB* genes and maps between the *HLA-DQ* and *HLA-DP* loci (Fig. 2.1). Its expression has only been detected at the mRNA level in B cell lines.[235] The HLA-DOB molecule has no DOA partner, but rather combines with the A molecule of the DNA locus. The *HLA-DNA* gene (previously *DOα*, *DZα*)[576] is located centromeric to *HLA-DOB*.[577-579] These genes appear to be expressed only in the thymus. The roles of the HLA-DOB and HLA-DNA gene products in the immune system still remain to be elucidated, as well as those of the nonpolymorphic murine Oa and Ob counterparts.

HLA-DM

HLA-DM is the most recent family of MHC class II molecules discovered.[580] The *HLA-DMA* and *-DMB* genes have been mapped between the *HLA-DN* and *HLA-DO* loci on chromosome 6. Like other genes which encode α and β-chains of MHC class II molecules, they are organized in 'tandem'. Their upstream genetic regions contain sequences homologous to known regulatory motifs of class *II* genes.[580-582] The number of exons encoding *HLA-DMA* and *HLA-DMB* correlates with that in other α- and β-chain encoding class *II* genes (Fig. 2.9).[582] Despite these class II features, DMA and DMB share only 30% overall amino acid sequence homology with other class II molecules. The α2 and β2 domain sequences suggest that they are equally related to immunoglobulin chains, class I heavy chains and β2-microglobulin as well as to classical class II molecules. HLA-DM exhibits only limited polymorphism.[580-584] The expression of *HLA-DMA* and *-DMB* is coregulated with classical class *II* genes and is under the control of the *MHC* class *II* transactivators RFX5 and CIITA.[585,586] Recent work has led to an understanding of DM as one of the key players in intracellular selection and loading of antigenic peptides onto classical MHC class II molecules in endosomal/lysosomal compartments (reviewed in Kropshofer et al).[587] In contrast to the human *HLA-DM* loci the murine *H2-M* region contains one *Ma* gene and two *Mb* genes, termed *Mb1* and *Mb2*.[588] Like their human counterparts the three *H2-M* genes display a very limited degree of polymorphism.[589,590] In addition, certain *H2-M* alleles could exclusively be identified in autoimmune prone mouse strains.[590] Segregation of certain *H2-M* alleles within haplotypes susceptible to autoimmune diseases suggests that besides classical class II molecules additional genes operating at different levels of the antigen presentation pathway are required to mount autoimmune responses.[590] Rat homologs have also been identified.[591]

Other Loci in the Class *II* Subregion

The clustering of genes with related functions is most marked within the class *II* region. Actually, to date the function of only one gene in the class *II* region, *RING3*, has nothing to do with the immune system. It is a homolog of the *Drosophila* female sterile homeotic (*fsh*) gene and seems widely expressed. It has also been mapped to the mouse and *Xenopus* class *II* regions.[592-593] Its exact tissue specificity and properties have not yet been assigned.[594,592] All of the other genes are expressed in particular tissues and most of them respond to induction with γ-interferon.[563,570,595-598]

Genes involved in processing antigens for the MHC class I antigen presentation, such as the ATP-binding cassette (ABC) transporter loci and two proteasome components also map to the class *II* region.[595,599-603]

The *LMP2* and *LMP7* (low molecular weight proteins) genes encode components for the protease complex which degrades cytosolic proteins. They may be involved in generating antigenic peptides.[604] *LMP7* maps between the two transporter genes, *LMP2* maps within 500 bp centromeric to the *TAP1* locus, with the 5' promotor ends of the two genes adjacent.[598,605] The two genes encode subunits of the proteasome which presumably translocates peptides into an exocytic compartment where they associate with class I molecules.[597,606] The mouse counterpart of *LMP2* (*Lmp-2*) is mapped to the *MHC* class *II* region on chromosome 17 and has six exons.[607-609]

Many of the peptides presented by class I molecules are derived from cytosolic proteins and must therefore cross a lipid bilayer membrane in order to assemble with newly synthesized class I molecules in the lumen of the ER. To get peptides there, the cell has adapted ABC transporters.

The TAP (transporter associated with antigen processing) is composed of the two homologous proteines, TAP1 and TAP2, with approximately 12 membrane-spanning domains and two hydrophilic ATP-binding domains.[610-612] Specificity for peptide length (8-13 AA) and a certain selectivity for peptide sequence has been observed, more in mouse and rat than in humans.[613,614] The mouse homologs *Ham1* and *Ham2* are also located within the class *II* region and are functionally and structurally homologous to *TAP1* and *TAP2*.[615]

The *TAP* and *LMP* gene clusters form a tightly linked cluster of interferon-inducible genes.[616,606,617] Induction of LMP2/LMP7 expression by IFNγ alters the composition of the proteasome via a displacement mechanism that exchanges two homologous structural subunits (X and Y) for the *MHC*-encoded LMPs.

Expression of Class *II* Genes

In comparison to class I molecules there is a striking difference in class II with respect to their cellular expression on different cell types and their reaction upon cytokine modulation. The range of tissue expression of class II molecules is much more limited than that of class I molecules. They are constitutively expressed on macrophages, B cells, dendritic cells and the thymic epithelium and in humans by activated T cells that are all antigen-presenting cells for T lymphocytes. Their expression can be induced on other cell types, including fibroblasts and epithelial cells, in response to stimulation with agonists such as IFNγ.[549,550] The expression of class *II* genes is furthermore regulated in a tissue-specific manner.[618]

Class II expression can be constitutive or inducible and varies with differentiation stages and growth conditions. For the constitutive expression of class *II* genes in B cells several transacting factors need to interact with conserved promotor elements.[549,550,619] Some—though not all—class *II* promotors have a *TATA* box which does not always—even if present—influence initiation of transcription. Not all promotors have a *CCAAT* box, which is apparently functionally not important. The main control element regulating transcription is a highly conserved 150 bp promoter proximal region situated upstream of the transcription intitiation site. This promoter proximal region contains sequence motifs called the *S*, X_1, X_2 and *Y* boxes (Fig. 2.8). Their sequences, orientations, relative positions, and spacing are conserved in all of the α and β chain genes in all species that have been examined as well as in *HLA-DM* and invariant (Ii) chain genes.[549,550,620-622] The *X* and *Y* boxes are separated from each other by 18-20 bp and are necessary for both constitutive and cytokine-mediated expression.[549,550,623,624] The *Y* box is a 10 bp motif located 40-90 bp 5' of the transcription start site and contains a reverse *CCAAT* sequence. The *X* box is located further upstream and consists of two subunits, X_1, which is located at position -108 to -95, and X_2, located at position -96 to -90. Depending on the gene, the X_2 box resembles either a cAMP responsive element (*CRE*) or a TPA responsive element (*TRE*). Still further upstream is the *S* box (also called *H* box) which consists of 7 bp and is embedded in a larger *W* (or *Z*) region.[624,549,550] Three MHC-II promoter binding complexes, RFX, NF-Y, and X2BP are particularly relevant to the regulation of *MHC II* genes: RFX binds to the X box, NF-Y is a heteromeric *CCAAT* binding protein, X2BP binds to the X_2 box.[625-628] Chromatin structure, promotor accessibility and negative regulatory proteins may furthermore determine tissue-specific class II expression.[550] A review on *MHC* class *II* regulation has recently been published by Mach et al.[629]

Among antigen presenting cells, the mononuclear phagocytes do not express class II molecules, unless they are triggered by IFNγ or other cytokines. Interleukin-10 functions as antagonist. The mechanism of class II induction by IFNγ had for a long time been obscure since class *II* promotors lack *ICS/IRS* and *IRF*. Later, the indirect regulation of *MHC* class *II* gene transcription via IFNγ induction of the *CIITA* gene expression was proposed.[630]

CIITA does not bind DNA but rather functions through the trans-activation of a conserved set of DNA binding proteins in the class *II* promotor region.[630-633] Induction of cell surface MHC class II molecules by IFNγ is accompanied by an increase in the steady state class II mRNA levels; this is largely due to an increase in the rate of transcription.[634] Recent data suggest the existence of an intragenic promoter driving an IFNγ inducible expression of CIITA.[635] *HLA-DR, -DP, -DQ, -DMA,-DMB* and the invariant chain gene have been shown to be activated by CIITA.[634,636] Recently, a mouse class II transactivator has been described, which has domains as conserved as in humans.[637]

There are also differences in expression of DR, DQ, and DP: DR seems to be present in much greater quantities on the cell surface than DQ and DP. A far smaller number of DQ and DP allomorphs has to date been identified (Table 2.5 and 2.6). *DQ* and *DP* might not be as widely used as *DR* genes.[618] Certain *HLA* class *II* alleles are strongly associated with susceptibility to autoimmune disease (also see Table 5.8).[638] Moreover, differences in the regulation of transcription of alleles at these loci—as demonstrated for *DQB1* and *DRB1*—may contribute to the onset and/or perpetuation of these diseases.[639-642] Although DQ molecules have a pattern of tissue distribution and inducibility similar to that of DR and DP, their regulation is not strictly coordinated with DR and DP.[643,644] Their promotor regions are polymorphic, with some of the nucleotide sequence polymorphisms being located in the *X* and *Y* motifs essential for the regulation of *HLA* class *II* gene expression. They carry, however, sequence motifs not found in other *MHC* class *II* gene promotors, such as a putative NFκB site.[645-647]

Class *III* Region

The class *III* region of the human *MHC* spans about 1.100 kb on chromosomal region 6p21.3 and contains genes such as *TNF*, *HSP70*, 21-hydroxylase as well as genes encoding the complement proteins C2, C4 and Factor B (Bf) and represents the region with the highest number of genes unrelated to antigen presentation. The unrelated genes are usually grouped in four categories:[513]

1) Genes whose products function in immune reactions seemingly distinct from antigen presentation, e.g., the complement components C4, C2, Bf and TNF.

2) Genes whose products function in antigen presentation, such as TAP, LMP and HSP70.

3) Genes whose products have no immunological function, e.g., G7a (valyl-tRNA synthetase).
4) Genes without known function. They represent the largest group.

The complement region is most densely populated with genes—estimates lie around 63 genes/Mbp; the number of genes in the class *II* region is estimated to about 34/Mbp; the number of class *I* genes is still difficult to determine.[570,648,572,6] The most centromeric genes within the region are those encoding CYP21 and C4 (Fig. 2.1) These two genes are tandemly repeated in most haplotypes.[649-651] The *CYP21* genes are each located 3' to the *C4A* and *C4B* genes. C2 is the most telomeric gene in the complement region.[652] Between the genes for *C2* and *HLA-B* map the genes for the tumor necrosis factor (TNFα and TNFβ) and the heat-shock protein HSP70.[653]

CYP21

CYP21 (steroid 21-hydroxylase) is a cytochrome P-450 enzyme consisting of 494 amino acid residues which hydroxylates progesterone at the 21 position in the synthetic pathway of cortisol. Deficiency of this enzyme results in the syndrome of congenital adrenal hyperplasia and the salt-wasting syndrome. The *CYP21* (also called *CYP21B*) gene encodes the functional enzyme; *CYP21P* (or *CYP21A*) is a pseudogene and therefore not transcribed.[654,655,650] These genes are located downstream from the genes for complement proteins *C2* and *Bf*, between *HLA-B* and *DR*.

In the typical 21-hydroxylase deficiency, about 25% of the disease alleles result from a deletion spanning the *CYP21* as well as the *C4B* gene. Other 21-hydroxylase deficiencies may have resulted from gene conversion events. The *CYP21* pseudogene, e.g., lies close to the functional gene *CYP21* and this genomic organization seems to predispose the functional gene to mutation through gene conversion or through deletion by homologous recombination and unequal crossing-over.[649,650]

C4

C4A and *C4B* are functional genes which code for the fourth component of complement. It is a 200 kD serum protein synthesized as a single precursor molecule, the mature protein has three domains—α, β, γ—of 75, 95 and 30 kD, respectively. It participates in the classical pathway of complement activation, i.e., upon activation by the C1 component C4 activates another member of the complement cascade (C2). The C4A component binds efficiently to proteins in antigen-antibody complexes and thus facilitates their solubilization and clearance, the C4B component binds preferentially to cell surfaces and thus participates in cell lysis. The C4A and C4B proteins are encoded in two separate loci which are members of a family that includes two other complement-encoding loci C3 and C5, as well as the α2-macroglobulin gene.[656] The *C4A* gene is approximately 22 kb long, the *C4B* gene is polymorphic in size, i.e., either 22 or 16 kb. This size variation is due to the presence of a 7 kb intron located approximately 2.5 kb from the 5' end of the *C4* genes.[657-659] There are multiple alleles of each *C4* locus, with differences between *C4A* and *C4B* residing within a stretch of 90 amino acids in the α chain. The gene frequencies of allelic variants differ.

C4 deficiency is associated with autoimmune diseases. Homozygous deficiency of *C4A* is associated with systemic lupus erythematosus (SLE) and with type I diabetes mellitus; the homozygous deficiency of *C4B* is associated with susceptibility to bacterial meningitis.[660]

C2 and Bf

The factor B locus and C2 deficiency loci are close together, and are 3-5 cM from the *HLA-A* and *B* loci.[661] The order is centromere; *DR; CYP21; C2; TNFA; TNFB; HLA-B*.[6,662] The most telomeric of the complement genes is *C2*. C2 and Factor B are members of the serine protease family of proteins and play an important role in activation of the complement cascade. Both proteins possess the typical serine protease domain at their C-terminal, which has the characteristic triad of active site residues histidine, aspargine and serine at specific positions with the domain. The *Bf* gene is 6 kb in size and encodes a protein of 739 amino acids.[663] *C2* is 18 kb in size and possesses larger introns. Both genes are polymorphic in the population but the number of common alleles in the population is much lower than for *C4*.

TNFA and TNFB

The genes for the tumor necrosis factor (*TNFA* and *TNFB*) are located between *HLA-B* and *C2*, about 600 kb centromeric to *HLA-B*.[653] Both genes are expressed and their products (TNFα: 156 amino acids, TNFβ: 171 amino acids) are secreted from activated macrophages, monocytes, neutrophils, NK cells and activated T lymphocytes in the course of the inflammatory response. CD4-positive cells secrete TNFα while CD8 positive cells secrete little or no TNFα. They have pleiotropic effects on many cell types including other lymphocytes, neutrophils, and vascular endothelium.[664,665]

The synthesis of TNF is induced by many different stimuli, including cytokines such as IL2, GM-CSF, SP, PAF. Its production is, for example, inhibited by IL6, TGFβ and vitamin D3. The *TNFA* and *TNFB* genes are approximately 3.6 kb long and contain 4 exons. The primary transcript comprises 2762 nucleotides. The *A* and *B* genes are regulated independently. The murine counterparts also lie close to each other on chromosome 17.

Other cytokines, such as lymphotoxin (LT) and lymphotoxin β (LT-β) map between the complement and the class *I* region.

RD

The *RD* gene, initially identified in the mouse, is located between the *C4* and *Bf* genes of the *H2* and *HLA* complexes of mouse and humans, respectively.[666] It contains 10 exons spread over approximately 6 kb of DNA and encodes a 42 kD polypeptide with no hydrophobic leader sequence. Neither does it bear a recognizable relation to known protein families, which suggests that the protein is not destined to penetrate the endoplasmic reticulum.[667] It seems to be, however, a nucleic acid binding protein. The observed high degree of homology between the human and mouse genes indicates functional importance. The name is derived from R (the single letter code for arginine) and D (the single letter code for aspartic acid) since there is a 58 amino acid segment in the central portion of the RD protein that consists almost entirely of alternating arginine and aspartic acid residues. The RD protein contains the so-called RNP consensus sequence which is present in many different nuclear RNA-binding proteins.

HSP70

The HSP70 family of heat-shock proteins constitutes the major proteins synthesized in response to elevated temperatures and other forms of stress. They may be involved in the delivery of denatured proteins to the proteasome for degradation. Harrison et al demonstrated that functional genes encoding HSP70 map to chromosome 6, in the region 6p22-6p21.3, to chromosome 14 and at least one more other chromosome.[668] Later it was shown that a duplicated *HSP70* locus exists between the complement and tumor necrosis factor genes, 12 kb apart from each other and 92 kb telomeric of the *C2* gene.[669] The bovine *HSP70-1* and *HSP70-2* genes are homologous to human *HSPA1* and *HSPA1L*, since they are located on bovine chromosome 23 and show synteny with loci on 6p in the human.

Related Genes Unlinked to the MHC

There are several proteins which belong to the MHC superfamily but which are encoded by genes that are unlinked to the *MHC*, e.g., CD1, IgG, Fc receptor and zinc finger-binding proteins. In humans, there are five *CD1* genes (A-D) which also function in antigen presentation to T cells (though they do not present peptide antigen). In mouse, 2 homologous proteins (mCD1.1 and mCD1.2) have been characterized which map to mouse chromosome 3.[519,670]

The human *CD1* genes are located on chromosome 1q21-q23 in the order *CD1D, CD1A, CD1C, CD1B, CD1E* from the centromere in a 190 kb segment of DNA.[671,670] With the exeption of *CD1B*, they are all in the same transcriptional orientation. They are evenly spaced in the complex except for the distance between *CD1D* and *CD1A*, which is two to three times greater than the average. The products of the *CD1A, -B* and *-C* genes have been serologically defined; the products of *CD1D* and *CD1E* are unknown. They share a highly conserved exon, which is homologous to the β2m-binding domain (α3) of MHC class I antigens.[672]

The CD molecules are not polymorphic and—apart from CD1D—noncovalently associated with β2m.[673] In cells infected with mycobacteria, the CD1 molecule is able to bind and present a mycobacterial membrane component, mycolic acid. Whether CD1 molecules can also present peptide antigens still remains unclear, although this has been shown at least for one member of the CD1 family.[674]

Another member of the immunoglobulin gene superfamily is β2-microglobulin (β2m) which is noncovalently associated with all class I molecules and constitutes the light chain. It is, however, not located on chromosome 6 but on chromosome 15 (15q21).[675] In contrast to the HLA class I heavy chain, there is no polymorphism in β2m. The sequence of β2m is rather similar to the constant region of immunoglobulin, the membrane-proximal domain of the class I heavy chain and the class II α and β chains.

MHC Gene Organization in Other Species

The mouse, rat, bovine, chicken and primate *MHCs* are among those studied in most detail, but genes of the class *I* and class *II* regions have been sequenced and described in a large number of vertebrates. Selected class *I* and *II* alleles of a number of species are shown in Figure 2.17 and 2.18. The putative peptide binding regions are indicated.

Interspecific sequence comparisons of human and primate class *I* and *II* alleles show a high similarity and indicate that humans diverged from their nearest ape-like relatives just a few million years ago. Chromosome binding patterns of primates studied so far are remarkably similar and some human alloantisera crossreact on nonhuman primates.[1] The genomic organization is also similar throughout the primates, although the two infraorders of anthropoid primates, New World Monkeys (*Platyrrhini*) and Old Word Monkeys/Hominoids (*Catarrhini*), diverged from a common ancestor 37 million years ago. The MHC polymorphism is not only found in the alleles but also in the different haplotypes.[387,713-718] The existence of similar haplotypes in different human populations and primates implies that the observed haplotype polymorphism is as old as the allelic polymorphism. Some regions are rather constant, e.g., the *DP* region is conserved in size and organization as well as in gene orientation. Even most of the *Alu* and other repeat sequences have been maintained.[719] This is in contrast to the *C4-CYP21* and the *DR* regions that show evolutionary instability.[720-722]

In the sequence comparisons of class *I* and class *II* genes (Figs. 2.17 and 2.18), selected alleles of *Platyrrhini* and *Catarrhini* are included, e.g., chimpanzee (*Pan troglodytes*),[678,50,676,696] pygmy chimpanzee (*Pan paniscus*),[676] orang-utan (*Pongo pygmaeus*),[678] Rhesus macaques (*Macaca mulatta, M. fascicularis, M. nemestrina*),[679,698,699] tamarins (*Saguinus oedipus*),[680,723] lemurs (*Galago senegalensis/Galago garnetti*),[699] and loris (*Loris tardigradus*).[700]

The *MHC* class *I* and *II* genes of lagomorphs (*Oryctolagus cuniculus*)[724,685] is rather similar to the organization in the primate *MHC* (Fig. 2.19).[725-727] The class *II* region contains representatives of *DP, DQ, DR* and *DO* genes in a order similar to that in humans. There are, however, hints that at least one class *I* gene may be linked to *DRA* without any intervening class *III* genes.[728]

Among carnivores the *MHC* of cat (*Felis catus*)[729,681,730] and dog (*Canis familiaris*)[731,682] have been investigated. Some 20 and 5 feline class *I* and class *II* genes, respectively, have been identified. The organization of the canine *MHC* region is similar to that of humans and exhibits allele polymorphism.[732,733]

Among rodents the *MHC* of mouse and rat have been studied most extensively; there are however, also data available for squirrels (*Sciurus aberti*),[689,734] hamster (*Mesocritetus auratus*)[735] and beavers (*Castor fiber*).[736]

The mouse *MHC* (*H2*) is situated on chromosome 17 and is in many respects organized like the human *MHC* region (Fig. 2.19).[1,737] There is, however, a striking difference: not all class *I* loci are located within the same DNA stretch. The class *I* *H2-K* locus is situated at the proximal end of the class *II* region, which seems to be a direct insertion of about 60 kb of DNA since flanking markers *KE-3* and *RING1* are adjacent in the equivalent human region.[738] It has been difficult to relate the mouse and human regions, but it appears that *HLA-C* corresponds to the *H2-Q* region (*S* gene), *HLA-E* to *T24* in the *H2-T* region (*R1* gene) and the *HLA-A* cluster to the *M4-M6* genes with the *H2-M* region.[513] A comparison of different haplotypes of the *K*, *D*, and *L* genes is shown in Figure 2.20. A comparison of mouse class I α and β sequences is shown in Figures 2.21 and 2.22.

The mouse genome has between 40 to 60 described class *Ib* genes which are found in the *Q* (formerly *Qa*), *T* (*Tla*) or *M* (*Hmt*) regions and all telomeric to the classical *Ia* loci.[519,776,777] The *H2-Q* region is adjacent to the *H2-D/L* cluster and contains some 10 different loci. Some of them, e.g., *Q4* and the *Qa-2* genes (*Q6/Q9*) are expressed in many different tissues *Q2*, *Q5* and *Q10* are more tissue specific.[519] The mouse *Q* region genes are more similar to the classical Iα molecules than to the other nonclassical antigens and tend to be expressed as phosphatidyl-inositol linked proteins.[777,519] Most of these molecules associate with β2m.

The *H2-T* region lies telomeric of the *Q* region and contains some 24 genes which are expressed as transmembrane proteins. They have a limited tissue distribution.[777,778] For example, TL is a transplantation antigen eliciting an α/β cytotoxic T cell response and which is expressed efficiently in the absence of a functional TAP2 molecule.[779,780]

The *H2-M* region is telomeric to the T region and contains eight class *I* genes (*H2-M1-8*).[513,519,776,781,756,782,754] One of these genes is a restriction element for the maternally transmitted antigen (Mta) of mice that consists of a peptide, MTF, which is presented on the cell surface by the *MHC*-linked class Ib molecule H2-M3.[519,562,776]

The *RING3* gene, *TAP* and *LMP* genes also have their mouse counterparts. The *UC* region also shows a high similarity in organization (Fig. 2.19), the gene clusters are, however, smaller in places probably due to shorter introns and smaller intragenic regions. The distance between the *Mb* and *LMP2* genes in mice is less than 30 kb, in the *HLA* region the distance amounts to 75 kb.[783,648,784] The nonclassical human class *I* genes have no orthologous relationships with nonclassical mouse class *I* genes. These genes have species-specific characteristics. In mouse, the nonclassical class *I* genes comprise several clusters which differ markedly in numbers of members between different strains.

Apart from the mouse the most extensively studied rodent is the rat. The *MHC* organization is similar to that of the mouse but additional important phenotypes map to the rat *MHC* (Fig. 2.19).[785,570] The *grc-G/C* region (mouse equivalent is Q/T region) has no equivalent in other species and contains genes such as *rcc* (resistance to chemical carcinogenesis), *ft* (fertility) and *dw-3* (dwarf).[786] *RT1.A* is the main polymorphic class *I* locus and is located at the proximal end of the MHC, next to the class *II* region. The direct equivalent of the mouse *T* loci is called *N* in the rat, the mouse *Q* is referred to as *O*, and *M* is designated identically. The rat transporter is unique in the sense that different alleles of *TAP* have functional consequences. Two different forms of the rat transporter, which differ by 25 amino acids, are based on two allelic versions of the rat TAP2 molecule. They are presented through RT1.A.[787] In contrast, the human *TAP* alleles are rather uniform.[788,601,789,603] Since rats have only one major expressed polymorphic class *I* locus, the different *TAP* alleles may provide an alternative way of diversifying the immune repertoire.[787,570] The rat TAP1/TAP2^a (cim^a) heterodimer resembles human TAP since it does not have a preference for a particular amino acid at the C terminus. The TAP1/TAP2 (cim^b) heterodimer resembles mouse TAP since it prefers peptides with hydrophobic residues at the C terminus.[790-793]

Recently *RING1*, *RING2*, *KE6*, *RXRB* and *Col11a2* have been mapped to the rat *MHC*. The relative order and transcriptional orientation are the same as in their human and murine homologs. The distances are also similar, except for the *Col11a2*-class *II* interval which is clearly shorter in rat and mouse compared with humans.[794]

Cattle (*Bos taurus*),[705,795,796,688] horse (*Equus equus*),[797,683,702] sheep (*Ovar aries*),[512,706] pig (*Sus scrofa*),[703] moose (*Alces alces*),[704] deer (*Cervus elaphus*)[701] and goat (*Capra hircus*)[798] have also been investigated. The bovine and sheep *MHC* class *II* region carry no *DP* loci and the respective haplotypes may differ in the number of *DQ* genes. The sheep *MHC* contains at least three expressed class *I* genes as well as *DRA*, *DNA* and *DOB* genes, the *DRB*, *DQA* and *DQB* loci have been duplicated. The *DY* subregion of sheep contains a class *II A/B* gene pair, of which only one is present when both are transcribed.[799]

The bovine major histocompatibility complex differs from that of other species in that it has a second group of class *II* genes that are separated from the classical class *I*/class *II* complex by 15 to 20 cM (Fig. 2.19).[800-802] These are referred to as class *IIb*. The bovine *MHC* is therefore divided into four regions: class *I*, class *IIa*, class *IIb* and class *III* (Fig. 2.19).[570] The class *IIa* region encodes the class II molecules known to be functional. The expression states of *IIb* genes are not yet known. The *IIb* cluster also contains the *TCP1* gene which corresponds to the mouse t-complex. In humans the *TCP1* gene is positioned on the long arm of chromosome 6 (6q27).[803] Two class *I* genes have been found that are expressed, *Bota-A* and *Bota-B*.[804,805] These two genes are less than 210 kb apart. To the class *II* region map one *DRA* gene and three *DRB* genes with variable degrees of polymorphism. The number of *DQ* genes varies between *MHC* haplotypes there may be 1 *DQA* and 1 *DQB* gene, or 1 *DQA* and 2 *DQB*, or two of each. The class *IIb* region contains also the *LMP7* gene. There is also a bovine counterpart of *HLA-DM* genes.[806]

The amphibian *MHC* was first described by Du Pasquier and coworkers in *Xenopus*, which shared a common ancestor with humans and mice about 350 million years ago.[807] Later, class *I* and class *II* genes were described in the same species.[808-811] *Xenopus* is tetraploid, but despite that its *MHC* seems to be diploidized and the second set of genes has been either silenced or deleted. Only one expressed *MHC* class *I* locus seems to exist. Non-*MHC*-linked class *I* genes have also been described.[693] Evidence exists for two or three inducible *HSP70* genes and a factor B gene, as well as the *RING3* gene with as yet unknown function.[812,813,593] The class *I* genes apparently fit into both classical and nonclassical families[810] with the nonclassical genes being on a different chromosome from the one harboring the MHC.[693] Like their mammalian counterpart, the frog class *Ib* genes are minimally polymorphic and lack some of the invariant amino acids essential for anchoring of peptide-ligands in the classic class I groove.[693,513] Other data show linkage of *Bf* and *LMP7* to the *MHC* and a likely separation of *LMP7*/class *II* from class *III* and *I* in a recombinant.[570]

The chicken *B*-complex has been under thorough investigation because it controls resistance to neoplastic diseases of viral origin.[814,690] It is located on a minichromosome and has a completely different organization than *HLA* and *H2* (Fig. 2.19).[707,690,815-817] First of all, the avian *MHC* is extremely compact, the gene clusters cover only about 400 kb and the introns in class *I* (*B-F*) and class *II* (*B-L*) are very small, the intergenic distances are very short (10-20 kb).[814,534,513] The *B*-complex does not contain well defined class *I* and class *II* regions since *B-F* and *B-L* beta genes are closely associated with unrelated genes. Class *II* genes are very closely linked to class *I* genes in two clusters and to the *NOR* (nucleolus organizer region). Three loci have been identified: genes which code for B-F and B-L molecules homologous to class *I* and *II*, as well as *B-G*. The latter contain multiple heptad repeats at their C-termini and code for the highly polymorphic IV antigens which have a wide tissue distribution but no mammalian equivalent, although the human MOG gene product has similarities to B-G antigens and cattle butyrophilin.[535-537,531] Five *B-L* locus genes have been identified and at least two *B-F* locus genes. Other estimates for class genes range up to six. So far, no class *III* gene analogs to the mammalian genes encoding the complement factors, steroid 21-hydroxlyase or TNF have been found linked to the *MHC*.[814,534,815,818] Class *I* and class *II* genes are close to each other and tightly linked with other genes, such as a GTP-binding protein gene, 12.3 cM upstream of the most telomeric *B-G* gene.[534] The human equivalent of this protein is neither in the *MHC* nor on chromosome 6. A class *I* and class *II* gene cluster, not linked to the *B-F* and *B-L* regions, *Rfp-Y*, has been identified.[819,820] This genetic region represents the first instance when *MHC* class *I* and class *II* genes have been shown to be linked outside of the *MHC* proper. The organization of DNA elements regulating avian class *II B* genes differs from that in mammalian species, though the *S*, *X* and *Y* boxes are well conserved in sequence and location. They do not seem, however, to have a significant effect on promoter activity.[821]

The *MHC* class *II DB* genes of the red-necked wallaby (*Macropus rufogriseus*),[822] belong to new families that are not orthologous to eutherian *DB* families. This indicates the possibility that the *DB* genes of marsupials have an ancestor different from the *DB* gene ancestors of mammals.

In the last few years, extensive studies have been undertaken on fish *MHC*. There are three major groups of extant fish. The *Agnatha* class (jawless fish) includes lampreys and hagfish, the *Chondrichthyes* (cartilaginous fish) include sharks[823-825] and *Osteichthyes* (bony fish) which includes teleost species such as *carp (Cyprinus carpio)*,[826,711,694,827] Atlantic salmon (*Salmo salar*),[828] trout (*Oncorhynches gorbuschi*)[829], perch, catfish, cichlids,[569] the zebrafish (*Brachydanio rerio*),[620,830-832] guppy *(Poecilia reticulata)*,[833] the goldfish (*Carassius auratus*),[827] as well as several species of lungfish and the single extant coelacanth *Latimeria chalumnae.*[834] The lungfishes and the coelacanth have large amounts of DNA comparable to that of amphibians; puffer fish (Fugu) and zebrafish have extremely small genes and genomes.[835] Class *IA* genes have been cloned from dogfish, carp, zebrafish, Atlantic salmon and the coelacanth; class *IIA* genes from the nurse shark and the zebrafish and class *IIB* genes from the nurse shark, carp, zebrafish, Atlantic salmon, rainbow trout and cichlids. At least in zebrafish some *IIA* class and *B* genes are linked to each other; class *I* and class *II* are not.[570] As in mammals, the *MHC* genes also seem to be polymorphic in fishes.[832,825]

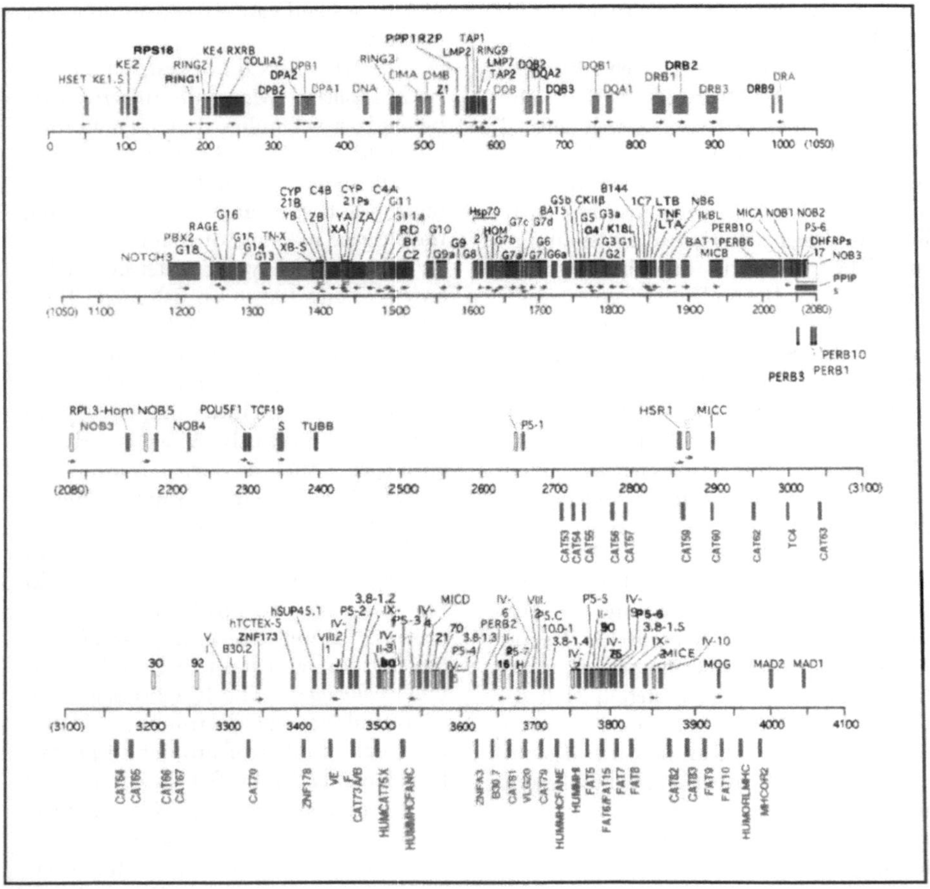

Fig. 2.1. Map of the human chromosome 6. Reprinted with permission from: Campbell RD, Trowsdale J. Immunol Today 1997; 18:Centerfold ©1997 Elsevier Trends Journals. (Please see color insert.)

Fig. 2.2. Comparison of HLA-A α1 and α2 domain amino acid sequences

The AA are given in the international single-letter code. The consensus sequence is derived from all, at the time of writing, available *HLA-A, HLA-B,* and *HLA-C* amino acid sequences. Identity with the consensus is indicated by hyphens; unavailability of information is indicated by a dot, indels introduced for optimal homology are indicated by a slash. See also Table 2.1. Sequences of which only the nucleotides were available, the AA sequence was deferred. AA residues involved in putative peptide binding regions are marked with an asterisk (*).[499]

α1 Domain

	1	11	21	31	41	51	61	71	81 90
	* * *		**	*	*	*	* ** *	** * *	* *
CONSENSUS	GSHSMRYFYT	SVSRPGRGEP	RFIAVGYVDD	TQFVRFDSDA	ASPRMEPRAP	WIEQEGPEYW	DRETQIVKAN	TQTDRESLRN	LRGYYNQSEA
A*0101	--------F-	----------	----------	----------	--QK------	----------	-Q--RNM--H	S----AN-GT	---------D
A*0102	--------S-	------S---	----------	----------	--QK------	----------	-Q--RNM--H	S----AN-GT	---------D
A*0201	--------F-	----------	----------	----------	--Q-------	----------	-G--RK---H	S--H-VD-GT	----------
A*0202	.-------F-	----------	----------	----------	--R-------	----------	-G--RK---H	S--H-VD-GT	----------
A*0203	--------F-	----------	----------	----------	--Q-------	----------	-G--RK---H	S--H-VD-GT	----------
A*0204	--------F-	----------	----------	----------	--Q-------	----------	-G--RK---H	S--H-VD-GT	----------
A*0205	----------	----------	----------	----------	--R-------	----------	-G--RK---H	S--H-VD-GT	----------
A*0206	----------	----------	----------	----------	--Q-------	----------	-G--RK---H	S--H-VD-GT	----------
A*0207	--------F-	----------	----------	----------	--Q-------	----------	-G--RK---H	S--H-VD-GT	----------
A*0208	----------	----------	----------	----------	--R-------	----------	-G--RN---H	S--H-VD-GT	----------
A*0209	--------F-	----------	----------	----------	--Q-------	----------	-G--RK---H	S--H-VD-GT	----------
A*0210	----------	----------	----------	----------	--Q-------	----------	-G--RK---H	S--H-VD-GT	----------
A*0211	--------F-	----------	----------	----------	--Q-------	----------	-G--RK---H	S-I--VD-GT	----------
A*0212	--------F-	----------	----------	----------	--Q-------	----------	-G--RK---H	S--H-VD-GT	----------
A*0213	--------F-	----------	----------	----------	--Q-------	----------	-G--RK---H	S--H-VD-GT	----------
A*0214	.---------	----------	----------	----------	--R-------	----------	-G--RK---H	S--H-VD-GT	----------
A*0215N	--------F-	----------	----------	----------	--Q-------	----------	-G--RK---H	S--H-VD-GT	----------
A*0216	--------F-	----------	----------	----------	--Q-------	----------	-G--RK---H	S--H-VD-GT	----------
A*0217	--------F-	----------	----------	----------	--Q-------	----------	-G--RK---H	S--H-VD-GT	----------
A*0218	--------F-	----------	----------	----------	--Q-------	----------	-G--RK---H	S--H-VD-GT	----------
A*0219	.-------F-	----------	----------	----------	--Q-------	----------	-G--RK---H	S--H-VD-GT	----------
A*0220	.-------F-	----------	----------	----------	--Q-------	----------	-G--RN---H	S--H-VD-GT	----------
A*0221	--------Y-	----------	---------N	----------	--Q-------	----------	-G--RK---H	S--H-VD-GT	----------
A*0222	.-------F-	----------	----------	----------	--Q-------	----------	-G--RK---H	S--H-VD-GT	----------
A*0301	--------F-	----------	----------	----------	--Q-------	----------	-Q--RN---Q	S----VD-GT	----------
A*0302	--------F-	----------	----------	----------	--Q-------	----------	-Q--RN---Q	S----VD-GT	----------
A*0303N	--------F-	----------	----------	----------	--Q-------	----------	-Q--RN---Q	S----VD-GT	----------

Fig. 2.2. (con't)

CONSENSUS	GSHSMRYFYT	SVSRPGRGEP	RFIAVGYVDD	TQFVRFDSDA	ASPRMEPRAP	WIEQEGPEYW	DRETQIVKAN	TQTDRESLRN	LRGYYNQSEA
A*1101	----------	----------	----------	----------	--Q-------	----------	-Q--RN---Q	S----VD-GT	---------D
A*1102	----------	--------K-	----------	----------	--Q-------	----------	-Q--RN---Q	S----VD-GT	---------D
A*1103	.---------	----------	----------	----------	--Q-------	----------	-Q--RN---Q	S----VD-GT	---------D
A*1104	----------	----------	----------	----------	--Q-------	----------	-Q--RN---Q	S----VD-GT	---------D
A*2301	--------S-	----------	----------	----------	--Q-------	----------	-E--GK---H	S-----N--I	ALR-------
A*2402	--------S-	----------	----------	----------	--Q-------	----------	-E--GK---H	S-----N--I	ALR-------
A*2403	--------S-	----------	----------	----------	--Q-------	----------	-E--GK---H	S-----N--I	ALR-------
A*2404	--------S-	----------	----------	----------	--Q-------	----------	-E--GK---H	S----AN-GT	----------
A*2405	.-------S-	----------	----------	----------	--Q-------	----------	-E--GK---H	S-----N--I	ALR-------
A*2406	.-------S-	----------	----------	----------	--Q-------	----------	-E--GK---H	S-----N--I	ALR-------
A*2407	--------S-	----------	----------	----------	--Q-------	----------	-E--GK---Q	S-----N--I	ALR-------
A*2408	.-Q-----S-	----------	----------	----------	--Q-------	----------	-G--RK---H	S-----N--I	ALR-------
A*2409N	--------S-	----------	----------	----------	--Q-------	----------	-E--GK---H	S-----N--I	ALR-------
A*2410	.-------S-	----------	----------	----------	--Q-------	----------	-E--GK---H	S-----N--I	ALR-------
A*2413	.-------S-	----------	----------	----------	--Q-------	----------	-E--GK---H	S-----N--I	ALR-------
A*2414	.-------S-	----------	----------	----------	--Q-------	----------	-E--GK---H	S-----N--I	ALR-------
A*2501	----------	----------	----------	----------	--Q-------	----------	--N-RN---H	S--------I	ALR------D
A*2502	----------	----------	----------	----------	--Q-------	----------	--N-RN---Q	S--------I	ALR------D
A*2601	----------	----------	----------	----------	--Q-------	----------	--N-RN---H	S----AN-GT	---------D
A*2602	----------	----------	----------	----------	--Q-------	----------	--N-RN---H	S----AN-GT	---------D
A*2603	----------	----------	----------	----------	--Q-------	----------	--N-RN---H	S--H-VD-GT	---------D
A*2604	----------	----------	----------	----------	--Q-------	----------	--N-RN---H	S----AN-GT	---------D
A*2605	----------	----------	----------	----------	--Q-------	----------	--N-RN---H	S-----N-GT	---------D
A*2606	.---------	----------	----------	----------	--Q-------	----------	--N-RN---H	S--H-VD-GT	---------D
A*2607	----------	----------	----------	----------	--Q-------	----------	-G--RK---H	S----AN-GT	---------D
A*2608	----------	----------	----------	----------	--Q-------	----------	--N-RN---H	S----AN-GT	---------D
A*2901	--------T-	----------	----------	----------	--Q-------	----------	-LQ-RN---Q	S----AN-GT	----------
A*2902	--------T-	----------	----------	----------	--Q-------	----------	-LQ-RN---Q	S----AN-GT	----------
A*2903	..------T-	----------	----------	----------	--Q-------	----------	-LQ-RN---Q	S----AN-GT	----------
A*3001	--------S-	------S---	----------	----------	--Q-------	-----R----	-Q--RN---Q	S----VD-GT	----------
A*3002	--------S-	------S---	----------	----------	--Q-------	-----R----	-Q--RN---H	S-----N-GT	----------
A*3003	--------S-	------S---	----------	----------	--Q-------	----------	-Q--RN---H	S-----N-GT	----------
A*3004	.-------S-	------S---	----------	----------	--Q-------	-----R----	-Q--RN---H	S-----N-GT	----------
A*3005	..------S-	------S---	----------	----------	----------	-----R----	-R--RN---H	S-----N-GT	----------
A*31012	--------T-	----------	----------	----------	--Q-------	-----R----	-Q--RN---H	S-I--VD-GT	----------
A*3201	--------F-	----------	----------	----------	--Q-------	----------	-Q--RN---H	S--------I	ALR-------
A*3202	--------F-	----------	----------	----------	--Q-------	----------	-Q--RN---H	S--------I	ALR-------
A*3301	--------T-	----------	----------	----------	--Q-------	----------	--N-RN---H	S-I--VD-GT	----------
A*3302	--------T-	------S---	----------	----------	--Q-------	----------	--N-RN---H	S-I--VD-GT	----------
A*3303	--------T-	----------	----------	----------	--Q-------	----------	--N-RN---H	S-I--VD-GT	----------
A*3401	----------	----------	----------	----------	--Q-------	----------	--N-RK---Q	S----VD-GT	---------D

```
A*3402     ---------- ---------- ---------- ---------- --Q------- ---------- --N-RN---Q S----VD-GT ---------D
A*3601     --------F- ---------- ---------- ---------- --QK------ ---------- -Q--RNM--H S----AN-GT ---------D
A*4301     ---------- ---------- ---------- ---------- --Q------- ---------- -LQ-RN---H S----AN-GT ---------D
A*6601     ---------- ---------- ---------- ---------- --Q------- ---------- --N-RN---Q S----VD-GT ---------D
A*6602     ---------- ---------- ---------- ---------- --Q------- ---------- --N-RN---Q S----VD-GT ----------
A*6603     .--------- ---------- ---------- ---------- --Q------- ---------- --N-RN---H S----VD-GT ----------
A*68011    ---------- ---------- ---------- ---------- --Q------- ---------- --N-RN---Q S----VD-GT ----------
A*68012    ---------- ---------- ---------- ---------- --Q------- ---------- --N-RN---Q S----VD-GT ----------
A*6802     ---------- -M-------- ---------- ---------- --Q------- ---------- --N-RN---Q S----VD-GT ----------
A*6803     .--------- ---------- ---------- ---------- --Q------- ---------- --N-RN---H S----VD-GT ----------
A*6901     ---------- ---------- ---------- ---------- --Q------- ---------- --N-RN---Q S----VD-GT ----------
A*7401     --------F- ---------- ---------- ---------- --Q------- ---------- -Q--RN---H S----VD-GT ----------
A*7402     --------F- ---------- ---------- ---------- --Q------- ---------- -Q--RN---H S----VD-GT ----------
A*7403     --------F- ---------- ---------- ---------- --Q------- ---------- -Q--RN---H S----VD-AT ----------
A*8001     --------F- ---------- ---------- S--Q------ --Q------- -----E---- -E--RN---H S--N-AN-GT ---------D
CONSENSUS  GSHSMRYFYT SVSRPGRGEP RFIAVGYVDD TQFVRFDSDA ASPRMEPRAP WIEQEGPEYW DRETQIVKAN TQTDRESLRN LRGYYNQSEA

α2 Domain  91         101        111        121        131        141        151        161        171        181
           * *                **  *       *                        *  **       *  **  **  *    *     *

CONSENSUS  GSHTLQRMYG CDVGPDGRLL RGYDQYAYDG KDYIALNEDL RSWTAADTAA QITQRKWEAA RVAEQLRAYL EGTCVEWLRR YLENGKETLQ RA
A*0101     ----I-I--- --------F- ---R-D---- ---------- -------M-- ---K-----V HA---R-V-- --R--DG--- ---------- -T
A*0102     ----I-I--- --------F- ---R-D---- ---------- -------M-- ---K-----V HA---R-V-- --R--DG--- ---------- -T
A*0201     ----V----- ----S-W-F- ---H------ ------K--- -------M-- -T-KH----- H--------- ---------- ---------- -T
A*0202     ---------- ----S-W-F- ---H------ ------K--- -------M-- -T-KH----- H----W---- ---------- ---------- -T
A*0203     ----V----- ----S-W-F- ---H------ ------K--- -------M-- -T-KH---T- HE---W---- ---------- ---------- -T
A*0204     ----V-M--- ----S-W-F- ---H------ ------K--- -------M-- -T-KH----- H--------- ---------- ---------- -T
A*0205     ---------- ----S-W-F- ---H------ ------K--- -------M-- -T-KH----- H----W---- ---------- ---------- -T
A*0206     ----V----- ----S-W-F- ---H------ ------K--- -------M-- -T-KH----- H--------- ---------- ---------- -T
A*0207     ----V---C- ----S-W-F- ---H------ ------K--- -------M-- -T-KH----- H--------- ---------- ---------- -T
A*0208     ---------- ----S-W-F- ---H------ ------K--- -------M-- -T-KH----- H----W---- ---------- ---------- -T
A*0209     ----V----- ----S-W-F- ---H------ ------K--- -------M-- -T-KH----- H--------- ---------- ---------- -T
A*0210     ----V---F- ----S---F- ---H------ ------K--- -------M-- -T-KH----- H--------- ---------- ---------- -T
A*0211     ----V----- ----S-W-F- ---H------ ------K--- -------M-- -T-KH----- H--------- ---------- ---------- -T
A*0212     ----V----- ----S-W-F- ---H------ ------K--- -------M-- -T-KH----- H----Q---- ---------- ---------- -T
A*0213     ----V----- ----S-W-F- ---H------ ------K--- -------M-- -T-KH----- HE---Q---- ---------- ---------- -T
A*0214     ---------- ----S-W-F- ---H------ ------K--- -------M-- -T-KH----- H--------- ---------- ---------- -T
A*0215N    ----V---C- ----S-W-F- ---H------ ------K--- -------M-- -T-KH----- H--------- ---------- ---------- -T
A*0216     ----V----- ----S-W-F- ---H------ ------K--- -------M-- -T-KH----- H--------- --E------- ---------- -T
A*0217     ------M-F- ----S-W-F- ---H------ ------K--- -------M-- -T-KH----- H--------- ---------- ---------- -T
A*0218     ----V---C- ----S-W-F- ---H------ ------K--- -------K-- -T-KH----- H--------- ---------- ---------- -T
```

Fig. 2.2. (con't)

ISENSUS	GSHTLQRMYG	CDVGPDGRLL	RGYDQYAYDG	KDYIALNEDL	RSWTAADTAA	QITQRKWEAA	RVAEQLRAYL	EGTCVEWLRR	YLENGKETLQ	RA
A*0219	----V-----	----S-W-F-	---H------	------K---	-------M--	---K------	H----Q----	-----DG---	----------	-T
A*0220	----V-----	----S-W-F-	---H------	------K---	-------M--	-T-KH-----	H---------	----------	----------	-T
A*0221	----V-----	----S-W-F-	---H------	------K---	-------M--	-T-KH-----	H---------	----------	----------	-T
A*0222	----V-----	----S-W-F-	---H------	------K---	-------M--	-T-KH-----	H----W----	------W---	----------	-T
A*0301	----I-I---	----S---F-	---R-D----	----------	-------M--	---K------	HE--------	D---------	----------	-T
A*0302	----I-I---	----S---F-	---R-D----	----------	-------M--	---K------	H----Q----	D---------	----------	-T
A*0303N	----I-I---	//--S---F-	---R-D----	----------	-------M--	---K------	HE--------	D---------	----------	-T
A*1101	----I-I---	--------F-	---R-D----	----------	-------M--	---K------	HA---Q----	--R-------	----------	-T
A*1102	----I-I---	--------F-	---R-D----	----------	-------M--	---K------	HA---Q----	--R-------	----------	-T
A*1103	----I-I---	--------F-	---R-D----	----------	-------M--	---K------	-E---Q----	--R-------	----------	-T
A*1104	----I-I---	--------F-	---R-D----	----------	-------M--	---K------	HA---Q----	----------	----------	-T
A*2301	------M-F-	----S---F-	---H------	------K---	-------M--	----------	----------	-----DG---	----------	-T
A*2402	------M-F-	----S---F-	---H------	------K---	-------M--	---K------	H----Q----	-----DG---	----------	-T
A*2403	------M-F-	----S---F-	---H------	------K---	-------M--	---K------	H----Q----	----------	----------	-T
A*2404	------M-F-	----S---F-	---H------	------K---	-------M--	---K------	H----Q----	-----DG---	----------	-T
A*2405	------M-F-	----S---F-	---H------	------K---	-------M--	----------	H----Q----	-----DG---	----------	-T
A*2406	------M-F-	----S---F-	---H------	------K---	-------M--	---K------	H----W----	-----DG---	----------	-T
A*2407	------M-F-	----S---F-	---H------	------K---	-------M--	---K------	H----Q----	-----DG---	----------	-T
A*2408	------M-F-	----S---F-	---H------	------K---	-------M--	---K------	H----Q----	-----DG---	----------	-T

A*2413	------M-F-	----S---F-	---H------	------K---	-------M--	---K------	H---------	-----DG---	----------	-T
A*2414	----R-----	----S-W-F-	---H------	------K---	-------M--	---K------	H---------	-----DG---	----------	-T
A*2501	----I-----	--------F-	---Q-D----	----------	-------M--	--------T-	HE---W----	--R-------	----------	-T
A*2502	----I-----	--------F-	---Q-D----	----------	-------M--	--------T-	HE---W----	--R-------	----------	-T
A*2601	----I-----	--------F-	---Q-D----	----------	-------M--	--------T-	HE---W----	--R-------	----------	-T
A*2602	----I-----	--------F-	---Q-N----	----------	-------M--	--------T-	HE---W----	--R-------	----------	-T
A*2603	----I-----	--------F-	---Q-D----	----------	-------M--	--------T-	HE---W----	--R-------	----------	-T
A*2604	----I-----	--------F-	---Q-D----	----------	-------M--	--------T-	HE---W----	--L-------	----------	-T
A*2605	----I-----	--------F-	---Q-D----	----------	-------M--	--------T-	HE---W----	--R-------	----------	-T
A*2606	----I-----	--------F-	---QRD----	----------	-------M--	--------T-	HE---W----	--R-------	----------	-T
A*2607	----I-----	--------F-	---Q-D----	----------	-------M--	--------T-	HE---W----	--R-------	----------	-T
A*2608	----I-----	--------F-	---Q-D----	----------	-------M--	--------T-	HE---Q----	--R-------	----------	-T
A*2901	----I-M---	-H--S---F-	---R-D----	----------	-------M--	----------	----------	----------	----------	-T
A*2902	----I-M---	----S---F-	---R-D----	----------	-------M--	----------	----------	----------	----------	-T
A*2903	----I-M---	----S---F-	---R-D----	----------	-------M--	----------	----------	-----DG---	----------	-T
A*3001	----I-I---	----S---F-	---E-H----	----------	-------M--	----------	-W--------	----------	----------	-T
A*3002	----I-I---	----S---F-	---E-H----	----------	-------M--	----------	-R--------	----------	----------	-T
A*3003	----I-I---	----S---F-	---E-H----	----------	-------M--	----------	-R--------	----------	----------	-T
A*3004	----I-I---	----S---F-	---E-H----	----------	-------M--	----------	H----W----	----------	----------	-T
A*3005	----I-I---	----S---F-	---E-H----	----------	-------M--	----------	H----W----	----------	----------	-.
A*31012	----I-M---	----S---F-	---Q-D----	----------	-------M--	----------	----------	----------	----------	-T
A*3201	----I-M---	----------	---Q-D----	----------	-------M--	----------	----------	----------	----------	-T
A*3202	----I-M---	----------	---Q-D----	----------	-------M--	----------	H----Q----	----------	----------	-T
A*3301	----I-M---	----S---F-	---Q-D----	----------	-------M--	----------	----------	----------	H---------	-T
A*3302	----I-M---	----S---F-	---Q-D----	----------	-------M--	----------	----------	----------	----------	-T
A*3303	----I-M---	----S---F-	---Q-D----	----------	-------M--	----------	----------	----------	----------	-T
A*3401	----I-----	--------F-	---Q-D----	----------	-------M--	--------T-	HE---W----	----------	----------	-T
A*3402	----I-I---	----S---F-	---R-D----	----------	-------M--	--------T-	HE--------	----------	----------	-T
A*3601	----I-I---	--------F-	---R-D----	----------	-------M--	---K-----V	HA---R-V--	----------	----------	-T
A*4301	----I-----	--------F-	---Q-D----	----------	-------M--	--------T-	HE---W----	--R-------	----------	-T
A*6601	----I-----	--------F-	---Q-D----	----------	-------M--	--------T-	HE---W----	--R-------	----------	-T
A*6602	----I-----	--------F-	---Q-D----	----------	-------M--	--------T-	HE---W----	--E-------	----------	-T
A*6603	----I-----	--------F-	---Q-D----	----------	-------M--	--------T-	HE---W----	--E-------	----------	-T
A*68011	----I-M---	----S---F-	---R-D----	------K---	-------M--	-T-KH-----	H----W----	----------	----------	-T
A*68012	----I-M---	----S---F-	---R-D----	------K---	-------M--	-T-KH-----	H----W----	----------	----------	-T
A*6802	----I-----	--------F-	---H------	------K---	-------M--	-T-KH-----	H----W----	----------	----------	-T
A*6803	----I-M---	----S---F-	---R-D----	------K---	-------M--	-T-KH-----	H----W----	----------	----------	-T
A*6901	----V-----	----S-W-F-	---H------	------K---	-------M--	-T-KH-----	H---------	----------	----------	-T
A*7401	----I-M---	----------	---Q-D----	----------	-------M--	----------	----------	----------	----------	-T
A*7402	----I-M---	----------	---Q-D----	----------	-------M--	----------	----------	----------	----------	-T
A*7403	----I-M---	----------	---Q-D----	----------	-------M--	----------	----------	----------	----------	-T
A*8001	----I-I---	----S---F-	---R-D----	----------	-------M--	---K------	-R--------	--E--DG---	----------	-T
CONSENSUS	GSHTLQRMYG	CDVGPDGRLL	RGYDQYAYDG	KDYIALNEDL	RSWTAADTAA	QITQRKWEAA	RVAEQLRAYL	EGTCVEWLRR	YLENGKETLQ	RA

Fig. 2.3. Comparison of *HLA-B* α1 and α2 domain amino acid sequences

The AA are given in the international single-letter code. The consensus sequence is derived from all, at the time of writing, available *HLA-A*, *HLA-B*, and *HLA-C* amino acid sequences. Identity with the consensus is indicated by hyphens; unavailability of information is indicated by a dot, indels introduced for optimal homology are indicated by a slash. See also Table 2.2. Sequences of which only the nucleotides were available, the AA sequence was deferred. AA residues involved in putative peptide binding regions are marked with an asterisk (*).[499]

α1 Domain

```
           1          11         21         31         41         51         61         71         81        90
               * * *                 **        *           *              *  *  **  *   **  *  * *  *
CONSENSUS  GSHSMRYFYT SVSRPGRGEP RFIAVGYVDD TQFVRFDSDA ASPRMEPRAP WIEQEGPEYW DRETQIVKAN TQTDRESLRN LRGYYNQSEA
B*0702     ---------- ---------- ---S------ ---------- ----E----- ---------- --N---Y--Q A--------- ----------
B*0703     ---------- ---------- ---S------ ---------- ----E----- ---------- --N---Y-T- ---------- ----------
B*0704     ---------- ---------- ---S------ ---------- ----E----- ---------- --N---Y--Q A--------- ----------
B*0705     ---------- ---------- ---S------ ---------- ----E----- ---------- --N---Y--Q A--------- ----------
B*0706     ---------- ---------- ---S------ ---------- ----E----- ---------- --N---Y--Q A--------- ----------
B*0707     .--------- ---------- ---S------ ---------- ----E----- ---------- --N---Y--Q A--------- ----------
B*0801     --------D- AM-------- ---S------ ---------- ----E----- ---------- --N---F-T- ---------- ----------
B*0802     --------D- AM-------- ---S------ ---------- ----E----- ---------- --N---F-T- ------N--T ALR-------
B*0803     .......-D- AM-------- ---S------ ---------- ----E----- ---------- --N---F-T- ---Y--N--I ALR-------
B*1301     ---------- AM-------- ---T------ ---------- T----A---- ---------- ------S-T- ---Y--N--T ALR-------
B*1302     ---------- AM-------- ---T------ ---------- T----A---- ---------- ------S-T- ---Y--N--T ALR-------
B*1303     ---------- AM-------- ---T------ ---------- T----A---- ---------- ------S-T- ---Y--N--T ALR-------
B*1401     ---------- ---------- ---S------ ---------- ----E----- ---------- --N---C-T- ---------- ----------
B*1402     ---------- A--------- ---S------ ---------- ----E----- ---------- --N---C-T- ---------- ----------
B*1501     ---------- AM-------- ---------- ---------- -----A---- ---------- ------S-T- ---Y------ ----------
B*1502     ---------- AM-------- ---------- ---------- -----A---- ---------- --N---S-T- ---Y------ ----------
B*1503     ---------- AM-------- ---S------ ---------- ----E----- ---------- ------S-T- ---Y------ ----------
B*1504     ---------- AM-------- ---------- ---------- -----A---- ---------- ------S-T- ---Y------ ----------
B*1505     ---------- AM-------- ---------- ---------- -----A---- ---------- ------S-T- ---Y------ ----------
B*1506     ---------- AM-------- ---------- ---------- -----A---- ---------- ------S-T- ---Y------ ----------
B*1507     ---------- AM-------- ---------- ---------- -----A---- ---------- ------S-T- ---Y------ ----------
B*1508     ---------- AM-------- ---------- ---------- -----A---- ---------- --N---F-T- ---Y------ ----------
B*1509     ---------- AM-------- ---S------ ---------- ----E----- ---------- --N---C-T- ---Y------ ----------
B*1510     ---------- AM-------- ---S------ ---------- ----E----- ---------- --N---C-T- ---Y------ ----------
B*1511     ---------- AM-------- ---------- ---------- -----A---- ---------- --N---Y-T- ---Y------ ----------
B*1512     ---------- AM-------- ---------- ---------- -----A---- ---------- ------S-T- ---Y------ ----------
B*1513     ---------- AM-------- ---------- ---------- -----A---- ---------- --N---S-T- ---Y--N--I ALR-------
B*1514     ---------- AM-------- ---------- ---------- -----A---- ---------- ------S-T- ---Y------ ----------
```

```
B*1515   ---------- AM-------- ---------- ---------- -----A---- ---------- --N---S-T- ---Y------ ----------
B*1516   ---F------ AM-------- ---------- ---------- -----A---- ---------- ----RNM--S A--Y--N--I ALR-------
B*1517   ---------- AM-------- ---------- ---------- -----A---- ---------- ----RNM--S A--Y--N--I ALR-------
B*1518   ---------- AM-------- ---S------ ---------- ----E----- ---------- --N---C-T- ---Y------ ----------
B*1519   ---------- AM-------- ---------- ---------- -----A---- ---------- ------S-T- ---Y------ ----------
B*1520   ---------- AM-------- ---------- ---------- -----A---- ---------- ------S-T- ---Y------ ----------
B*1521   ---------- AM-------- ---------- ---------- -----A---- ---------- --N---C-T- ---Y------ ----------
B*1522   ---------- AM-------- ---------- ---------- ----T----- ---------- --N---F-T- ---Y------ ----------
B*1523   ---------- AM-------- ---S------ ---------- ----E----- ---------- --N---C-T- ---Y--N--I ALR-------
B*1524   .--------- AM-------- ---------- ---------- -----A---- ---------- ------S-T- ---Y--N--I ALR-------
B*1525   ---------- AM-------- ---------- ---------- -----A---- ---------- ------S-T- ---Y------ ----------
B*1526N  ---------- AM-------- ---------- ---------- -----A---- ---------- ------S-T- ---Y------ ----------
B*1527   ....------ AM-------- ---------- ---------- -----A---- ---------- ------S-T- ---Y------ ----------
B*1528   ---------- AM-------- ---------- ---------- -----A---- ---------- ---I--S-T- ---Y------ ----------
B*1529   ---------- AM-------- ---S------ ---------- ----E----- ---------- --N---F-T- ---Y------ ----------
B*1530   ....------ AM-------- ---------- ---------- -----A---- ---------- ------S-T- ---Y------ ----------
B*1531   ....------ AM-------- ---------- ---------- -----A---- ---------- --N---S-T- ---Y------ ----------
B*1532   .--------- AM-------- ---------- ---------- -----A---- ---------- ------S-T- ---Y------ ----------
B*1533   .--------- AM-------- ---------- ---------- -----A---- ---------- ------S-T- ---Y------ ----------
B*1534   .--------- AM-------- ---------- ---------- -----A---- ---------- ------S-T- ---Y------ ----------
B*1535   .--------- AM-------- ---------- ---------- -----A---- ---------- ------S-T- ---Y------ ----------
B*1537   .--------- AM-------- ---S------ ---------- ----E----- ---------- --N---C-T- ---Y------ ----------
B*1801   --------H- ---------- ---S-----G ---------- ----T----- ---------- --N---S-T- ---Y------ ----------
B*1802   --------H- ---------- ---S-----G ---------- ----T----- ---------- --N---S-T- ---Y------ ----------
B*1803   .-------H- ---------- ---S-----G ---------- ----T----- ---------- --N---S-T- ---------- ----------
B*1805   .-------H- ---------- ---S-----G ---------- ----T----- ---------- --N---S-T- ---Y------ ----------
B*2701   --------H- ---------- ---T------ -L-------- ----E----- ---------- ------C--K A--Y--N--T ALR-------
B*2702   --------H- ---------- ---T------ -L-------- ----E----- ---------- ------C--K A-----N--I ALR-------
B*2703   --------H- ---------- ---T------ -L-------- ----E----- --------H- ------C--K A-----D--T -LR-------
B*2704   -----.--H- ---------- ---T------ -L-------- ----E----- ---------- ------C--K A--------T -LR-------
B*27052  --------H- ---------- ---T------ -L-------- ----E----- ---------- ------C--K A-----D--T -LR-------
B*27053  .......... .......... ......---- -L-------- ----E----- ---------- ------C--K A-----D--T -LR-------
B*2706   --------H- ---------- ---T------ -L-------- ----E----- ---------- ------C--K A--------T -LR-------
B*2707   --------H- ---------- ---T------ -L-------- ----E----- ---------- ------C--K A-----D--T -LR-------
B*2708   --------H- ---------- ---T------ -L-------- ----E----- ---------- ------C--K A--------- ----------
B*2709   --------H- ---------- ---T------ -L-------- ----E----- ---------- ------C--K A-----D--T -LR-------
B*2710   --------H- ---------- ---T------ -L-------- ----E----- ---------- ------C--K A-----D--T -LR-------
B*3501   ---------- AM-------- ---------- ---------- ----T----- ---------- --N---F-T- ---Y------ ----------
B*3502   ---------- AM-------- ---------- ---------- ----T----- ---------- --N---F-T- ---Y------ ----------
B*3503   ---------- AM-------- ---------- ---------- ----T----- ---------- --N---F-T- ---Y------ ----------
```

Fig. 2.3. (con't)

```
CONSENSUS  GSHSMRYFYT SVSRPGRGEP RFIAVGYVDD TQFVRFDSDA ASPRMEPRAP WIEQEGPEYW DRETQIVKAN TQTDRESLRN LRGYYNQSEA
 B*3504    ---------- AM-------- ---------- ---------- ----T----- ---------- --N---F-T- ---Y------ ----------
 B*3505    ---------- AM-------- ---------- ---------- ----T----- ---------- --N---F-T- ---Y------ ----------
 B*3506    ---------- AM-------- ---------- ---------- ----T----- ---------- --N---F-T- ---Y------ ----------
 B*3507    ---------- AM---V---- ---------- ---------- ----T----- ---------- --N---F-T- ---Y------ ----------
 B*3508    ---------- AM-------- ---------- ---------- ----T----- ---------- --N---F-T- ---Y------ ----------
 B*35091   ---------- AM-------- ---------- ---------- ----T----- ---------- --N---F-T- ---Y------ ----------
 B*35092   .--------- AM-------- ---------- ---------- ----T----- ---------- --N---F-T- ---Y------ ----------
 B*3510    ---------- AM-------- ---------- ---------- ----T----- ---------- ------F-T- ---Y------ ----------
 B*3511    ---------- AM-------- ---------- ---------- ----T----- ---------- --N---F-T- ---Y------ ----------
 B*3512    ---------- AM-------- ---------- ---------- ----T----- ---------- --N---F-T- ---Y------ ----------
 B*3513    ---------- AM-------- ---------- ---------- ----T----- ---------- ------F-T- ---Y------ ----------
 B*3515    ---------- AM-------- ---------- ---------- ----T----- ---------- --N---F-T- ---Y------ ----------
 B*3516    ---------- AM-------- ---------- ---------- ----T----- ---------- ------F-T- ---Y------ ----------
 B*3517    ---------- AM-------- ---------- ---------- ----T----- ---------- --N---F-T- ---Y------ ----------
 B*3518    ---------- AM-------- ---------- ---------- ----T----- ---------- --N---F-T- ---Y------ ----------
 B*3519    .--------- AM-------- ---------- ---------- ----K----- ---------- --N---F-T- ---Y------ ----------
 B*3520    .--------- AM-------- ---------- ---------- ----T----- ---------- --N---S-T- ---Y------ ----------
 B*3521    .--------- AM-------- ---------- ---------- ----T----- ---------- --N---F-T- ---Y-----N ----------
 B*3701    --------H- ---------- ---S------ ---------- ----T----- ---------- ------S-T- ---Y--D--T -LR-------
 B*3702    --------H- ---------- ---S------ ---------- ----T----- ---------- ------S-T- ---Y--D--T -LR-------
 B*3801    ---------- ---------- ---S------ ---------- ----E----- ---------- --N---C-T- ---Y--N--I ALR-------
 B*3802    ---------- ---------- ---S------ ---------- ----E----- ---------- --N---C-T- ---Y--N--T ALR-------
 B*39011   ---------- ---------- ---S------ ---------- ----E----- ---------- --N---C-T- ---------- ----------
 B*39013   ---------- ---------- ---S------ ---------- ----E----- ---------- --N---C-T- ---------- ----------
 B*39021   ---------- ---------- ---S------ ---------- ----E----- ---------- ------S-T- ---------- ----------
 B*39022   ---------- ---------- ---S------ ---------- ----E----- ---------- ------S-T- ---------- ----------
 B*3903    ---------- ---------- ---S------ ---------- ----E----- ---------- --N---C-T- ---------- ----------
 B*3904    ---------- AM-------- ---S------ ---------- ----E----- ---------- --N---C-T- ---------- ----------
 B*3905    ---------- ---------- ---S------ ---------- ----E----- ---------- --N---C-T- ---Y------ ----------
 B*39061   ---------- ---------- ---S------ ---------- ----E----- ---------- --N---C-T- ---------- ----------
 B*39062   ---------- ---------- ---S------ ---------- ----E----- ---------- --N---C-T- ---------- ----------
 B*3907    .......... .......... .......... .....----- ----E----- ---------- --N---C-T- ---Y------ ----------
 B*3908    ---------- ---------- ---S------ ---------- ----E----- ---------- ------S-T- ---Y------ ----------
 B*3909    ---------- ---------- ---S------ ---------- ----E----- ---------- --N---C-T- ---------- ----------
 B*3910    ---------- ---------- ---S------ ---------- ----E----- ---------- --N---Y-T- ---------- ----------
 B*3911    ........-- ---------- ---S------ ---------- ----E----- ---------- --N---C-T- ---Y------ ----------
 B*3912    .-------D- A--------- ---S------ ---------- ---RE----- ---------- --N---C-T- ---------- ----------
 B*40011   --------H- AM-------- ---T------ -L-------- T---K----- ---------- ------S-T- ---Y------ ----------
 B*40012   --------H- AM-------- ---T------ -L-------- T---K----- ---------- ------S-T- ---Y------ ----------
 B*4002    --------H- ---------- ---T------ -L-------- T---K----- ---------- ------S-T- ---Y------ ----------
 B*4003    --------H- ---------- ---T------ -L-------- T---K----- ---------- ------S-T- ---Y------ ----------
 B*4004    --------H- ---------- ---T------ -L-------- T---K----- ---------- ------S-T- ---Y------ ----------
 B*4005    --------H- ---------- ---T------ -L-------- T---K----- ---------- ------S-T- ---Y------ ----------
 B*4006    --------H- ---------- ---T------ -L-------- T---K----- ---------- ------S-T- ---Y------ ----------
```

```
B*4007   --------H- AM-------- ---T------ -L-------- T---K----- ---------- ------F-T- ---Y------ ----------
B*4008   --------H- ---------- ---T------ -L-------- T---K----- ---------- --N---F-T- ---Y------ ----------
B*4009   .-------H- ---------- ---T------ -L-------- T---K----- ---------- ------S-T- ---Y------ ----------
B*4101   --------H- AM-------- ---T------ -L-------- T---K----- ---------- ------S-T- ---Y------ ----------
B*4102   --------H- AM-------- ---T------ -L-------- T---K----- ---------- ------S-T- ---Y------ ----------
B*4201   ---------- ---------- ---S------ ---------- ----E----- ---------- --N---Y--Q A--------- ----------
B*4402   ---------- AM-------- ---T------ -L-------- T---K----- ---------- ------S-T- ---Y--N--T ALR-------
B*44031  ---------- AM-------- ---T------ -L-------- T---K----- ---------- ------S-T- ---Y--N--T ALR-------
B*44032  .--------- AM-------- ---T------ -L-------- T---K----- ---------- ------S-T- ---Y--N--T ALR-------
B*4404   ---------- AM-------- ---T------ -L-------- T---K----- ---------- ------S-T- ---Y--N--T ALR-------
B*4405   ---------- AM-------- ---T------ -L-------- T---K----- ---------- ------S-T- ---Y--N--T ALR-------
B*4406   ---------- AM-------- ---------- ---------- ----T----- ---------- --N---F-T- ---Y--N--I ALR-------
B*4407   ---------- AM-------- ---T------ -L-------- ----K----- ---------- ------S-T- ---Y--N--T ALR-------
B*4408   ---------- AM-------- ---T------ -L-------- -----A---- ---------- ------S-T- ---Y--N--T ALR-------
B*4410   .--------- AM-------- ---T------ -L-------- T---K----- ---------- ------S-T- ---Y--N--T ALR-------
B*4501   --------H- AM-------- ---T------ -L-------- T---K----- ---------- ------S-T- ---Y------ ----------
B*4601   ---------- AM-------- ---------- ---------- -----A---- ---------- -----KY-RQ A----V---- ----------
B*4701   ---------- AM-------- ---T------ -L-------- T---K----- ---------- ------S-T- ---Y--D--T -LR-------
B*4702   ---------- AM-------- ---T------ -L-------- T---K----- ---------- ------S-T- ---Y------ ----------
```

Fig. 2.3. (con't)

CONSENSUS	GSHSMRYFYT	SVSRPGRGEP	RFIAVGYVDD	TQFVRFDSDA	ASPRMEPRAP	WIEQEGPEYW	DRETQIVKAN	TQTDRESLRN	LRGYYNQSEA
*B*4801*	----------	----------	---S------	----------	----E-----	----------	------S-T-	---Y------	----------
*B*4802*	----------	----------	---S------	----------	----E-----	----------	------S-T-	---Y------	----------
*B*4803*	.---------	----------	---S------	----------	----E-----	----------	------S-T-	---Y------	----------
*B*4901*	--------H-	AM--------	---T------	-L--------	T---K-----	----------	------S-T-	---Y--N--I	ALR-------
*B*5001*	--------H-	AM--------	---T------	-L--------	T---K-----	----------	------S-T-	---Y------	----------
*B*51011*	----------	AM--------	----------	----------	----T-----	----------	--N---F-T-	---Y--N--I	ALR-------
*B*51012*	.---------	AM--------	----------	----------	----T-----	----------	--N---F-T-	---Y--N--I	ALR-------
*B*51021*	----------	AM--------	----------	----------	----T-----	----------	--N---F-T-	---Y--N--I	ALR-------
*B*51022*	----------	AM--------	----------	----------	----T-----	----------	--N---F-T-	---Y--N--I	ALR-------
*B*5103*	----------	AM--------	----------	----------	----T-----	----------	--N---F-T-	---Y--N--I	ALR-------
*B*5104*	----------	AM--------	----------	----------	----T-----	----------	--N---F-T-	---Y--N--I	ALR-------
*B*5105*	----------	AM--------	----------	----------	----T-----	----------	--N---F-T-	---Y--N--I	ALR-------
*B*5106*	----------	AM--------	----------	----------	----T-----	----------	--N---F-T-	---Y--N--I	ALR-------
*B*5107*	.---------	AM--------	----------	----------	----T-----	----------	--N---S-T-	---Y--N--I	ALR-------
*B*5108*	....	AM--------	----------	----------	----T-----	----------	--N---F-T-	---Y--N--I	ALR-------
*B*52011*	----------	AM--------	----------	----------	----T-----	----------	------S-T-	---Y--N--I	ALR-------
*B*52012*	----------	AM--------	----------	----------	----T-----	----------	------S-T-	---Y--N--I	ALR-------
*B*5301*	----------	AM--------	----------	----------	----T-----	----------	--N---F-T-	---Y--N--I	ALR-------
*B*5401*	----------	AM--------	----------	----------	----G-----	-V--------	--N---Y--Q	A---------	----------
*B*5501*	----------	AM--------	----------	----------	----E-----	----------	--N---Y--Q	A---------	----------
*B*5502*	----------	AM--------	----------	----------	----E-----	----------	--N---Y--Q	A---------	----------
*B*5503*	.---------	AM--------	----------	----------	----E-----	----------	--N---Y--Q	A----V----	----------
*B*5504*	.---------	AM--------	----------	----------	----E-----	----------	--N---Y--Q	A---------	----------
*B*5505*	----------	AM--------	----------	----------	----E-----	-------A--	--N---Y--Q	A---------	----------
*B*5601*	----------	AM--------	----------	----------	----E-----	----------	--N---Y--Q	A---------	----------
*B*5602*	----------	AM--------	----------	----------	----E-----	----------	--N---Y--Q	A---------	----------
*B*5603*	.---------	AM--------	----------	----------	----E-----	----------	--N---Y--Q	A---------	----------
*B*5701*	----------	AM--------	----------	----------	-----A----	----------	-G--RNM--S	A--Y--N--I	ALR-------
*B*5702*	----------	AM--------	----------	----------	-----A----	----------	-G--RNM--S	A--Y--N--I	ALR-------
*B*5703*	----------	AM--------	----------	----------	-----A----	----------	-G--RNM--S	A--Y--N--I	ALR-------
*B*5704*	----------	AM--------	----------	----------	-----A----	----------	-G--RNM--S	A--Y--N--I	ALR-------
*B*5801*	----------	AM--------	----------	----------	----T-----	----------	-G--RNM--S	A--Y--N--I	ALR-------
*B*5802*	----------	AM--------	----------	----------	----T-----	----------	-G--RNM--S	A--Y--N--I	ALR-------
*B*5901*	----------	AM--------	----------	----------	----E-----	----------	--N---F-T-	---Y--N--I	ALR-------
*B*67011*	----------	----------	---S------	----------	----E-----	----------	--N---Y--Q	A---------	----------
*B*67012*	.---------	----------	---S------	----------	----E-----	----------	--N---Y--Q	A---------	----------
*B*7301*	--------H-	----------	---T------	----------	----E-----	----------	--N---C--K	A----VG---	---------D
*B*7801*	----------	AM--------	----------	----------	----T-----	----------	--N---F-T-		----------
*B*78021*	----------	AM--------	----------	----------	----T-----	----------	--N---F-T-	---Y------	----------
*B*78022*	.---------	AM--------	----------	----------	----T-----	----------	--N---F-T-	---Y------	----------
*B*8101*	----------	----------	---S------	----------	----E-----	----------	--N---Y--Q	A---------	----------
*B*8201*	----------	AM--------	---S------	----------	----E-----	----------	--N---Y--Q	A---------	----------
CONSENSUS	GSHSMRYFYT	SVSRPGRGEP	RFIAVGYVDD	TQFVRFDSDA	ASPRMEPRAP	WIEQEGPEYW	DRETQIVKAN	TQTDRESLRN	LRGYYNQSEA

α2 Domain

	91	101	111	121	131	141	151	161	171	181
	* *		** *	*		* **	* ** **	* *	*	
CONSENSUS	GSHTLQRMYG	CDVGPDGRLL	RGYDQYAYDG	KDYIALNEDL	RSWTAADTAA	QITQRKWEAA	RVAEQLRAYL	EGTCVEWLRR	YLENGKETLQ	RA
*B*0702*	------S---	----------	--H-------	----------	----------	----------	-E---R----	--E-------	------DK-E	--
*B*0703*	------S---	----------	--H-------	----------	----------	----------	-E---R----	--E-------	------DK-E	--
*B*0704*	------S---	----------	--H-------	----------	----------	----------	-E---D----	--E-------	------DK-E	--
*B*0705*	------S---	----------	--HN------	----------	----------	----------	-E---R----	--E-------	------DK-E	--
*B*0706*	------S---	----------	--HN------	----------	----------	----------	-E---R----	--E-------	------DK-E	--
*B*0707*	----------	----------	--H-------	----------	----------	----------	-E---R----	--E-------	------DK-E	--
*B*0801*	------S---	----------	--HN------	----------	----------	----------	-----D----	----------	------D--E	--
*B*0802*	------S---	----------	--HN------	----------	----------	----------	-----D----	----------	------D--E	--
*B*0803*	------S---	----------	--HN------	----------	----------	----------	-----D----	----------	------D--E	--
*B*1301*	---II-----	--L-------	--HN-L----	----------	S---------	----L-----	----------	--E-------	----------	--
*B*1302*	----W-T---	--L-------	--HN-L----	----------	S---------	----L-----	----------	--E-------	----------	--
*B*1303*	----W-T---	--L-------	--HN-L----	----------	S---------	----------	----------	--L-------	----------	--
*B*1401*	------W---	----------	---N-F----	----------	S---------	----------	-E--------	----------	H---------	--
*B*1402*	------W---	----------	---N-F----	----------	S---------	----------	-E--------	----------	H---------	--
*B*1501*	----------	----------	--H--S----	----------	S---------	----------	-E---W----	--L-------	----------	--
*B*1502*	---II-----	----------	-----S----	----------	S---------	----------	-E--------	--L-------	----------	--
*B*1503*	----------	----------	--H--S----	----------	S---------	----------	-E--------	--L-------	----------	--
*B*1504*	----W-T---	----------	--H--S----	----------	S---------	----------	-E---W----	--L-------	----------	--
*B*1505*	----------	----------	--H--S----	----------	S---------	----------	----------	--L-------	----------	--
*B*1506*	--------F-	----------	-----S----	----------	S---------	----------	-E--------	--L-------	----------	--
*B*1507*	------S---	----------	--H--S----	----------	S---------	----------	-E---W----	--L-------	----------	--
*B*1508*	----------	----------	--H--S----	----------	S---------	----------	-E---W----	--L-------	----------	--
*B*1509*	----------	----------	--HN------	----------	S---------	----------	-E--------	--L-------	----------	--
*B*1510*	----------	----------	--H-------	----------	S---------	----------	-E--------	--L-------	----------	--
*B*1511*	----------	----------	--H--S----	----------	S---------	----------	-E---W----	--L-------	----------	--
*B*1512*	----------	----------	--H--S----	----------	S---------	----------	-E---W----	--L--DG---	----------	--
*B*1513*	---II-----	----------	-----S----	----------	S---------	----------	-E--------	--L-------	----------	--
*B*1514*	----------	----------	--H--S----	----------	S---------	----------	-E---W----	--L---S---	----------	--
*B*1515*	----------	----------	--H--S----	----------	S---------	----------	-E---W----	--L-------	----------	--
*B*1516*	----W-----	--L-------	--H--S----	----------	S---------	----------	-E--------	--L-------	----------	--
*B*1517*	----------	----------	---H-D----	----------	S---------	----------	-E--------	--L-------	----------	--
*B*1518*	----------	----------	--H--S----	----------	S---------	----------	-E--------	--L-------	----------	--
*B*1519*	----------	----------	--H--S----	----------	S---------	----------	-E---W----	--L--DG---	----------	--
*B*1520*	---II-----	--L-------	--H--S----	----------	S---------	----------	----------	--L-------	----------	--
*B*1521*	---II-----	----------	-----S----	----------	S---------	----------	-E--------	--L-------	----------	--
*B*1522*	----------	----------	--H--S----	----------	S---------	----------	-E---W----	--L-------	----------	--
*B*1523*	----------	----------	--H--S----	----------	S---------	----------	-E--------	--L-------	----------	--
*B*1524*	----------	----------	--H--S----	----------	S---------	----------	-E---W----	--L-------	----------	--

Fig. 2.3. (con't)

CONSENSUS	GSHTLQRMYG	CDVGPDGRLL	RGYDQYAYDG	KDYIALNEDL	RSWTAADTAA	QITQRKWEAA	RVAEQLRAYL	EGTCVEWLRR	YLENGKETLQ	RA
*B*1525*	---II-----	----------	-----S----	----------	S---------	----------	-E--------	--L-------	----------	--
*B*1526N*	--------/-	----------	--H--S----	----------	S---------	----------	-E---W----	--L-------	----------	--
*B*1527*	--------F-	----------	--H--S----	----------	S---------	----------	-E---W----	--L-------	----------	--
*B*1528*	----------	----------	--H--S----	----------	S---------	----------	-E---W----	--L-------	----------	--
*B*1529*	----------	----------	--H--S----	----------	S---------	----------	-E--------	--L-------	----------	--
*B*1530*	----------	----------	--HN------	----------	S---------	----------	-E---W----	--L-------	----------	--
*B*1531*	----------	----------	-----S----	----------	S---------	----------	----------	--L-------	----------	--
*B*1532*	--------S-	----------	--H--S----	----------	S---------	----------	-E---W----	--L-------	----------	--
*B*1533*	----------	----------	--H--S----	----------	-------K--	----------	-E---W----	--L-------	----------	--
*B*1534*	----------	--L-------	--H--S----	----------	S---------	----------	-E---W----	--L-------	----------	--
*B*1535*	------T---	----------	--H--S----	----------	S---------	----------	-E---W----	--L-------	----------	--
*B*1537*	----------	----------	--H-------	----------	S---------	----------	-E--------	--L-------	H---------	--
*B*1801*	----------	----------	--H--S----	----------	S---------	----------	----------	----------	H---------	--
*B*1802*	------N---	----------	--H--S----	----------	S---------	----------	----------	----------	H---------	--
*B*1803*	----------	----------	--H--S----	----------	S---------	----------	----------	----------	H---------	--
*B*1805*	----------	----------	--H--S----	------K---	S---------	----------	----------	--T-------	H---------	--
*B*2701*	------N---	----------	---H-D----	----------	S---------	----------	----------	--E-------	----------	--
*B*2702*	------N---	----------	---H-D----	----------	S---------	----------	----------	--E-------	----------	--
*B*2703*	------N---	----------	---H-D----	----------	S---------	----------	----------	--E-------	----------	--
*B*2704*	------N---	----------	---H-D----	----------	S---------	----------	-E--------	--E-------	----------	--
*B*27052*	------N---	----------	---H-D----	----------	S---------	----------	----------	--E-------	----------	--
*B*27053*	------N---	----------	---H-D----	----------	S---------	----------	----------	--E---....	....	..
*B*2706*	------N---	----------	----------	----------	S---------	----------	-E--------	--E-------	----------	--
*B*2707*	------S---	----------	--HN------	----------	----------	----------	----------	--E-------	----------	--
*B*2708*	------N---	----------	---H-D----	----------	S---------	----------	----------	--E-------	----------	--
*B*2709*	------N---	----------	---H-H----	----------	S---------	----------	----------	--E-------	----------	--
*B*2710*	------N---	----------	---H-D----	----------	S---------	----------	-E--------	--E-------	----------	--
*B*3501*	---II-----	--L-------	--H--S----	----------	S---------	----------	----------	--L-------	----------	--
*B*3502*	---II-----	--L-----F-	--HN------	----------	S---------	----------	----------	--L-------	----------	--
*B*3503*	---II-----	--L-------	--H--F----	----------	S---------	----------	----------	--L-------	----------	--
*B*3504*	---II-----	--L-------	--HN------	----------	S---------	----------	----------	--L-------	----------	--
*B*3505*	------S---	--L-------	--H--S----	----------	S---------	----------	----------	--L-------	----------	--
*B*3506*	---II-----	--L-------	--HN-F----	----------	S---------	----------	----------	--L-------	----------	--
*B*3507*	---II-----	--L-------	--H--S----	----------	S---------	----------	----------	--L-------	----------	--
*B*3508*	---II-----	--L-------	--H--S----	----------	S---------	----------	-----R----	--L-------	----------	--
*B*35091*	---II-----	--L-------	--HN------	----------	----------	----------	----------	--L-------	----------	--
*B*35092*	---II-----	--L-------	--HN------	----------	----------	----------	----------	--L-------	----------	--
*B*3510*	---II-----	--L-------	--H--S----	----------	S---------	----------	----------	--L-------	----------	--
*B*3511*	---II-----	--L-------	--H--S----	----------	S---------	----------	-E--------	--L-------	----------	--
*B*3512*	---II-----	----------	--HN------	----------	S---------	----------	----------	--L-------	----------	--
*B*3513*	---II-----	--L-------	--H--F----	----------	S---------	----------	----------	--L-------	----------	--
*B*3515*	---II-----	--L-------	--H--S----	----------	S---------	----------	----------	--E-------	----------	--

```
B*3516   ---II-S--- ---------- --H--S---- ---------- S--------- ---------- ---------- --L------- ---------- --
B*3517   ---II-S--- ---------- --H--S---- ---------- S--------- ---------- ---------- --L------- ---------- --
B*3518   ---II----- --L------- --HN------ ---------- ---------- ---------- -----R---- --L------- ---------- --
B*3519   ---II----- --L------- --H--S---- ---------- S--------- ---------- ---------- --L------- ---------- --
B*3520   ---II----- --L------- --H--S---- ---------- S--------- ---------- ---------- --L------- ---------- --
B*3521   ---II----- --L------- --H--S---- ---------- S--------- ---------- -E-------- --L------- H--------- --
B*3701   ----I---S- ---------- ---N-F---- ---------- S--------- ---------- -----D---- ---------- ---------- --
B*3702   ------N--- ---------- ---H-D---- ---------- S--------- ---------- ---------- --E------- ---------- --
B*3801   ---------- ---------- --HN-F---- ---------- S--------- ---------- -------T-- ---------- ---------- --
B*3802   ---------- ---------- --HN-F---- ---------- S--------- ---------- -------T-- ---------- ---------- --
B*39011  ---------- ---------- --HN-F---- ---------- S--------- ---------- -------T-- ---------- ---------- --
B*39013  ---------- ---------- --HN-F---- ---------- S--------- ---------- -------T-- ---------- ---------- --
B*39021  ---------- ---------- --HN-F---- ---------- S--------- ---------- -------T-- ---------- ---------- --
B*39022  ---------- ---------- --HN-F---- ---------- S--------- ---------- -------T-- ---------- ---------- --
B*3903   ------S--- ---------- --HN-F---- ---------- S--------- ---------- -------T-- ---------- ---------- --
B*3904   ---------- ---------- --HN-F---- ---------- S--------- ---------- -------T-- ---------- ---------- --
B*3905   ---------- ---------- --HN-F---- ---------- S--------- ---------- -------T-- ---------- ---------- --
B*39061  ----W-T--- ---------- --HN-F---- ---------- S--------- ---------- -------T-- ---------- ---------- --
B*39062  ----W-T--- ---------- --HN-F---- ---------- S--------- ---------- -------T-- ---------- ---------- --
B*3907   ---------- ---------- --H--S---- ---------- S--------- ---------- -------T-- ---------- --........ ..
B*3908   ---------- ---------- --HN-F---- ---------- S--------- ---------- -----R-T-- ---------- ---------- --
B*3909   --------S- ---------- --HN-F---- ---------- S--------- ---------- -------T-- ---------- ---------- --
B*3910   ---------- ---------- --HN-F---- ---------- S--------- ---------- -------T-- ---------- ---------- --
B*3911   ---------- ---------- --HN-F---- ---------- S--------- ---------- -----R-T-- ---------- ---------- --
B*3912   ---------- ---------- --HN-F---- ---------- S--------- ---------- -------T-- ---------- ---------- --
B*40011  ---------- ---------- --HN------ ---------- ---------- --S---L--- ---------- --E------- ------DK-E --
B*40012  ---------- ---------- --HN------ ---------- ---------- --S---L--- ---------- --E------- ------DK-E --
B*4002   ------S--- ---------- --HN------ ---------- ---------- ---------- ---------- --E------- ---------- --
B*4003   ------S--- ---------- --H--S---- ---------- ---------- ---------- ---------- --E------- ---------- --
B*4004   ---II----- --L------- --HN------ ---------- ---------- ---------- ---------- --E------- ---------- --
B*4005   ------S--- ---------- --HN------ ---------- ---------- ---------- -E-------- --L------- ---------- --
B*4006   ----W-T--- ---------- --HN------ ---------- ---------- ---------- ---------- --E------- ---------- --
B*4007   ---------- ---------- --HN------ ---------- ---------- --S---L--- ---------- --E------- ------DK-E --
B*4008   ------S--- ---------- --HN------ ---------- ---------- ---------- ---------- --E------- ---------- --
B*4009   ------S--- ---------- ---------- ---------- ---------- ---------- ---------- --E------- ---------- --
B*4101   ----W----- ---------- --HN------ ---------- ---------- ---------- -----D---- ---------- ------D--E --
B*4102   ------S--- ---------- --HN------ ---------- ---------- ---------- -----D---- ---------- ------D--E --
B*4201   ------S--- ---------- --HN------ ---------- ---------- ---------- -----D---- ---------- ------D--E --
B*4402   ---II----- ---------- -----D---- ---------- S--------- ---------- -----D---- --L---S--- ---------- --
B*44031  ---II----- ---------- -----D---- ---------- S--------- ---------- ---------- --L---S--- ---------- --
B*44032  ---II----- ---------- -----D---- ---------- S--------- ---------- ---------- --L---S--- ---------- --
```

Fig. 2.3. (con't)

CONSENSUS	GSHTLQRMYG	CDVGPDGRLL	RGYDQYAYDG	KDYIALNEDL	RSWTAADTAA	QITQRKWEAA	RVAEQLRAYL	EGTCVEWLRR	YLENGKETLQ	RA
*B*4404*	---II-----	----------	-----D----	----------	S---------	----------	-----R----	------S---	----------	--
*B*4405*	---II-----	----------	----------	----------	S---------	----------	-----D----	--L---S---	----------	--
*B*4406*	---II-----	----------	-----D----	----------	S---------	----------	-----D----	--L---S---	----------	--
*B*4407*	---II-----	----------	-----D----	----------	S---------	----------	----------	--L---S---	----------	--
*B*4408*	---II-----	----------	-----D----	----------	S---------	----------	-----D----	--L---S---	----------	--
*B*4410*	---II---F-	--L-------	--HN-L----	----------	S---------	----------	----------	--L---S---	----------	--
*B*4501*	----W-----	--L-------	---N-L----	----------	S---------	----------	-----D----	--L---S---	----------	--
*B*4601*	----------	----------	--H--S----	----------	S---------	----------	-E---W----	--L-------	----------	--
*B*4701*	--------F-	----------	---H-D----	----------	S---------	----------	----------	--E-------	----------	--
*B*4702*	--------F-	----------	---H-D----	----------	S---------	----------	----------	----------	----------	--
*B*4801*	------S---	----------	--HN------	----------	----------	--S---L---	----------	--E-------	------DK-E	--
*B*4802*	---II-----	--L-------	--H--S----	----------	S---------	----------	----------	--L-------	----------	--
*B*4803*	----------	----------	--HN------	----------	----------	--S---L---	----------	--E-------	------DK-E	--
*B*4901*	----W-----	--L-------	---N-L----	----------	S---------	----------	-E--------	--L-------	----------	--
*B*5001*	----W-----	--L-------	---N-L----	----------	S---------	----------	-E--------	--L-------	----------	--
*B*51011*	----W-T---	----------	--HN------	----------	S---------	----------	-E--------	--L-------	H---------	--
*B*51012*	----W-T---	----------	--HN------	----------	S---------	----------	-E--------	--L-------	H---------	--
*B*51021*	----W-T---	----------	--HN------	----------	S---------	----------	-E--------	--L-------	----------	--
*B*51022*	----W-T---	----------	--HN------	----------	S---------	----------	-E--------	--L-------	----------	--
*B*5103*	----W-T---	----------	--HN------	----------	S---------	----------	-E--------	--L---G---	H---------	--
*B*5104*	---II-----	----------	--HN------	----------	S---------	----------	-E--------	--L-------	H---------	--
*B*5105*	----W-T---	----------	--HN------	----------	S---------	----------	-----R----	--L-------	----------	--
*B*5106*	----------	----------	--HN------	----------	S---------	----------	-E--------	--L-------	H---------	--
*B*5107*	----W-T---	----------	--HN------	----------	S---------	----------	-E--------	--L-------	H---------	--
*B*5108*	----W-T---	----------	--HN------	----------	S---------	----------	-----D----	--L-------	H---------	--
*B*52011*	----W-T---	----------	--HN------	----------	S---------	----------	-E--------	--L-------	H---------	--
*B*52012*	----W-T---	----------	--HN------	----------	S---------	----------	-E--------	--L-------	H---------	--
*B*5301*	---II-----	--L-------	--H--S----	----------	S---------	----------	----------	--L-------	----------	--
*B*5401*	----W-T---	--L-------	--HN-L----	----------	S---------	----------	----------	----------	----------	--
*B*5501*	----W-T---	--L-------	--HN-L----	----------	S---------	----------	-E--------	----------	----------	--
*B*5502*	----W-T---	--L-------	--HN-L----	----------	S---------	----------	----------	----------	----------	--
*B*5503*	----W-T---	--L-------	--HN-L----	----------	S---------	----------	-E--------	----------	----------	--
*B*5504*	------S---	----------	--HN------	----------	----------	----------	----------	----------	----------	--
*B*5505*	----W-T---	--L-------	--HN-L----	----------	S---------	----------	-E--------	--T-------	----------	--
*B*5601*	----W-T---	--L-------	--HN-L----	----------	S---------	----------	----------	--L-------	----------	--
*B*5602*	----------	--L-------	--HN-L----	----------	S---------	----------	----------	--L-------	----------	--
*B*5603*	----------	----------	--H--S----	----------	S---------	----------	-E---W----	--L-------	----------	--
*B*5701*	---II-V---	----------	--H--S----	----------	S---------	----------	----------	--L-------	----------	--
*B*5702*	---II-V---	----------	--HN------	----------	S---------	----------	-----R----	--L-------	----------	--
*B*5703*	---II-V---	----------	--HN------	----------	S---------	----------	----------	--L-------	----------	--

```
B*5704     ---II-V--- ---------- -----D---- ---------- S--------- ---------- -----R---- --L------- ---------- --
B*5801     ---II----- --L------- --H--S---- ---------- S--------- ---------- ---------- --L------- ---------- --
B*5802     ------W--- --L------- --H--S---- ---------- S--------- ---------- ---------- --L------- ---------- --
B*5901     ----W-T--- --L------- --HN-L---- ---------- S--------- ---------- ---------- ---------- ---------- --
B*67011    ---------- ---------- --HN-F---- ---------- S--------- ---------- -------T-- ---------- ---------- --
B*67012    ---------- ---------- --HN-F---- ---------- S--------- ---------- -------T-- ---------- ---------- ..
B*7301     ----W-T--- --M------- ---N-F---- ---------- ---------- ---------- ---------- --E------- H--------- --
B*7801     ----W-T--- ---------- --HN------ ---------- S--------- ---------- -E-------- --L------- H--------- --
B*78021    ----W-T--- ---------- --HN------ ---------- S--------- ---------- -E-------- --L------- H--------- --
B*78022    ----W-T--- ---------- --HN------ ---------- S--------- ---------- -E-------- --L------- H--------- --
B*8101     ------S--- ---------- --HN------ ---------- ---------- --S---L--- ---------- --E------- ------DK-E --
B*8201     --------F- --L------- --HN-L---- ---------- S--------- ---------- -----D---- -DL---S--- ---------- --
CONSENSUS  GSHTLQRMYG CDVGPDGRLL RGYDQYAYDG KDYIALNEDL RSWTAADTAA QITQRKWEAA RVAEQLRAYL EGTCVEWLRR YLENGKETLQ RA
```

Fig. 2.4. Comparison of *HLA-C* α1 and α2 domain amino acid sequences (see following pages)

The AA are given in the international single-letter code. The consensus sequence is derived from all, at the time of writing, available *HLA-A*, *HLA-B*, and *HLA-C* amino acid sequences. Identity with the consensus is indicated by hyphens, unavailability of information is indicated by a dot. See also Table 2.3. Sequences of which only the nucleotides were available, the AA sequence was deferred. AA residues involved in putative peptide binding regions are marked with an asterisk (*).[499]

Fig. 2.4. (con't)

α1 domain

```
            1          11         21         31         41         51         61         71         81        90
               * * *                **         *          *              *     *  **  *    **  *   *  *  *
CONSENSUS   GSHSMRYFYT SVSRPGRGEP RFIAVGYVDD TQFVRFDSDA ASPRMEPRAP WIEQEGPEYW DRETQIVKAN TQTDRESLRN LRGYYNQSEA
  Cw*0102   C----K--F- ---------- ---S------ ---------- ----G----- -V-------- -----KY-RQ A----V---- ----------
  Cw*0103   C----K--F- ---------- ---S------ ---------- ----G----- -V-------- -----KY-RQ A----V---- ----------
  Cw*02021  C--------- A----S---- H--------- ---------- ----G----- -V-------- -----KY-RQ A----VN--K ----------
  Cw*02022  C--------- A----S---- H--------- ---------- ----G----- -V-------- -----KY-RQ A----VN--K ----------
  Cw*02023  .--------- A----S---- H--------- ---------- ----G----- -V-------- -----KY-RQ A----VN--K ----------
  Cw*0302   ---------- A--------- H--------- ---------- ----G----- -V-------- -----KY-RQ A----V---- ----------
  Cw*0303   ---------- A--------- H--------- ---------- ----G----- -V-------- -----KY-RQ A----V---- ----------
  Cw*0304   ---------- A--------- H--------- ---------- ----G----- -V-------- -----KY-RQ A----V---- ----------
  Cw*0401   --------S- ---W------ ---------- ---------- ----G---E- -V-------- -----KY-RQ A-A--VN--K ---------D
  Cw*0402   --------S- ---W------ ---------- ---------- ----G---SR -V-------- -----KYNRQ A-A--VN--K ---------D
  Cw*0403   ---------- A----S---- H--------- ---------- ----G----- -V-------- -----KY-RQ A-A--VN--K ---------D
  Cw*0501   C--------- A--------- H--------- ----Q----- ----G----- -V-------- -----KY-RQ A----VN--K ----------
  Cw*0602   C-------D- A--------- ---S------ ---------- ----G----- -V-------- -----KY-RQ A-A--VN--K ---------D
  Cw*0701   C-------D- A--------- ---S------ ---------- ----G----- -V-------- -----NY-RQ A-A--V---- ---------D
  Cw*0702   --------D- A--------- ---S------ ---------- ----G----- -V-------- -----KY-RQ A-A--V---- ---------D
  Cw*0703   C-------D- A-----A--- ---S------ ---------- ----G----- -V-------- -----KY-RQ A-A--V---- ---------D
  Cw*0704   C-------D- A--------- ---S------ ---------- ----G----- -V-------- -----KY-RQ A-A--V---- ---------D
  Cw*0705   .-------D- A--------- ---S------ ---------- ----G----- -V-------- -----KY-RQ A-A--V---- ---------D
  Cw*0706   C-------D- A--------- ---S------ ---------- ----G----- -V-------- -----NY-RQ A-A--V---- ---------D
  Cw*0707   .-------D- A--------- ---S------ ---------- ----G----- -V-------- -----NY-RQ A-A--VN--K ----------
  Cw*0801   C--------- A--------- ---------- ----Q----- ----G----- -V-------- -----KY-RQ A----V---- ----------
  Cw*0802   C--------- A--------- ---------- ----Q----- ----G----- -V-------- -----KY-RQ A----V---- ----------
  Cw*0803   C--------- A--------- ---------- ----Q----- ----G----- -V-------- -----KY-RQ A----V---- ----------
  Cw*12021  C--------- A--------- ---------- ---------- ----G----- -V-------- -----KY-RQ A-A--V---- ----------
  Cw*12022  C--------- A--------- ---------- ---------- ----G----- -V-------- -----KY-RQ A-A--V---- ----------
  Cw*1203   C--------- A--------- ---------- ---------- ----G----- -V-------- -----KY-RQ A-A--V---- ----------
  Cw*1204   C--------- A--------- ---------- ---------- ----G----- -V-------- -----KY-RQ A-A--VN--K ----------
  Cw*1301   C--------- A--------- H--------- ---------- ----G----- -V-------- -----KY-RQ A-A--V---- ----------
  Cw*1402   C-------S- ---------- ---------- ---------- ----G----- -V-------- -----KY-RQ A----V---- ----------
  Cw*1403   C-------S- ---------- H--------- ---------- ----G----- -V-------- -----KY-RQ A----V---- ----------
  Cw*1502   C--------- A--------- H--------- ---------- ----G----- -V-------- -----NY-RQ A----VN--K ----------
  Cw*1503   C--------- A--------- H--------- ---------- ----G----- -V-------- -----NY-RQ A-A--VN--K ----------
  Cw*1504   C--------- A--------- H--------- ---------- ----G----- -V-------- -----NY-RQ A----VN--K ----------
  Cw*15051  C--------- A--------- H--------- ---------- ----G----- -V-------- -----NY-RQ A----VN--K ----------
  Cw*15052  C--------- A--------- H--------- ---------- ----G----- -V-------- -----NY-RQ A----VN--K ----------
  Cw*1601   C--------- A--------- ---------- ---------- ----G----- -V-------- -----KY-RQ A----V---- ----------
  Cw*1602   C--------- A--------- ---------- ---------- ----G----- -V-------- -----KY-RQ A----VN--K ----------
  Cw*1701   ---------- A--------- ---------- ---------- ----G----- -V-------- -----KY-RQ A-A--VN--K ----------
  Cw*1702   ---------- A--------- ---------- ---------- ----G----- -V-------- -----KY-RQ A-A--VN--K ----------
  Cw*1801   C-------D- A--------- ---S------ ---------- ----G----- -V-------- -----KY-RQ A-A--VN--K ---------D
  Cw*1802   C-------D- A--------- ---S------ ---------- ----G----- -V-------- -----KY-RQ A-A--VN--K ---------D
CONSENSUS   GSHSMRYFYT SVSRPGRGEP RFIAVGYVDD TQFVRFDSDA ASPRMEPRAP WIEQEGPEYW DRETQIVKAN TQTDRESLRN LRGYYNQSEA
```

α2 Domain

```
           91         101        111        121        131        141        151        161        171        181
                 * *              ** *        *                       *  **     *  **  **   *   *    *
CONSENSUS  GSHTLQRMYG CDVGPDGRLL RGYDQYAYDG KDYIALNEDL RSWTAADTAA QITQRKWEAA RVAEQLRAYL EGTCVEWLRR YLENGKETLQ RA
Cw*0102    ------W-C- --L------- ---------- ---------- ---------- ---------- -E---R---- ---------- ---------- --
Cw*0103    ------W-C- --L------- ---N-F---- ---------- ---------- ---------- -E---R---- ---------- ---------- --
Cw*02021   ---------- --L------- -----S---- ---------- ---------- ---------- -E---W---- --E------- ---------- --
Cw*02022   ---------- --L------- -----S---- ---------- ---------- ---------- -E---W---- --E------- ---------- --
Cw*02023   ---------- --L------- -----S---- ---------- ---------- ---------- -E---W---- --E------- ---------- --
Cw*0302    ---I------ ---------- -----S---- ---------- ---------- ---------- -E-------- --L------- --K------- --
Cw*0303    R--II----- ---------- ---------- ---------- ---------- ---------- -E-------- --L------- --K------- --
Cw*0304    ---II----- ---------- ---------- ---------- ---------- ---------- -E-------- --L------- --K------- --
Cw*0401    --------F- --L------- ---N-F---- ---------- ---------- ---------- -E---R---- ---------- ---------- --
Cw*0402    --------F- --L------- ---N-F---- ---------- ---------- ---------- -E--ER---- ---------- ---------- --
Cw*0403    --------F- --L------- ---N-F---- ---------- ---------- ---------- -E---R---- ---------- ---------- --
Cw*0501    ---------- --L------- ---N-F---- ---------- -------K-- ---------- -E---R---- ---------- ------K--- --
Cw*0602    ------W--- --L------- -----S---- ---------- ---------- ---------- -E---W---- ---------- ---------- --
Cw*0701    ---------- --L------- -----S---- ---------- ---------- ------L--- -A-------- ---------- ---------- --
Cw*0702    --------S- --L------- -----S---- ---------- ---------- ------L--- -A-------- ---------- ---------- --
Cw*0703    --------S- --L------- -----S---- ---------- ---------- ---------- -A-------- --L------- ---------- --
Cw*0704    ----F----- --L------- -----F---- ---------- ---------- ------L--- -A---D---- ---------- ------K--- --
Cw*0705    ------N--- --L------- -----S---- ---------- ---------- ------L--- -A-------- ---------- ---------- --
Cw*0706    ---------- --L------- -----S---- ---------- ---------- ------L--- -A-------- ---------- ---------- --
Cw*0707    ---------- --L------- -----S---- ---------- ---------- ------L--- -A-------- ---------- ---------- --
Cw*0801    ---------- --L------- ---N-F---- ---------- ---------- ---------- -T-------- ---------- ------K--- --
Cw*0802    ---------- --L------- ---N-F---- ---------- -------K-- ---------- -E---R---- ---------- ------K--- --
Cw*0803    ---------- --L------- ---N-F---- ---------- ---------- ---------- -T-------- ---------- ----R-K--- --
Cw*12021   ---------- --L------- -----S---- ---------- ---------- ---------- -E---W---- ---------- ---------- --
Cw*12022   ---------- --L------- -----S---- ---------- ---------- ---------- -E---W---- ---------- ---------- --
Cw*1203    ------W--- --L------- -----S---- ---------- ---------- ---------- -E---W---- ---------- ---------- --
Cw*1204    ------W--- --L------- -----S---- ---------- ---------- ---------- -E---W---- ---------- ---------- --
Cw*1301    ---------- --L------- -----S---- ---------- ---------- ---------- -E---W---- ---------- ---------- --
Cw*1402    ------W-F- --L------- -----S---- ---------- ---------- ---------- -E---R---- ---------- ---------- --
Cw*1403    ------W-F- --L------- -----S---- ---------- ---------- ---------- -E---R---- ---------- ---------- --
Cw*1502    ---II----- --L------- --H--L---- ---------- ---------- ---------- -E-------- ---------- ---------- --

Cw*1503    ---II----- --L------- --H--L---- ---------- ---------- ---------- -E-------- ---------- ---------- --
Cw*1504    ---II----- --L------- -----S---- ---------- ---------- ---------- -E-------- ---------- ---------- --
Cw*15051   ---II----- --L------- --H--F---- ---------- ---------- ---------- -E-------- ---------- ---------- --
Cw*15052   ---II----- --L------- --H--F---- ---------- ---------- ---------- -E-------- ---------- ---------- --
Cw*1601    ------W--- --L------- -----S---- ---------- ---------- ---------- -A---Q---- ---------- ---------- --
Cw*1602    ------W--- --L------- -----S---- ---------- ---------- ---------- -A---Q---- ---------- ---------- --

Cw*1701    ----I----- --L------- ---N-F---- ---------- ---------- --S---L--- -E-------- --E------G ---------- --
Cw*1702    ----I----- --L------- ---N-F---- ---------- ---------- --S---L--- -E-------- --E------G ---------- --
Cw*1801    --------F- --L------- ---N-F---- ---------- ---------- ---------- -E---R---- ---------- ---------- --
Cw*1802    --------F- --L------- ---N-F---- ---------- ---------- ---------- -E---R---- ---------- ---------- --
CONSENSUS  GSHTLQRMYG CDVGPDGRLL RGYDQYAYDG KDYIALNEDL RSWTAADTAA QITQRKWEAA RVAEQLRAYL EGTCVEWLRR YLENGKETLQ RA
```

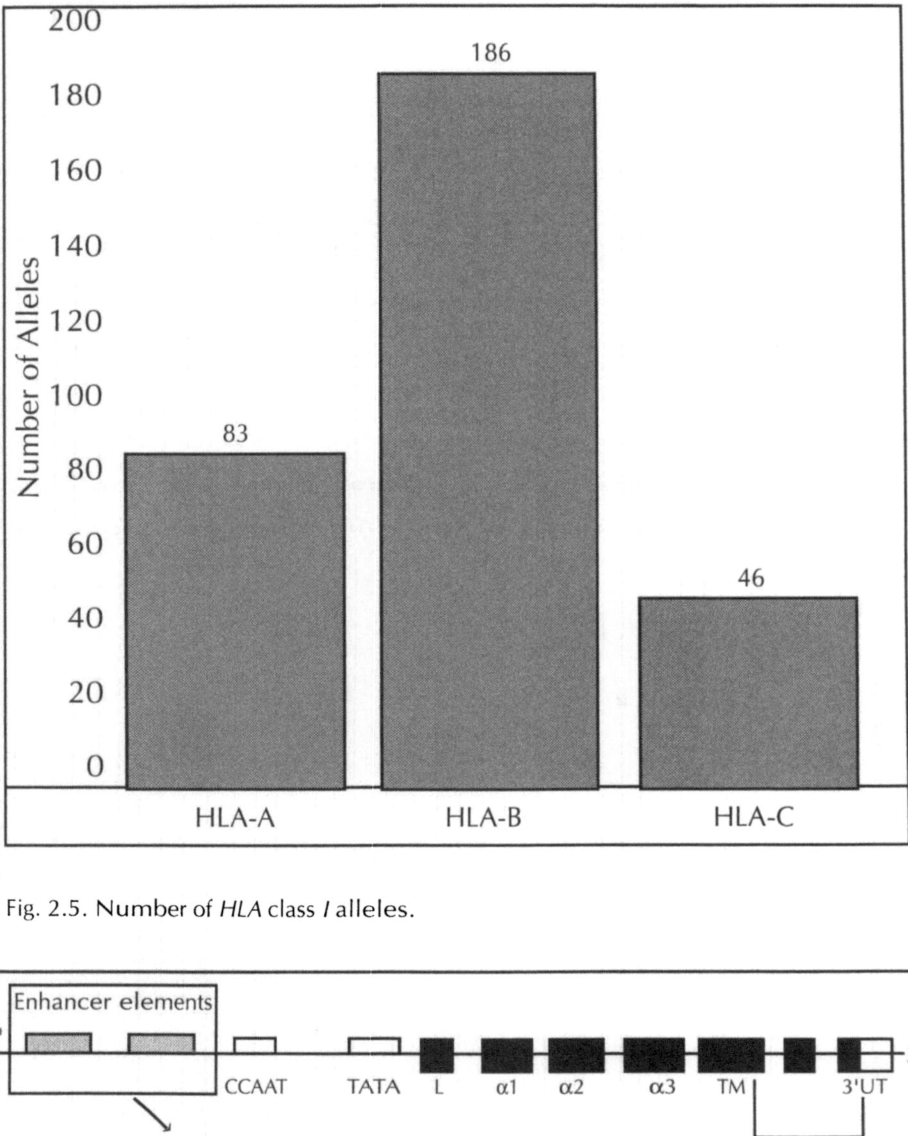

Fig. 2.5. Number of *HLA* class *I* alleles.

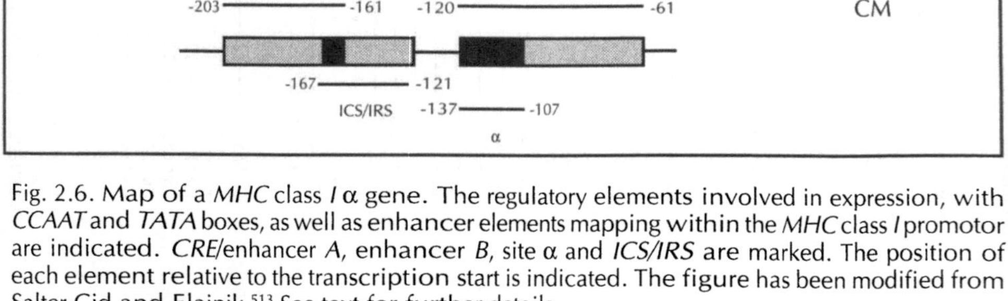

Fig. 2.6. Map of a *MHC* class *I* α gene. The regulatory elements involved in expression, with *CCAAT* and *TATA* boxes, as well as enhancer elements mapping within the *MHC* class *I* promotor are indicated. *CRE*/enhancer *A*, enhancer *B*, site α and *ICS/IRS* are marked. The position of each element relative to the transcription start is indicated. The figure has been modified from Salter-Cid and Flajnik.[513] See text for further details.

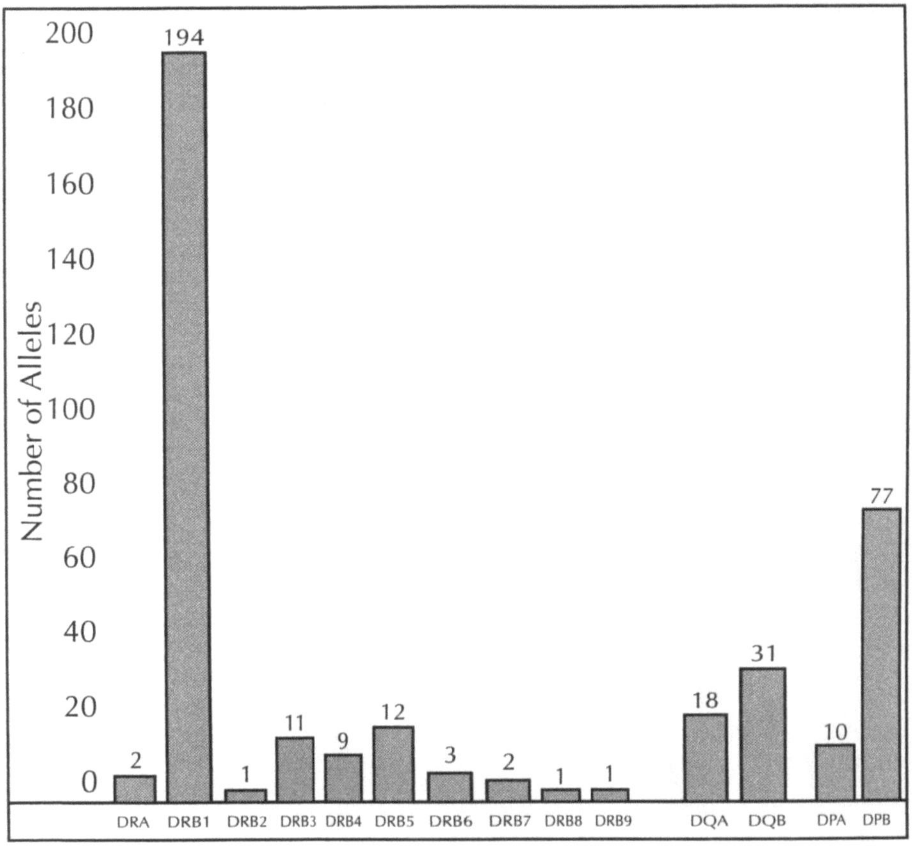

Fig. 2.7. Number of *HLA* class *II* alleles.

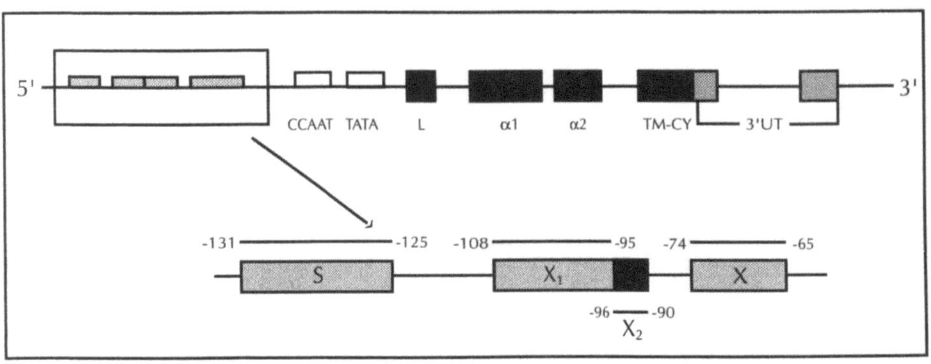

Fig. 2.8. Map of a *MHC* class *II* a gene. The regulatory elements in the 5′ promoter proximal region are also shown. The *S*, X_1, X_2 and *Y* elements are identified and the position of each element relative to the transcription site is indicated. The figure has been modified from Salter-Cid and Flajnik.[513] See text for further details.

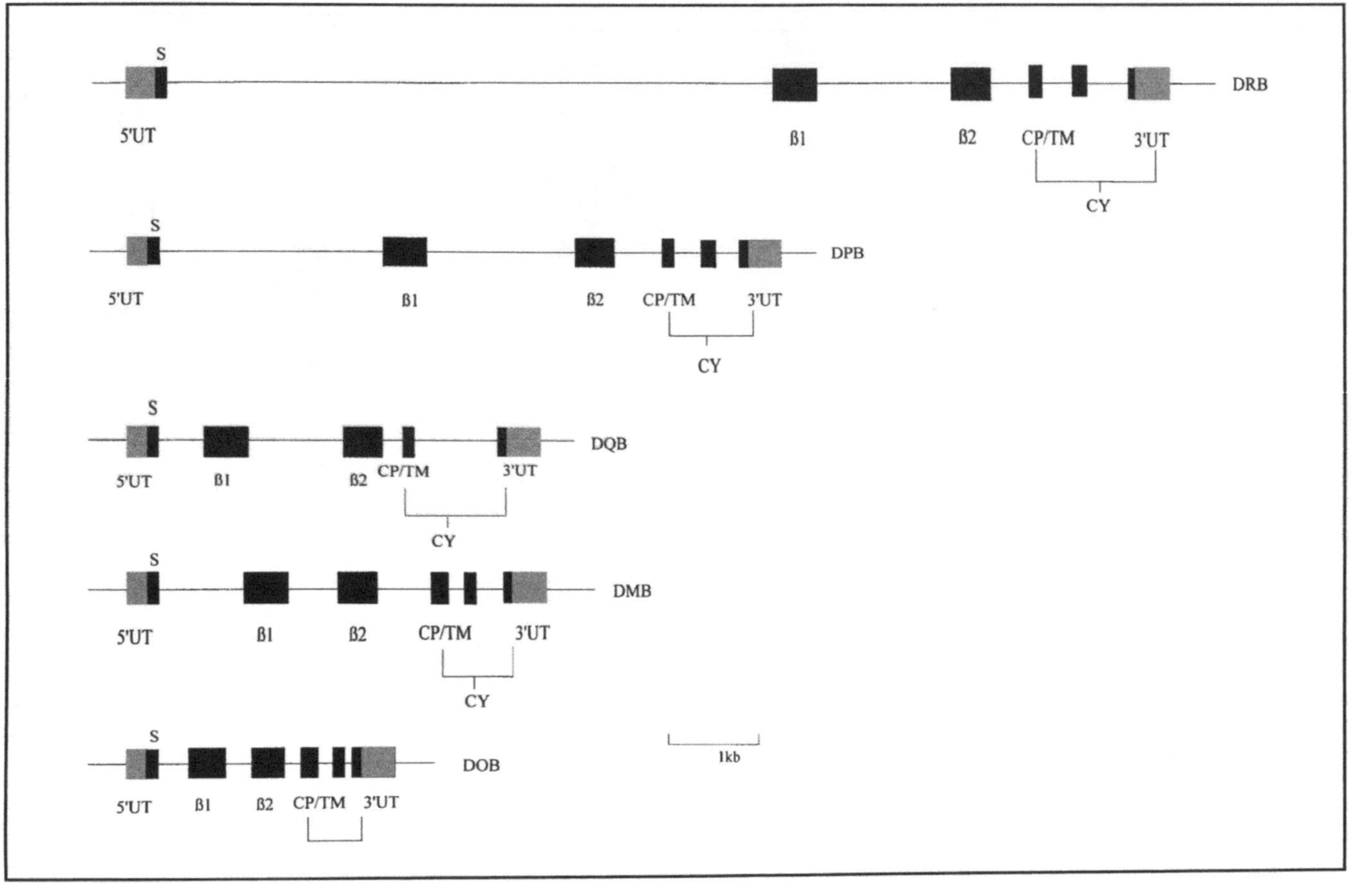

Fig. 2.9. Organization of *HLA* class *II* genes. All genes, except *DQB*, have six exons. The figure has been modified from Trowsdale.[570]

Fig. 2.10. Comparison of *HLA-DRA* α1 and α2 domain amino acid sequences

The AA are given in the international single-letter code. Identity with *DRA1*0101* is indicated by hyphens, unavailability of information is indicated by a dot. The residues involved in formation of the peptide binding groove as given by Stern et al are indicated by asterisks.[571]

α1 domain

```
             1          11         21         31         41         51         61         71         81
                   * *  *                     ** *         *                    *  **  *   **  *
DRA*0101     IKEEHVIIQA EFYLNPDQSG EFMFDFDGDE IFHVDMAKKE TVWRLEEFGR FASFEAQGAL ANIAVDKANL EIMTKRSNYT PITN
DRA*0102     ...------- ---------- ---------- ---------- ---------- ---------- ---------- ---------- ----
```

α2 domain

```
                    91         101        111        121        131        141        151        161        171
DRA*0101     VPPEVT VLTNSPVELR EPNVLICFID KFTPPVVNVT WLRNGKPVTT GVSETVFLPR EDHLFRKFHY LPFLPSTEDV YDCRVEHWGL DEPLLKHW
DRA*0102     ------ ---------- ---------- ---------- ---------- ---------- ---------- ---------- ---------- --------
```

αTM-CY domain

```
                181        191        201        211        221
DRA*0101     EF DAPSPLPETT ENVVCALGLT VGLVGIIIGT IFIIKGVRKS NAAERRGPL
DRA*0102     -- ---------- ---------- ---------- ------L--- ---------
```

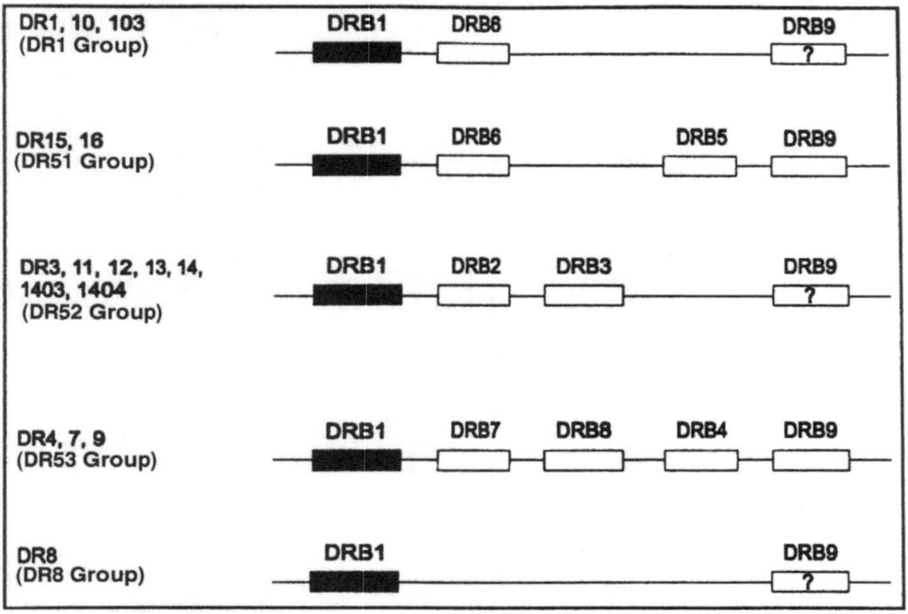

Fig. 2.11. *DRB* gene variation in the five major haplotypes. The figure has been modified from Campbell and Trowsdale.[572] ? means that the existance of *DRB9* in these haplotypes needs to be confirmed.

Fig. 2.12. Comparison of *HLA-DRB* amino acid sequences

The AA are given in the international single letter code. Identity with the consensus sequence is indicated by hyphens, Unavailability of information is indicated by dots. See also Table 2.4. The amino acid residues involved in peptide binding are marked with an asterisk (*).[571]

ß1 domain

	1	11	21	31	41	51	61	71	81	91
	*	* *	*		*	*	* * *	** * *	** **	
CONSENSUS	GDTRPRFLEY	STSECHFFNG	TERVRFLDRY	FYNQEESVRF	DSDVGEYRAV	TELGRPDAEY	WNSQKDLLED	RRAAVDTYCR	HNYGVGESFT	VQRRV
*DRB1*0101*	--------WQ	LKF-------	-----L-E-C	I---------	----------	----------	---------Q	----------	----AV----	-----
*DRB1*01021*	--------WQ	LKF-------	-----L-E-C	I---------	----------	----------	---------Q	----------	----AV----	-----
*DRB1*01022*	.....---WQ	LKF-------	-----L-E-C	I---------	----------	----------	---------Q	----------	----AV----	---..
*DRB1*0103*	--------WQ	LKF-------	-----L-E-C	I---------	----------	----------	------I---	E---------	----------	-----
*DRB1*0104*	....	..F-------	-----L-E-C	I---------	----------	----------	---------Q	------N---	-----V-...	.....
*DRB1*03011*	----------	----------	-----Y----	-H----N---	------F---	----------	---------Q	K-GR--N---	-----V----	-----
*DRB1*03012*	.....-----	----------	-----Y----	-H----N---	------F---	----------	---------Q	K-GR--N---	-----V----	--...
*DRB1*03021*	----------	----------	-------E--	-H----N---	----------	----------	---------Q	K-GR--N---	----------	-----
*DRB1*03022*	----------	----------	-------E--	-H----N---	----------	----------	---------Q	K-GR--N---	----------	-----
*DRB1*0303*	.........-	----------	-------E--	-H----N---	----------	----------	---------Q	K-GR--N---	-----V----	----.
*DRB1*0304*	.......---	----------	-----Y----	-H--------	------F---	----------	---------Q	K-GR--N---	-----V-...	.....
*DRB1*0305*	....	....	-----Y----	-H----N---	------F---	----------	---------Q	K-GR--N---	----------	--...
*DRB1*0306*	.....-----	----------	-----Y----	-H----N---	----------	----------	---------Q	K-GR--N---	-----V----	--...
*DRB1*0307*	----------	----------	----------	-H----N---	------F---	----------	---------Q	K-GR--N---	-----V----	-----
*DRB1*0308*	----------	----------	-----Y----	-H----N---	------F---	-------E--	---------Q	K-GR--N---	-----V----	-----
*DRB1*0311*	.....-----	----------	-----Y----	-H----N---	------F---	----------	---------Q	K-GQ--N---	-----V----	----.
*DRB1*04011*	---------Q	VKH-------	----------	--H---Y---	----------	----------	---------Q	K---------	----------	-----
*DRB1*04012*	.....----Q	VKH-------	----------	--H---Y---	----------	----------	---------Q	K-----T---	----------	----.
*DRB1*0402*	---------Q	VKH-------	----------	--H---Y---	----------	----------	------I---	E---------	-----V----	----.
*DRB1*0403*	---------Q	VKH-------	----------	--H---Y---	----------	----------	---------Q	---E------	-----V----	-----
*DRB1*0404*	---------Q	VKH-------	----------	--H---Y---	----------	----------	---------Q	----------	-----V----	-----
*DRB1*04051*	---------Q	VKH-------	----------	--H---Y---	----------	------S---	---------Q	----------	----------	----.
*DRB1*04052*	....	...-------	----------	--H---Y---	----------	------S---	---------Q	----------	----------	----G
*DRB1*0406*	---------Q	VKH-------	----------	--H-------	----------	----------	---------Q	---E------	-----V----	-----
*DRB1*0407*	---------Q	VKH-------	----------	--H---Y---	----------	----------	---------Q	---E------	----------	----.
*DRB1*0408*	....	...-------	----------	--H---Y---	----------	----------	---------Q	----------	-------...	.....
*DRB1*0409*	....	...-------	----------	--H---Y---	----------	------S---	---------Q	K---------	-------...	.....
*DRB1*0410*	......---Q	VKH-------	----------	--H---Y---	----------	------S---	---------Q	----------	-----V----	.....
*DRB1*0411*	---------Q	VKH-------	----------	--H---Y---	----------	------S---	---------Q	---E------	-----V----	-----
*DRB1*0412*	......---Q	VKH-------	----------	--H---Y---	----------	------S---	------I---	---L------	-----V----	---..

Fig. 2.12. (con't)

CONSENSUS	GDTRPRFLEY	STSECHFFNG	TERVRFLDRY	FYNQEESVRF	DSDVGEYRAV	TELGRPDAEY	WNSQKDLLED	RRAAVDTYCR	HNYGVGESFT	VQRRV
DRB1*0413	....	..H-------	----------	--H---Y---	----------	----------	---------Q	K---------	-----V----	.....
DRB1*0414	....	...-------	----------	--H---Y---	----------	----------	------I---	E---------	-------...	.....
DRB1*0415	.....----Q	VKH-------	----------	--H---Y---	----------	-------E--	------F---	----------	-----V-...	.....
DRB1*0416	....	...-------	----------	--H---Y---	----------	--------Q-	---------Q	K---------	------....	.....
DRB1*0417	....	...-------	----------	--H---Y---	----------	------S---	---------Q	---E------	------....	.....
DRB1*0418	....	........--	----------	--H---Y---	----------	----------	------I---	---L------	-----V----	-....
DRB1*0419	....	..H-------	----------	--H-------	----------	----------	---------Q	----------	----------	-....
DRB1*0420	....	...-------	----------	--H-------	----------	----------	---------Q	---E------	------....	.....
DRB1*0421	........-Q	VKH-------	----------	--H-------	----------	----------	---------Q	K---------	----------	-....
DRB1*0422	........-Q	VKH-------	----------	--H---Y---	----------	----------	---------Q	K-GR--N---	-----V----	.....
DRB1*0423	.....----Q	VKH-------	----------	--H---Y---	----------	----------	---------Q	----------	-----V-R--	----.
DRB1*0701	---Q----WQ	GKYK------	----Q--E-L	------F---	----------	------V--S	------I---	--GQ---V--	----------	-----
DRB1*0801	----------	--G--Y----	----------	------Y---	----------	------S---	------F---	---L------	------....	.....
DRB1*08021	----------	--G--Y----	----------	------Y---	----------	----------	------F---	---L------	----------	-----
DRB1*08022	.....-----	--G--Y----	----------	------Y---	----------	----------	------F---	---L------	----------	-----
DRB1*08031	.....-----	--G--Y----	----------	------Y---	----------	------S---	------I---	---L------	----------	-----
DRB1*08032	----------	--G--Y----	----------	------Y---	----------	------S---	------I---	---L------	----------	----.
DRB1*08041	----------	--G--Y----	----------	------Y---	----------	----------	------F---	---L------	-----V----	-----
DRB1*08042	....	.......---	----------	------Y---	----------	----------	------F---	---L------	-----V----	---..
DRB1*0805	.....-----	--G--Y----	----------	------Y---	----------	------S---	------F---	----------	------....	.....
DRB1*0806	....------	--G--Y----	----------	------Y---	----------	------S---	------F---	---L------	-----V----	.....
DRB1*0807	....	..G--Y----	----------	------Y---	----------	------V---	------F---	---L------	----------	-....
DRB1*0808	.......---	--G--Y----	----------	------Y---	----------	------A--H	------F---	---L------	-------...	.....
DRB1*0809	....	...--Y----	----------	-H----F---	----------	----------	------F---	---L------	------....	.....
DRB1*0810	.....-----	--G--Y----	----------	------Y---	----------	------S---	------I---	---L------	-----V----	----.
DRB1*0811	........--	--G--Y----	----------	------Y---	----------	------A---	------F---	---L------	-----.....	.....
DRB1*0812	.....-----	--G--Y----	----------	------Y---	----------	------S---	------I---	---L------	----AV----	----.
DRB1*0813	.......---	--G--Y----	----------	------Y---	----------	----------	----------	---L------	-------...	.....
DRB1*0814	.....-----	-RG--Y----	----------	------Y---	----------	------S---	------I---	---L------	----------	-....
DRB1*0815	......----	--G--Y----	----------	------Y---	----------	---------H	------I---	---L------	----------	.....
DRB1*0816	.....-----	--G--Y----	----------	------D---	----------	------S---	------F---	---L------	------....	.....
DRB1*09011	....	.......---	-----Y-H-G	I-----N---	----------	------V--S	------F--R	---E---V--	----------	-----
DRB1*09012	---Q----KQ	DKF-------	-----Y-H-G	I-----N---	----------	------V--S	------F--R	---E---V--	------....	.....
DRB1*1001	---------E	VKF-------	-----L-E-R	VH----YA-Y	----------	----------	---------R	----------	----------	-----
DRB1*11011	----------	----------	----------	------Y---	------F---	-------E--	------F---	----------	----------	-----
DRB1*11012	----------	----------	----------	------Y---	------F---	-------E--	------F---	----------	----------	-----
DRB1*11013	.........-	----------	----------	------Y---	------F---	-------E--	------F---	----------	---------.	.....
DRB1*1102	----------	----------	----------	------Y---	------F---	-------E--	------I---	E---------	-----V----	-----
DRB1*1103	----------	----------	----------	------Y---	------F---	-------E--	------F---	E---------	-----V----	-----
DRB1*11041	----------	----------	----------	------Y---	------F---	-------E--	------F---	----------	-----V----	----.
DRB1*11042	----------	----------	----------	------Y---	------F---	-------E--	------F---	----------	-----V----	-----

```
DRB1*1105   ....------ --G------- ---------- ------Y--- ------F--- -------E-- ------F--- ---------- ---------- ----.
DRB1*1106   .....----- ---------- ---------- ------Y--- ------F--- -------E-- ------F--- ---------- ----AV---- .....
DRB1*1107   ......---- ---------- ---------- ------Y--- ------F--- -------E-- ---------Q K-GR--N--- -----V---- ----.
DRB1*11081  .......... ..-------- ---------- ------Y--- ------F--- -------E-- ---------- ---------- ---------- -....
DRB1*11082  .......... ..-------- ---------- ------Y--- ------F--- -------E-- ---------- ---------- ---------- -....
DRB1*1109   .......... .....----- ---------- -H----N--- ------F--- -------E-- ------F--- ---------- ---------- --...
DRB1*1110   .......... ...------- ---------- -H----F--- ------F--- -------E-- ------F--- ---------- ------.... .....
DRB1*1111   .......... ..-------- ---------- ------Y--- ------F--- -------E-- ------F--- E--------- ---------- -....
DRB1*1112   .......... ...------- ---------- ------F--- ------F--- -------E-- ------F--- ---------- ------.... .....
DRB1*1113   ---------- ---------- ---------- -H----F--- ------F--- -------E-- ---------R ---------- -----V---- ----.
DRB1*1114   ---------- ---------- ---------- ------Y--- ------F--- -------E-- ------I--- E--------- ---------- ---..
DRB1*1115   ---------- ---------- ---------- ------DL-- ------F--- -------E-- ------F--- ---------- ---------- -----
DRB1*1116   .......... ..-------- ---------- -H----N--- ------F--- -------E-- ------I--- E--------- -----V.... .....
DRB1*1117   ---------- ---------- ---------- -H----F--- ---------- -------E-- ---------R ---E------ -----V---- -----
DRB1*1118   .....----- ---------- ---------- ------Y--- ------F--- -------E-- ------I--- ---------- -----V---- ----.
DRB1*1119   .....----- ---------- ---------- ------Y--- ------F--- -------E-- ------I--- ---------- ---------- ----.
DRB1*1120   .......--- ---------- ---------- -H----N--- ------F--- -------E-- ------I--- E--------- ---------- --...
DRB1*1121   .......--- ---------- ---------- ------Y--- ------F--- -------E-- ------I--- E--------- ----AV-... .....
DRB1*1122   ....-----Q VKH------- ---------- ------Y--- ------F--- -------E-- ------F--- ---------- -------... .....
DRB1*1123   .......... ..-------- ---------- ------Y--- ------F--- -------E-- ------F--- ---L------ ------.... .....
DRB1*1124   .......... ..-------- ---------- ------D--- ------F--- -------E-- ------F--- ---L------ ------.... .....
DRB1*1125   ....------ ---------- ---------- ------Y--- ------F--- -------E-- ------F--- ---L------ -----V---- ----.
DRB1*1126   .......--- ---------- ---------- ------Y--- ------F--- -------E-- ---------Q ---------- -------... .....
DRB1*1127   ......---- ---------- ---------- ------Y--- ------F--- -------E-- ------F--- ------N--- -------... .....
DRB1*1129   .....----- ---------- ---------- ---------- ------F--- -------E-- ------F--- ---------- ------.... .....
DRB1*1130   ....-----L LK-------- ---------- ------Y--- ------F--- -------E-- ------F--- ---------- ---------- ----.
DRB1*1201   ---------- --G--Y---- -----L-E-H -H----LL-- ------F--- ------V--S ------I--- ---------- ----AV---- -----
DRB1*12021  .....----- --G--Y---- -----L-E-H -H----LL-- ------F--- ------V--S ------F--- ---------- ----AV.... .....
DRB1*12022  ......---- --G--Y---- -----L-E-H -H----LL-- ------F--- ------V--S ------F--- ---------- ----AV-... .....
DRB1*12031  ---------- --G--Y---- -----L-E-H -H----LL-- ------F--- ------V--S ------I--- ---------- -----V---- ----.
DRB1*12032  ....------ --G--Y---- -----L-E-H -H----LL-- ------F--- ------V--S ------I--- ---------- -----V---- ---..
DRB1*1204   ........-- --G--Y---- -----L-E-H -H----LL-- ------F--- -------E-- ------I--- ---------- ----AV.... .....
DRB1*1205   .....----- --G--Y---- -----L-E-H -H----FL-- ------F--- ------V--S ------I--- ---------- ----AV---- ----.
DRB1*1301   ---------- ---------- ---------- -H----N--- ------F--- ---------- ------I--- E--------- -----V---- -----
DRB1*1302   ---------- ---------- ---------- -H----N--- ------F--- ---------- ------I--- E--------- ---------- ----.
DRB1*13031  ---------- ---------- ---------- ------Y--- ---------- ------S--- ------I--- K--------- ---------- -----
DRB1*13032  .....----- ---------- ---------- ------Y--- ---------- ------S--- ------I--- K--------- ---------- ----G
DRB1*1304   ---------- ---------- ---------- ------Y--- ------F--- ------S--- ------I--- E--------- -----V---- -----
DRB1*1305   .....----- ---------- ---------- -H----N--- ------F--- ---------- ------F--- ---------- ---------- .....
DRB1*1306   .......... ....------ ---------- -H----N--- ------F--- ---------- ------I--- ---------- -----V---- .....
DRB1*1307   ......---- ---------- ---------- ------Y--- ---------- ---------- ------F--- ---------- ---------- .....
```

Fig. 2.12. (con't)

CONSENSUS	GDTRPRFLEY	STSECHFFNG	TERVRFLDRY	FYNQEESVRF	DSDVGEYRAV	TELGRPDAEY	WNSQKDLLED	RRAAVDTYCR	HNYGVGESFT	VQRRV
*DRB1*1308*	......----	----------	----------	-H----F---	----------	----------	------I---	E---------	-----V----	-....
*DRB1*1309*	......----	----------	----------	-H----N---	------F---	----------	------I--Q	A---------	-----V----	-....
*DRB1*1310*	.......---	----------	----------	-H----N---	------F---	----------	------I---	K---------	-----V-...	.....
*DRB1*1311*	.......---	----------	----------	------Y---	------F---	----------	------F---	----------	-----V----	---..
*DRB1*1312*	.....-----	----------	----------	------Y---	----------	------S---	------I---	----------	----------	----.
*DRB1*1313*	.....-----	----------	----------	------Y---	----------	------S---	------I---	---L------	----------	-....
*DRB1*1314*	....	.---------	----------	------Y---	------F---	----------	------F---	----------	------....	.....
*DRB1*1315*	....	...-------	-------E--	-H----N---	------F---	----------	------I---	E---------	-----V....	.....
*DRB1*1316*	........--	----------	----------	-H----N---	------F---	----------	------I---	E---------	-----D----	.....
*DRB1*1317*	----------	--G--Y----	----------	------Y---	------F---	----------	------I---	E---------	-----V----	-----
*DRB1*1318*	.......---	----------	----------	-H----N---	------F---	----------	------F---	---L------	-----V----	----.
*DRB1*1319*	----------	----------	-------E--	-H----F---	----------	----------	------I---	E---------	-----V----	-----
*DRB1*1320*	.....-----	----------	----------	-H----N---	------F---	----------	----------	E---------	-----V----	---..
*DRB1*1321*	----------	----------	----------	------Y---	------F---	------S---	------F---	----------	----------	-----
*DRB1*1322*	.....-----	----------	----------	------Y---	------F---	----------	------I---	E---------	-----V----	----.
*DRB1*1323*	.....-----	----------	----------	------Y---	------F---	----------	------I---	E---------	----------	---..
*DRB1*1324*	.....-----	----------	----------	------Y---	------F---	----------	------F---	E---------	-----V----	---..
*DRB1*1326*	.......---	----------	-------E--	-H----N---	----------	----------	------F---	----------	-------...	.....
*DRB1*1327*	....	..--------	-----Y----	-H----N---	------F---	----------	------I---	E---------	-----V....	.....
*DRB1*1328*	.......---	----------	----------	-H----N---	------F---	----------	------I---	E---------	---R-V----	.....
*DRB1*1329*	.....-----	----------	----------	-H----N---	------F---	----------	----------	E---------	----------	----.
*DRB1*1330*	.....-----	----------	----------	------Y---	------F---	------S---	------I---	----------	----------	.....
*DRB1*1401*	----------	----------	----------	-H----F---	----------	------A--H	---------R	---E------	-----V----	----.
*DRB1*1402*	----------	----------	-------E--	-H----N---	----------	----------	---------Q	----------	----------	----.
*DRB1*1403*	----------	----------	-------E--	-H----N---	----------	----------	----------	---L------	----------	----.
*DRB1*1404*	.....-----	--G--Y----	----------	-H----F---	----------	------A--H	---------R	---E------	-----V----	----.
*DRB1*1405*	......----	-----Q----	----------	-H----F---	----------	----------	---------R	---E------	-----V....	.....
*DRB1*1406*	........--	----------	-------E--	-H----N---	----------	----------	---------Q	----------	-----V----	.....
*DRB1*1407*	........--	----------	----------	-H----F---	----------	------A--H	---------R	---E------	------....	.....
*DRB1*1408*	......----	----------	----------	-H----F---	----------	---------H	---------R	---E------	-----V----	---..
*DRB1*1409*	......----	----------	----------	-H----N---	----------	----------	---------Q	----------	----------	---..
*DRB1*1410*	......---Q	VKH-------	----------	-H----F---	----------	------A--H	---------R	---E------	-----V----	---..
*DRB1*1411*	........--	--G--Y----	----------	-H----F---	----------	-------E--	---------R	---E------	-----V....	.....
*DRB1*1412*	....	..--------	-------E--	-H----N---	----------	----------	----------	---L------	-----V....	.....
*DRB1*1413*	........--	----------	-------E--	-H----N---	----------	------S---	---------Q	----------	------....	.....
*DRB1*1414*	......----	----------	----------	-H----F---	----------	----------	---------R	---E------	----------	-....
*DRB1*1415*	....	--G--Y----	----------	-H----F---	----------	----------	------F---	---L------	-----V----	--...
*DRB1*1416*	.......---	----------	----------	-H----F---	----------	------A--H	------I---	E---------	-----V-...	.....
*DRB1*1417*	.....-----	----------	----------	-H----N---	------F---	----------	---------Q	----------	-----V----	---..
*DRB1*1418*	....	...-------	-------E--	-H----N---	----------	----------	---------R	---E------	-----V----	----.
*DRB1*1419*	----------	----------	-------E--	-H----N---	----------	----------	---------O	K---------	----------	.....

```
DRB1*1420    .......--- ---------- -------E-- -H----F--- ---------- ---------- ---------Q ---------- -----V-... .....
DRB1*1421    .......--- ---------- ---------- -H----N--- ------F--- ---------- ---------Q K--------- -----V-... .....
DRB1*1422    .....----- ---------- ---------- -H----F--- ---------- ------A--H ------F--- ---------- ---------- ----.
DRB1*1423    .....----- ---------- ---------- -H----F--- ---------- ---------- ---------R ---E------ -----V---- ----.
DRB1*1424    .......... ..-------- -------E-- -H----N--- ---------- ---------- ------I--Q A--------- ---------- -----
DRB1*1425    ........-- ---------- ---------- ------Y--- ---------- ------A--H ------F--- ---------- ------.... .....
DRB1*1426    .....----- ---------- ----Q----- -H----F--- ---------- ------A--H ---------R ---E------ -----V---- ----.
DRB1*1427    .....----- ---------- -------E-- -H----N--- ---------- ---------- ------F--- ---L------ ---------- ----.
DRB1*1428    .....----- --G--Y---- ---------- -H----F--- ---------- ------A--H ---------R ---E------ ----AV.... .....
DRB1*1429    .....----- ---------- -------E-- -H----N--- ---------- ---------- ---------Q ---------- ----AV---- ----.
DRB1*15011   --------WQ PKR------- ---------- ---------- ------F--- ---------- ------I--Q A--------- -----V---- -----
DRB1*15012   .....---WQ PKR------- ---------- ---------- ------F--- ---------- ------I--Q A--------- -----V---- ---..
DRB1*15021   --------WQ PKR------- ---------- ---------- ------F--- ---------- ------I--Q A--------- ---------- -----
DRB1*15022   .......... ...------- ---------- ---------- ------F--- ---------- ------I--Q A--------- ------.... .....
DRB1*1503    .....---WQ PKR------- ---------H ---------- ------F--- ---------- ------I--Q A--------- -----V---- ----.
DRB1*1504    .......... ...------- ---------- ---------- ------F--- ---------- ------F--Q A--------- -----V.... .....
DRB1*1505    ......--WQ PKR------- ---------- ---------- ------F--- ---------- ---------Q A--------- -----V---- ---..
DRB1*1506    .......... ...------- ---------- ---------- -----EF--A ---------- ------I--Q A--------- -----V.... .....
DRB1*16011   --------WQ PKR------- ---------- ---------- ---------- ---------- ------F--- ---------- ---------- -----
DRB1*16012   .....---WQ PKR------- ---------- ---------- ---------- ---------- ------F--- ---------- ---------- .....
DRB1*16021   --------WQ PKR------- ---------- ---------- ---------- ---------- ---------- ---------- ---------- -----
DRB1*16022   .......... ..R------- ---------- ---------- ---------- ---------- ---------- ---------- ------.... .....
DRB1*1603    --------WQ PKR------- ---------- ---------- ---------- ---------- ------F--- -A-------- ---------- -----
DRB1*1604    ........WQ PKR------- ---------- ---------- ---------- ---------- ------F--- ---L------ ------.... .....
DRB1*1605    .......... ....------ ---------- ---------- ---------- ---------- ------I--- ---------- ------.... .....
DRB1*1606    .......-WQ PKR------- ---------- ---------- ---------- ---------- ------I--- -A-------- -------... .....
DRB1*1608    .....---WQ PKR------- ---------- ------N--- ---------- ---------- ------F--- ---------- ---------- --...
DRB3*01011   ---------L RKS------- -----Y---- -H----FL-- ---------- ------V--S ---------Q K-GR--N--- ---------- -----
DRB3*01013   .......... RK-------- -----Y---- -H----FL-- ---------- ------V--S ---------Q K-GR--N--- --------.. .....
DRB3*0102    ......---L CK-------- -----Y---- -H----FL-- ---------- ------V--S ---------Q K-GR--N--- --------.. .....
DRB3*0201    ---------L LK-------- -------E-H -H----YA-- ---------- R--------- ---------Q K-GQ--N--- -----V---- -----
DRB3*0202    ---------L LK-------- -------E-H -H----YA-- ---------- R--------- ---------Q K-GQ--N--- ---------- -----
DRB3*0203    .......--L LK-------- -------E-H -H-------- ---------- R--------- ---------Q K-GQ--N--- ---------- ----.
DRB3*0204    .....----L LK-------- -------E-H -H----YA-- ---------- R--------- ---------Q K-GR--N--- -----V---- ----.
DRB3*0205    .....----L LK-------- -------E-- -H----YA-- ---------- R--------- ---------Q K-GQ--N--- ---------- --...
DRB3*0206    .....----L LK-------- -------E-H -H----NA-- ---------- R--------- ---------Q K-GQ--N--- ------.... .....
DRB3*0301    ---------L LK-------- -------E-- -H----F--- ---------- ------V--S ---------Q K-GQ--N--- -----V---- -----
DRB4*0101101 ---Q-----Q AKC----L-- ----WN-I-- I-----YA-Y N--L---Q-- ---------- ---------R ---E------ Y----V---- -----
DRB4*0102    .......... .......... .---WN-I-- I-----YA-Y N--L---Q-- ---------- ---------R ---E-G---- Y----V---- --...
DRB4*0103101 ---Q-----Q AKC----L-- ----WN-I-- I-----YA-Y N--L---Q-- ---------- ---------R ---E------ Y----V---- -----
DRB4*0104    .....----O AKC----L-- ----WN-I-- I-----YA-Y N--L---Q-- ---------- ---------R ---E--N--- Y----V---- ----.
```

Fig. 2.12. (con't)

CONSENSUS	GDTRPRFLEY	STSECHFFNG	TERVRFLDRY	FYNQEESVRF	DSDVGEYRAV	TELGRPDAEY	WNSQKDLLED	RRAAVDTYCR	HNYGVGESFT	VQRRV
*DRB4*0201N*	.....----Q	AKC----L--	--PDQIHL..	....	....	....	....	....	....	.....
*DRB5*0101*	--------QQ	DKY-------	-------H-D	I-----DL--	----------	----------	------F---	----------	----------	-----
*DRB5*0102*	--------QQ	DKY-------	-------H-G	I-----N---	----------	----------	------F---	----------	----------	-----
*DRB5*0103*	.......-QQ	DKY-------	-------H-G	I-----N---	----------	----------	------F---	T---------	----------	----.
*DRB5*0104*	--------QQ	DKY-------	-------H-D	I-----DL--	----------	----------	------F---	---L------	----------	-----
*DRB5*0105*	....----QQ	DKY-------	-------H-D	I-----D---	----------	----------	------F---	----------	----------	---..
*DRB5*0201*	-----C--QQ	DKY-------	-------H-G	I-----N---	----------	----------	------I--Q	A---------	----AV----	-----
*DRB5*0202*	-----C--QQ	DKY-------	-------H-G	I-----N---	----------	----------	------I--Q	A---------	----AV----	-----
*DRB5*0203*	......--QQ	DKY-------	-------H-G	I-----N---	----------	----------	------I--Q	A---------	----------	---..
*DRB5*0204*	.....C--QQ	DKY-------	-------H-G	I-----N---	----------	----------	------F--Q	A---------	----AV----	.....
*DRB6*0101*	....	.KC---I---	MK--QY-N--	IHKR--NLPF	----E-FQ--	------V--N	-----GI--E	N-DK------	YS---F-...	.....
*DRB6*0201*	........-Q	AKC---I---	MK--QY-N--	IHKR--NL--	--N-E-FQ--	------V--N	-----GIP-E	K-DKM-D---	Y----F....	.....
*DRB6*0202*	....	.KC---I---	MK--QY-N--	IHKR--NL--	--N-E-FQ--	------V--N	-----GIP-E	K-DKM-D---	Y--R-F....	.....
*DRB7*01011*	......---Q	AK--------	---YL///--	------Y---	N--M--F---	----------	------I--Q	K--E--N/-.	....	.....
*DRB7*01012*	......---O	AK--------	---YL///--	------Y---	N--M--F---	----------	------I--Q	K--E--N/-.	....	.....

ß2 domain

```
                 101        111        121        131        141        151        161        171        181
Consensus  HPKVT VYPSKTQPLQ HHNLLVCSVS GFYPGSIEVR WFRNGQEEKA GVVSTGLIQN GDWTFQTLVM LETVPRSGEV YTCQVEHPSV TSPLTVEW
DRB1*0101  E---- ---------- ---------- ---------- ---------- ---------- ---------- ---------- ---------- --------
DRB1*0102  E---- ---------- ---------- ---------- ---------- ---------- ---------- ---------- ---------- --------
DRB1*0103  E---- ---------- ---------- ---------- ---------- ---------- ---------- ---------- ---------- --------
DRB1*03021 ----- ---------- ---------- ---------- ---------T --------H- ---------- ---------- ---------- --------
DRB1*03022 ----- .......... .......... .......... .......... .......... .......... .......... .......... ........
DRB1*0307  ----- --........ .......... .......... .......... .......... .......... .......... .......... ........
DRB1*0308  ----- --........ .......... .......... .......... .......... .......... .......... .......... ........
DRB1*0311  ----- ---------- ---------- ---------- ---------T --------H- ---------- ---------- ---------- --------
DRB1*04011 Y-E-- ---A------ ---------N ---------- ---------T ---------- ---------- ---------- ---------L --------
DRB1*0403  Y-E-- ---A------ ---------N ---------- ---------T ---------- ---------- ---------- ---------L --------
DRB1*0404  Y-E-- ---A------ ---------N ---------- ---------T ---------- ---------- ---------- ---------L --------
DRB1*04052 E.... .......... .......... .......... .......... .......... .......... .......... .......... ........
DRB1*0406  Y-E-- ---A------ ---------N ---------- ---------T ---------- ---------- ---------- ---------L --------
DRB1*0411  Y-E-- ---A------ ---------N ---------- ---------T ---------- ---------- ---------- ---------L --------
DRB1*0701  --E-- ---A------ ---------- ---------- ---------- ---------- ---------- ---------- ---------- M-------
DRB1*08021 ----- ---------- ---------- ---------- ---------T --------H- ---------- ---------- ---------- --------
DRB1*08022 ----- ---------- ---------- ---------- ---------T --------H- ---------- ---------- ---------- --------
DRB1*08031 ----- ---------- ---------- ---------- ---------T --------H- ---------- ---------- ---------- --------
DRB1*08041 ----- -......... .......... .......... .......... .......... .......... .......... .......... ........
DRB1*0813  ----- --........ .......... .......... .......... .......... .......... .......... .......... ........
DRB1*09011 --E-- ---A------ ---------- ---------- ---------- ---------- ---------- ---------- ---------- M-------
DRB1*1001  Q---- ---------- ---------N ---------- ---------T ---------- ---------- -----Q---- ---------- M-------
DRB1*11011 ----- ---------- ---------- ---------- ---------T --------H- ---------- ---------- ---------- --------
DRB1*11012 ----- -......... .......... .......... .......... .......... .......... .......... .......... ........
DRB1*1102  ----- ---------- ---------- ---------- ---------T --------H- ---------- ---F------ ---------- --------
DRB1*1103  ----- ---------- ---------- ---------- ---------T --------H- ---------- ---------- ---------- --------
DRB1*11042 ----- ---....... .......... .......... .......... .......... .......... .......... .......... ........
DRB1*1115  ----- ---------- --........ .......... .......... .......... .......... .......... .......... ........
DRB1*1117  ----- ---------- --........ .......... .......... .......... .......... .......... .......... ........
DRB1*1201  ----- ---------- ---------- ---------- ---------T --------H- ---------- P--------- ---------- --------
DRB1*1301  ----- ---------- ---------- ---------- ---------T --------H- ---------- ---------- ---------- --------
DRB1*13031 ----- -......... .......... .......... .......... .......... .......... .......... .......... ........
DRB1*13032 E.... .......... .......... .......... .......... .......... .......... .......... .......... ........
DRB1*1304  ----- -......... .......... .......... .......... .......... .......... .......... .......... ........
DRB1*1317  ----- ---------- ----...... .......... .......... .......... .......... .......... .......... ........
DRB1*1319  ----- --------.. .......... .......... .......... .......... .......... .......... .......... ........
DRB1*1321  ----- ---------- ---------. .......... .......... .......... .......... .......... .......... ........
DRB1*1424  ----- --........ .......... .......... .......... .......... .......... .......... .......... ........
```

Fig. 2.12. (con't)

Consensus	HPKVT	VYPSKTQPLQ	HHNLLVCSVS	GFYPGSIEVR	WFRNGQEEKA	GVVSTGLIQN	GDWTFQTLVM	LETVPRSGEV	YTCQVEHPSV	TSPLTVEW
*DRB1*15011*	Q----	----------	----------	----------	--L-------	-M--------	----------	----------	----------	--------
*DRB1*15021*	Q----	----------	----------	----------	--L-------	-M--------	----------	----------	----------	--------
*DRB1*1601*	Q----	----------	----------	----------	--L-------	-M--------	----------	----------	----------	--------
*DRB1*16021*	Q----	----------	----------	----------	--L-------	-M--------	----------	----------	----------	--------
*DRB1*1603*	Q----	----------	----------	----------	--L-------	-M--------	----------	----------	----------	--------
*DRB3*0101*	--Q--	---A------	----------	----------	----------	----------	----------	----------	----------	--A-----
*DRB3*0201*	--Q--	---A------	----------	----------	----------	----------	----------	---F------	----------	--------
*DRB3*0202*	--Q--	---A------	----------	----------	----------	----------	----------	----------	----------	--------
*DRB3*0301*	--Q--	---A------	----------	----------	---------T	--------H-	----------	----------	----------	--------
*DRB4*01011*	Q----	----------	---------N	----------	----S-----	----------	----------	----------	---------M	M-----Q-
*DRB4*0103*	Q----	----------	---------N	----------	----------	----------	----------	----------	---------M	M-----Q-
*DRB5*0101*	E----	---AR--T--	---------N	----------	----S-----	----------	----------	----------	----------	--------
*DRB5*0102*	E----	---AR--T--	---------N	----------	----S-----	----------	----------	----------	----------	--------
*DRB5*0104*	E----	---AR--T--	-.........	....	....	....	....	....	....	....
*DRB5*0201*	E----	---AR--T--	---------N	----------	----------	----------	------I---	----------	----------	--------
*DRB5*0202*	E----	---AR--T--	---------N	----------	----------	----------	------I---	----------	----------	--------

ß TM-CY domain

```
               191        201        211        221        231
Consensus   RA RSESAQSKML SGVGGFVLGL LFLGAGLFIY FRNQKGHSGL QPTGFLS
DRB1*0101   -- ---------- ---------- ---------- ---------- -------
DRB1*0102   -- ---------- ---------- ---------- ---------- -------
DRB1*0103   -- ---------- ---------- ---------- ---------- -------
DRB1*03011  -- ---------- ---------- ---------- ---------- --R----
DRB1*0302   -- ---------- ---------- ---------- ---------- --R----
DRB1*04011  -- ---------- ---------- ---------- ---------- -------
DRB1*0403   -- ---------- ---------- ---------- ---------- -------
DRB1*0404   -- ---------- ---------- ---------- ---------- -------
DRB1*0406   -- ---------- ---------- ---------- ---------- -------
DRB1*0411   -- ---------- ---------- ---------- ---------- -------
DRB1*0701   -- ---------- ---------- ---------- ---------- -------
DRB1*08021  S- ---------- ---------- ---------- ---------- -------
DRB1*09011  -- ---------- ---------- ---------- ---------- -------
DRB1*1001   -- ---------- ---------- ---------- ---------- P------
DRB1*11011  -- ---------- ---------- ---------- ---------- --R----
DRB1*1102   -- ---------- ---------- ---------- ---------- --R----
DRB1*1103   -- ---------- ---------- ---------- ---------- --R----
DRB1*1201   -- ---------- ---------- ---------- ---------- --R----
DRB1*1301   -- ---------- ---------- ---------- ---------- --R----
DRB1*15011  -- ---------- ---------- ---------- ---------- -------
DRB1*15021  -- ---------- ---------- ---------- ---------- -------
DRB1*1601   -- ---------- ---------- ---------- ---------- -------
DRB1*16021  -- ---------- ---------- ---------- ---------- -------
DRB1*1603   -- ---------- ---------- ---------- ---------- ---....
DRB3*0201   S- ---------- ---------- ---------- ---------- -------
DRB3*0202   S- ---------- ---------- ---------- ---------- -------
DRB4*01011  S- ---------- ---------- ----T----- ---------- ----L--
DRB4*0103   S- ---------- ---------- ----T----- ---------- ----L--
DRB5*0101   -- Q--------- ---------- ---------- -K-------- H---LV-
DRB5*0102   -- Q--------- ---------- ---------- -K-------- H---LV-
DRB5*0201   -- Q--------- ---------- ---------- -K-------- H---LV-
DRB5*0202   -- Q--------- --I------- ---------- -K-------- H---LV-
```

Fig. 2.13. Alignment of *HLA-DQA* α1 and α2 domain amino acid sequences

The AA are given in the international single letter code. Identity with *DQA1*0101* is indicated by hyphens, unavailability of information is indicated by dots, and slashes indicate indels. See also Table 2.5. Sequences of which only the nucleotides were available, the amino acid sequence was deferred.

α1 domain

```
             1          11         21         31         41         51         61         71         81
DQA1*0101    EDIVADHVAS CGVNLYQFYG PSGQYTHEFD GDEEFYVDLE RKETAWRWPE FSKFGGFDPQ GALRNMAVAK HNLNIMIKRY NSTAATN
DQA1*01021   ---------- ---------- ---------- ---Q------ ---------- ---------- ---------- ---------- -------
DQA1*01022   ---------- ---------- ---------- ---Q------ ---------- ---------- ---------- ---------- -------
DQA1*0103    ---------- ---------- ----F----- ---Q------ K--------- ---------- ---------- ---------- -------
DQA1*0104    -G-------- ---------- ---------- ---------- ---------- ---------- ---------- ---------- -------
DQA1*0105    -G-------- ---------- ---------- ---------- ---------- ---------- ---------- ---------- -------
DQA1*0201    ---------- Y------S-- ----F----- ---------- ----V-KL-L -HRL/R---- F--T-I--L- -----L---S -------
DQA1*03011   ---------- Y------S-- -----S---- ---------- ----V-QL-L -RR-RR---- F--T-I--L- -----V---S -------
DQA1*0302    ---------- Y------S-- -----S---- ---------- ----V-QL-L -RR-RR---- F--T-I--L- -----V---S -------
DQA1*0303    ---------- Y------S-- -----S---- ---------- ----V-QL-L -RR-RR---- F--T-I--L- -----V---S -------
DQA1*0401    ---------- Y------S-- ---------- ---Q-----G ----V-CL-V LRQ-/R---- F--T-I--T- -----L---S -------
DQA1*05011   ---------- Y------S-- ---------- ---Q-----G ----V-CL-V LRQ-/R---- F--T-I--L- ----SL---S -------
DQA1*05012   ---------- Y------S-- ---------- ---Q-----G ----V-CL-V LRQ-/R---- F--T-I--L- ----SL---S -------
DQA1*05013   ---------- Y------S-- ---------- ---Q-----G ----V-CL-V LRQ-/R---- F--T-I--L- ----SL---S -------
DQA1*0502    .......... .------S-- ---------- ---Q-----G ----V-CL-V LRQ-/R--R- F--T-I--L- ----SL---S ------.
DQA1*0503    ---------- Y------S-- ---------- ---Q-----G ----V-CL-V LRQ-/R---- F--T-I--L- ----SL---S -------
DQA1*0601    ---------- Y------S-- ----F----- ---Q-----G ----V-CL-V LRQ-/R---- F--T-I--T- -----L---S -------
```

α2 domain

```
                 91         101        111        121        131        141        151        161        171
DQA1*0101    EVP EVTVFSKSPV TLGQPNTLIC LVDNIFPPVV NITWLSNGQS VTEGVSETSF LSKSDHSFFK ISYLTFLPSA DEIYDCKVEH WGLDQPLLKH W
DQA1*01021   --- ---------- ---------- ---------- ---------- ---------- ---------- ---------- ---------- ---------- -
DQA1*01022   --- ---------- ---------- ---------- ---------- ---------- ---------- ---------- ---------- ---------- -
DQA1*0103    --- ---------- ---------- ---------- --------HA ---------- ---------- ---------- ---------- ---------- -
DQA1*0104    --- ---------- ---------- ---------- ---------- ---------- ---------- ---------- ---------- ---------- -
DQA1*0105    --- ---------- ---------- ---------- ---------- ---------- ---------- ---------- ---------- ---------- -
DQA1*0201    --- ---------- ---------- ---------- --------H- ---------- ---------- ---------- ---------- ----E----- -
DQA1*03011   --- ---------- ---------- ---------- --------H- ---------- ---------- ---------- ---------- ----E----- -
DQA1*0302    --- ---------- ---------- ---------- --------H- ---------- ---------- ---------D ---------- ----E----- -
DQA1*0303    --- ---------- ---------- ---------- --------H- ---------- ---------- ---------D ---------- ----E----- -
DQA1*0401    --- ---------- ---------- ---------- --------H- ---------- ---------- ---------- ---------- ----E----- -
```

```
DQA1*05011  --- ---------- ------I--- ---------- --------H- ---------- ---------- -----L---- E-S------- ----K----- -
DQA1*05013  --- ---------- ------I--- ---------- --------H- ---------- ---------- -----L---- E-S------- ----K----- -
DQA1*0503   --- ---------- ------I--- ---------- --------H- ---------- ---------- -----L---S E-S------- ----K----- -
DQA1*0601   --- ---------- ---------- ---------- --------H- ---------- ---------- ---------- ---------- ----E----- -
```

αTM-CY domain

```
                      191        201        211        221        231
DQA1*0101   EPEIPAPMS ELTETVVCAL GLSVGLVGIV VGTVFIIQGL RSVGASRHQG PL
DQA1*01021  --------- ---------- ------M--- ---------- ---------- --
DQA1*01022  --------- ---------- ------M--- ---------- ---------- --
DQA1*0103   --------- ---------- ---------- ---------- ---------- --
DQA1*0104   --------- --------T- ---------- ---------- ---------- --
DQA1*0105   --------- ---------- ---------- ---------- -------... ..
DQA1*0201   --------- ---------- ---------- ----L--R-- ---------- --
DQA1*03011  -----T--- ---------- ---------- ----L--R-- ---------- --
DQA1*0302   -----T--- ---------- ---------- ----L--R-- ---------- --
DQA1*0303   -----T--- ---------- ---------- ----L--R-- --------.. ..
DQA1*0401   --------- ---------- ---------- -------R-- ---------- --
DQA1*05011  --------- ---------- ---------- -------R-- ---------- --
DQA1*05013  --------- ---------- ---------- -------R-- ---------- --
DQA1*0503   --------- ---------- ---------- -------R-- ---------- --
DQA1*0601   --------- ---------- ---------- -------R-- ---------- --
```

Fig. 2.14. Alignment of *HLA-DQB* amino acid sequences

The AA are given in the international single letter code. Identity with the consensus sequence is indicated by hyphens, unavailability of information is indicatd by a dot. See also Table 2.5. Sequences of which only the nucleotides were available, the AA sequence was deferred.

ß1 domain

	1	11	21	31	41	51	61	71	81	91
Consensus	RDSPEDFVYQ	FKGMCYFTNG	TERVRLVTRY	IYNREEYARF	DSDVGVYRAV	TPQGRPDAEY	WNSQKEVLER	TRAEVDTVCR	HNYEVAYRGI	LQRRV
*DQB1*0201*	----------	----------	-------S-S	------IV--	-----EF---	-LL-L-A---	-----DI---	K--A--R---	---QLEL-TT	-----
*DQB1*0202*	----------	----------	-------S-S	------IV--	-----EF---	-LL-L-A---	-----DI---	K--A--R---	---QLEL-TT	-----
*DQB1*0203*	....	----------	-------S-S	------IV--	-----EF---	-LL-L-----	-----DI---	K--A--....	....	.....
*DQB1*0301*	----------	--A-------	-----Y----	----------	----E-----	--L-P-----	----------	----L-----	---QLEL-TT	-----
*DQB1*0302*	----------	----------	----------	----------	----------	--L-P-A---	----------	----L-----	---QLEL-TT	-----
*DQB1*03032*	----------	----------	----------	----------	----------	--L-P-----	----------	----L-----	---QLEL-TT	-----
*DQB1*0304*	----------	--A-------	-----Y----	----------	----E-----	--L-P-A---	----------	----L-----	---QLEL-TT	-----
*DQB1*0305*	....------	----------	-----G----	----------	----------	--L-P-A---	----------	----L-----	---QLEL-TT	-----
*DQB1*0306*	.....-----	----------	----------	----------	----------	--L-P-----	-----DI--E	D--S------	---QLEL-TT	----.
*DQB1*0401*	--------F-	----------	--L--G----	----------	----------	--L--L----	-----DI--E	D--S------	---QLEL-TT	-----
*DQB1*0402*	--------F-	----------	-----G----	----------	----------	--L--L----	-----DI--E	D--S------	---QLEL-TT	-----
*DQB1*0501*	----------	---L------	-----G---H	-------V--	----------	------V---	---------G	A--S--R---	----------	-----
*DQB1*0502*	----------	---L------	-----G---H	-------V--	----------	------S---	---------G	A--S--R---	----------	-----
*DQB1*05031*	----------	---L------	-----G---H	-------V--	----------	----------	---------G	A--S--R---	----------	-----
*DQB1*05032*	....	....	-----G---H	-------V--	----------	----------	---------.	....	....	.....
*DQB1*0504*	........--	---L------	-----G----	-------V--	----------	------S---	-----DI--E	D--S--R---	--........	.....
*DQB1*06011*	--P-----L-	--A-------	-----Y----	------DV--	----------	----------	-----DI---	----L-----	------F---	-----
*DQB1*06012*	....	..A-------	-----Y----	------DV--	----------	----------	-----DI---	----L-----	....	.....
*DQB1*0602*	--------F-	----------	----------	----------	----------	----------	---------G	----L-----	------F---	-----
*DQB1*0603*	----------	----------	---------H	----------	----------	----------	---------G	----L-----	------F---	-----
*DQB1*0604*	----------	----------	---------H	----------	----------	------V---	----------	----L-----	-----G----	-----
*DQB1*06051*	----------	---L------	----------	----------	----------	------V---	----------	----L-----	-----G----	-----
*DQB1*06052*	....	....	----------	----------	----------	------V---	----------	----L--...	....	.....
*DQB1*0606*	....	....	----------	----------	----------	------V---	----------	---A--R-..	....	.....
*DQB1*0607*	........--	----------	---------H	----------	----------	----------	----------	----L-----	--........	.....
*DQB1*0608*	........--	----------	---------H	----------	----------	------V---	---------G	----L-----	--........	.....
*DQB1*0609*	....------	----------	----------	----------	----------	------V---	----------	----L-----	-----G----	----.
*DQB1*0610*	.....---F-	----------	----------	----------	----------	------S---	---------G	----L-----	------F---	----.
*DQB1*0611*	........--	----------	----------	----------	----------	----------	---------G	----L-----	------F---	---..
*DQB1*0612*	----------	----------	----------	----------	----------	------V---	---------G	----L-----	-----G----	-----

ß2 domain

```
                   101        111        121        131        141        151        161        171        181
Consensus   EPTVT ISPSRTEALN HHNLLVCSVT DFYPAQIKVR WFRNDQEETA GVVSTPLIRN GDWTFQILVM LEMTPQRGDV YTCHVEHPSL QSPITVEW
DQB1*0201   ----- ---------- ---------- ---------- ---------- ---------- ---------- ---------- ---------- --------
DQB1*0202   ----- ---------- ---------- ---------- ----G----- ---------- ---------- ---------- ---------- --------
DQB1*0301   ----- ---------- ---------- ---------- ---------T ---------- ---------- -----H---- ---------- -N------
DQB1*0302   ----- ---------- ---------- ---------- ---------T ---------- ---------- ---------- ---------- -N--I---
DQB1*03032  ----- ---------- ---------- ---------- ---------T ---------- ---------- ---------- ---------- -N--I---
DQB1*0304   ----- ---------- ---------- ---------- ---------T ---------- ---------- -----H---- ---------- -N------
DQB1*0305   ----- ---------- ---------- ---------- ---------T ---------- ---------- ---------- ---------- -N--I---
DQB1*0401   ----- ---------- ---------- ---------- ---------T ---------- ---------- ---------- ---------- -N--I---
DQB1*0402   ----- ---------- ---------- ---------- ---------T ---------- ---------- ---------- ---------- -N--I---
DQB1*0501   ----- ---------- -----I---- ----S----- ---------- ---------- ---------- ---------- ---------- --------
DQB1*0502   ----- ---------- -----I---- ----SH---- ---------- ---------- ---------- ---------- ---------- --------
DQB1*05031  ----- ---------- -----I---- ----S----- ---------- ---------- ---------- ---------- ---------- --------
DQB1*06011  ----- ---------- ---------- ----G----- ---------- ---------- ---------- -----H---- ---------- --------
DQB1*0602   ----- ---------- ---------- ----G----- ---------- ---------- ---------- ---------- ---------- --------
DQB1*0603   ----- ---------- ---------- ----G----- ---------- ---------- ---------- ---------- ---------- --------
DQB1*0604   ----- ---------- ---------- ----G----Q ---------- ---------- ---------- ---------- ---------- --------
DQB1*06051  ----- --------.. .......... .......... .......... .......... .......... .......... .......... ........
DQB1*0612   ----- ---------- ---------- ----G----Q ---------- ---------- ---------- ---------- ---------- --------
```

ßTM-CY domain

```
               191        201        211        221
Consensus   RA QSESAQSKML SGIGGFVLGL IFLGLGLIIR QRSQKGLLH
DQB1*0201   -- ---------- ---------- ---------H H--------
DQB1*0202   -- ---------- ---------- ---------H H--------
DQB1*0301   -- ---------- ---------- ---------H H--------
DQB1*0302   -- ---------- ---------- ---------H H--------
DQB1*03032  -- ---------- ---------- ---------H H--------
DQB1*0304   -- ---------. .......... .......... .........
DQB1*0305   -- ---------. .......... .......... .........
DQB1*0401   -- ---------- ---------- ---------H H--------
DQB1*0402   -- ---------- ---------- ---------H H--------
DQB1*0501   -- ---------- --V------- ---------- ---R-----
DQB1*0502   -- ---------- --V------- ---------- ---R-----
DQB1*05031  -- ---------- --V------- ---------- ---R-----
DQB1*06011  -- ------N--- ---------- ---------- ---------
DQB1*0602   -- ---------- --V------- ---------- ---------
DQB1*0603   -- ---------- --V------- ---------- ---------
DQB1*0604   -- ---------- --V------- ---------- ---------
DQB1*0612   -- ---------- --V------- ---------- ---------
```

Fig. 2.15. Alignment of *HLA-DPA* domain amino acid sequences

The AA are given in the international single letter code. Identity with *DPA1*0103* is indicated by hyphens, unavailabiliy of information is indicated by dots. See also Table 2.6. Sequences of which only the nucleotides were available, the AA sequence was deferred.

α1 domain

```
             1          11         21         31         41         51         61         71         81
DPA1*0103    IKADHVSTYA AFVQTHRPTG EFMFEFDEDE MFYVDLDKKE TVWHLEEFGQ AFSFEAQGGL ANIAILNNNL NTLIQRSNHT QATN
DPA1*0104    .........- ---------- -------D-- ---------- ---------- ---------- ---------- ---------- ----
DPA1*0105    .........- ---------- ---------- ---------- ---------- ---------- ---------- ---------- --A-
DPA1*02011   ---------- ---------- ---------- Q--------- ---------R ---------- ---------- ---------- --A-
DPA1*02012   ...------- ---------- ---------- Q--------- ---------R ---------- ---------- ---------- --A-
DPA1*02021   .......--- M--------- ---------- Q--------- ---------R ---------- ---------- ---------- --A-
DPA1*02022   ...------- M--------- ---------- Q--------- ---------R ---------- ---------- ---------- --A-
DPA1*0301    .........- M--------- ---------- ---------- ---------- ---------- -----S---- ---------- ----
DPA1*0401    .........- -------T-- -------D-- ---------- ---------R ---------- ---------- -IA------- --A-
```

α2 domain

```
                    91         101        111        121        131        141        151        161        171
DPA1*0103    DPPEVT VFPKEPVELG QPNTLICHID KFFPPVLNVT WLCNGELVTE GVAESLFLPR TDYSFHKFHY LTFVPSAEDF YDCRVEHWGL DQPLLKHW
DPA1*0104    ------ ---------- ---------- ---------- ---------- ---------- ---------- ---------- ---------- --------
DPA1*02011   ------ ---------- ---------- R--------- ------P--- ---------- ---------- ---------V ---------- --------
DPA1*02021   ------ ---------- ---------- R--------- ------P--- ---------- ---------- ---------V ---------- --------
DPA1*02022   ------ ---------- ---------- R--------- ------P--- ---------- ---------- ---------V ---------- --------
DPA1*0301    ------ ---------- ---------- ---------- ---------- ---------- ---------- ---------- ---------- --------
DPA1*0401    ------ -----A---- ---------- ---------- ------P--- ---------- ---------- ---------V ---------- --------
```

αTM-CY domain

```
                181        191        201        211        221
DPA1*0103    EA QEPIQMPETT ETVLCALGLV LGLVGIIVGT VLIIKSLRSG HDPRAQGTL
DPA1*0104    -- ---------- ---------- ---------- ---------- ---------
DPA1*02011   -- ---------- ---------- ---------- ---------- -------P-
DPA1*02021   -- ---------- ---------- ---------- ---------- -------P-
DPA1*02022   -- ---------- ---------- ---------- ---------- -------P-
DPA1*0301    -- ---------- ---------- ---------- ---------- ---------
DPA1*0401    -- ---------A ---------- ---------- ---------- -------P-
```

Fig. 2.16. Alignment of *HLA-DPB* domain amino acid sequences

The AA are given in the international single letter code. Identity with *DPB1*01011* is indicated by hyphens, unavailability of information is indicated by dots, indels are indicated by a slash. See also Table 2.6.

β1 domain

```
              1          11         21         31         41         51         61         71         81         91
DPB1*01011    RATPENYVYQ GRQECYAFNG TQRFLERYIY NREEYARFDS DVGEFRAVTE LGRPAAEYWN SQKDILEEKR AVPDRVCRHN YELDEAVTLQ RRV
DPB1*01012    ....------ ---------- ---------- ---------- ---------- ---------- ---------- ---------- ---------- --.
DPB1*02011    -------LF- ---------- ---------- ----FV---- ---------- ----DE---- --------E- -----M---- ---GGPM--- ---
DPB1*02012    -------LF- ---------- ---------- ----FV---- ---------- ----DE---- --------E- -----M---- ---GGPM--- ---
DPB1*02013    ....---LF- ---------- ---------- ----FV---- ---------- ----DE---- --------E- -----M---- ---GGPM--- --
DPB1*0202     .....--LF- ---------- ---------- ----LV---- ---------- ----E----- --------E- -----M---- ---GGPM--- ...
DPB1*0301     ---------- L--------- ---------- ----FV---- ---------- ----DED--- ----L----- ---------- ---------- ---
DPB1*0401     -------LF- ---------- ---------- ----F----- ---------- ---------- ---------- -----M---- ---GGPM--- ---
DPB1*0402     -------LF- ---------- ---------- ----FV---- ---------- ----DE---- ---------- -----M---- ---GGPM--- ---
DPB1*0501     .....--LF- ---------- ---------- ----LV---- ---------- ----E----- ---------- -----M---- ---------- ...
DPB1*0601     ....------ L--------- ---------- ----FV---- ---------- ----DED--- ----L---E- -----M---- ---------- ...
DPB1*0801     .......LF- ---------- ---------- ----FV---- ---------- ----DE---- --------E- ---------- ---------- ...
DPB1*0901     .....---H- L--------- ---------- ----FV---- ---------- ----DED--- --------E- ---------- ---------- ...
DPB1*1001     .....---H- L--------- ---------- ----FV---- ---------- ----DE---- --------E- ---------- ---------- ...
DPB1*11011    .......--- L--------- ---------- --Q------- ---------- ---------- ----L---R- -----M---- ---------- ...
DPB1*11012    ....------ L--------- ---------- --Q------- ---------- ---------- ----L---R- -----M---- ---------- ...
DPB1*1301     ....------ L--------- ---------- ---------- ---------- ---------- --------E- -----I---- ---------- ...
DPB1*1401     .....---H- L--------- ---------- ----FV---- ---------- ----DED--- ----L----- ---------- ---------- ...
DPB1*1501     .....----- ---------- ---------- --Q------- ---------- ---------- ----L---R- -----M---- ---VGPM--- ...
DPB1*1601     .....--LF- ---------- ---------- ----FV---- ---------- ----DE---- --------E- -----M---- ---------- ...
DPB1*1701     .....---H- L--------- ---------- ----FV---- ---------- ----DED--- --------E- -----M---- ---------- ...
DPB1*1801     .......--- ---------- ---------- ----FV---- ---------- ----DE---- ---------- -----M---- ---VGPM--- ...
DPB1*1901     .....--LF- ---------- ---------- ----FV---- ---------- ----E----- --------E- -----I---- ---------- ...
DPB1*20011    ....------ L--------- ---------- ----FV---- ---------- ----DED--- ----L----- -----M---- ---------- --.
DPB1*20012    ....------ L--------- ---------- ----FV---- ---------- ----DED--- ----L----- -----M---- ---------- --.
DPB1*2101     ....------ L--------- ---------- ----LV---- ---------- ----E----- --------E- -----M---- ---------- --.
DPB1*2201     ....---LF- ---------- ---------- ----LV---- ---------- ----E----- --------E- -----M---- ---------- --.
DPB1*2301     ....---LF- ---------- ---------- ----FV---- ---------- ---------- ---------- -----M---- ---GGPM--- --.
DPB1*2401     ....---LF- ---------- ---------- ----F----- ---------- ----E----- ---------- -----M---- ---GGPM--- --.
DPB1*2501     ....------ L--------- ---------- ----FV---- ---------- ----DE---- ----L----- ---------- ---------- --.
DPB1*26011    .......--- L--------- ---------- ---------- ---------- ---------- ---------- ---------- ---------- --.
```

Fig. 2.16. (con't)

```
CONSENSUS    RATPENYVYQ GRQECYAFNG TQRFLERYIY NREEYARFDS DVGEFRAVTE LGRPAAEYWN SQKDILEEKR AVPDRVCRHN YELDEAVTLQ RRV
DPB1*26012   .......--- L--------- ---------- ---------- ---------- ---------- ---------- ---------- ---------- --.
DPB1*2701    ....------ L--------- ---------- ---------- ---------- ---------- ---------- -----M---- ---------- --.
DPB1*2801    ....---LF- ---------- ---------- ----F----- ---------- ----DE---- ----L----- -----M---- ---VGPM--- --.
DPB1*2901    ....------ L--------- ---------- ----FV---- ---------- ----DED--- ----L---E- ---------- ---------- --.
DPB1*3001    ....----H- L--------- ---------- ----FV---- ---------- ----E----- --------E- -----M---- ---------- ...
DPB1*3101    ....---LF- ---------- ---------- ----F----- ---------- ---------- ----L----- -L---M---- ---------- --.
DPB1*3201    ....---LF- ---------- ---------- ----FV---- ---------- ----DEV--- --------E- -----M---- ---GGPM--- --.
DPB1*3301    ....---LF- ---------- ---------- ----F----- ---------- ---------- --------E- -----M---- ---GGPM--- ...
DPB1*3401    ....---LF- ---------- ---------- ----LV---- ---------- ---------- ----L----- -L---M---- ---VGPM--- ...
DPB1*3501    ....----H- L--------- ---------- ----FV---- ---------- ----DED--- ---------- ---------- ---------- ...
DPB1*3601    ....------ L--------- ---------- ----LV---- ---------- ----E----- ---------- -----M---- ---------- --.
DPB1*3701    .......--- L--------- ---------- ----FV---- ---------- ----DE---- --------E- ---------- ---------- --.
DPB1*3801    .......LF- ------P--- ---------- ----LV---- ---------- ----E----- ---------- -----M---- ---------- ...
DPB1*3901    ....---LF- ---------- ---------- ---------- ---------- ---------- ---------- -----M---- ---GGPM--- --.
DPB1*4001    ....---LF- ---------- ---------- ---------- ---------- ---------- ---------- -----M---- ---VGPM--- --.
DPB1*4101    .....--LF- ---------- ---------- ----FV---- ---------- ----DE---- ----F---E- -----M---- ---GGPM--- --.
DPB1*4401    ....------ L--------- ---------- ----LV---- ---------- ----DED--- ----L---E- ---------- ---------- --.
DPB1*4501    .......-H- L--------- ---------- ----FV---- ---------- ----DE---- ----L----- ---------- ---------- ...
DPB1*4601    .....--LF- ---------- ---------- ----FV---- ---------- ----DED--- --------E- -----M---- ---GGPM--- --.
DPB1*4701    .....--LF- ---------- ---------- ----FV---- ---------- ----E----- --------E- -----M---- ---GGPM--- --.
DPB1*4801    .....--LF- ---------- ---------- ----LV---- ---------- ----DE---- --------E- -----M---- ---GGPM--- ...
DPB1*4901    .....--LF- ---------- ---------- ---------- ---------- ----DE---- ---------- -----M---- ---GGPM--- ...
DPB1*5001    ....------ ---------- ---------- ----FV---- ---------- ----DED--- ----L----- ---------- ---------- ...
DPB1*5101    ....---LF- ---------- ---------- ----F----- ---------- ----DE---- ---------- -----M---- ---GGPM--- --.
DPB1*5201    ....------ L--------- ---------- ----FV---- ---------- ---------- ----L----- ---------- ---------- ...
DPB1*5301    .....--LF- ---------- ---------- ---------- ---------- ----DE---- ---------- -----M---- ---VGPM--- ...
DPB1*5401    ....----H- L--------- ---------- ----FV---- ---------- ----E----- --------E- ---------- ---------- ...
DPB1*5501    ....----H- L--------- ---------- ----FV---- ---------- ---------- --------E- -----M---- ---------- ...
DPB1*5601    .......--- L--------- ---------- ----F----- ---------- ---------- ----L----- ---------- ---------- ...
DPB1*5701    .......LF- ---------- ---------- ----FV---- ---------- ----DED--- ----L----- ---------- ------.... ...
DPB1*5801    .....---H- L--------- ---------- ----LV---- ---------- ---------- --------E- -----M---- ---------- ...
DPB1*5901    .....--LF- ---------- ---------- ----FV---- ---------- ----DE---- ----L----- -----M---- ---GGPM--- ...
DPB1*6001    ....---LF- ---------- ---------- ----FV---- ---------- ----DE---- ----N----- -----M---- ---GGPM--- ...
DPB1*6101N   ....------ L--------- ---------- ----FV---- ---------- ----DED--- ----L--/-- ---------- ---------- ...
DPB1*6201    ....---LF- ---------- ---------- ----LV---- ---------- ---------- ---------- -----M---- ---VGPM--- ...
DPB1*6301    .....--LF- ---------- ---------- ----LV---- ---------- ---------- ---------- -----M---- ---------- ...
DPB1*6401N   .....-/-Y- L--------- ---------- ----FV---- ---------- ----DED--- ----L---E- -----M---- ---------- ...
DPB1*6501    .....--LF- ---------- ---------- ----YA---- ---------- ---------- ---------- ---------- ---------- --.
DPB1*6901    ....------ L--------- ---------- ----FV---- ---------- ----DED--- --------R- -----M---- --------.. ...
```

ß2 domain

```
                 101        111        121        131        141        151        161        171        181
DPB1*01011  QPKVNVS PSKKGPLQHH NLLVCHVTDF YPGSIQVRWF LNGQEETAGV VSTNLIRNGD WTFQILVMLE MTPQQGDVYI CQVEHTSLDS PVTVEW
DPB1*02011  --R---- ---------- ---------- ---------- ---------- ---------- ---------- ---------T ---------- ------
DPB1*02012  --R---- ---------- ---------- ---------- ---------- ---------- ---------- ---------T ---------- ------
DPB1*0301   ------- ---------- ---------- ---------- ---------- ---------- ---------- ---------- ---------- ------
DPB1*0401   --R---- ---------- ---------- ---------- ---------- ---------- ---------- ---------T ---------- ------
DPB1*0402   --R---- ---------- ---------- ---------- ---------- ---------- ---------- ---------T -------M-- ------
```

ßTM-CY domain

```
                 191        201        211        221
DPB1*01011  KAQS DSAQSKTLTG AGGFVLGLII CGVGIFMHRR SKKVQRGSA
DPB1*02011  ---- ---R------ ---------- ---------- ---------
DPB1*02012  ---- ---R------ ---------- ---------- ---------
DPB1*0301   ---- ---R------ ---------- ---------- ---------
DPB1*0401   ---- ---R------ ---------- ---------- ---------
DPB1*0402   ---- ---R------ ---------- ---------- ---------
```

Fig. 2.17. Comparison of class I α1 domain amino acid sequenes of selected species

Identity to the human *HLA-A*0101* is indicated by a dash, unavailability of information by dots, and indels introduced for optimal alignment by a slash (/). Residues involved in putative peptide binding as given by Saper et al for *HLA-A*0201* are marked with an asterisk (*).[499]
HLA is from Girdlestone et al,[18] chimpanzee (*Patr*) from McAdam et al,[676] gorilla (*Gogo*) from Lawlor et al,[677] orang-utan (*Popy*) from Lawlor et al[678,] rhesus monkey (*Mamu*) from Miller et al,[679] cotton-top mandarin (*Saoe*) from Watkins et al,[680] long-haired spider monkey (*Atbe*), common marmoset (*Caja*) and brown-headed tamarin (*Safu*) from Cadavid et al (unpublished), cat (*Feca*) from Yuhki and O'Brien,[681] dog (*Cafa*) from Burnett and Geraghty,[682] horse (*Eqca*) from Ellis et al,[683] pig (*Susc*) from Frels et al,[684] rabbit (*Orcu*) from Tykocinski et al,[685] rat (*RT1*) from Salgar et al,[686] mouse (*H2*) from Duran et al[687] cattle (*Bota*) from Brown et al,[688] sheep (*Ovar*) from Grossberger et al,[512] squirrel (*Scab*) from Wettstein et al,[689] chicken (*Gaga*) from Kroemer et al,[690] lizard (*Amam*) from Grossberger and Parham,[691] axolotl (*Amme*) from Sammut et al,[692] clawed frog (*Xela*) from Flajnik et al,[693] carp (*Cyca*) from Hashimoto et al.[694]

```
              1          11         21         31         41         51         61         71         81         91
                  * * *                 **         *           *              *    *  **   *  **  *   **  *
HLA-X55710    GSHSMRYFFT SVSRPGRGEP RFIAVGYVDD TQFVRFDSDA ASQKMEPRAP WI/EQEGPEY WDQETRNMKA HSQTDRANLG TLRGYY/NQS ED
Patr-U10537   --------S- ---------- ---------- ---------- ---R------ --/------- --R---SV-- GA-IY----- ------/--- --
Gogo-P30375   --------S- ---------- ---------- ---------- ---R------ --/------- --RN---V-- ------VD-- ------/--- --
Popy-M30680   --------S- ---------- ---------- ---------- ---R----T- -M/------- --R---SV-- -A--N-VD-- ------/--- DG
Mamu-U50836   -----K--Y- -M------Q- ---------- ---------- ---R------ -V/------- --R------T ET-NAPV--R --LR--/--- -A
Saoe-M33475   --------E- ---------- -Y-S------ ---------- --PR------ -M/------- -EE---KG-- DA--F-VD-Q --L---/--- -A
Atbe-U59647   --------D- A--------- H-F------- ---------- --PR-----R -M/------- -EE---RS-- QA--H-VS-R N-----/--- -A
Caja-U59637   --------Y- ---------- ---I------ ---------- -NPR------ -V/------- -EEQ--RA-- -A----VD-R ------/--- DA
Safu-U59634   --------S- T--------- -Y-E------ ---------- --PR----S- -V/------- -EE---RA-R NA--F-V--Q --L---/--- -A
Feca-JH0291   ----L---Y- A-----L--- ---S------ ---------- PNPR------ -V/------- --R------N TA-IF-VD-N -MLR--/--- GS
Cafa-Z25418   ----L-FLN- V-----H--- -HW--A---- -P-E--N-ER EGRRP--LVR -L/------- -EER-L-SRT CT-VL-RT-N EVSQD-S--- RT
Eqca-X71809   --------L- A--------- ---S------ ---------- --PR------ -M/------- -ERN--TA-D NA-AF-VS-N N-----/--- -A
Susc-A60369   -P--L---D- A----D--K- ---E------ ---------- PNPR----V- --/-K--Q-- --K--E-AMG SA--F-V--K N-----/--- -A
Orcu-K02441   --------Y- ------L--- ---I------ ---------- --PR--Q--- -M/G-VE--- ---Q-QIA-D TA--F-V--N -ALR--/--- AA
H2-A30547     -P------E- A-----LE-- -Y-S-----N KE-------- ENPRY----- -M/------- -ER--QKA-G QE-WF-VS-R N-L---/--- AG
RT1-L26224    --------DI A-----L--- -Y-S-----H -E-------- ENPRY----- -M/-R---D- -ER--QKA-G NE-NY-VS-R N-----/--- -G
Bota-M24090   --------S- A-----L--- -YLE------ ---------- PNPR-----R -V/------- ------KA-G TA--F----N IAL---/--- -A
Ovar-M34676   -P------S- A---A-A--- -YLE------ ---------- PDP---Q-E- -M/K-V---- --RN---P-G NA--F-VG-T I-----/--- -T
Scab-M97617   -----W--E- ---------- -YL------- ---------- -TPR------ -M/--Q--D- -ER--QKA-G NA--H-VS-N -ALR--/--- -G
Amme-U83137   ----F-G-YS -L-EEVP-V- --S---F--- VPIEGYS--T //RRW----- -MRKI-D-Q- -ER--ERARG TEPVE---V- IVMERL/--T RG
Amam-M81094   P---LQ--Y- G--E--Q-L- Q--V-----G QL--QY--NT RE//-L--VS --KDN-DSK- -EGQ-Q-LQG AEPVF-G-IN -AMNR-/--T GG
Gaga-M31012   EL-TL--IQ- AMTD--P-Q- W-VT-----G EL--HYN-T- RRY//V--TE --AAKADQQ- --GQ-QIGQG NE-I--E--- I-QRR-/--T GG
Xela-M58019   R--TLHFHI- LA-A-IP-LS QYAIIV-M-G V-YG-YN--I RRAQFYS/// /ASLNPLSV- L-MQ-KFAQT FEVWQ-HR-N F-M-VF/-TT NG
Cyca-M37107   .K-YL--M-- /-MLKADTL- V-S---ES-H I-ISHYSIEE Q////////V -MR-NLTEDD ---APEGPPG TRDWYLDLIK I-SN/////C TE
```

Fig. 2.18. Comparison of selected class II β1 domain sequences of different species

Dashes indicate identity with *HLA-DRB1*0101*[235], dots unavailability of information, and a slash indels introduced for optimal alignment. Residues involved in putative peptide binding as given by Stern et al for HLA-DR are marked with an asterisk.[571] Rat (*RT1*) is from Eccles and McMaster,[695] mouse (*H2*) from Nygard et al (unpublished), chimpanzee (*Patr*) from Kenter et al,[696] common marmoset (*Caja*), dusky titi (*Camo*), cotton-top mandarin (*Saoe*), common squirrel monkey (*Sasc*) and brown capuchin (*Ceap*) from Trtkova et al,[697] pigtail macaque (*Mane*) from Zhu et al,[698] rhesus monkey (*Mamu*) from Knapp et al (U57955), crab-eating macaque (*Mafa*), lemur (*Lefs*), otolemur (*Gaga*), from Gaur and Nepom,[699] yellow baboon (*Paca*) from Gaur et al (unpublished), slender lori (*Lota*) and bushbaby (*Gamo*) from Figueroa et al,[700] red deer (*Ceel*) from Swarbrick et al,[701] horse (*Eqca*) from Gustafsson and Andersson,[702] pig (*Susc*) from Vage et al,[703] moose (*Alal*) from Mikko and Andersson,[704] cattle (*Bota*) from Fraser et al,[705] sheep (*Ovar*) from Ballingall et al,[706] dog (*Cafa*) from Francino et al (unpublished), chicken (*Gaga-B-LBII*) from Zoorob et al,[707] clawed frog (*Xela*) from Kobari et al,[708] red-necked wallaby (*Maru*) from Schneider et al,[709] alligator (*Almi*) from Edwards et al,[710] carp (*Cyca*) from van Erp et al,[711] pink salmon (*Ongo*) from Miller and Withler.[712] In several cases only the database designations could be given.

```
               5          15         25         35         45         55         65         75         85
                   * * *                *                     *          *   *      * ** *       *      ** **
HLA-DRB1*0101  PRFLWQLKFE CHFFNGTERV RLLERCIYNQ EESVRFDSDV GEYRAVTELG RPDAEYWNSQ KDLLEQRRAA VDTYCRHNYG VGESFTVQRR
Patr-DRB1*0302 .---EYSTS- ---------- -F-D-YFH-- --Y------- ---------- --V--S---- --I--D--GQ --N------- -----.....
Caja-DRB1*0301 .---EYSTS- ---------- -F-D-YFF-- --NL------ --F------- -----S---- --F--D---E ---V-----E ILDR-L-P--
Camo-DRB1*0301 .---EYSTS- -Y-------- -F-D-YFH-- --L------- --F------- --------G- E-F--RK-GQ --N------- -F--------
Saoe-DRB1*0301 .---EYSTS- --H------- -F-D-YFH-- --FL------ W-------R- -RS--HF--R -NYM-DA--- --S/-----E IS-R-L-L--
Sasc-DRB*w1201 .---E---G- --H--R---- ---A-L---- --F------- --F------- --I--NL--R -EV--YM--- ---F-----K GF-M-L-P--
Ceap-DRB*w1301 .---E-A-S- ---L------ -F-D-YF--- --Y------- --F------- --S------- --I--DA-GQ --N------- ----------
Mane-DRB1*01   ----EYSTS- ---------- -F-D-YF--- --Y------- ------S--- -RS-----G- --I--DA--- ---------R I---------
Mamu-DRB1*0315 ...-EYSTS- -------A-- -Y-D-YF--- --Y---N--- --FQ------ --A-----G- --I---K--R --N------- -----.....
Mafa-DRB1*03a  ..--EYSTS- ---------- -Y-D-YF--- --N------- ---------- ---------- --I---K--R --N------- -F-.......
Lefs-DRB*01    ..--E-F-S- ---Y------ LY-H-YF--R --Y------- --F------- ---------- --F---K--N ---....... ..........
Gaga-DRB*01    ..--E-V-H- ---L---Q-- -F-D-YF--R --W------L ---------- -RV--S---- -NI--EA--- ---------- ---.......
Lota-DRB*w2002 .---E-R-A- ---Y---Q-- -Y-D-YF--R Q-Y------- ---------- ---------L ---M-RK-T- --WF--VS-Q IPDG......
Gamo-DRB       .---E-A-S- ---------- -F-D-Y-H-- --NL------ --F------- ---------- --F------- ---------- AV--------
Paca-DRB1*13a  ..--EYSTS- ---------- -F-D-YF--- --Y------- --F---S--- -RS------R --Y--DE--- ------Y--- -V-.......
Ceel-DRB1      -H--EYA-R- ---P---Q-- GF-D-YF--G --Y------W ---------- ----K----- -EYM-RA--- ---------. ..........
Eqca-DRB*1     ....EYSTS- ---------- -Y-D-YF--G K-Y------- -----L---- --------G- Q-I---K--K ---------A -S---L-...
Susc-DRB1      .H--YLL-F- ---------- -----QY--G --Y------- ---------- --V-KD---- ---------E ---------R TSDT......
Alal-DRB1*2    ....EYH-S- ---------- -F-D-Y---R --Y------- ---------- ----K----- E-I------E ---------- --------..
Bota-DRB       -H--EYS-S- ---------- -F-D-YYT-G --T------W --F------- WQ-------- --F--EK--E --RV------ GM--------
Ovar-DRB       .H--EYH-S- -R-S------ -Y-D-YF--G --Y----N-W ------A--- ----K----- --F---T-TE ------/--- -I---S----
Cafa-DRB1*10   ...VY-F-P- ---T------ -FV--Y-H-R --F------- ----P----- --V--S--G- -E----E--T ---------- -I........
Gaga-B-LBII    AF-FCGAIS- --YL------ -Y-Q-Y---R QQFTH----- -KFV-DSP-- E-Q------N AE---N-MNE --RF------ GV-------S
H2I-Aβd        .H-VV-F-G- -YYT---Q-I --VT-Y---R --Y--Y---- ---------- ---------- PEI--RT--E ---A-----E GP-TS-SL--
RT1.Aβ         .D-VY-F-GL -YYT---Q-I -SVD-RF--- --FL-Y---- --F--L---- -SW-DD---- -EI---K--E M--V--Y--E ET-VP-SL--
Maru-DAB2      KH-TE-F-S- -D-V---QH- -FMD-Y---R --N------- ---V-L---- ---------- -E--DL---- --WF--VC-E IS-P-L-R--
Xela-DAB       .DYVY-Y-AQ -Y-R---DN- ---W-HY--L --TDY----- -LFI-K---- K-S-D----- -ET---K--- ---V-----P FDKP--ID-K
Almi-B         .......... .........- -Y-D-HVWDR QQFMH---N- -V-V-D---- E-T-K----- --V--N--G- -......... ..........
Ongo-34b       .......... ........GI EFIDSYVF-- V-YI--N-T- -R-VGY--HA VKN--A---D AGI-G-EQ-E LER--K--DA NYY-AILDKT
Cyca-DAB3*01   .YYEYMTFDC VYSASDYSDM -Y-LS-SF-- GLDAQ-N-S- -KFVGY--K- MK------NN PAE-Q----E --------AQ ILD-SVRDKT
```

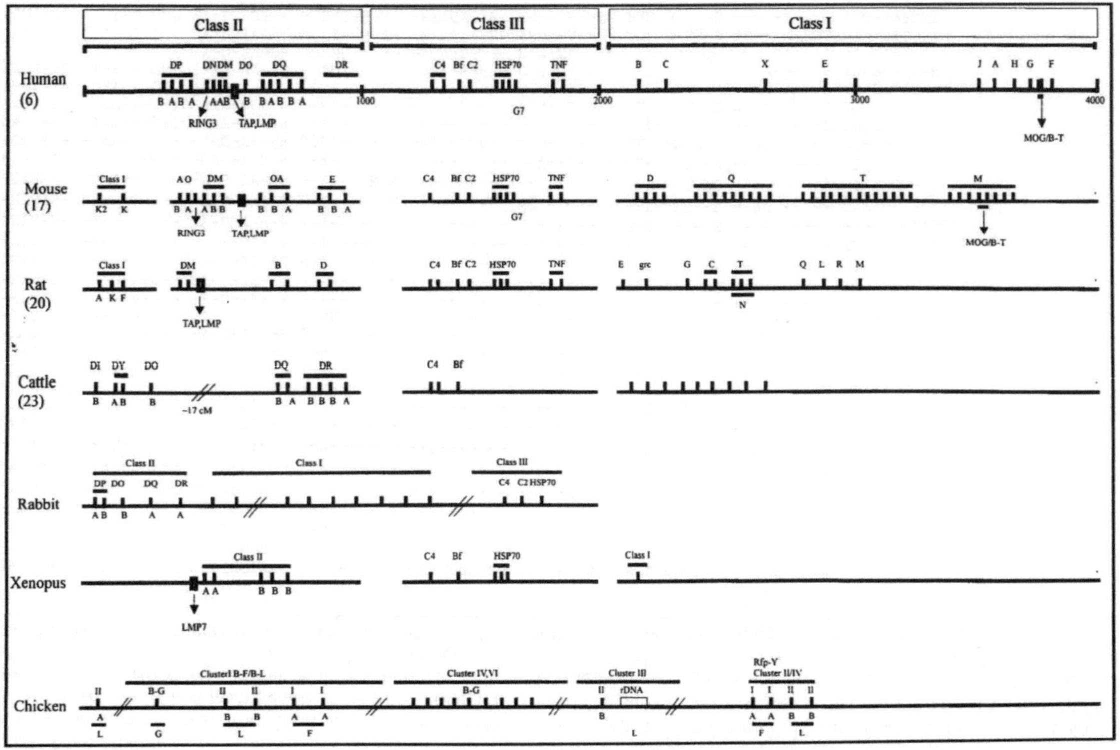

Fig. 2.19. Map of the human, mouse, rat, bovine, rabbit, *Xenopus* and chicken major histocompatibility complex. The map is modified from figures made by Trowsdale and Salter-Cid and Flajnik.[570,513] The maps are only very roughly to scale. The analogous class I, II and III regions are situated below each other, in chicken and rat the differently organized gene clusters are designated individually. Not all *MHC* genes are shown. MHC-related genes may map to two or more different chromosomes. See text for further details.

Fig. 2.20. Alignment of H2 class I α1, α2 domain amino acid sequences

Identiity with *H2-D^{b}* is indicated by hyphens, unavailability of information by dots and indels by a slash. *H2-K^{b}* from Weiss et al,[739] *H2-K^{d}* from Kvist et al,[740] *H2-K^{f}* from Horton et al,[741] *H2-K^{k}* is from Watts et al,[742] *H2-K^{q}* from W. Walter (pers. Comm.), *H2-K^{tw32}* from Jaulin et al,[743] *H2-K^{w28}* from Morita et al,[744] *H2-D^{b}* is from Duran et al.[687] *H2-D^{d}* is from Nairn et al.[745] *H2-D^{dx}* is from Cai and Pease,[746] *H2-D^{f}* is from Hildebrand et al,[747] *H2-D^{k}* is from Watts et al,[742] *H2-D^{p}* is from Schepart et al,[748] *H2-D^{q}* is from Lee et al,[749] *H2-D^{r}* and *H2-D^{s}* are from Cai and Pease,[750] *H2-D^{Bm14}* and *H2-D^{Bm24}* from Hemmi et al,[751] *H2-D^{37}*, *H2-D^{24}* and *H2-D^{33}* from Lalanne et al,[752-754] *H2-L^{d}* from Moore et al,[755] *H2-L^{q}* from Rubocki et al.[756] The putative peptide binding sites as given by Matsumura et al[757] are indicated by asterisks.

α1 domain

	1	11	21	31	41	51	61	71	81
	* * *		* *	*	*	*	* * *	* *	*
H2-D^{b}	GPHSMRYFET	AVSRPGLEEP	RYISVGYVDN	KEFVRFDSDA	ENPRYEPRAP	WMEQEGPEYW	ERETQKAKGQ	EQWFRVSLRN	LLGYYNQSAG
H2-D^{d}	-S--L---V-	------FG--	--ME------	T---------	---------R	-I--------	----RR---N	--S---D--T	A-R-------
H2-D^{dx}	----L---V-	-------GK-	--ME------	T---------	----MK---R	----------	-GQ--N--SN	--I---N--T	----------
H2-D^{f}	----L-----	-------G--	-F-A------	----------	----------	----------	-P--------	------N--I	----------
H2-D^{k}	----L-----	V------G--	-F--------	T---------	----D---VR	----------	-----I---N	--S---D--T	--R-----E-
H2-D^{p}	----L---V-	-------GK-	--ME------	T---------	----MK--VR	----------	-Q---N--DH	--S-------	--------K-
H2-D^{q}	----------	-------G--	----------	----------	-------Q--	----------	--I--I--DN	---------T	A-A-------
H2-D^{r}	-R--L---V-	-------G--	---E-----D	T---------	----V---VR	----VE----	--N--I---N	--I---N--T	--S-----K-
H2-D^{s}	-R--L---V-	-------G--	---E------	T---------	----V---VR	----VE----	--N--I---N	--S---N--T	A-R-----K-
H2-D^{Bm14}	.---------	----------	----------	----------	----------	----------	---------H	----------	----------
H2-D^{Bm24}	.---------	----------	----------	----------	----------	----------	---------N	--S---D--T	----------
H2-D^{24}	----L/////	//////////	//////////	///////---	D---F-----	----------	-EQ--R--SD	---------T	AQR-----K-
H2-D^{33}	----L---V-	-------G--	-F-A-----D	TQ--------	D---F-----	----------	-EQ--R--SD	---------T	AQR-----K-
H2-D^{37}	S---L---T-	-------G--	-F-I-----D	TQ--------	----M----R	-I--------	----W--RDM	GRN---N--T	--------ND
H2-K^{b}	----L---V-	-------G--	--ME-----D	T---------	---------R	----------	---------N	--S---D--T	--------K-
H2-K^{d}	----L---V-	-------G--	-F-A-----D	TQ--------	D---F-----	----------	-EQ--R--SD	---------T	AQR-----K-
H2-K^{f}	----L-----	-------G--	----------	T---------	----F---VR	----------	-----R----	--S---D--T	--------ES
H2-K^{k}	----L---H-	-------GK-	-F-------D	TQ--------	--------VR	----VE----	--N--I---N	--I---N--T	A-R-------
H2-K^{q}	----L---H-	-------GK-	-F-------D	T---------	---------R	----VE----	--N--I--DN	--SS--D--T	--R-------
H2-K^{tw32}	----L---H-	-------GK-	-F-------D	T---------	---------R	----VE----	--N--I--DN	--SS--D--T	--R-------
H2-K^{w28}	----L---H-	-------GK-	-F-------D	T---------	---------R	----VE----	--N--I--DN	--SS--D--T	--R-------
H2-L^{d}	----------	----R--G--	----------	----------	----------	----------	--I--I----	------N--T	----------
H2-L^{q}	----------	-------G--	----------	----------	-------Q--	----------	--I--I----	------N--T	----------

Fig. 2.20. (con't)

α2 domain

	91	101	111	121	131	141	151	161	171	181
	* * *		* * *	**		* *	* * **		*	
H2-D^b	GSHTLQQMSG	CDLGSDWRLL	RGYLQFAYEG	RDYIALNEDL	KTWTAADMAA	QITRRKWEQS	GAAEHYKAYL	EGECVEWLHR	YLKNGNATLL	RT
H2-D^d	------W-A-	--VE--G---	---W----D-	C---------	----------	---------A	----RDR---	--------R-	----------	--
H2-D^dx	----F-R-Y-	----------	---E-S--D-	---L------	----------	---------G	-E--RFR---	--T-----R-	--EL------	--
H2-D^f	----I-R-Y-	--V-------	---E-Y--D-	C---------	----------	---------A	-D----R---	--A-----R-	--QL------	--
H2 D^k	----I-RL--	--V-------	---E----D-	C---------	----------	L--KH----A	----RDR---	--T-----R-	--EL------	H-
H2-D^p	----I-G-R-	--V-------	---E----D-	P---------	----------	---------A	----TLR---	--A-----R-	--EL------	C-
H2-D^q	----I-R-Y-	--V-L-G---	---E----D-	L---------	----------	---------G	----------	----------	----------	--
H2-D^r	----I-W-F-	--VE--G---	---Q-Y--D-	C---------	-------T--	---------A	----RKR---	--T-----L-	H-----E---	--
H2-D^s	----V-V---	--V---G---	---Q-H--D-	----------	-------T--	---------G	-D--------	--T-----L-	--EL--E---	--
H2-D^{Bm14}	----------	----------	----------	----------	----------	----------	----------	----------	----------	--
H2-D^{Bm24}	----------	----------	----------	----------	----------	----------	----------	----------	----------	--
H2-D^{24}	----F-R-F-	--V-------	---Q----D-	----------	-------T--	L--------A	-D--Y-R---	--------R-	--EL--E---	--
H2-D^{33}	----F-R-F-	--V-------	---H----D-	----------	-------T--	L--------A	-D--Y-R---	--------R-	--EL--E---	--
H2-D^{37}	E-----W-Y-	--V-P-G---	---C-E--D-	Q---S-----	RS---N-I-S	--SKH-S-AV	DE-HQQR---	Q-P-----H-	--RL--E--Q	-S
H2-K^b	----I-VI--	-EV---G---	---Q-Y--D-	C---------	----------	L--KH----A	-E--RLR---	--T-----R-	----------	--
H2-K^d	----F-R-F-	--V-------	---Q----D-	----------	-------T--	L--------A	-D--Y-R---	--------R-	--EL--E---	--
H2-K^f	------V-Y-	--V-------	---Q-H--D-	----------	----------	L--KQ----A	----RLR---	--A-----R-	--ER------	--
H2-K^k	----F-R-Y-	-EV-------	---E-Y--D-	C---------	----------	L--KH----A	-D--RDR---	--T-----R-	--QL-----P	--
H2-K^q	----I-R-Y-	--V---G---	---E-V--D-	C---------	----------	L--KH----A	----RRR---	--A-----S-	H---------	--
H2-K^{tw32}	----I-R-Y-	--V---G---	---E-V--D-	C---------	----------	L--KH----A	----RRR---	--A-----S-	H---------	--
H2-K^{w28}	----I-R-Y-	--V---G---	---E-V--D-	C---------	----------	L--KH----A	----RRR---	--A-----S-	H---------	--
H2-L^d	-T----W-Y-	--V---G---	---E----D-	C---------	----F---SS	---------A	----Y-R---	----------	----------	--
H2-L^q	-T--I-R-Y-	--V-------	---E-Y--D-	C---------	----------	---------A	----------	----------	----------	--

Fig. 2.21. Comparison of selected mouse class *II* α amino acid sequences.

Unavailability of information is indicated by a dot; slashes have been introduced for optimal alignment. *H2-A*$_\alpha^k$ is from Landais et al,[758] *H2-A*$_\alpha^b$, *H2-A*$_\alpha^f$, *H2-A*$_\alpha^u$, *H2-A*$_\alpha^d$, *H2-A*$_\alpha^q$ *and H2-E*$_\alpha^u$ from Benoist et al,[759] *H2-A*$_\alpha^s$ and *H2-A*$_\alpha^r$ from Landais et al,[758] *H2-E*$_\alpha^k$ from Mathis et al,[760] *H2-E*$_\alpha^d$ from Hyldig-Nielsen et al,[761] *H2-E*$_\alpha^{w28}$ from Kasahara et al.[762]

α1 domain

	1	11	21	31	41	51	61	71	81
H2-A$_\alpha^k$	EDDIEADHVG	SYGITVYQSP	GDIGQYTFEF	DGDELFYVDL	DKKETVWMLP	EFAQLRRFEP	QGGLQNIATG	KHNLEILTKR	SNSTPATN
H2-A$_\alpha^b$	EDDIEADHVG	TYGISVYQSP	GDIGQYTFEF	DGDELFYVDL	DKKETVWMLP	EFGQLASFDP	QGGLQNIAVV	KHNLGVLTKR	SNSTPATN
H2-A$_\alpha^f$	EDDIEADHVG	FYGISVYQSP	GDIGQYTFEF	DGDEWFYVDL	DKKETVWRLP	EFGQLTSFDP	QGGLQEIATG	KHNLGILTKR	SNFTPATN
H2-A$_\alpha^u$	.....ADHVG	SYGIVVYQSP	GDIGQYTFEF	DGDELFYVDL	DKKETIWMLP	EFAQLRSFDP	QGGLQNIATG	KHNLGVLTKR	SNSTPATN
H2-A$_\alpha^d$	EDDIEADHVG	FYGTTVYQSP	GDIGQYTHEF	DGDELFYVDL	DKKKTVWRLP	EFGQLILFEP	QGGLQNIAAE	KHNLGILTKR	SNFTPATN
H2-A$_\alpha^s$	EDDIEADHVG	VYGTTVYQSP	GDIGQYTHEF	DGDEWFYVDL	DKKETIWMLP	EFGQLTSFDP	QGGLQNIATG	KYTLGILTKR	SNSTPATN
H2-A$_\alpha^r$	EDDIEADHVG	VYGTTVYQSP	GDIGQFTHEF	DGDEWFYVDL	DKKETVWMLP	EFGQLTSFDP	QGGLQNIAVV	KHNLEILTKR	SNFTPAAN
H2-A$_\alpha^q$	....	..GIVVYQSP	GDIGQYTHEF	DGDEWFYVDL	DKKETVWMLP	EFGQLTSFDP	QGGLQNIATG	KHNLGGWTKR	SNFTPATN
H2-E$_\alpha^k$	...IKEEHTI	I/QAEFYLLP	DKRGEFMFDF	DGDEIFHVDI	EKSETIWRLE	EFAKFASFEA	QGALANIAVD	KANLDVMKER	SNNTPDAN
H2-E$_\alpha^d$	...IKEEHTI	I/NAEFYLLP	DKRGEFMFDF	DGDEIFHVDI	EKSETIWRLE	EFAKFASFEA	QGALANIAVD	KANLDVMKER	SNNTPDAN
H2-E$_\alpha^u$	....KEEHTI	I/QAEFYLLP	DKRGEYMFDF	DGDEIFHVDI	EKSETIWRLE	EFAKFASFEA	QGALANIAVD	KANLDVMKKR	SNNTPDAN
H2-E$_\alpha^{w28}$	......EHTI	I/QAEFYLLP	DKRGEFMFDF	DGDEIFHVDI	EKSETIWRLE	EFAKFASFEA	QGALANIAVD	KANLDVMKER	SNNTPDAN

α2 domain

		91	101	111	121	131	141	151	161	171	181
H2-A$_\alpha^k$	EA	PQATVFPKSP	VLLGQPNTLI	CFVDNIFPPV	INITWLRNSK	SVTDGVYETS	FFVNRDYSFH	KLSYLTFIPS	DDDIYDCKVE	HWGLEEPVLK	HW
H2-A$_\alpha^b$	EA	PQATVFPKSP	VLLGQPNTLI	CFVDNIFPPV	INITWLRNSK	SVADGVYETS	FFVNRDYSFH	KLSYLTFIPS	DDDIYDCKVE	HWGLEEPVLK	HW
H2-A$_\alpha^f$	EA	PQATVFPKSP	VLLGQPNTLI	CFVDNIFPPV	INITWLRNSK	SVTDGVYETS	FLVNRDHSFH	KLSYLTFIPS	DDDIYDCKVE	HWGLEEPVLK	HW
H2-A$_\alpha^u$	EA	PQATVFPKSP	VLLGQPNTLI	CFVDNIFPPV	INITWLRNSK	SVADGVYETS	FFVNRDYSFH	KLSYLTFIPS	DDDIYDCKVE	HWGLEEPVLK	HW
H2-A$_\alpha^d$	EA	PQATVFPKSP	VLLGQPNTLI	CFVDNIFPPV	INITWLRNSK	SVTDGVYETS	FLVNRDHSFH	KLSYLTFIPS	DDDIYDCKVE	HWGLEEPVLK	HW
H2-A$_\alpha^s$	EA	PQATVFPKSP	VLLGQPNTLI	CFVDNIFPPV	INITWLRNSK	SVTDGVYETS	FLVNRDHSFH	KLSYLTFIPS	DDDIYDCKVE	HWGLEEPVLK	HW
H2-A$_\alpha^r$	EA	PQATVFPKSP	VLLGQPNTLI	CFVDNIFPPV	INITWLRNSK	SVTDGVYETS	FLVNRDHSFH	KLSYLTFIPS	DDDIYDCKVE	HWGLEEPVLK	HW
H2-A$_\alpha^q$	EA	PQATVFPKSP	VLLGQPNTLI	CFVDNIFPPV	INITWLRNSK	SVTDGVYETS	FLVNRDHSFH	KLSYLTFIPS	DDDIYDCKVE	HWGLDEPVLK	HW
H2-E$_\alpha^k$	VA	PEVTVLSRSP	VNLGEPNILI	CFIDKFSPPV	VNVTWLRNGR	PVTEGVSETV	FLPRDDHLFR	KFHYLTFLPS	TDDFYDCEVD	HWGLEEPLRK	HW
H2-E$_\alpha^d$	VA	PEVTVLSRSP	VNLGEPNILI	CFIDKFSPPV	VNVTWLRNGR	PVTTGVSETV	FLPRDDHLFR	KFHYLTFLPS	TDDFYDCEVD	HWGLEEPLRK	AW
H2-E$_\alpha^u$	VA	PEVTVLSRSP	VNLGEPNILV	CFIDKFSPPV	VNVTWLRNGQ	PVTEGVSETV	FLPRDDHLFR	KFHYLTFLPS	TDDFYDCEVD	HWGLEEPLRK	HW
H2-E$_\alpha^{w28}$	VA	PEVTVLSRSP	VNLGEPNILI	CFIDKFSPPV	VNVTWLRNGR	PVTEGVSETV	FLPRDDHLFR	KFHFLTFLPS	TDDFYDCEVD	HWGLEEPLRK	HW

Fig. 2.21. (continued)

α TM-CY domain		191	201	211	221	231
H2-A$_{\alpha}^{k}$	EPEIPAPM	SELTETVVCA	LGLSVGLVGI	VVGTIFIIQG	LRSGGTS/RH	PGPL
H2-A$_{\alpha}^{b}$	EPEIPAPM	SELTETVVCA	LGLSVGLVGI	VVGTIFIIQG	LRSGGTS/RH	PGPL
H2-A$_{\alpha}^{f}$	EPEIPAPM	SELTETVVCA	LGLSVGLVGI	VVGTIFIIQG	LRSGGTS/RH	PGPL
H2-A$_{\alpha}^{u}$	EPEIPAPM	SELTETVVCA	LGLSVGLVGI	VVGTIFIIQG	LRSGGTS/RH	PGPL
H2-A$_{\alpha}^{d}$	EPEIPAPM	SELTETVVCA	LGLSVGLVGI	VVGTIFIIQG	LRSGGTS/RH	PGPL
H2-A$_{\alpha}^{s}$	EPEIPAPM	SELTETVVCA	LGLSVGLVGI	VVGTIFIIQG	LRSGGTS/RH	PGPL
H2-A$_{\alpha}^{r}$	EPEIPAPM	SELTETVVCA	LGLSVGLVGI	VVGTIFIIQG	LRSGGTS/RH	PGPL
H2-A$_{\alpha}^{q}$	EPEIPAPM	SELTETVVCA	LGLSVGLVGI	VVGTIFIIQG	LRSGGTS/RP	PGPL
H2-E$_{\alpha}^{k}$	EFEEKTLL	PETKENVVCA	LGLFVGLVGI	VVGIILIMKG	IKKRNVVERR	QGAL
H2-E$_{\alpha}^{d}$	EFEEKTLL	PETKENVMCA	LGLFVGLVGI	VVGIILIMKG	IKKRNVVERR	QGAL
H2-E$_{\alpha}^{u}$	EFEEKTLL	PETKENVVCA	LGLFVGLVGI	VVGIILIMKG	IKKRNVVERR	QGAL
H2-E$_{\alpha}^{w28}$	EFEEKTLL	PETKENVVCA	LGLFVGLVGI	VVGIILIMTG	IKKRNVVERR	QGAL

Fig. 2.22. Comparison of selected mouse class *II* β amino acid sequences.

Unavailability of information is indicated by a dot, slashes have been introduced for optimal alignment. *H2-A$_\beta{}^r$* is from She et al,[763] *H2-A$_\beta{}^p$* from Holmdahl et al and She et al,[763,764] *H2-A$_\beta{}^d$* from Malissen et al,[765] H2-A$_\beta{}^b$ from Choi et al,[766] *H2-A$_\beta{}^p$* from Janitz et al (unpubl.) and Holmdahl et al,[765] *H2-A$_\beta{}^u$*, *H2-A$_\beta{}^f$*, *H2-A$_\beta{}^s$* and *H2-A$_\beta{}^k$* from Estess et al,[767] *H2-E$_\beta{}^d$* from Nygard et al (unpubl), *H2-E$_\beta{}^u$* from Ayane et al,[768] *H2-E$_\beta{}^z$* from Ogawa et al,[769] *H2-E$_\beta{}^b$* from Widera and Flavell,[770] *H2-E$_\beta{}^s$* from Padgett et al,[771] *H2-E$_\beta{}^k$* from King et al,[772] *H2-E$_{\beta2}{}^{a/k}$* and *H-E$_{\beta2}{}^d$* from Braunstein and Germain,[773] *H2-E$_\beta{}^q$* and *H2-E$_\beta{}^f$* from Begovich et al,[774] *H2-E$_\beta{}^r$* and *H2-E$_\beta{}^p$* from Wei et al.[775]

β1 domain

	1	11	21	31	41	51	61	71	81	91
H2-A$_\beta{}^k$	.....HFVHQ	FQPFCYFTNG	TQRIRLVIRY	IYNREEYVRF	DSDVGEYRAV	TELGRPDAEY	WNKQ/Y/LER	TRAELDTVCR	HNYEKTETPT	SLRRLE
H2-A$_\beta{}^u$	GDSERHFLVQ	FQPFCYFTNG	TQRIRYVTRY	IYNREEYLRF	DSDVGEYRAV	TELGRPDAEY	YNKQ/Y/LER	TRAELDTVCR	YNYEETEVPT	SLRRLE
H2-A$_\beta{}^r$	.....HFVYQ	FKGACYFTNG	TQRIRLVTRY	IYNREEYLRY	DSDVGEYRAV	TELGRPDPEY	YNKQ/Y/LER	TRAELDTVCR	HNYEGLETHT	V/////
H2-A$_\beta{}^p$	.....HFVAQ	LKGECYFTNG	TQRIRSVNRY	IYNREEWVRF	DSDVGEYRAV	TELGRPDAEY	WNSQPEILER	TRAEVDTVCR	HNYEETEVPT	SLRRL/
H2-A$_\beta{}^d$	GNSERHFVVQ	FKGECYYTNG	TQRIRLVTRY	IYNREEYVRY	DSDVGEYRAV	TELGRPDAEY	WNSQPEILER	TRAEVDTACR	HNYEGPETST	SLRRLE
H2-A$_\beta{}^b$	GDSERHFVYQ	FMGECYFTNG	TQRIRYVTRY	IYNREEYVRY	DSDVGEHRAV	TELGRPDAEY	WNSQPEILER	TRAELDTVCR	YNYEGPETHT	SLRRLE
H2-A$_\beta{}^q$	GNSERHFVAQ	LKGECYFTNG	TQRIRSVNRY	IYNREEWVRF	DSDVGEYRAV	TELGRPDAEY	WNSQPEILER	TRAEVDTVCR	HNYEGVETHT	SLRRL/
H2-A$_\beta{}^s$	GDSERHFVFQ	FKGECYFTNG	TQRIRSVDRY	IYNREEYLRF	DSDVGEYRAV	TELGRPDAEY	YNKQ/Y/LEQ	TRAELDTVCR	HNYEGVETHT	SLRRL/
H2-A$_\beta{}^f$	GNSERHFVSQ	FKGECYFTNG	TQRIRSVDRY	IYNREEYLRF	DSDVGEYRAV	TELGRSDAEY	YNKQ/Y/LER	TRAELDTVCR	HNYEGVETPT	SLRRL/
H2-E$_\beta{}^d$	VRDTRPRFLEY	VTSECHFYNG	TQHVRFLERF	IYNREENLRF	DSDVGEYRAV	TELGRPDAEN	WNSQPEILED	ARASVDTYCR	HNYEISDKFL	VRRRV/
H2-E$_\beta{}^u$	VRDSRPRFLGY	STSECHFYNG	TQRVRFLDRY	FYNREEWVRF	DSDVGEYRAV	TELGRPEAEN	WNSQPEILEQ	RRAAVDTYCR	HNYEISDKFL	VRRRV/
H2-E$_\beta{}^z$	VRDSRPRFLGY	STSECHFYNG	TQRVRFLDRY	FYNREEWVRF	DSDVGEYRAV	TELGRPEAEN	WNSQPEILEQ	RRAAVDTYCR	HNYEISDKFL	VRRRV/
H2-E$_\beta{}^b$	VRDSRPWFLEY	CKSECHFYNG	TQRVRLLERY	FYNLEENLRF	DSDVGEFRAV	TELGRPDAEN	WNSQPEFLEQ	KRAEVDTVCR	HNYEISDKFL	VRRRV/
H2-E$_\beta{}^s$	......WFLEY	STSECHFYNG	TQRVRLLERY	FYNLEENLRF	DSDVGEFRAV	TELGRPDAEN	WNSQPEFLEQ	RRAAVDTYCR	HNYEILDKFL	VPRRV/
H2-E$_\beta{}^k$	.ASFRPWFLEY	CKSECHFYNG	TQRVRLLVRY	FYNLEENLRF	DSDVGEFRAV	TELGRPDAEN	WNSQPEFLEQ	KRAEVDTVCR	HNYEIFDNFL	VPRRV/
H2-E$_{\beta2}{}^{a/k}$	VRDPRPRFLEQ	LKAECHYFNG	KERVWSVTRF	IYNQEEFARF	NSDFGKFLAV	TELGRPIVEY	LNTQKDMLDN	YRASVDR/CR	NNYDLVDIFM	LNLKA/
H2-E$_{\beta2}{}^d$	......RFLEQ	LKAECHYFNG	KERVWSVTRF	IYNQEEFARF	NSDFGKFLAV	TELGRPIVEY	LNTQKDMLDN	YRASVDR/CR	NNYDLVDIFM	LNLKA/
H2-E$_\beta{}^q$	VRDSRPWFLEY	CKSECHFYNG	TQRVRFLKRY	FYNLEENLRF	DSDVGEFRAV	TELGRPDAEN	WNSQPEILEQ	KRAAVDTYCR	HNYEIFDNFL	VRRRV/
H2-E$_\beta{}^f$	VRDSRPWFLEY	CKSECHFYNG	TQRVRFLKRY	FYNLEENLRF	DSDVGEFRAV	TELGRPDAEN	WNSQPEILED	ARAAVDTYCR	YNYEILDKFL	VRRRV/
H2-E$_\beta{}^r$	VRDSRPWFLEY	STSECHFYNG	TQRVRLLERY	FYNLEENLRF	DSDVGEFRAV	TELGRPDAEN	WNSQPEFLEE	RRAAVDTYCR	HNYEISDKFL	VRRRV/
H2-E$_\beta{}^p$	VRDTRPRFMEQ	FKSECHFYNG	TQRVRHLVRF	IYNREEYVCF	DSDLGEHRAV	TELGRPDAEY	WNNQKELLER	RRAEVDTVCR	HNYEIFDNFL	VPRRV/

ß2 domain

		101	111	121	131	141	151	161	171	181
$H2\text{-}A_{\beta}^{k}$	QPSV	VISLSRTEAL	NHHNTLVCSV	TDFYPAKIKV	RWFRNGQEET	VGVSSTQLIR	NGDWTFQVLV	MLEMTPRRGE	VYTCHVEHPS	LKSPITVEW
$H2\text{-}A_{\beta}^{u}$	QPNV	VISLSRTEAL	NHHNTLVCSV	TDFYPAKIKV	RWFRNGQEET	VGVSSTQLIR	NGDWTFQVLV	MLEMTPRRGE	VYTCHVEHPS	LKSPITVEW
$H2\text{-}A_{\beta}^{r}$	PPEV	TVYPERTPLL	QQHNLLLCSV	TGFYPGDISV	KWFRNGQEER	SGVMSTGLVR	NGDWTFQTTV	MLEMIPELGD	IYSCLVEHPG	LLRPVSVAW
$H2\text{-}A_{\beta}^{d}$	QPNV	AISLSRTEAL	NHHNTLVCSV	TDFYPAKIKV	RWFRNGQEET	VGVSSTQLIR	NGDWTFQVLV	MLEMTPHQGE	VYTCHVEHPS	LKSPITVEW
$H2\text{-}A_{\beta}^{b}$	QPNV	VISLSRTEAL	NHHNTLVCSV	TDFYPAKIKV	RWFRNGQEET	VGVSSTQLIS	NGDWTFQVLV	MLEMTPRRGE	VYTCHVEHPS	LKSPITVEW
$H2\text{-}E_{\beta}^{d}$	EPTV	TVYPTKTQPL	EHHNLLVCSV	SDFYPGNIEV	RWFRNGKEEE	TGIVSTGLVR	NGDWTFQTLV	MLETVPQSGE	VYTCQVEHPS	LTDPVTVEW
$H2\text{-}E_{\beta}^{u}$	EPTV	TVYPTKTQPL	EHHNLLVCSV	SDFYPGNIEV	RWFRNGKEEK	TGIVSTGLVR	NGDWTFQTLV	MLETVPQGGE	VYTCQVEHPS	LTDPVTVEW
$H2\text{-}E_{\beta}^{r}$	EPTV	TVYPTKTQPL	EHHNLLVCSV	SDFYPGNIEV	RWFRNGKEEK	TGIVSTGLVR	NGDWTFQTLV	MLETVPQGGE	VYTCQVEHPS	LTDPVTVEW
$H2\text{-}E_{\beta}^{b}$	EPTV	TVYPTKTQPL	EHHNLLVCSV	SDFYPGNIEV	RWFRNGKEEK	TGIVSTGLVR	NGDWTFQTLV	MLETVPQSGE	VYTCQVEHPS	LTDPVTVEW
$H2\text{-}E_{\beta}^{s}$	EPTV	TVYPTKTQPL	EHHNLLVCSV	SDFYPGNIEV	RWFRNGKEEK	TGIVSTGLVR	NGDWTFQTLV	MLETVPQSGE	VYTCQVEHPS	LTDPVTVEW
$H2\text{-}E_{\beta}^{k}$	EPTV	TVYPTKTQPL	EHHNLLVCSV	SDFYPGNIEV	RWFRNGKEEK	TGIVSTGLVR	NGDWTFQTLV	MLETVPQSGE	VYTCQVEHPS	LTDPVTVEW
$H2\text{-}E_{\beta 2}^{a/k}$	EPKV	TVYPAKTQPL	EHHNLLVCSV	IDFYPGSIEV	RWFRNGEEEK	TGVVSTGLIQ	NGDWTYQTLV	MLETVPRGGE	VYTCQVEHPS	LTSPVTVEW
$H2\text{-}E_{\beta 2}^{d}$	EPKV	TVYLAKTQPL	EHHNLLVCSV	IDFYPGSIEV	RWFRNGEEEK	TGVVSTGLIQ	NGDWTYQTLV	MLETVPRGGE	VYTCQVEHLS	LTSPVTVEW
$H2\text{-}E_{\beta}^{q}$	EPTV	TVYPTKTQPL	EHHNLLVCSV	SDFYPGNIEV	RWFRNGKEEK	TGIVSTGLVR	NGDWTFQTLV	MLETVPQSGE	VYTCQVEHPS	LTDPVTVEW
$H2\text{-}E_{\beta}^{f}$	EPTV	TVYPTKTQPL	EHHNLLVCSV	SDFYPGNIEV	RWFRNGKEEK	TGIVSTGLVR	NGDWTFQTLV	MLETVPQSGE	VYTCQVEYPS	LTDPVTVEW
$H2\text{-}E_{\beta}^{r}$	EPTV	TVYPTKTQPL	EHHNLLVCSV	SDFYPGNIEV	RWFRNGKEEK	TGIVSTGLVR	NGDWTFQTLV	MLETVPQSGE	VYTCQVEHPS	LTDPVTVEW
$H2\text{-}E_{\beta}^{p}$	EPTV	TVYPTKTQPL	EHHNLLVCSV	SDFYPGNIEV	RWFRNGKEEK	TGIVSTGLVR	NGDWTFQTLV	MLETVPQSGE	VYTCQVEHPS	LTDPVTVEW

ß TM-CY domain

		191	201	211	221	231
$H2\text{-}A_{\beta}^{k}$	R	AQSESARSKM	LSGIGGCVLG	VIFLGLGLFI	RHRSQKGPRG	PPPA....
$H2\text{-}A_{\beta}^{u}$	R	AQSESARSKM	LSGIGGCVLG	VIFLGLGLFI	RHRSQKGPRG	PPPAGLLQ
$H2\text{-}A_{\beta}^{r}$	M	AQSEYSWKKI	LSGAAVFLLG	LIVFLVGVVI	HLKAQKASVE	TQPGNESR
$H2\text{-}A_{\beta}^{d}$	R	AQSESARSKM	LSGIGGCVLG	VIFLGLGLFI	RHRSQKGPRG	PPPAGLLQ
$H2\text{-}A_{\beta}^{b}$	R	AQSESARSKM	LSGIGGCVLG	VIFLGLGLFI	RHRSQKGPRG	PPPAGLLQ
$H2\text{-}A_{\beta 2}$	R	AQSESARSKM	LSGIGGCVLG	VIFLGLGLFI	RHRSQKGPRG	PPPAGLLQ
$H2\text{-}E_{\beta}^{d}$	K	AQSTSAQNKM	LSGVGGFVLG	LLFLGAGLFI	YFRNQKGQSG	LQPTGLLS
$H2\text{-}E_{\beta}^{u}$	K	AQSTSAQNKM	LSGVGGFVLG	LLFLGAGLFI	YFRNQKGQSG	LQPTGLLS
$H2\text{-}E_{\beta}^{r}$	K	AQSTSAQNKM	LSGVGGFVLG	LLFLGAGLFI	Y.........	....
$H2\text{-}E_{\beta}^{b}$	K	AQSTSAQNKM	LSGVGGFVLG	LLFLGAGLFI	YFRNQKGQSG	LQPTGLLS
$H2\text{-}E_{\beta}^{s}$	K	AQSTSAQNKM	LSGVGGFVLG	LLFLGAGLFI	YFRNQKGQSG	LQPTGLLS
$H2\text{-}E_{\beta}^{k}$	K	AQSTSAQNKM	LSGVGGFVLG	LLFLGAGLFI	YFRNQKGQSG	LQPTGLLS
$H2\text{-}E_{\beta 2}^{a/k}$	R	ARSTSAQNKL	LSGVMGMALG	LFILAVGLFF	YLRNLR....	....
$H2\text{-}E_{\beta 2}^{d}$	R	TRSTSAQSKL	LSGAMGMALG	LFILAVGLFF	YLRNLR....	....
$H2\text{-}E_{\beta}^{q}$	K	AQSTSAQNKM	LSGVGGFVLG	LLFLGAGLFI	YFRNQKGQSG	LQPTGLLS
$H2\text{-}E_{\beta}^{f}$	K	AQSTSAQNKM	LSGVGGFVLG	LLFLGAGLFI	YFRNQKGQSG	LQPTGLLS
$H2\text{-}E_{\beta}^{r}$	K	AQSTSAQNKM	LSGVGGFVLG	LLFLGAGLFI	YFRNQKGQSG	LQPTGLLS
$H2\text{-}E_{\beta}^{p}$	K	AQSTSAQNKM	LSGVGGFVLG	LLFLGAGLFI	YFRNQKGQSG	LQPTGLLS

***Table 2.1. List of* HLA-A *alleles recognized at the last WHO Nomenclature Committee meeting in Paris 1996*[17]**

The sequence designations *A*2401, A*2412, A*3005, A*31011, A*3302* have been dropped for reasons of sequence identity to others or sequencing errors. Where possible HLA specificity, previous equivalents, accession numbers, selected references or submitting authors are given. In some cases correcting sequences are given (indicated by *).

Allele	HLA specificity	Accession numbers	Previous equivalents	References or submitting authors	Notes
*A*0101*	A1	M24043, X55710	-	18, 19	
*A*0102*	A1	U07161	-	20	
*A*0201*	A2	M32322, K02883, M84379, X02457	A2.1	21, 22, 23, 24, 25	
*A*0202*	A2	M17566, M17568, X94566	A2.2F	26, R. Blasczyk	
*A*0203*	A203	U03863, M17567, M19670, X94567	A2.3	27, 26, R. Blasczyk	
*A*0204*	A2	M86404, X57954, X94568	-	28, 29, R. Blasczyk	
*A*0205*	A2	U03862, L76290, X94569	A2.2Y	27, P. Parham, R. Blasczyk	
*A*0206*	A2	M24042, X94570	A2.4a	30, 31, R. Blasczyk	
*A*0207*	A2	D50458	A2.4b	32, K. Tokunaga	
*A*0208*	A2	X94571	A2.4c	33, R. Blasczyk	
*A*0209*	A2	L76936	A2-OZB	34	
*A*0210*	A210	Z23071, X94572	A2-LEE	35, R. Blasczyk	
*A*0211*	A2	M84377, X60764, X94573	A2.5	36, 24, R. Blasczyk	
*A*0212*	A2	M84378	-	24	
*A*0213*	A2	Z27120	A2SLU	37	
*A*0214*	A2	Z30341	A2'1S'	38	
*A*0215N*	A'Blank'	D38525	HLA-Anull	39	
*A*0216*	A2	Z46633	A2'TUB'	40	
*A*0217*	A2	U18930, L43526, L43527, X89707, X89708	A*New	41, 42, R. Blasczyk	
*A*0218*	A2	D83515	A*2K	43	
*A*0219*	-.	L76936	A-02X09	P. Stastny	
*A*0220*	A2	X96724	-	44	
*A*0221*	A2	U56825	A206W331R	45	
*A*0222*	A2	U76398, U76399	A-02x28	P. Stastny	
*A*0301*	A3	K02057, X00492, U32184	A3.1	46, W. Hildebrand*	
*A*0302*	A3	U56434, U56435	A3.2	47, C. Hurley	
*A*0303N*	A'Blank'	L77702	A3blank	48	two AA deletions (pos. 101/102 in alignment)
*A*1101*	A11	M16007, M16008, X13111, D16841	A11E, A11.1	49, 50, 51	
*A*1102*	A11	D16842, X13112	A11K, A11.2	50, 51	

Table 2.1. (con't)

Allele	HLA specificity	Accession numbers	Previous equivalents	References or submitting authors	Notes
*A*1103*	A11	X91399	-	H. Tijssen	
*A*1104*	A11	U50574, U59701, U59702	-	52, D. Bugawan	
*A*2301*	A23(9)	M64742, L76288	-	53, P. Parham	
*A*2401*	-	M15497	-	54	thought to contain errors, designation was dropped
*A*2402101*	A24(9)	M64740, M84376, L47206, Z72423	A2402, A24	53, 24, P. Parham, M Laforet	
*A*2402102L*	-	L76291, Z72422	A2402LOW, APET	P. Parham, M. Laforet	
*A*2403*	A2403	M64741	A9.3	53	
*A*2404*	A24(9)	D26550, L43532, L43533	A24AK	55, 42	
*A*2405*	A24(9)	X82161, X82189	A24New	56	
*A*2406*	A24(9)	U18987, U19733	A*24YM	X. Gao	
*A*2407*	A24(9)	U25971, L43530, L43531, U36914	A#46	42, A. Sevalkumar, M. Chopek	
*A*2408*	A24(9)	L43528, L43529, D83516	A*9HH	57,42, K. Tokunaga	previously A*2412
*A*2409N*	A'Blank'	L47231	A24Null	P. Parham	
*A*2410*	A9	U37110, U37111, U59699, U59700	A*24JV	58, D. Bugawan	
*A*2411N*	A'Blank'	L76289	A*24LM	P. Parham	
*A*2413*	A24(9)	U37112, U37113	A*24YM2	X. Gao	
*A*2414*	A24(9)	U37114, U37115	A*24SA	X. Gao	
*A*2501*	A25(10)	M32321	-	22	
*A*2502*	A10	X97802	A66var	P. Krausa	
*A*2601*	A26(10)	M24095, U03697, D16843, D32130, D32131	A26.1, A26.3	21, 59, 60, 61	
*A*2602*	A26(10)	M98453, D14350	A26.2, A26.1	60, 61	
*A*2603*	A26(10)	D14351, D32129	A26.4	61	
*A*2604*	A26(10)	D14354	A10SA	61	
*A*2605*	A26(10)	D50068, L43536, L43537	A26KY	42, 62	
*A*2606*	A26(10)	L43534, L43535	-	42	
*A*2607*	A26(10)	L48341	A26mic	63	
*A*2608*	A26(10)	U45480, U52429, X99733	A26RMH	64, W. Hildebrand,D. Middleton	
*A*2901*	A29(19)	M23739	-	65	
*A*2902*	A29(19)	X60108	A29.2	66	
*A*2903*	-	Y09218	-	A-M. Little	
*A*3001*	A30(19)	M30576, M28414, U07234	A30.3, A30RSH	67, 68	

*A*3002*	A30(19)	X61702	A30.2	69	
*A*3003*	A30(19)	M93657	A30JS	70	
*A*3004*	A30(19)	U18988, U19734, Z34921, X83770, X83771	A*30AD, A30W7, A30JW	71*, 72, X. Gao	
*A*3005*	A30(19)	X83770, X83771	A30JW	R. Blasczyk	identical to A*3004, designation was dropped
*A*31011*	A31(19)	M30578, M28416	-	67	identical to A*31012, designation was dropped
*A*31012*	A31(19)	M84375, M86405, L78918, M30578, M28416	-	29, 24, 73*	
*A*3201*	A32(19)	P10314	-	74	
*A*3202*	A32(19)	X97120	-	75	
*A*3301*	A33(19)	M30580, M28415, U18989, U19735, X83004-5	Aw33.1	67, 76, X. Gao	
*A*3302*	A33(19)	L06440	Aw33.2	77	new name: A*3303
*A*3303*	A33(19)	U09740, U18990, U19736, X83002-3, L06440	A33NC, A33MK	76, 78, X. Gao	
*A*3401*	A34(10)	X61704	-	60	
*A*3402*	A34(10)	X61705	-	60	
*A*3601*	A36	X61700	-	79	
*A*4301*	A43	X61703	-	60	
*A*6601*	A66(10)	U17571, X61711	-	69, 60, C. Hurley	
*A*6602*	A66(10)	X61712, X51745	-	69, 80	
*A*6603*	A10	X96638	A66KA	81	
*A*68011*	A68(28)	X03070, X03071	Aw68.1	81	
*A*68012*	A68(28)	L06425	Aw68.1	P. Parham	
*A*6802*	A68(28)	U03861	Aw68.2	27	
*A*6803*	A28	U41057, U56436, U56437	-	W. Hildebrand, C. Hurley	
*A*6901*	A69(28)	X03158, X03159	-	82	
*A*7401*	A74(19)	U17569, U17570, X61701		79, C. Hurley	
*A*7402*	A74(19)	X95409	A*74dc	83	
*A*7403*	A19	X95561	A*74pb	83	
*A*8001*	A80	M94880, L18898, L19403, U03754	AX"BG", A-new	84, 85, 86, 87	

***Table 2.2. List of* HLA-B *alleles recognized at the last WHO Nomenclature Committee meeting, 1996*[17]**

The sequence designations *B*0702, B*27051, B*39012, B*4401, B*7901* have been dropped for reasons of sequence identity to others or sequencing errors. Where possible *HLA* specificity, previous equivalents, accession numbers, selected references or submitting authors are given. In some cases correcting sequences are given (indicated by *).

Allele	HLA specificity	Accession numbers	Previous equivalents	References and submitting authors	Notes
*B*0701*	-		B7.1	88	thought to contain errors, designation was dropped
*B*0702*	B7	M16102, M32317, M35444, P01889, L47338, U29057, U49904, U49905	B7.2, B*07L	22, 89, 90, W. Hildebrand, A. Arnaiz-Villena, C. Hurley	
*B*0703*	B703	X64454, U21053	BPOT	91, 92	
*B*0704*	B7	U04245	B7E	93	
*B*0705*	B7	L33922, U18661, U21052	B*07ZEL	92, 94, 95	
*B*0706*	B7	X91749	B7-L79	96	
*B*0707*	B7	Z70315	-	97	
*B*0708*	-	X99735	-	D. Middleton	
*B*0801*	B8	M59841, M24036, M28204, L76093	-	99, 19, 98, P. Stastny	
*B*0802*	B8	U04244	B8V, B8JON	100	
*B*0803*	B8	U28759		E. Petersdorf	
*B*0804*	-	U67330, U67331, U74386	B*08New-UW	101, C. Hurley	
*B*1301*	B13	M24075, D50290	B13.1	103, 102	
*B*1302*	B13	M19757, M24041, D50291	B13.2, B13N	31, 103, 104	
*B*1303*	-	U14943	B New	105	
*B*1304*	-	U75533	B*15X21	W. Hildebrand	
*B*1401*	B64(14)	M24040, X94574	-	19, 106, R. Blasczyk	
*B*1402*	B65(14)	M59840, M24032	-	98, 19	
*B*1501*	B62(15)	M28203, M83193, U03859, D50292, L48400	-	99, 107, 108, 109, 110 A. Arnaiz-Villena	
*B*1502*	B75(15)	M75138, M83192, D50293	B15N	110, 107, 111	
*B*1503*	B72(70)	X61709	-	112	
*B*1504*	B62(15)	M84382, M86402	Bw62-G	29, 24	
*B*1505*	B62(15)	M83191	Bw62.1	107	
*B*1506*	B62(15)	M83194	Bw62.4	107	
*B*1507*	B62(15)	M83195	Bw62.5	107	

*B*1508*	B62(15)	L11666	B62variant	108	
*B*1509*	B70	L11571	B70.1	112	
*B*1510*	B71(70)	L11570, U11262, U11264, U11269	B70.2	112, 113	
*B*1511*	B15	L11604, D50294	B15variant, B75v	108, 110	
*B*1512*	B76(15)	L11603	B76	108	
*B*1513*	B77(15)	L15005, D50295	B77	108, 110	
*B*1514*	B76(15)	L19937	B76	108	
*B*1515*	B62(15)	L22027, L49343	B62s	108, A. Arnaiz-Villena	
*B*1516*	B63(15)	L09735	B63.1, 8W66	108	
*B*1517*	B63(15)	U01848, U35431	B63	108, 114	
*B*1518*	B71(70)	U11266, U11268, D50296, U57966	B*7901, B"X"-HS	115, 110, C. Hurley, W. Hildebrand	originally named B*7901
*B*1519*	B76(15)	U03027	B76	108	
*B*1520*	B62(15)	U06862	-	109	
*B*1521*	B75(15)	L32862, D44500, U32678	B15Ab	116, 110, C. Hurley	
*B*1522*	-	U14756, L42506, U34619	B15UW1, B35V2	117, 118, 119	
*B*1523*	-	L37881	B'NM5'	W. Hildebrand	
*B*1524*	B62(15)	U16309, L42146	B*15ZEL, 1501-B4a, B1501-Bw4	95, P. Stastny	
*B*1525*	B62(15)	U18660, U50710, U52177, U52178	B*15AOH	95, C. Hurley	
*B*1526N*	B'Blank'	D49824	B-null	H. Mine	
*B*1527*	B62(15)	L42144, L40182	-	P. Stastny	
*B*1528*	B15	D44499	B15v1	110	
*B*1529*	B15	D44501	B15v3	110	
*B*1530*	B75(15)	L42296, U49900, U49901, U52171, U52172	B*1501V1	P. Stastny, C. Hurley	
*B*1531*	B75(15)	L42145, U52173, U52174	B*1502V	P. Stastny, C. Hurley	
*B*1532*	B62(15)	X95410	-	R. Blasczyk	
*B*1533*	B15	U49898, U49899	-	C. Hurley	
*B*1534*	B15	U49902, U49903	-	C. Hurley	
*B*1535*	B15	U52167, U52168	-	C. Hurley	
*B*1536*	-	U58315, U58316	B*15MD	X. Gao	
*B*1537*	-	U55022, U55023	-	C. Hurley	
*B*1801*	B18	M24039	-	19, 31	
*B*1802*	B18	D25275	B18PE	120	
*B*1803*	B18	X94480, Y07824	-	121, R. Blasczyk	
*B*1804*	-	U38792, U38793	B*18IM	X. Gao	

Table 2.2. (con't)

Allele	HLA specificity	Accession numbers	Previous equivalents	References and submitting authors	Notes
*B*1805*	B18	Y07710	B*18GSW	R. Blasczyk	
*B*2701*	B27	L76935	27f	122, P. Stastny	
*B*2702*	B27	X03664, X03667, L38504*, U18659*	27e, 27K, B27.2	95, 123, 124	
*B*2703*	B27	M54883, M37272	27d, 27J	125, 126	
*B*2704*	B27	U27608	27b, 27C, B27.3	127, 128	
*B*27051*	B27				identical to B*27052, designation was dropped
*B*27052*	B27	X03945, M12967, L20086, M14013, M12678	27a, 27W, B27.1	123, 129, 130, 131	
*B*27053*	B27	X83727, X83737	B27MW	R. Blasczyk	
*B*2706*	B27	X73578, U35734	27D, B27.4	132, 133, 128	
*B*2707*	B27	M62852	B27-HS	115	
*B*2708*	B2708	L19923	B27Qui	134	
*B*2709*	B27	Z33453	B27-ci	135	
*B*2710*	B27	L76095	B2705v	P. Stastny	
*B*2711*	B27	D83043	B27KH	136	
*B*3501*	B35	U11265, M28109-12, L63544	-	137, C. Hurley, A. Arnaiz-Villena	
*B*3502*	B35	M63454	-	138	
*B*3503*	B35	M81798, D50299	-	139, K. Tokunaga	
*B*3504*	B35	M86403, U30936, L47986	-	29, W. Hildebrand, A. Arnaiz-Villena	
*B*3505*	B35	M84385, L76930	B35-G	24, P. Stastny	
*B*3506*	B35	M84381	B35-K	24	
*B*3507*	B35	L04695	-	140	
*B*3508*	B35	L04696, Z22651	B35TL	140, 141	
*B*35091*	B35	U17107	-	L. Satz	
*B*35092*	B35	L76932	-	P. Stastny	
*B*3510*	-	L36979	-	142	
*B*3511*	B35	L40599	B35v	P. Parham	
*B*3512*	B35	L42281, L76094, L49342	B-3504v	143, P. Stastny, A. Arnaiz-Villena	
*B*3513*	B35	X87268	2993	144	
*B*3514*	B35	L42545	B*35M	145	
*B*3515*	B35	U30904	-	114	
*B*3516*	-	U29880	B*35GAR	146	
*B*3517*	B35	U34618, L75941, L49341	B35V1, B*35PNS, B-3505v	119, 147, P. Stastny	
*B*3518*	B35	L75942	B-3508v	P. Stastny	

*B*3519*	B35	L76933	B-40X35	P. Stastny	
*B*3520*	B35	U76392, U76393	B-3501V	P. Stastny	
*B*3521*	-	U76390, U76391	B-3511H	P. Stastny	
*B*3701*	B37	M32320, U11267	-	22, C. Hurley	
*B*3702*	-	U31971	B27-37	148	
*B*3801*	B38(16)	M29864, L36591, U40498	B16.1	149, 150, V. Brichard	
*B*3802*	B38(16)	L22028	-	151	
*B*39011*	B3901	M94052, M29865	B39.1, B16.2	29, 152, 149	
*B*39012*	-			29	identical to B*39011, designation was dropped
*B*39013*	B3901	M94051	B39.1J	152, 151	
*B*39021*	B3902	M94053	B39.2	152	
*B*39022*	B3902	U04243	B39.2	150	
*B*3903*	B39(16)	L20088	-	29	
*B*3904*	B39(16)	L22649	B39N	153	
*B*3905*	B16	U15638, L36318, L36980	ST-16, B*39UW1, B*39JAI	117, 150, A. Arnaiz-Villena	
*B*39061*	B39(16)	U15639, L42024, L76639, U76396, L76640	B*39UW2	117, 154, A. Arnaiz-Villena	
*B*39062*	B39(16)	U16298, L40562, U29083, U32660	B*39DBU, B39G	95, 155, A. Arnaiz-Villena, W. Hildebrand	
*B*3907*	-	U15640	B*39UW3	117	
*B*3908*	B39(16)	L42280	-	143	
*B*3909*	B39(16)	U29480, L76088	B39-143.2	156, P. Stastny	
*B*3910*	B39(16)	U56246, U52175, U52176, Y09058	B39.ZU47	157, 158, C. Hurley	
*B*3911*	-	U74387	-	M. Eberle	
*B*3912*	B39(16)	U76394, U76395	B-3901V	P. Stastny	
*B*40011*	B60(40)	P01890, U03698	-	159, 160	
*B*40012*	B60(40)	M95530, L41628	B60Ut	161, 151	
*B*4002*	B61(40)	L09736, D14343, L76089	B40*	162, 163, 159, P. Stastny	
*B*4003*	B40	M84383	B40-G1	24	
*B*4004*	B40	M84384, L76090	B40-G2	24, P. Stastny	
*B*4005*	B4005	M84694	BN21	164	
*B*4006*	B61(40)	M95531	B61	161	
*B*4007*	-	D31816	B'Fu'	165	
*B*4008*	-	L41353	-	166	
*B*4009*	B61(40)	L76934	B-4003V	P. Stastny	
*B*4010*	B60(40)	U58644, U58643	B*40MD	X. Gao	
*B*4101*	B41	M24035	-	19	
*B*4102*	B41	X81363, U17572, X86704	B41.2	167, 144	
*B*4201*	B42	M24034	-	19	
*B*4202*	B42	D50709	B42ANDO	168	

Table 2.2. (con't)

Allele	HLA specificity	Accession numbers	Previous equivalents	References and submitting authors	Notes
*B*4401*	-	M15470		169	identical to B*4402, designation was dropped
*B*4402*	B44(12)	M24038, M15470	B44.1, B44.2	19	
*B*44031*	B44(12)	X64366, L42283	B44.1:New	170, 143	
*B*44032*	B44(12)	L42282, U58469, U58470	-	143, C. Hurley	
*B*4404*	B44(12)	X75953, X78426, X78427	B44.4	171, 172	
*B*4405*	B44(12)	X78849, X78850, L31798	B44WJG, B44KB	173, 174	
*B*4406*	B44(12)	X83400, X83401-3, L42345	-	175, 176	
*B*4407*	B44(12)	X90391	B*44GB	177	
*B*4408*	B44(12)	U64801	B44bo	P. Parham	
*B*4409*	B12	X99734	-	D. Middleton	
*B*4410*	-	U63559, U63560	-	C. Hurley	
*B*4501*	B45(12)	X61710	-	164	
*B*4601*	B46	M24033	-	31	
*B*4701*	B47	M19756	-	104	
*B*4702*	B47	Y09118	-	178	
*B*4801*	B48	M 84380	-	24, 151	
*B*4802*	B48	L20089	-	29	
*B*4803*	-	L76931	B-48.3	P. Stastny	
*B*4901*	B49(21)	M24037, U11263	-	31, C. Hurley	
*B*5001*	B50(21)	X61706, U11261	-	164, C. Hurley	
*B*5002*	-	U58317, U58318, Y08995	B*50IM, B*45v	X. Gao, C. Vilches	
*B*51011*	B51(5)	M32319, M21035, M22786-8, M28205, Z46808, L47985	-	22, 99, 179,180 A. Arnaiz-Villena	
*B*51012*	B51(5)	U52169, U52170, L76091	-	C. Hurley, P. Stastny	
*B*51021*	B5102	M68964	B5.35	181	
*B*51022*	B5102	L41925	-	182	
*B*5103*	B5103	M80670	BTA	183	
*B*5104*	B51(5)	Z15143	-	24	
*B*5105*	B51(5)	U06697	B51v	184	
*B*5106*	B5	U31334, U32661	-	114	
*B*5107*	B51(5)	X94481	B5101v	185	
*B*5108*	B51(5)	X96473, U52815, U52816, Y08994	B*51FA, B*51GAC	R. Blasczyk, C. Hurley, C. Vilches	

*B*5109*	B51(5)	U58319, U58320, U76400, U76401	B*51IM	X. Gao, P. Stastny	
*B*52011*	B52(5)	M21036, M22793-9	-	179, 186	
*B*52012*	B52(5)	L20090, L47984, L76091	-	29, A. Arnaiz-Villena, P. Stastny	
*B*5301*	B53	M33574, M58636	-	187, 188	
*B*5302*	-	U63561, U63562	-	C. Hurley	
*B*5401*	B54(22)	M77774	-	189	
*B*5501*	B55(22)	M77778	-	189	
*B*5502*	B55(22)	M77777	-	189	
*B*5503*	-	X94482	B5501v	190	
*B*5504*	B55(22)	L76225, D85761	B-4201v, B55.2	191, P. Stastny	
*B*5505*	B22	U63653	B5501 W669R	192	
*B*5601*	B56(22)	M77776	-	189	
*B*5602*	B56(22)	M77775	-	189	
*B*5603*	B22	D85762, U67746, U67747, U67749, U73113	B22N, B56/46	191, 193, C. Hurley	
*B*5701*	B57(17)	M32318, X55711	-	18, 22	
*B*5702*	B57(17)	X61707	Bw57.2	79	
*B*5703*	B57(17)	U18790, U39088, Y09157	B*57SAU	95, 114, 158	
*B*5704*	B57(17)	L76096	B-5702v	P. Stastny	
*B*5801*	B58(17)	M11799, U52813, U52814, U65395, U65396	-	194, 20, C. Hurley	
*B*5802*	-	L33923, X86703	B58v	20, 144	
*B*5901*	B59	L07743, D50300	-	195, K. Tokunaga	
*B*67011*	B67	L17005, L76252	-	151, A. Arnaiz-Villena	
*B*67012*	B67	U18789	B*67LAV	94	
*B*7301*	B73	U04787, L24373, X77658	-	186, 196, 197	
*B*7801*	B78	M33573, X61708	B'SNA', Bx1	198, 79	
*B*78021*	B78	L41214	-	182	
*B*78022*	B78	X96534, X96533	B78Hen	199	
*B*7901*	B71(70)			115	renamed B*1518
*B*8101*	B81	L37880, X90390, U34810	B'DT', B*7x48GB, B56b	177, M. Chopek	
*B*8201*	-	U29241, U38800, U36492	B22x45	114, 200	

***Table 2.3. List of* HLA-C *alleles recognized by the WHO Nomenclature Committee, 1996*[17]**

The sequence designations *Cw*0101, Cw*0201, Cw*0301, Cw*0601, Cw*1101, Cw*1201, Cw*1401, Cw*1501, Cw*1603* have been dropped for reasons of sequence identity to others or sequencing errors. Where possible *HLA* specificity, previous equivalents, accession numbers, selected references or submitting authors are given. In some cases correcting sequences are given (indicated by *).

Allele	HLA specificity	Accession numbers	Previous equivalents	References or submitting authors	Notes
*Cw*0101*	Cw1	M16272	Cw1.1	201	identical to Cw*0102, designation was dropped
*Cw*0102*	Cw1	M84171, Z46809, D50852	Cw1.2, C1J1	180, 202, 203	
*Cw*0103*	Cw1	D64145	C1J2	K. Tokunaga	
*Cw*0201*	Cw2	M16273	Cw2.1	201	identical to Cw*02022, designation was dropped
*Cw*02021*	Cw2	M24030	Cw2.2	19	
*Cw*02022*	Cw2	M26712, D83029, M16273	Cw2.2	204, K. Tokunaga	
*Cw*02023*	Cw2	Z72007	-	J-M. Tiercy	
*Cw*0301*	-	K02058		205	identical to Cw*0304, designation was dropped
*Cw*0302*	Cw10(w3)	M84172	-	202, 205	
*Cw*0303*	Cw9(w3)	M99390, D50853	C3J1	203	
*Cw*0304*	Cw10(w3)	M99389, U44064, U31372, U31373, D64150	C3J2	203, 206	
*Cw*0401*	Cw4	M84386, X58536, D83030	C4J1	24, 207, 203	
*Cw*0402*	Cw4	M26432	BeWo C.1	208	
*Cw*0403*	-	L54059	Cw4NM	209	
*Cw*0501*	Cw5	M58630, M34290, L24491, D64148, D83742	Cw5N	210, 203, 211	
*Cw*0601*	-				identical to Cw*0602, designation was dropped
*Cw*0602*	Cw6	Z22752-4, M28206, X70857, M28160, D64147	Cw6(W), C6J1	99, 212, 213, 214, 203	
*Cw*0701*	Cw7	M28207, Z46810	-	99, 180	
*Cw*0702*	Cw7	D38526, Z49112	JY328, Cw7J1, Cw7.5	215, J-M. Tiercy, 218	
*Cw*0703*	Cw7	M11886	HLA-4	216	
*Cw*0704*	Cw7	U09853, X83394, D49552, U38976	Cw7/8v	218, 217, M. Chopek	
*Cw*0705*	-	U38975	39C	M. Chopek	

*Cw*0706*	Cw7	X97321	Cw*07GB	219	
*Cw*0707*	-	Z79751	Cw7v	J-M. Tiercy	
*Cw*0801*	Cw8	M84174, D64151	C8J1	203, 31, 202	
*Cw*0802*	Cw8	M59865, M84173	-	98, 202	
*Cw*0803*	Cw8	Z15144, D50854	C8J2	24, 203	
*Cw*1101*	-				sequencing artefact, designation was dropped
*Cw*1201*	-	M21963, D12471-2	Cx52	220	identical to Cw*12022, designation was dropped
*Cw*12021*	-	M28172, M28174, M28176, M28178	Cb-2	221	
*Cw*12022*	-	X70856, D64152, D83741, M21963, D12471-2	Cw*1202gyp, C12J1	214, 203	
*Cw*1203*	-	U06695, U06696, X82122, D64146	Cw12New, C12J12	222, 203, R. de Pablo	
*Cw*1204*	-	X99704	Sy/9-2	Z. Tatari	
*Cw*1301*	-	M58631, M34291	CwBL18	210	
*Cw*1401*	-	M28171, M28173, M28175, M28177	Cb-1	221	identical to Cw*1402, designation was dropped
*Cw*1402*	-	U06487, U41386, Z47377, D49820, M28171, M28175, M28173, M28177	Cw14New	221, 184, 223*, M. Laforet, W. Hildebrand	
*Cw*1403*	-	D31817, L38251	Cx44	224, W. Hildebrand	
*Cw*1501*	-	M24096	Cl.9	21	identical to Cw*1502, designation was dropped
*Cw*1502*	-	L20091, X67818, D83031, M24096	C*X, Cw*6.2, C1.9, Cw15J1	29, 214, 203	
*Cw*1503*	-	M99388	-	P. Parham	
*Cw*1504*	-	X73518	Cw*15Sp	225	
*Cw*15051*	-	X78343	Cw*15v	226	
*Cw*15052*	-	X87841	Cw*1505v	96	
*Cw*1601*	-	M24097, U56259, U56260, U41420	Cl.10	21, M. Chopek*, W. Hildebrand*	
*Cw*1602*	-	X76189	Cw*16v	227	
*Cw*1603*	-	L38251	Cw*16New	W. Hildebrand	identical to Cw*1403, sequencing artefact
*Cw*1604*	-	Z75172	Cw*16New	J-M. Tiercy	
*Cw*1701*	-	U06835, X98742	Cw16New	229*, 228*, P. Parham	
*Cw*1702*	-	D64149	Cw17N	230	
*Cw*1801*	-	X96582, Z80227,	Cw*04GB, Cw4x6	219, J-M. Tiercy	
*Cw*1802*	-	Y09156	Cw*18GB	158	

Table 2.4. ***List of* HLA-DR *alleles recognized by the WHO Nomenclature Committee, 1996*[17]**

Where possible HLA specificity, previous equivalents, accession numbers, selected references or submitting authors are given. In some cases correcting sequences are given (indicated by *).

Alleles	HLA-DR serological specificities	HLA-D-associated (T cell-defined) specificities	Previous equivalents	Accession numbers	Notes	References/Submitting authors
*DRA1*0101*	-	-	Drα, PDR-α-2	J00194, J00196, J00203		233, 231, 232
*DRA1*0102*	-	-	DR-H	J00201		234
*DRB1*0101*	DR1	Dw1	-	X03069, M11161		236, 235
*DRB1*01021*	DR1	Dw20	DR1-NASC	-		238, 237
*DRB1*01022*	DR1	Dw20	DRB1*01DMT	Z50871		S. Hashemi
*DRB1*0103*	DR103	Dw'BON'	DR1-CETUS, DRB1*BON	M33600		240, 239
*DRB1*0104*	DR1	-	DRB1*01New	X70261		241
*DRB1*03011*	DR17(3)	Dw3	-	M17379, X04054		242, 243, 244, 245, 246
*DRB1*03012*	DR17(3)	Dw3	DRB1*IMR	M91807, L07767		248, 247
*DRB1*03021*	DR18(3)	Dw'RSH'	-	M27689		250, 249
*DRB1*03022*	DR18(3)	Dw'RSH'	-	U29342, U82403		250, M. Taylor
*DRB1*0303*	DR18(3)	-	-	M81743		251
*DRB1*0304*	DR17(3)	-	03MIT	X75441		252
*DRB1*0305*	DR17(3)	-	DR3New	L29807, U26557		253, S. Bowman
*DRB1*0306*	DR3	-	-	X90644		254
*DRB1*0307*	-	-	-	U37433		250
*DRB1*0308*	-	-	-	U47028		250
*DRB1*0309*	-	-	-	X93315		255
*DRB1*0310*	-	-	-	U65585		256
*DRB1*0311*	-	-	-	U79028		C. Hurley
*DRB1*04011*	DR4	Dw4	-	K02776, M17381, M20548-50, M19556		257, 242, 258, 259
*DRB1*04012*	DR4	Dw4	-	X96851		260
*DRB1*0402*	DR4	Dw10	-	M15068		245, 246, 259
*DRB1*0403*	DR4	Dw13	DR4 Dw13A, 13.1	-		262, 261
*DRB1*0404*	DR4	Dw14	DR4 Dw14A, 14.1	X02902, M15069, M15073, M15074		246, 259, 262
*DRB1*04051*	DR4	Dw15	-	M15070, L13875		263, 259
*DRB1*04052*	DR4	Dw15	DRB1*KOM	D50889, D49952		264
*DRB1*0406*	DR4	Dw'KT2'	-	-		261

*DRB1*0407*	DR4	Dw13	DR4, Dw13B,13.2	M37771		266, 265
*DRB1*0408*	DR4	Dw14	DR4-CETUS, Dw14B,14.2	M37770, L78169		266, B. Lo
*DRB1*0409*	DR4	-	-	M37769, M64794		267
*DRB1*0410*	DR4	-	DR4.CB	M81670, M36879		269, 268
*DRB1*0411*	DR4	-	DR4.EC	M81700, M55615, L42143, L79973		269, 268, P. Stastny A. Arnaiz-Villena
*DRB1*0412*	DR4	-	AB2	M77672		268
*DRB1*0413*	DR4	-	DRB1*LEV	M94460		270
*DRB1*0414*	DR4	-	DR4 Dw10.2	X65031		271
*DRB1*0415*	DR4	-	-	X68272		272
*DRB1*0416*	DR4	-	DR4-BELF	X70788		273
*DRB1*0417*	DR4	-	DRB1*04SAM	L14481		274
*DRB1*0418*	DR4	-	DRB1*04.N	X71610, U38974		275, M. Chopek
*DRB1*0419*	DR4	-	DR4FK	L21985		276
*DRB1*0420*	DR4	-	DRB1*04MC	L27217		277
*DRB1*0421*	DR4	-	DR4New	X80288		278
*DRB1*0422*	DR4	-	DR4New	U17014		M. Varney
*DRB1*0423*	DR4	-	-	Z68503		279
*DRB1*0424*	DR4	-	DRB1*Mi	Z71541		A. Dormoy
*DRB1*0701*	DR7	Dw17, Dw'DB1'	-	M16941, M17384, U09201		280, 281, 283, 282, 242
*DRB1*0702*					identical to DRB1*0701, designation dropped	
*DRB1*0801*	DR8	Dw8.1	-	M17386, L78166		242, B. Lo
*DRB1*08021*	DR8	Dw8.2	DRw8-SPL	-		284
*DRB1*08022*	DR8	Dw8.2	DRw8b	-		285
*DRB1*08031*	DR8	Dw8.3	DRw8-TAB	-		285
*DRB1*08032*	DR8	Dw8.3	-	M27511		286, 287, 288
*DRB1*08041*	DR8	-	RB1066-1, DR8-V86	M84446, M34315		289, 290
*DRB1*08042*	DR8	-	-	L10402		291
*DRB1*0805*	DR8	-	DR8-A74	M84357		290
*DRB1*0806*	DR8	-	DR8.6	M87543, M86590, Z32685, L78165		292, 251, 293, B. Lo
*DRB1*0807*	DR8	-	DR8BZ	L22341, L28096		294, 299
*DRB1*0808*	DR8	-	08New	X75443		252

Table 2.4. (con't)

Alleles	HLA-DR serological specificities	HLA-D-associated (T cell-defined) specificities	Previous equivalents	Accession numbers	Notes	References/Submitting authors
*DRB1*0809*	DR8	-	DR8.7,DRB1*8.2V	L23987, D45046		295
*DRB1*0810*	DR8	-	LP10-1	L19054, X82553		296, M. McGinnis
*DRB1*0811*	DR8	-	DR8TL, DR8New	L29082, L32810		297
*DRB1*0812*	DR8	-	DRB#52	X88854, U36836		298, M. Chopek
*DRB1*0813*	-	-	DRB#47	U36571		M. Chopek
*DRB1*0814*	DR8	-	DR8WE	U24179		299
*DRB1*0815*	-	-	DRB1*08Taree	U63802		300
*DRB1*0816*	-	-	DRB1*08JST	X99840		S. Hashemi
*DRB1*09011*	DR9	Dw23	-		Designation dropped,named DR1*09012	283
*DRB1*09012*	DR9	Dw23	-	M17387, U66826, D89917		242,301, A. Arnaiz-Villena
*DRB1*1001*	DR10	-	-	M20138		238, 244
*DRB1*11011*	DR11(5)	Dw5	DRw11.1	M11867		302
*DRB1*11012*	DR11(5)	Dw5	-	M34316		303
*DRB1*11013*	DR11(5)	Dw5	DR11.MD, DRB1*11DCT	X86803, Y07590		304, S. Hashemi
*DRB1*1102*	DR11(5)	Dw'JVM'	DRw11.2	M17382		242
*DRB1*1103*	DR11(5)	-	DRw11.3	M21966, M22047-49		305
*DRB1*11041*	DR11(5)	Dw'FS'	-	-		306
*DRB1*11042*	DR11(5)	-	-	M34317		303
*DRB1*1105*	DR11(5)	-	-	M84188		307
*DRB1*1106*	DR11(5)	-	DR11.CCY, 11PMH	M98436, D14352		309, 308
*DRB1*1107*	-	-	DR11+3	X73027, X82507		310, M. McGinnis
*DRB1*11081*	DR11(5)	-	DR11JL	L21984		276
*DRB1*11082*	DR11(5)	-	DR11HW	L21983		276
*DRB1*1109*	DR11(5)	-	DRB1*MON	X75347		311
*DRB1*1110*	-	-	DR11.5	L23986		312
*DRB1*1111*	-	-	DR11.6, DR11BRA	L23990, L26306		312, 313
*DRB1*1112*	-	-	DR11.7	L23988		312
*DRB1*1113*	DR11(5)	-	DR11-14, DR11+14	X76194, L29081, U09200, U03291, Z37162, X87677		314, 252, R. Blasczyk
*DRB1*1114*	DR11(5)	-	F1363, 115T, 94-09865	U08932, Z37161, D25639, Z50187		252, 314, A. Dormoy, 315

*DRB1*1115*	DR11(5)	-	DR1101v	Z34824, U17380		317, 316
*DRB1*1116*	-	-	DRB1*OULA, DR11+13	U13009, X87200		318, G. Mersch
*DRB1*1117*	-	-	UCSF-D3152, DR11-14N, 0104D0335	X77776, U17379, U33474		316, 319
*DRB1*1118*	-	-	RMS16	X82211		320
*DRB1*1119*	-	-	RMS117, DR11Loel	X82210, Z47353, U26558		320, 299
*DRB1*1120*	DR11(5)	-	-	U25442		321
*DRB1*1121*	DR11(5)	-	-	X86976		322
*DRB1*1122*	-	-	-	Z49113		323
*DRB1*1123*	DR11(5)	-	DRB1*11OS	D49468		N. Nagao
*DRB1*1124*	-	-	7CGCE	X89193, Z50746		324, G. Fischer
*DRB1*1125*	DR11(5)	-	DR11x08	X91823, X97291		325, E. Albert
*DRB1*1126*	DR11(5)	-	DRB.W11	X94350		W. Verduyn
*DRB1*1127*	DR11(5)	-	2166/1018	X95656		326
*DRB1*1128*	-	-	-	X97722		F. Guignier
*DRB1*1129*	-	-	DRB1*11PBT	X99841		S. Hashemi
*DRB1*1130*	-	-	-	U79027		C. Hurley
*DRB1*1201*	DR12(5)	Dw'DB6'	-	M27635, M27509		327, 287
*DRB1*12021*	DR12(5)	-	DRw12b	M27510		287
*DRB1*12022*	DR12(5)	-	DRB1*1202X	L34353		328
*DRB1*12031*	DR12(5)	-	DRw12POPE	S48645	new name: DRB1*1201	288
*DRB1*12032*	DR12(5)	-	DRB1*12JBT	X83455		242
*DRB1*1204*	-	-	MHT#12v	U39087		329
*DRB1*1205*	DR12(5)	-	-	D86503		K. Tokunaga
*DRB1*1301*	DR13(6)	Dw18	DRw6a I	M17383, X04056		243
*DRB1*1302*	DR13(6)	Dw19	DRw6c I	L76133		245, 330, A. Arnaiz-Villena
*DRB1*13031*	DR13(6)	Dw'HAG'	-	X52451, X16649, M59798, M34320, M57599, M35182		331, 332, 333, 334, 335
*DRB1*13032*	DR13(6)	Dw'HAG'	-	U41634, U34602		Y. Chen
*DRB1*1304*	DR13(6)	-	RB1125-14	M34324		333
*DRB1*1305*	DR13(6)	-	DRw6'PEV'	M57600, L78167		335, 336, B. Lo
*DRB1*1306*		-	DRB1*13.MW	M61899		337
*DRB1*1307*	DR13(6)	-	DRB1*JJY, DRB1*SHN	L06847, D13189		339, 338
*DRB1*1308*	DR13(6)	-	-	L03531		340
*DRB1*1309*	DR13(6)	-	DRB1*YUN	L23534		341
*DRB1*1310*	DR13(6)	-	13NEW	X75442		252
*DRB1*1311*	DR13(6)	-	1303-Like	X74313, X75445		252, 342
*DRB1*1312*	-	-	DR13BRA, DR13.7	L25427, L23989, D29836, L27216, X82508		312, 313
*DRB1*1313*	-	-	-	U79025, U79026	Deleted then reinstated	C. Hurley

Table 2.4. (con't)

Alleles	HLA-DR serological specificities	HLA-D-associated (T cell-defined) specificities	Previous equivalents	Accession numbers	Notes	References/Submitting authors
*DRB1*1314*	DR13(6)	-	1101A58, 13New	U08274, X82239		343
*DRB1*1315*	-	-	83-7601	U08276, U32325		344, C. Hurley
*DRB1*1316*	DR13(6)	-	DRB1*D86	U08277, U25638		345, 344
*DRB1*1317*	DR13(6)	-	RB1194 13/12	U03721		346
*DRB1*1318*	DR13(6)	-	DRB1*13HZ	Z36884, X82549, Z48631		347
*DRB1*1319*	DR13(6)	-	DR1308V	U17381		316
*DRB1*1320*	DR13(6)		DRB1*13VHT	Z48803		348
*DRB1*1321*	-	-	DR13TAS	L41992		D. H. Maurer
*DRB1*1322*	-	-	-	X86326, X87886		M.Tilanus, F. Dufossé
*DRB1*1323*	-	-	-	U36827		F-M. Robbins
*DRB1*1324*	-	-	-	U36825		F-M. Robbins
*DRB1*1325*	-	-	-	X93924		349
*DRB1*1326*	-	-	DRB1*16WIL	X96396		350
*DRB1*1327*	DR13(6)	-	DRB1*13MS, DRB1 *13NW	Z71289, U59691, X97601		351,G. Fischer, M. Tilanus
*DRB1*1328*	-	-	-	X97407		M. Varney
*DRB1*1329*	DR6	-	-	D87822		K. Tokunaga
*DRB1*1330*	-	-	DRB1*13DAS	U72264		W. Greville
*DRB1*1401*	DR14(6)	Dw9	DRw6b I	X04057		352, 243
*DRB1*1402*	DR14(6)	Dw16	-	-		352
*DRB1*1403*	DR1403	-	JX6	-		353
*DRB1*1404*	DR1404	-	DRB1*LY10, DRw6b.2	M34372		355, 354
*DRB1*1405*	DR14(6)	-	DRB1*14c	M33693, M60209, L78168		356, B. Lo
*DRB1*1406*	DR14(6)	-	DRB1*14.GB, 14.6	M63927, M74032, L78164		357, 337, B. Lo
*DRB1*1407*	DR14(6)	-	14.7	M74030		357
*DRB1*1408*	DR14(6)	-	AO1.14.8	M77673, M74031		357, 268
*DRB1*1409*	DR14(6)	-	AB4	M77671		268
*DRB1*1410*	-	-	AB3	M77670		268
*DRB1*1411*	DR14(6)	-	DRw14x11	M84238		358
*DRB1*1412*	-	-	DRB1*YOS	D16110		359
*DRB1*1413*	-	-	-	L21755		360
*DRB1*1414*	-	-	DRB1*14N	L17044		361
*DRB1*1415*	DR14(6)	-	DRB1*14af	U02561		362
*DRB1*1416*	-	-	DR13+14	X76195		252
*DRB1*1417*	DR14(6)	-	1412T	X76938		363
*DRB1*1418*	-	-	81-4641	U08275, X82552, U37264		299, 344, M. McGinnis

*DRB1*1419*	DR14(6)	-	DRB1*14MA, DRB.14a	Z38072, X86973		292, 322
*DRB1*1420*	DR14(6)	-	DRB.14o	X86974		322
*DRB1*1421*	-	-	DRB.14t	X86975		322
*DRB1*1422*	-	-	DRB1*BA	Z50730, Z71275		364, A. Dormoy
*DRB1*1423*	-	-	-	X91640		E. Albert
*DRB1*1424*	-	-	BY14V	U41489		C. Hurley
*DRB1*1425*	-	-	HL14V	U41490, U41491		C. Hurley
*DRB1*1426*	DR14(6)	-	-	D86502, D50865		K. Tokunaga
*DRB1*1427*	DR14(6)	-	-	D86504		K. Tokunaga
*DRB1*1428*	-	-	DRB1*14DKT	X99839		S. Hashemi
*DRB1*1429*	DR14(6)	-	-	D88310		K. Tokunaga
*DRB1*15011*	DR15(2)	Dw2	DR2B Dw2	M17378, M16957, M20430		366, 242, 365
*DRB1*15012*	DR15(2)	Dw2	DRB1*15MT	Z48359		365, 348
*DRB1*15021*	DR15(2)	Dw12	DR2B Dw12	M16958, M30180, M28584		368, 367
*DRB1*15022*	DR15(2)	Dw12	DR2MU	L23964		Smith et al.
*DRB1*1503*	DR15(2)	-	-	M35159		369
*DRB1*1504*	DR15(2)	-	DR2DAI	L23963, L34025		371, 370
*DRB1*1505*	DR15(2)	-	DRB1*15KY	D49823		372
*DRB1*1506*	DR15(2)	-	-	D63586, U45999, X98256		373, N. Nagao, D. Sese
*DRB1*16011*	DR16(2)	Dw21	DR2B Dw21	M16959, M30179, M28583, U56640		366, 365, 374*, 368*
*DRB1*16012*	DR16(2)	Dw21	-	U59686		C. Hurley
*DRB1*16021*	DR16(2)	Dw22	DR2B Dw22	M20504		375
*DRB1*16022*	DR16(2)	Dw22	DRB1*16MADANG	U38520		376
*DRB1*1603*	-	-	-	L02545		377
*DRB1*1604*	DR16(2)	-	DRB1*16x8	L14852		378
*DRB1*1605*	DR2	-	16PRET	X74343, X75444		379, 380*,
*DRB1*1606*	DR2	-	16PRET	X75444	identical to DRB1*1605, designation was dropped	252
*DRB1*1607*	-	-	DR2Mut	U26659		381
*DRB1*1608*	-	-	DRB1*(Gi+Pi)	Z72424		A. Dormoy
*DRB3*01011*	DR52	Dw24	DR3 III, DRw6a III	X04055, X04058		246, 245, 382, 243
*DRB3*01012*	DR52	Dw24	-	U66825		256
*DRB3*01013*	DR52	Dw24	DRB3*MOBD	X99771		M. Guttridge
*DRB3*0102*	-	-	DRB3*N409	Y08063		M. Guttridge
*DRB3*0201*	DR52	Dw25	DRw6b III	M17380, V00522		242, 243, 383
*DRB3*0202*	DR52	Dw25	pDR5b.3	X99690		384, M.Tilanus
*DRB3*0203*	DR52	-	DRB3.02p	X86977		322
*DRB3*0204*	-	-	-	X91639		E. Albert

Table 2.4. (con't)

Alleles	HLA-DR serological specificities	HLA-D-associated (T cell-defined) specificities	Previous equivalents	Accession numbers	Notes	References/Submitting authors
*DRB3*0205*	-	-	DRB3-02-3v	U36826		F-M. Robbins
*DRB3*0206*	-	-	DRB3*02MT	X95760		S. Hashemi
*DRB3*0301*	DR52	Dw26	-	-		245, 382, 385
*DRB4*01*	DR53	-	-	M17385, M17388, M15071-2, K02775		
*DRB4*0101101*	DR53	-	-	M16942	intron polymorphism	282
*DRB4*0101102N*	-	Dw11	DRB4 null		renamed DRB4*0103102N	386
*DRB4*0102*	DR53	-	DRB4*ICML	L08621		247
*DRB4*0103101*	DR53	-	-	M15178, M20555, M19556		387, 257
*DRB4*0103102N*	DR'Blank'	-	DRB4null	D89918		301*
*DRB4*0104*	-	-	DRB4*CR210	X92712		388
*DRB4*0105*	DR53	-	DRB4New	Y09313		389
*DRB4*0201N*	DR'Blank'	-	DRB4*VI	U50061, U70543, U70544		F-M. Robbins
*DRB4*0301N*	DR'Blank'	-	DRB4*v2	U70542		F-M. Robbins
*DRB5*01011*	DR51	Dw2	DR2A Dw2	M17377, M16954, M20429		365, 242, 366
*DRB5*01012*	DR51	Dw2	-	U66721		C. Hurley
*DRB5*0102*	DR51	Dw12	DR2A Dw12	M16955, M30182, M16086		365, 367*, 368
*DRB5*0103*	-	-	DRB5.Oli	X86978		322
*DRB5*0104*	-	-	DRB5*0101V	U31770		F.-M. Robbins
*DRB5*0105*	-	-	-	X87210		390
*DRB5*0106*	-	-	DRB5*New	Z83201		J-M. Tiercy
*DRB5*0107*	-	-	DRB5*01CBT	Y09342		S.Hashemi
*DRB5*0201*	DR51	Dw21	DR2A Dw21	M16956, M30181		365, 367
*DRB5*0202*	DR51	Dw22	DR2A Dw22	M20503, M15992, M32578		375, 391, 368
*DRB5*0203*	DR51	-	DRB5*HK	M91001		392
*DRB5*0204*	-	-	-	U59685		C. Hurley
*DRB6*0101*	-	-	DRBΣ*0101, DRBX11	X53357, M83892		393
*DRB6*0201*	-	-	DRBX21, DRBVI	M77284-7, X53358, M83893		394
*DRB6*0202*	-	-	DRBΣ*0201, DRBX22, DRB6 III	M83204, M83894		395
*DRB7*01011*	-	-	DRBΨ1	K02772-4, L31617		396, Day et al.
*DRB7*01012*	-	-	-	L31618		Day et al.

Table 2.5. List of HLA-DQ alleles recognized by the WHO Nomenclature Committee, 1996[17]

Where possible HLA specificity, previous equivalents, accession numbers, selected references or submitting authors are given.

Alleles	HLA-DQ serological specificities	HLA-D-associated (T cell defined) specificities	Previous equivalents	Accession numbers	Notes	References/Submitting authors
*DQA1*0101*	-	Dw1	DQA1.1, 1.9	L34082		246, 245, 397
*DQA1*01021*	-	Dw2, w21, w19	DQA1.2, 1.19, 1.AZH	M20431, L34083		245, 398, 246, 399, 397
*DQA1*01022*	-	Dw21	-	L34084		397
*DQA1*0103*	-	Dw18, w12, w8, Dw'FS'	DQA 1.3, 1.18, DRw8-DQw1	M34323, L34085		333, 246, 398
*DQA1*0104*	-	Dw9	-	M34314, L34086		400, 397, 401
*DQA1*0105*	-	-	-	L42625, L46877		397
*DQA1*0201*	-	Dw7, w11	DQA2, 3.7	L34087		246, 402
*DQA1*03011*	-	Dw4, w10, w13, w14, w15	DQA 3, 3.1, 3.2	M29613, M29616, L34088		246, 403, 245, 397,404,398
*DQA1*03012*	-	-	-		identical to DQA1 *0302, designation was dropped	
*DQA1*0302*	-	Dw23	DQA 3, 3.1, 3.2, DR9-DQw3	M11124, L34089		397, 405, 246, 406, 398
*DQA1*0303*	-	-	-	L34089, L46878		397
*DQA1*0401*	-	Dw8, DW'RSH'	DQA 4.2, 3.8	M33906, L34090		246, 407, 397, 398, 408
*DQA1*0501*	-	Dw3, w5, w22	DQA 4.1, 2	-	partial	398
*DQA1*05011*	-	Dw3	DQA 4.1, 2	X00370, K01160, L34091		409, 245, 397
*DQA1*05012*	-	Dw5	DQA 4.1, 2	-		246, 405
*DQA1*05013*	-	Dw22	DQA 4.1, 2	M20506, L34092		375, 397
*DQA1*0502*	-	-	-	U03675		410
*DQA1*0503*	-	Dw16	-	L34093		397
*DQA1*0601*	-	Dw8	DQA 4.3	L34094		397, 398
*DQB1*0201*	DQ2	Dw3	DQB2	K02405, M65043, M81140, L40179		246, 398, 245, 412,411,397
*DQB1*0202*	DQ2	Dw7	DQB2	M81141, U07848, L34095		411, 397, D. Monos
*DQB1*0203*	DQ2	-	DQB1*02DL	Z35099, U33329, U39089, U39090		414, 413, I. Fajardy
*DQB1*0301*	DQ7(3)	Dw4, w5, w8, w13	DQB 3.1	M65040, L34096		398, 415, 246,
*DQB1*0302*	DQ8(3)	Dw4, w10, w13, w14	DQB 3.2	M65038, K01499, L34097		398, 416, 245, 246, 397

Table 2.5. (con't)

Alleles	HLA-DQ serological specificities	HLA-D-associated (T cell defined) specificities	Previous equivalents	Accession numbers	Notes	References/Submitting authors
*DQB1*03031*	-	-	-	-	identical to DQB1 *03012, designation was dropped	
*DQB1*03032*	DQ9(3)	Dw23, w11	DQB 3.3	M65039, M60028, L34098		405, 418, 417, 398, 246, 397
*DQB1*0304*	DQ7(3)	-	DQB1*03HP, *03new	M74842, M83770, X76553		421, 419, 420
*DQB1*0305*	DQ8(3)	-	DQB1*03KC	X69169, X76554		421, 422
*DQB1*0306*	DQ3	-	DQB1*MAT	D78569		423
*DQB1*0307*	-	-	DQB1*D4	Z49215		424
*DQB1*0401*	DQ4	Dw15	DQB 4.1, Wa	M13279, L34099		259, 397
*DQB1*0402*	DQ4	Dw8, Dw'RSH'	DQB 4.2, Wa	M33907, M65042, L34100		397, 407, 246 398
*DQB1*0501*	DQ5(1)	Dw1	DQB1.1, DRw10-DQw1.1	X03068,M65044, L34101		397, 246, 236, 235, 398
*DQB1*0502*	DQ5(1)	Dw21	DQB 1.2, 1.21	L34102		426,425,397
*DQB1*05031*	DQ5(1)	Dw9	DQB 1.3, 1.9, 1.3.1	M65047, L34103, L40180		398, 246, 405, 397
*DQB1*05032*	DQ5(1)	Dw9	DQB 1.3, 1.9, 1.3.2	-		427
*DQB1*0504*	DQ5(1)	-	DQB 1.9	M65046, M94773		420, 428
*DQB1*06011*	DQ6(1)	Dw12, w8	DQB 1.4, 1.12	L34104, X89194, L40181		397,425, 398, 429, 430
*DQB1*06012*	DQ6(1)	Dw12, w8	DQB1*0601var.	M86740		431
*DQB1*0602*	DQ6(1)	Dw2	DQB 1.5, 1.2	M20432, M65048, L34105		426, 246, 428, 425, 408, 366
*DQB1*0603*	DQ6(1)	Dw18, Dw'FS'	DQB 1.6, 1.18	M65050, M34322, L34106		397, 333, 246, 398
*DQB1*0604*	DQ6(1)	Dw19	DQB 1.7, 1.19	M65051, L34107		245, 246, 397, 432, 398
*DQB1*06051*	DQ6(1)	Dw19	DQB 1.8, DQBSLE, 1.19b, 2013-24	M36472, M34321, M65052		333, 427, 433
*DQB1*06052*	DQ6(1)	Dw19	DQB1*MDvR-1	L26325		434
*DQB1*0606*	-	-	DQB1*WA1	M86226		435
*DQB1*0607*	-	-	DQB1*06BRI1	M87041		420
*DQB1*0608*	-	-	DQB1*06BRI2	M87042		420
*DQB1*0609*	DQ6(1)	-	DQB1*06AA, DQB1New	L19951, L27345, D29918, L42626		436, S. Yasunaga, 291
*DQB1*0610*	-	-	DQB1Mc	X86327		437
*DQB1*0611*	DQ1	-	UNM-95-228	U39086		438
*DQB1*0612*	DQ1	-	DQB1*06GB	X96420		439

***Table 2.6. List of* HLA-DP *alleles recognized by the WHO Nomenclature Committee, 1996*[17]**

Where possible HLA specificity, previous equivalents, accession numbers, selected references or submitting authors are given.

Alleles	Associated HLA-DP specificities	Previous equivalents	Accession numbers	Notes	References/Submitting authors
*DPA1*0101*				identical to DPA1*0103, designation was dropped	
*DPA1*0102*				identical to DPA1*0103, designation was dropped	
*DPA1*0103*	-	DPw4a1	X03100, X82390, X82392, X82389		440, 441, 442, 443, 444, 399, 445
*DPA1*0104*	-	01New	X78198, X81348, X82391		440
*DPA1*0105*	-	DPA1*RK	X96984		446
*DPA1*02011*	-	DPA2, pDAa13B	X82394, X82393, X78199		444, 442, 440
*DPA1*02012*	-	DPA1*TF	L31624, X83610		11, 447
*DPA1*02021*	-	2.21	M83906, L11642, X79475, X80482, X79479		440, 448, 449
*DPA1*02022*	-	2.22	M83907, L11641, X79476, X80484, X79480		448, 440, 449
*DPA1*0203*	-	DPA1*TC48	Z48473		450
*DPA1*0301*	-	3.1	M83908, X79477, X81347, X79481		440, 449
*DPA1*0401*	-	4.1	M83909, L11643, X79478, X80483, X78200		440, 448, 449
*DPB1*01011*	DPw1	DPB1, DPw1b	M83129, M83664, M62338, X72070		451, 444, 452, M.Tilanus
*DPB1*01012*	DPw1	DPB1*WA6	L19220, L27662		453, A. Begovich
*DPB1*0201*	DPw2	DPB2.1	X01426		454, 455
*DPB1*02012*	DPw2	DPB2.1	M62328, X03067,X99689		235, 444,M. Tilanus
*DPB1*02013*	DPw2	DPB2.1	X94078		456
*DPB1*0202*	DPw2	DPB2.2	M62329, X72071		444, M. Tilanus
*DPB1*0301*	DPw3	DPB3	M62334, X02964, X03023, X78044		454, M. Tilanus
*DPB1*0401*	DPw4	DPB4.1, DPw4a	M62326, M23675, X03022, X030025-8, X02228, X00532 K01615, N00010, M23906-9, X72072		457, 458, 444, 441, 454, 459, M. Tilanus
*DPB1*0402*	DPw4	DPB4.2, DPw4b	M62327, M21886		460, 444
*DPB1*0501*	DPw5	DPB5	M62333, X72073		444, M.Tilanus
*DPB1*0601*	DPw6	DPB6	M62335, X72074		444, M. Tilanus

Table 2.6. (con't)

Alleles	Associated HLA-DP specificities	Previous equivalents	Accession numbers	Notes	References/Submitting authors
DPB1*0801	-	DPB8	M62331		444
DPB1*0901	-	DPB9, DP'Cp63'	M62341, X72075		444, M. Tilanus
DPB1*1001	-	DPB10	M85223, M62342, X72076		444, M. Tilanus, A. Kimura
DPB1*11011	-	DPB11	M62336, X78046		444, M. Tilanus
DPB1*11012	-	-	L23399		461
DPB1*1301	-	DPB13	M62337, X72077		462, M. Tilanus
DPB1*1401	-	DPB14	M31778, M62343, X72078		463, M. Tilanus
DPB1*1501	-	DPB15	M31779, M62339, X72079		463, M. Tilanus
DPB1*1601	-	DPB16	M31780, M62332, X72080		463, M. Tilanus
DPB1*1701	-	DPB17	M31781, M62344, X72082		463,, M. Tilanus
DPB1*1801	-	DPB18	M62340		462
DPB1*1901	-	DPB19	M62330, X72081		462, M.Tilanus
DPB1*20011	-	Oos, DPB-JA	M58608, M63508		464, 465, 466
DPB1*20012	-	DPB*BR16	M97685		467
DPB1*2101	-	DPB-GM, DPB30, NewD	M77659, M83915, M84621, M80300		468, 464, 469, A. Kimura
DPB1*2201	-	DPB*AB1, NewH	M77674, M83919		470, A. Kimura
DPB1*2301	-	DPB32, NewB	M83913, M84014		471, 448, 461, A. Kimura
DPB1*2401	-	DPB33, NewC	M83914		A. Kimura
DPB1*2501	-	DPB34, NewE	M83916		A. Kimura
DPB1*26011	-	DPB31, WA2	M86229		472
DPB1*26012	-	DPB1*WA8	L24387		473
DPB1*2701	-	DPB23, WA3	M84619, M86230		472, 469
DPB1*2801	-	DPB21, JAVA2	M84617, L00599		474, 469
DPB1*2901	-	DPB27, NewG	M84625, M83918, L01467		475, 469, A. Kimura
DPB1*3001	-	DPB28	M84620, X78045		469, M. Tilanus
DPB1*3101	-	DPB22, NewF, JAVA1	M84618, M83917, L00598		474, 469, A. Kimura
DPB1*3201	-	DPB24, NewI	M84622, M85222		469, A. Kimura
DPB1*3301	-	DPB25	M84623		469
DPB1*3401	-	DPB26	M84624		469
DPB1*3501	-	DPB29	M84626		469
DPB1*3601	-	New A, SSK2	M83912, D10479, D10882		476, 477, A. Kimura
DPB1*3701	-	DPB1*WA4	M87046		478
DPB1*3801	-	SSK1	D10478		477

*DPB1*3901*	-	DPB1*BRI4	M97686, X78043		467, M. Tilanus
*DPB1*4001*	-	DPB1*BRI5, WA5	M97684, L19219, L23400		461, 453, 467
*DPB1*4101*	-	DPB2.3	D13174		479
*DPB1*4201*				identical to DPB1*3101, designation was dropped	
*DPB1*4301*				identical to DPB1*3101, designation was dropped	
*DPB1*4401*	-	STCZ	L01466		480
*DPB1*4501*	-	DPB1*NM	L09236		481
*DPB1*4601*	-	DPB1*NIB	L07768, L31817		482, 247
*DPB1*4701*	-	DPB1*02KY, *SUT	D14344, D10834		483, 484
*DPB1*4801*	-	-	L17314		461
*DPB1*4901*	-	-	L17313		461
*DPB1*5001*	-	-	L17311		461
*DPB1*5101*	-	DPB1*WA7, *EA1, *JYO	L17310, L19219, L27073, D28809		485, 486, 487, 461
*DPB1*5201*	-	-	L22076		461
*DPB1*5301*	-	-	L22077		461
*DPB1*5401*	-	DPB1New2	X78042		M.Tilanus
*DPB1*5501*	-	DPB1New3, DPBGUY	X78041, X80331		M.Tilanus
*DPB1*5601*	-	DPB1-R90	L31816		482
*DPB1*5701*	-	DPBMYT4220	X80752		488
*DPB1*5801*	-	DPB1newAW	X82123, X85966		489, 490
*DPB1*5901*	-	-	Z47806, U29534, U59422		491, 492, A. Dormoy
*DPB1*6001*	-	-	U22313		493
*DPB1*6101N*	DP'Blank'	-	U22312		493
*DPB1*6201*	-	-	U22311		493
*DPB1*6301*	-	DPB1*IsOr	U34033		494
*DPB1*6401N*	DP'Blank'	DPB1*IsAr	U34032		494
*DPB1*6501*	-	-	X91886		495
*DPB1*6601*	-	DPB*BR	X96986		496
*DPB1*6701*	-	DPB1*TF	X96985		497
*DPB1*6801*	-	DPB1*BAC	Z70731, U59440		492, A. Dormoy
*DPB1*6901*	-	-	X97406		M. Varney
*DPB1*7001*	-	-	U59441		492
*DPB1*7101*	-	-	U59438		492
*DPB1*7201*	-	-	U59439		492
*DPB1*7301*	-	-	U59437		492

References

1. Klein J. Natural History of the Major Histocompatibility Complex. New York:J. Wiley & Sons; 1986.
2. Klein J. Of HLA, tryps, and selection: an essay on coevolution of MHC and parasites. Hum Immunol 1991; 30:247-58.
3. Darden AG, Streilein JW. Syrian hamsters express two monomorphic class I major histocompatibility complex molecules. Immunogenetics 1984; 20:603-22.
4. Yunis JJ. Mid-prophase human chromosomes. The attainment of 2000 bands. Hum Genet 1981; 56:293-8.
5. Campbell RD, Trowsdale J. Map of the human MHC. Immunol Today 1997;18.
6. Dunham I, Sargent CA, Kendall E et al. Characterization of the class III region in different MHC haplotypes by pulsed-field gel electrophoresis. Immunogenetics 1990; 32:175-82.
7. Hardy DA, Bell JI, Long EO et al. Mapping of the class II region of the human major histocompatibility complex by pulsed-field gel electrophoresis. Nature 1986; 323:453-5.
8. Sargent CA, Dunham I, Campbell RD. Identification of multiple HTF-island associated genes in the human major histocompatibility complex class III region. EMBO J 1989; 8:2305-12.
9. Spies T, Bresnahan M, Strominger JL. Human major histocompatibility complex contains a minimum of 19 genes between the complement cluster and HLA-B. Proc Natl Acad Sci U S A 1989; 86:8955-8.
10. Spies T, Blanck G, Bresnahan M et al. A new cluster of genes within the human major histocompatibility complex. Science 1989; 243:214-7.
11. Versluis LF, Verduyn W, van der Zwan A et al. A complete exon 2 sequence of the HLA-DPA1*02012 allele. Tissue Antigens 1995; 46:206-7.
12. Bodmer JG, Marsh SG, Albert ED et al. Nomenclature for factors of the HLA system, 1990. Tissue Antigens 1991; 37:97-104.
13. Bodmer JG, Marsh SG, Albert ED et al. Nomenclature for factors of the HLA system, 1991. WHO Nomenclature Committee for factors of the HLA system. Tissue Antigens 1992; 39:161-73.
14. Bodmer JG, Marsh SG, Albert ED et al. Nomenclature for factors of the HLA system, 1994. Tissue Antigens 1994; 44:1-18.
15. Bodmer JG, Marsh SG, Albert ED et al. Nomenclature for factors of the HLA system, 1995. Tissue Antigens 1995; 46:1-18.
16. Klein J, Bontrop RE, Dawkins RL et al. Nomenclature for the major histocompatibility complexes of different species: a proposal. Immunogenetics 1990; 31: 217-9.
17. Bodmer JG, Marsh SGE, Albert ED et al. Nomenclature for factors of the HLA system, 1996. Tissue Antigens 1997; 49 (Part 2):297-321.
18. Girdlestone J. Nucleotide sequence of an HLA-A1 gene. Nucleic Acids Res 1990; 18:6701
19. Parham P, Lomen CE, Lawlor DA et al. Nature of polymorphism in HLA-A, -B, and -C molecules. Proc Natl Acad Sci U S A 1988; 85:4005-9.
20. Browning MJ, Madrigal JA, Krausa P et al. The HLA-A,B,C genotype of the class I negative cell line Daudi reveals novel HLA-A and -B alleles. Tissue Antigens 1995; 45:177-87.
21. Cianetti L, Testa U, Scotto L et al. Three new class I HLA alleles: structure of mRNAs and alternative mechanisms of processing. Immunogenetics 1989; 29: 80-91.
22. Ennis PD, Zemmour J, Salter RD et al. Rapid cloning of HLA-A,B cDNA by using the polymerase chain reaction: frequency and nature of errors produced in amplification. Proc Natl Acad Sci U S A 1990; 87:2833-7.
23. Koller BH, Orr HT. Cloning and complete sequence of an HLA-A2 gene: analysis of two HLA-A alleles at the nucleotide level. J Immunol 1985; 134: 2727-33.
24. Belich MP, Madrigal JA, Hildebrand WH et al. Unusual HLA-B alleles in two tribes of Brazilian Indians. Nature 1992; 357:326-9.
25. Krangel MS. Unusual RNA splicing generates a secreted form of HLA-A2 in a mutagenized B lymphoblastoid cell line. EMBO J 1985; 4:1205-10.
26. Mattson DH, Handy DE, Bradley DA et

al. DNA sequences of the genes that encode the CTL-defined HLA-A2 variants M7 and DK1. Immunogenetics 1987; 26:190-2.
27. Holmes N, Ennis P, Wan AM et al. Multiple genetic mechanisms have contributed to the generation of the HLA-A2/A28 family of class I MHC molecules. J Immunol 1987; 139:936-41.
28. Castaño AR, López de Castro JA. Structure of the HLA-A*0204 antigen, found in South American Indians. Spatial clustering of HLA-A2 subtype polymorphism. Immunogenetics 1991; 34:281-5.
29. Watkins DI, McAdam SN, Liu X et al. New recombinant HLA-B alleles in a tribe of South American Amerindians indicate rapid evolution of MHC class I loci. Nature 1992; 357:329-33.
30. Ezquerra A, Doménech N, van der Poel J et al. Molecular analysis of an HLA-A2 functional variant CLA defined by cytolytic T lymphocytes. J Immunol 1986; 137:1642-9.
31. Parham P, Lawlor DA, Lomen CE et al. Diversity and diversification of HLA-A,B,C alleles. J Immunol 1989; 142: 3937-50.
32. Doménech N, Ezquerra A, Castaño R et al. Structural analysis of HLA-A2.4 functional variant KNE. Implications for the mapping of HLA-A2-specific T-cell epitopes. Immunogenetics 1988; 27: 196-202.
33. Doménech N, Castaño R, Goulmy E et al. Molecular analysis of HLA-A2.4 functional variant KLO: close structural and evolutionary relatedness to the HLA-A2.2 subtype. Immunogenetics 1988; 28: 143-52.
34. Castaño R, Ezquerra A, Doménech N et al. An HLA-A2 population variant with structural polymorphism in the alpha 3 region. Immunogenetics 1988; 27:345-55.
35. Epstein H, Kennedy LJ, Holmes N. An Oriental HLA-A2 subtype is closely related to a subset of Caucasoid HLA-A2 alleles. Immunogenetics 1989; 29:112-6.
36. Castaño AR, López de Castro JA. Structure of the HLA-A*0211 (A2.5) subtype: further evidence for selection-driven diversification of HLA-A2 antigens. Immunogenetics 1992; 35:344-6.
37. Barber DF, Fernandez JM, Guttridge MG et al. Primary structure of a new HLA-A2 subtype: HLA-A*0213. Immunogenetics 1994; 39:378.
38. Krausa P, Barouch D, Bodmer JG et al. Characterization of a novel HLA-A2 variant, A*0214, by ARMS-PCR and DNA sequencing. Immunogenetics 1995; 41:50.
39. Ishikawa Y, Tokunaga K, Tanaka H et al. HLA-A null allele with a stop codon, HLA-A*0215N, identified in a homozygous state in a healthy adult. Immunogenetics 1996; 43:1-5.
40. Barouch D, Krausa P, Bodmer J et al. Identification of a novel HLA-A2 subtype, HLA-A*0216. Immunogenetics 1995; 41:388.
41. Selvakumar A, Granja CB, Salazar M et al. A novel subtype of A2 (A*0217) isolated from the South American Indian B-cell line AMALA. Tissue Antigens 1995; 45:343-7.
42. Dale Y, Kimura A, Sasazuki T. DNA typing of the HLA-A gene: population study and identification of four new alleles in Japanese. Tissue Antigens 1996; 47: 93-101.
43. Kashiwase K, Ishikawa Y, Tokunaga K et al. Sequence of a new HLA-A allele (A*0218) encoding a serological variant, HLA-A2K, observed in Japanese. Tissue Antigens 1996; 48:329-30.
44. Fleischhauer K, Zino E, Mazzi B et al. HLA-A*02 tissue distribution in caucasians from northern Italy: identification of A*0220. Tissue Antigens 1996; 48:673-9.
45. Szmania S, Gasque-Carter P, Baxter-Lowe L. Nucleotide sequence for A*0221 which encodes a novel HLA class I polymorphic residue. Tissue Antigens 1996; 48:720-4.
46. Strachan T, Sodoyer R, Damotte M et al. Complete nucleotide sequence of a functional class I HLA gene, HLA-A3: implications for the evolution of HLA genes. EMBO J 1984; 3:887-94.
47. Cowan EP, Jordan BR, Coligan JE. Molecular cloning and DNA sequence analysis of genes encoding cytotoxic T lymphocyte-defined HLA-A3 subtypes: the E1 subtype. J Immunol 1985; 135: 2835-41.
48. Lienert K, Russ G, Lester S et al. Stable inheritance of an HLA-A "BLANK" phe-

notype associated with a structural mutation on the HLA-A*0301 gene. Tissue Antigens 1996; 48:187-91.
49. Cowan EP, Jelachich ML, Biddison WE et al. DNA sequence of HLA-A11: remarkable homology with HLA-A3 allows identification of residues involved in epitopes recognized by antibodies and T cells. Immunogenetics 1987; 25:241-50.
50. Mayer WE, Jonker M, Klein D et al. Nucleotide sequences of chimpanzee MHC class I alleles: evidence for trans-species mode of evolution. EMBO J 1988; 7:2765-74.
51. Lin L, Tokunaga K, Ishikawa Y et al. Sequence analysis of serological HLA-A11 split antigents, A11.1 and A11.2. Tissue Antigens 1994; 43:78-82.
52. Bettinotti MP, Mitsuishi Y, Lau M et al. HLA-A*1104: a new allele found in a Laotian family. Tissue Antigens 1996; 48:717-9.
53. Little AM, Madrigal JA, Parham P. Molecular definition of an elusive third HLA-A9 molecule: HLA-A9.3. Immunogenetics 1992; 35:41-5.
54. N'Guyen C, Sodoyer R, Trucy J et al. The HLA-AW24 gene: sequence, surroundings and comparison with the HLA-A2 and HLA-A3 genes. Immunogenetics 1985; 21:479-89.
55. Kashiwase K, Tokunaga K, Ishikawa Y et al. A new HLA-A9 subtype lacking the Bw4 epitope. Ancestral or revertant allele? Hum Immunol 1995; 42:221-6.
56. Blasczyk R, Wehling J, Kubens BS et al. A novel HLA-A24 allele (A*2405) identified by single-strand conformation polymorphism analysis and confirmed by solid-phase sequencing and isoelectric focusing. Tissue Antigens 1995; 46:54-8.
57. Kashiwase K, Tokunaga K, Ishikawa Y et al. A new A9 sequence HLA-A9HH from Japanese. MHC 1996; 3:9-14.
58. Gao X, Matheson B. A novel HLA-A*24 (A*2410) allele identified in a Javanese population. Tissue Antigens 1996; 48: 711-3.
59. Zinszner H, Masset M, Bourge JF et al. Nucleotide sequence of the HLA-A26 class I gene: identification of specific residues and molecular mapping of public HLA class I epitopes. Hum Immunol 1990; 27:155-66.
60. Madrigal JA, Hildebrand WH, Belich MP et al. Structural diversity in the HLA-A10 family of alleles: correlations with serology. Tissue Antigens 1993; 41:72-80.
61. Ishikawa Y, Tokunaga K, Lin L et al. Sequences of four splits of HLA-A10 group. Implications for serologic cross-reactivities and their evolution. Hum Immunol 1994; 39:220-4.
62. Maruya E, Ishikawa Y, Lin Y et al. Allele typing of HLA-A10 group by nested-PCR-low ionic strength single stranded conformational polymorphism and a novel A26 allele (A26KY, A*2605). Hum Immunol 1996; 50:140-7.
63. Arnett KL, Moses JM, Williams F et al. HLA-A*2607: Sequence of a novel A*26 subtype predicted by DNA typing which shares the MA2.1 epitope with A*02, B*57 and B*58. Tissue Antigens 1996; 47:422-5.
64. Szmania S, Baxter-Lowe LA. Nucleotide sequence of a novel HLA-A26 gene encoding glutamine at codon 156. Tissue Antigens 1996; 48:210-2.
65. Trapani JA, Mizuno S, Kang SH et al. Molecular mapping of a new public HLA class I epitope shared by all HLA-B and HLA-C antigens and defined by a monoclonal antibody. Immunogenetics 1989; 29:25-32.
66. Tabary T, Prochnicka Chalufour A, Cornillet P et al. HLA-A29 sub-types and "Birdshot" choroido-retinopathy susceptibility: a possible "resistance motif" in the HLA-A29.1 molecule. C R Acad Sci III 1991; 313:599-605.
67. Kato K, Trapani JA, Allopenna J et al. Molecular analysis of the serologically defined HLA-Aw19 antigens. A genetically distinct family of HLA-A antigens comprising A29, A31, A32, and Aw33, but probably not A30. J Immunol 1989; 143:3371-8.
68. Olerup O, Daniels T, Baxter-Lowe LA. Correct sequence of the A*3001 allele obtained by PCR-SSP typing and automated nucleotide sequencing. Tissue Antigens 1994; 44:265-7.
69. Madrigal JA, Belich MP, Benjamin RJ et al. Molecular definition of a polymorphic antigen (LA45) of free HLA-A and -B heavy chains found on the surfaces of

activated B and T cells. J Exp Med 1991; 174:1085-95.
70. Choo SY, Starling GC, Anasetti C et al. Selection of an unrelated donor for marrow transplantation facilitated by the molecular characterization of a novel HLA-A allele. Hum Immunol 1993; 36:20-6.
71. Blasczyk R, Wehling J, Passler M et al. A novel HLA-A30 allele (A*3004) identified by single-strand conformation polymorphism analysis and confirmed by solid-phase sequencing. Tissue Antigens 1995; 46:322-6.
72. Krausa P, Carcassi C, Orru S et al. Defining the allelic variants of HLA-A30 in the Sardinian population using amplification refractory mutation system—polymerase chain reaction. Hum Immunol 1995; 44:35-42.
73. Arnett KL, Adams EJ, Parham P. On the sequence of A*3101. Tissue Antigens 1996; 47:428-30.
74. Wan AM, Ennis P, Parham P et al. The primary structure of HLA-A32 suggests a region involved in formation of the Bw4/Bw6 epitopes. J Immunol 1986; 137:3671-4.
75. Zino E, Severini GM, Mazzi B et al. Sequencing of a new subtype of HLA-A*32. Immunogenetics 1996; 45:76-7.
76. Blasczyk R, Wehling J, Hahn U et al. Identification of a novel HLA-A33 subtype (A*3303) and correction of the A*3301 sequence. Tissue Antigens 1995; 45:348-52.
77. Kato N, Kikuchi A, Kano K et al. Molecular analysis of a novel HLA-A33 subtype associated with HLA-B44. Tissue Antigens 1993; 41:211-3.
78. Balas A, Garcia-Sanchez F, Vicario JL. Molecular characterization of a novel HLA-A33 allele (A*3303). Tissue Antigens 1995; 45:73-6.
79. Madrigal JA, Belich MP, Hildebrand WH et al. Distinctive HLA-A,B antigens of black populations formed by interallelic conversion. J Immunol 1992; 149:3411-5.
80. Schnabl E, Stockinger H, Majdic O et al. Activated human T lymphocytes express MHC class I heavy chains not associated with beta 2-microglobulin. J Exp Med 1990; 171:1431-42.
81. Binder T, Wehling J, Huhn D, Blasczyk R. Increased diversity within the HLA-A*66 group: Implications for matching in unrelated bone marrow transplantation. [In Press] Tissue Antigens 1997.
82. Holmes N, Parham P. Exon shuffling in vivo can generate novel HLA class I molecules. EMBO J 1985; 4:2849-54.
83. Blasczyk R, Wehling J, Önaldi-Mohr D et al. Structural definition of the A*74 group: Implications for matching in bone marrow transplantation with alternative donors. Tissue Antigens 1996; 48:205-9.
84. Starling GC, Witkowski JA, Speerbrecher LS et al. A novel HLA-A*8001 allele identified in an African-American population. Hum Immunol 1994; 39:163-8.
85. Wagner AG, Hughes AL, Iandoli ML et al. HLA-A*8001 is a member of a newly discovered ancient family of HLA-A alleles. Tissue Antigens 1993; 42:522-9.
86. Domena JD, Hildebrand WH, Bias WB et al. A sixth family of HLA-A alleles defined by HLA-A*8001. Tissue Antigens 1993; 42:156-9.
87. Balas A, Garcia-Sanchez F, Gomez-Reino F et al. Characterization of a new and highly distinguishable HLA-A allele in a Spanish family. Immunogenetics 1994; 39:452.
88. Taketani S, Krangel MS, Spits H et al. Structural analysis of an HLA-B7 antigen variant detected by cytotoxic T lymphocytes. J Immunol 1984; 133:816-21.
89. Orr HT, López de Castro JA, Lancet D et al. Complete amino acid sequence of a papain-solubilized human histocompatibility antigen, HLA-B7. 2. Sequence determination and search for homologies. Biochemistry 1979; 18:5711-20.
90. Fukumaki Y, Collins F, Kole R et al. Sequences of human repetitive DNA, nonalpha-globin genes, and major histocompatibility locus genes. Cold Spring Harb Symp Quant Biol 1983; 47 Pt 2:1079-86.
91. Bergmans AM, Tijssen H, Lardy N et al. Complete nucleotide sequence of HLA-B*0703, a B7 variant (BPOT). Hum Immunol 1993; 38:159-62.
92. Smith KD, Epperson DF, Lutz CT. Alloreactive cytotoxic T-lymphocyte-defined HLA-B7 subtypes differ in peptide

antigen presentation. Immunogenetics 1996; 43:27-37.
93. Kubens BS, Arnett KL, Adams EJ et al. Definition of a new HLA-B7 subtype (B*0704) by isoelectric focusing, family studies and DNA sequence analysis. Tissue Antigens 1995; 45:322-7.
94. Arnett KL, Adams EJ, Domena JD et al. Structure of a novel subtype of B7 (B*0705) isolated from a Chinese individual. Tissue Antigens 1994; 44:318-21.
95. Petersdorf EW, Hansen JA. A comprehensive approach for typing the alleles of the HLA-B locus by automated sequencing. Tissue Antigens 1995; 46:73-85.
96. Sanz L, Vilches C, de Pablo R et al. Haplotypic association of two new HLA class I alleles: Cw*15052 and B*0706: evolutionary relationships of HLA-Cw*15 alleles. Tissue Antigens 1996; 47:329-32.
97. Grundschober C, Rufer N, Adami N et al. Sequence of a new HLA-B7 variant, B*0707, that differs from the common B*0702 allele by one single residue in the peptide binding groove. Tissue Antigens 1997; 49:508-11.
98. Bronson SK, Pei J, Taillon-Miller P et al. Isolation and characterization of yeast artificial chromosome clones linking the HLA-B and HLA-C loci. Proc Natl Acad Sci U S A 1991; 88:1676-80.
99. Pohla H, Kuon W, Tabaczewski P et al. Allelic variation in HLA-B and HLA-C sequences and the evolution of the HLA-B alleles. Immunogenetics 1989; 29: 297-307.
100. Arnett KL, Adams EJ, Gumperz JE et al. Expression of an unusual Bw4 epitope by a subtype of HLA-B8 [B*0802]. Tissue Antigens 1995; 46:316-21.
101. Eberle M, Lorentzen D, Iwanaga KK, Hennes LF, Watkins DI. Identification of a new HLA-B*08 variant, HLA-B*0804. [In Press] Tissue Antigens 1997.
102. Kato K, Dupont B, Yang SY. Localization of nucleotide sequence which determines Mongoloid subtype of HLA-B13. Immunogenetics 1989; 29:117-20.
103. Lin L, Tokunaga K, Nakajima F et al. Both HLA-B*1301 and B*1302 exist in Asian populations and are associated with different haplotypes. Hum Immunol 1995; 43:51-6.
104. Zemmour J, Ennis PD, Parham P et al. Comparison of the structure of HLA-Bw47 to HLA-B13 and its relationship to 21-hydroxylase deficiency [published erratum appears in Immunogenetics 1989; 29:224]. Immunogenetics 1988; 27:281-7.
105. Balas A, Garcia-Sanchez F, Vicario JL. HLA-B*1303: a new example of poor correlation between serology and structure. Hum Immunol 1996; 45:32-6.
106. Domena JD, Azumi K, Bias WB et al. B*1401 encodes the B64 antigen: the B64 and B65 splits of B14 differ only at residue 11, a buried amino acid. Tissue Antigens 1993; 41:110-1.
107. Choo SY, Fan LA, Hansen JA. Allelic variations clustered in the antigen binding sites of HLA-Bw62 molecules. Immunogenetics 1993; 37:108-13.
108. Hildebrand WH, Domena JD, Shen SY et al. HLA-B15: a widespread and diverse family of HLA-B alleles. Tissue Antigens 1994; 43:209-18.
109. Domena JD, Little AM, Arnett KL et al. A small test of a sequence-based typing method: definition of the B*1520 allele. Tissue Antigens 1994; 44:217-24.
110. Lin L, Tokunaga K, Tanaka H et al. Further molecular diversity in the HLA-B15 group. Tissue Antigens 1996; 47:265-74.
111. Little AM, Parham P. The HLA-Bw75 subtype of B15: molecular characterization and comparison with crossreacting antigens. Tissue Antigens 1991; 38: 186-90.
112. Domena JD, Little AM, Madrigal AJ et al. Structural heterogeneity in HLA-B70, a high-frequency antigen of black populations. Tissue Antigens 1993; 42:509-17.
113. Rodriguez SG, Johnson AH, Hurley CK. Molecular characterization of HLA-B71 from an African American individual. Hum Immunol 1993; 37:192-4.
114. Hurley CK, Steiner NK, Hoyer RJ et al. Novel HLA-B alleles, B*8201, B*3515 and B*5106, add to the complexity of serologic identification of HLA types. Tissue Antigens 1996; 47:179-87.
115. Choo SY, Fan LA, Hansen JA. A novel HLA-B27 allele maps B27 allospecificity to the region around position 70 in the alpha 1 domain. J Immunol 1991; 147: 174-80.
116. Lienert K, McCluskey J, Bennett G et al.

HLA class I variation in Australian aborigines: characterization of allele B*1521. Tissue Antigens 1995; 45:12-7.

117. Garber TL, Butler LM, Trachtenberg EA et al. HLA-B alleles of the Cayapa of Ecuador: new B39 and B15 alleles [published erratum appears in Immunogenetics 1995; 42:308]. Immunogenetics 1995; 42:19-27.

118. Martinez-Laso J, Layrisse Z, Gomez-Casade E et al. A new HLA-B15 allele (B*1522) found in Bari-Motilones Amerindians in Venezuela: comparison of its intron 2 sequence with those of B*1501 and B*3504. Immunogenetics 1996; 43:108-9.

119. Cereb N, Kim C, Hughes AL et al. Molecular analysis of HLA-B35 alleles and their relationship to HLA-B15 alleles. Tissue Antigens 1997; 49:389-396.

120. Lin L, Tokunaga K, Ishikawa Y et al. A new B18 sequence (B*1802) from Asian individuals. Hum Immunol 1995; 42: 23-6.

121. Curran MD, Williams F, Middleton D. A novel HLA-B allele, HLA-B*1803. Tissue Antigens 1996; 48:708-10.

122. Rojo S, Aparicio P, Choo SY et al. Structural analysis of an HLA-B27 population variant, B27f. Multiple patterns of amino acid changes within a single polypeptide segment generate polymorphism in HLA-B27. J Immunol 1987; 139:831-6.

123. Seemann GH, Rein RS, Brown CS et al. Gene conversion-like mechanisms may generate polymorphism in human class I genes. EMBO J 1986; 5:547-52.

124. Moses JH, Marsh SG, Arnett KL et al. On the nucleotide sequences of B*2702 and B*2705. Tissue Antigens 1995; 46: 50-3.

125. Choo SY, St. John T, Orr HT et al. Molecular analysis of the variant alloantigen HLA-B27d (HLA-B*2703) identifies a unique single amino acid substitution. Hum Immunol 1988; 21:209-19.

126. Rojo S, Aparicio P, Hansen JA et al. Structural analysis of an HLA-B27 functional variant, B27d, detected in American blacks. J Immunol 1987; 139: 3396-401.

127. Vega MA, Wallace L, Rojo S et al. Delineation of functional sites in HLA-B27 antigens. Molecular analysis of HLA-B27 variant Wewak I defined by cytolytic T lymphocytes. J Immunol 1985; 135: 3323-32.

128. Rudwaleit M, Bowness P, Wordsworth P. The nucleotide sequence of HLA-B*2704 reveals a new amino acid substitution in exon 4 is also present in HLA-B*2706. Immunogenetics 1996; 43:160-2.

129. Weiss EH, Kuon W, Dorner C et al. Organization, sequence and expression of the HLA-B27 gene: a molecular approach to analyze HLA and disease associations. Immunobiology 1985; 170:367-80.

130. Coppin HL, McDevitt HO. Absence of polymorphism between HLA-B27 genomic exon sequences isolated from normal donors and ankylosing spondylitis patients. J Immunol 1986; 137:2168-72.

131. Szots H, Riethmüller G, Weiss E et al. Complete sequence of HLA-B27 cDNA identified through the characterization of structural markers unique to the HLA-A, -B, and -C allelic series. Proc Natl Acad Sci USA 1986; 83:1428-32.

132. Vega MA, Bragado R, Ivanyi P et al. Molecular analysis of a functional subtype of HLA-B27. A possible evolutionary pathway for HLA-B27 polymorphism. J Immunol 1986; 137:3557-65.

133. Vilches C, de Pablo R, Kreisler M. Nucleotide sequence of HLA-B*2706. Immunogenetics 1996; 43:114.

134. Hildebrand WH, Domena JD, Shen SY et al. The HLA-B7Qui antigen is encoded by a new subtype of HLA-B27 (B*2708). Tissue Antigens 1994; 44:47-51.

135. Del Porto P, D'Amato M, Fiorillo MT et al. Identification of a novel HLA-B27 subtype by restriction analysis of a cytotoxic gamma delta T cell clone. J Immunol 1994; 153:3093-100.

136. Hasegawa T, Ogawa A, Sugahara Y et al. Novel HLA-B27 allele (B*2711) encoding an antigen reacting with both B27 and B40 specific antisera. [In Press] Tissue Antigens 1997.

137. Ooba T, Hayashi H, Karaki S et al. The structure of HLA-B35 suggests that it is derived from HLA-Bw58 by two genetic mechanisms. Immunogenetics 1989; 30: 76-80.

138. Chertkoff LP, Herrera M, Fainboim L et al. Complete nucleotide sequence of a genomic clone encoding HLA-B35 iso-

lated from a Caucasian individual of Hispanic origin. Identification of a new variant of HLA-B35. Hum Immunol 1991; 31:153-8.
139. Zemmour J, Little AM, Schendel DJ et al. The HLA-A,B "negative" mutant cell line C1R expresses a novel HLA-B35 allele, which also has a point mutation in the translation initiation codon. J Immunol 1992; 148:1941-8.
140. Theiler G, Pando M, Delfino JM et al. Isolation and characterization of two new functional subtypes of HLA-B35. Tissue Antigens 1993; 41:143-7.
141. Steinle A, Reinhardt C, Nossner E et al. Microheterogeneity in HLA-B35 alleles influences peptide-dependent allorecognition by cytotoxic T cells but not binding of a peptide-restricted monoclonal antibody. Hum Immunol 1993; 38:261-9.
142. Gomez-Casado E, Montoya F, Martinez-Laso J et al. A new HLA-B35 allele (B*3510) found in isolated Jaidukama South American Indians. Immunogenetics 1995; 42:231-2.
143. Adams EJ, Little A, Arnett KL et al. Three new HLA-B alleles found in Mexican-Americans. Tissue Antigens 1995; 46:414-6.
144. Curran MD, Williams F, Middleton D. Long range PCR amplification as an alternative strategy to characterising novel HLA-B alleles. Eur J Immunogenetics 1996; 23:297-309.
145. Vargas-Alarcón G, Martinez-Laso J, Granados J et al. Description of a novel HLA-B35 (B*3514) allele found in a Mexican family of Nahua Aztec descent. Hum Immunol 1996; 45:148-51.
146. Vargas-Alarcón G, Alvarez M, Martinez-Laso J et al. A new HLA-B35 (B*3516) allele found in a Mexican of Nahua (Aztec) descent. Immunogenetics 1996; 43:244-5.
147. Vargas-Alarcón G, Martinez-Laso J, Gomez-Casado E et al. A novel HLA-B35 (B*3517) allele found in a Mexican of Otomi ascent. Tissue Antigens 1996; 47:547-50.
148. Santos S, Vicario JL, Merino JL et al. Characterization of a new HLA-B allele (B*3702) generated by an intronic recombination event. Immunogenetics 1996; 43:171-2.
149. Müller CA, Engler-Blum G, Gekeler V et al. Genetic and serological heterogeneity of the supertypic HLA-B locus specificities Bw4 and Bw6. Immunogenetics 1989; 30:200-7.
150. Adams EJ, Martinez-Naves E, Arnett KL et al. HLA-B16 antigens: sequence of the ST-16 antigen, further definition of two B38 subtypes and evidence for convergent evolution of B*3902. Tissue Antigens 1995; 45:18-26.
151. Little AM, Domena JD, Hildebrand WH et al. HLA-B67: a member of the HLA-B16 family that expresses the ME1 epitope. Tissue Antigens 1994; 43:38-43.
152. Kato N, Karaki S, Kashiwase K et al. Molecular analysis of HLA-B39 subtypes. Immunogenetics 1993; 37:212-6.
153. Ogawa A, Tokunaga K, Nakajima F et al. Identification of the gene encoding a novel HLA-B39 subtype. Two amino acid substitutions on the beta-sheet out of the peptide-binding floor form a novel serological epitope. Hum Immunol 1994; 41:241-7.
154. Zhao W, Fernandez-Vina MA, Lazaro AM et al. Full cDNA of a novel HLA-B39 subtype, B*39061. Tissue Antigens 1996; 47:435-7.
155. Garber TL, McAdam SN, Butler LM et al. HLA-B alleles of the Navajo: no evidence for rapid evolution in the Nadene. Tissue Antigens 1996; 47:143-6.
156. Ramos M, Postigo JM, Vilches C et al. Primary structure of a novel HLA-B39 allele (B*3909) from the Sarao Indians of Venezuela. Further evidence for local HLA-B diversification in South America. Tissue Antigens 1995; 46:401-64.
157. Wells RS, Parham P. A novel recombinant HLA-B*39 allele (B*3910) in a South African Zulu. Tissue Antigens 1996; 48:595-7.
158. Vilches C, Bunce M, de Pablo R et al. A novel HLA-Cw*1802-B*5703 haplotype detected in the Bubi population from Equatorial Guinea. [In Press] Tissue Antigens 1997.
159. Ways JP, Lawlor DA, Wan AM et al. A transposable epitope of HLA-B7, B40 molecules. Immunogenetics 1987; 25: 323-8.
160. López de Castro J, Bragado R, Strong DM et al. Primary structure of papain-

solubilized human histocompatibility antigen HLA-B40 (-Bw60). An outline of alloantigenic determinants. Biochemistry 1983; 22:3961-9.
161. Kawaguchi G, Kato N, Kashiwase K et al. Structural analysis of HLA-B40 epitopes. Hum Immunol 1993; 36:193-8.
162. Domena JD, Johnston-Dow L, Parham P. The B*4002 allele encodes the B61 antigen: B40* is identical to B61. Tissue Antigens 1992; 40:254-6.
163. Ling L, Watanabe Y, Tokunaga K et al. A common Japanese haplotype HLA-A26-Cw3-B61-DR9-DQ3 carries HLA-B*4002. Tissue Antigens 1992; 40:257-60.
164. Hildebrand WH, Madrigal JA, Belich MP et al. Serologic cross-reactivities poorly reflect allelic relationships in the HLA-B12 and HLA-B21 groups. Dominant epitopes of the alpha 2 helix. J Immunol 1992; 149:3563-8.
165. Lin L, Tokunaga K, Ishikawa Y et al. A new member of the HLA–B40 family of alleles, B*4007, coding for B'FU' serological specificity. Tissue Antigens 1995; 45:276-9.
166. Adams EJ, Little AM, Arnett KL et al. Identification of a novel HLA-B40 allele (B*4008) in a patient with leukemia. Tissue Antigens 1995; 46:204-5.
167. Rufer N, Roosnek E, Kressig R et al. Sequencing of a new HLA-B41 subtype (B*4102) that occurs with a high frequency in the Caucasoid population. Immunogenetics 1995; 41:333.
168. Ando H, Mizuku N, Ohno S et al. Identification of a novel HLA-B allele (B*4202) in a Saudi Arabian family with Behcet's disease. Tissue Antigens 1997; 49:526-8.
169. Kottmann AH, Seemann GH, Guessow HD et al. DNA sequence of the coding region of the HLA-B44 gene. Immunogenetics 1986; 23:396-400.
170. Fleischhauer K, Kernan NA, Dupont B et al. The two major subtypes of HLA-B44 differ for a single amino acid in codon 156. Tissue Antigens 1991; 37: 133-7.
171. Gauchat-Feiss D, Breur Vriesendorp BS, Rufer N et al. Sequencing of a novel functional HLA-B44 subtype differing in two residues in the alpha 2 domain. Tissue Antigens 1994; 44:261-4.
172. Yao Z, Keller E, Scholz S et al. Identification of two major HLA-B44 subtypes and a novel B44 sequence (B*4404). Oligotyping and solid phase sequencing of polymerase chain reaction products. Hum Immunol 1995; 42:54-60.
173. Yao Z, Volgger A, Scholz S et al. Nucleotide sequence of a novel HLA-B44 subtype B*4405. Immunogenetics 1994; 40:310.
174. Petersdorf EW, Setoda T, Smith AG et al. Analysis of HLA-B*44 alleles encoded on extended HLA haplotypes by direct automated sequencing. Tissue Antigens 1994; 44:211-6.
175. Yao Z, Lattermann A, Volgger A et al. A new HLA-B44 subtype, B*4406, differing in exon 2. Immunogenetics 1995; 41:387.
176. Zhao W, Fernandez-Vina MA, Lazaro AM et al. Complete cDNA sequence of B*4406, an HLA-B allele containing sequences of B*5101 and B*4402. Tissue Antigens 1996; 47:431-4.
177. Vilches C, Sanz L, de Pablo R et al. Molecular characterisation of the new alleles HLA-B*8101 and B*4407. Tissue Antigens 1996; 47:139-42.
178. Fischer GF, Broer F, Fae I et al. Nucleotide sequence analysis of an HLA-B47 variant (HLA-B*4702). [In Press] Tissue Antigens 1997.
179. Hayashi H, Ennis PD, Ariga H et al. HLA-B51 and HLA-Bw52 differ by only two amino acids which are in the helical region of the alpha 1 domain. J Immunol 1989; 142:306-11.
180. Steinle A, Schendel DJ. HLA class I alleles of LCL 721 and 174 x CEM.T2 (T2). Tissue Antigens 1994; 44:268-70.
181. Kawaguchi G, Hildebrand WH, Hiraiwa M et al. Two subtypes of HLA-B51 differing by substitution at position 171 of the alpha 2 helix. Immunogenetics 1992; 37:57-63.
182. Prilliman KR, Steiner N, Ellexson ME et al. Novel alleles HLA-B*7802 and B*51022: evidence for convergency in the HLA-B5 family. Tissue Antigens 1996; 47:49-57.
183. Kawaguchi G, Nakayama S, Nagao T et al. A single amino acid substitution at residue 167 forms a novel HLA-B51 subtype. Tissue Antigens 1993; 42:39-41.
184. Cereb N, Choi JW, Riu KZ et al. HLA-

B*5105, a newly identified B51 IEF variant. Tissue Antigens 1994; 44:271-3.
185. Curran MD, Williams F, Rima BK et al. A new HLA-B51 allele, B*5107 in RCE55 detected and characterised by PCR-SSOP, cloning and nucleotide sequence determination. Tissue Antigens 1996; 48: 228-30.
186. Parham P, Arnett KL, Adams EJ et al. The HLA-B73 antigen has a most unusual structure that defines a second lineage of HLA-B alleles. Tissue Antigens 1994; 43:302-13.
187. Allsopp CE, Hill AV, Kwiatkowski D et al. Sequence analysis of HLA-Bw53, a common West African allele, suggests an origin by gene conversion of HLA-B35. Hum Immunol 1991; 30:105-9.
188. Hayashi H, Ooba T, Nakayama S et al. Allospecificities between HLA-Bw53 and HLA-B35 are generated by substitution of the residues associated with HLA-Bw4/Bw6 public epitopes. Immunogenetics 1990; 32:195-9.
189. Hildebrand WH, Madrigal JA, Little AM et al. HLA-Bw22: a family of molecules with identity to HLA-B7 in the alpha 1-helix. J Immunol 1992; 148:1155-62.
190. Williams F, Curran MD, Vaughan RW et al. Identification of a new HLA-B*55 allele, HLA-B*5503. Tissue Antigens 1996; 48:598-9.
191. Bannai M, Tokunaga K, Tanaka H et al. Five HLA-B22 group alleles in Japanese. Tissue Antigens 1997; 49:376-82.
192. Szmania S, Seurynck K, Baxter-Lowe LA. Nucleotide sequence of HLA-B*5505 which expresses a unique HLA class I polymorphism. [In Press] Tissue Antigens 1997.
193. Barnardo MCNM, Bunce M, Lord CJ et al. HLA-B*5603: Sequence of a novel hybrid allele comprising B*56 and B*4601. Tissue Antigens 1997; 49:496-8.
194. Ways JP, Coppin HL, Parham P. The complete primary structure of HLA-Bw58. J Biol Chem 1985; 260:11924-33.
195. Hildebrand WH, Domena JD, Parham P. Primary structure shows HLA-B59 to be a hybrid of HLA-B55 and HLA-B51, and not a subtype of HLA-B8. Tissue Antigens 1993; 41:190-5.
196. Vilches C, de Pablo R, Herrero MJ et al. HLA-B73: an atypical HLA-B molecule carrying a Bw6-epitope motif variant and a B pocket identical to HLA-B27. Immunogenetics 1994; 40:166.
197. Hoffmann HJ, Kristensen TJ, Jensen TG et al. Antigenic characteristics and cDNA sequences of HLA-B73. Eur J Immunogenet 1995; 22:231-40.
198. Sekimata M, Hiraiwa M, Andrien M et al. Allodeterminants and evolution of a novel HLA-B5 CREG antigen, HLA-B DNA. J Immunol 1990; 144:3228-33.
199. Andrien M, Defleur V, De Canck I et al. B*78022, a new caucasian member within the B78 family. Tissue Antigens 1997; 49:79-83.
200. Ellexson M, Stewart D, Chretien P et al. A modified sequencing strategy for the molecular characterisation of HLA-B *8201. Tissue Antigens 1996; 47:438-41.
201. Gussow D, Rein RS, Meijer I et al. Isolation, expression, and the primary structure of HLA-Cw1 and HLA-Cw2 genes: evolutionary aspects [published erratum appears in Immunogenetics 1988; 27: 158]. Immunogenetics 1987; 25:313-22.
202. Zemmour J, Gumperz JE, Hildebrand WH et al. The molecular basis for reactivity of anti-Cw1 and anti-Cw3 alloantisera with HLA-B46 haplotypes. Tissue Antigens 1992; 39:249-57.
203. Wang H, Tokunaga K, Akaza T et al. Identification of HLA-C alleles using PCR-single stranded-conformation polymorphism and direct sequencing. Tissue Antigens 1997; 49:134-40.
204. Lutz CT, Jensen DA, Schiffenbauer J et al. Multiple mechanisms produce diversity of HLA-C alleles. Hum Immunol 1990; 28:27-31.
205. Sodoyer R, Damotte M, Delovitch TL et al. Complete nucleotide sequence of a gene encoding a functional human class I histocompatibility antigen (HLA-CW3). EMBO J 1984; 3:879-85.
206. Zarling A, Smith KD, Lutz CT et al. Correction of the HLA-Cw3 genomic sequence tentatively identifies it as HLA-Cw*0304. Immunogenetics 1996; 44: 82-3.
207. Grassi F, Meneveri R, Gullberg M et al. Human immunodeficiency virus type 1 gp120 mimics a hidden monomorphic epitope borne by class I major histocom-

patibility complex heavy chains. J Exp Med 1991; 174:53-62.
208. Ellis SA, Strachan T, Palmer MS et al. Complete nucleotide sequence of a unique HLA class I C locus product expressed on the human choriocarcinoma cell line BeWo. J Immunol 1989; 142: 3281-5.
209. Little A, Mason A, Marsh SGE et al. HLA-C typing of eleven Papua New Guineans: Identification of an HLA-Cw4/Cw2 hybrid allele. Tissue Antigens 1996; 48:113-7.
210. Tibensky D, DeMars R, Holowachuk EW et al. Sequence and gene transfer analyses of HLA-CwBL18 (HLA-C blank) and HLA-Cw5 genes. Implications for the control of expression and immunogenicity of HLA-C antigens. J Immunol 1989; 143:348-55.
211. Petersdorf EW, Stanley JF, Martin PJ et al. Molecular diversity of the HLA-C locus in unrelated marrow transplantation. Tissue Antigens 1994; 44:93-9.
212. Steinle A, Nossner E, Schendel DJ. Isolation and characterization of a genomic HLA-Cw6 clone. Tissue Antigens 1992; 39:134-7.
213. Mizuno S, Kang SH, Lee HW et al. Isolation and expression of a cDNA clone encoding HLA-Cw6: unique characteristics of HLA-C encoded gene products. Immunogenetics 1989; 29:323-30.
214. Vilches C, de Pablo R, Herrero MJ et al. Molecular cloning and polymerase chain reaction-sequence-specific oligonucleotide detection of the allele encoding the novel allospecificity HLA-Cw6.2 (Cw*1502) in Spanish gypsies. Hum Immunol 1993; 37:259-63.
215. Srivastava R, Duceman BW, Biro PA et al. Molecular organization of the class I genes of human major histocompatibility complex. Immunol Rev 1985; 84: 93-121.
216. Davidson WF, Kress M, Khoury G et al. Comparison of HLA class I gene sequences. Derivation of locus-specific oligonucleotide probes specific for HLA-A, HLA-B, and HLA-C genes. J Biol Chem 1985; 260:13414-23.
217. Vilches C, Bunce M, de Pablo R et al. Anchored PCR cloning of the novel HLA-Cw*0704 allele detected by PCR-SSP. Tissue Antigens 1995; 46:19-23.
218. Wang H, Tokunaga K, Ishikawa Y et al. Identification and DNA typing of two Cw7 alleles (Cw*0702 and Cw*0704) in Japanese, with the corrected sequence of Cw*0702. Hum Immunol 1996; 45:52-8.
219. Vilches C, Bunce M, Sanz L et al. Molecular cloning of two new HLA-C alleles: Cw*1801 and Cw*0706. Tissue Antigens 1996; 48:698-702.
220. Takata H, Inoko H, Ando A et al. Cloning and analysis of HLA class I cDNA encoding a new HLA-C specificity Cx52. Immunogenetics 1988; 28:265-70.
221. Takiguchi M, Nishimura I, Hayashi H et al. The structure and expression of genes encoding serologically undetected HLA-C locus antigens. J Immunol 1989; 143:1372-8.
222. Cereb N, Choi JW, Lee S et al. Identification of two new HLA-C alleles, Cw*1203 and Cw*1402, from the sequence analysis of seven HLA homozygous cell lines carrying HLA-C blank. Tissue Antigens 1994; 44:193-5.
223. Wang H, Tokunaga K, Ogawa A et al. DNA typing of Cw14 alleles in Japanese and the corrected sequence of Cw*1402. Tissue Antigens 1996; 47:442-6.
224. Wang H, Tokunaga K, Ishikawa Y et al. A new HLA-C allele, Cw*1403, associated with HLA-B44 in Japanese. Hum Immunol 1995; 43:295-300.
225. de Pablo MR, Vilches C, Moreno ME et al. A novel HLA-C allele (Cw*1504) related to the Cw6.2 phenotype. Immunogenetics 1994; 39:79.
226. Vilches C, de Pablo R, Herrero MJ et al. Cw*1505: a novel HLA-C allele isolated from a B*7301 haplotype. Immunogenetics 1994; 40:313.
227. Vilches C, Herrero MJ, de Pablo R et al. Molecular characterization of a novel, serologically detectable, HLA-C allele: Cw*1602. Hum Immunol 1994; 41: 167-70.
228. Cereb N, Hughes AL, Yang SY. Cw*1701, a new HLA-C allelic lineage with an unusual transmembrane domain. [In Press] Tissue Antigens 1997.
229. Herrero MJ, Vilches C, de Pablo R et al. The complete primary structure of

Cw*1701 reveals a highly divergent HLA class I molecule. Tissue Antigens 1997; 49:267-70.
230. Wang H, Tokunaga K, Akaza T et al. A novel allele, Cw*1702 with serological Cw2 specificity. Tissue Antigens 1997; 49:183-5.
231. Lee JS, Trowsdale J, Travers PJ et al. Sequence of an HLA-DR alpha-chain cDNA clone and intron-exon organization of the corresponding gene. Nature 1982; 299:750-2.
232. Larhammar D, Gustafsson K, Claesson L et al. Alpha chain of HLA-DR transplantation antigens is a member of the same protein superfamily as the immunoglobulins. Cell 1982; 30:153-61.
233. Das HK, Lawrance SK, Weissman SM. Structure and nucleotide sequence of the heavy chain gene of HLA-DR. Proc Natl Acad Sci USA 1983; 80:3543-7.
234. Korman AJ, Auffray C, Schamboeck A et al. The amino acid sequence and gene organization of the heavy chain of the HLA-DR antigen: homology to immunoglobulins. Proc Natl Acad Sci USA 1982; 79:6013-7.
235. Tonnelle C, DeMars R, Long EO. DO beta: a new beta chain gene in HLA-D with a distinct regulation of expression. EMBO J 1985; 4:2839-47.
236. Bell JI, Estess P, St. John T et al. DNA sequence and characterization of human class II major histocompatibility complex beta chains from the DR1 haplotype. Proc Natl Acad Sci U S A 1985; 82: 3405-9.
237. Hurley CK, Ziff BL, Silver J et al. Polymorphism of the HLA-DR1 haplotype in American blacks. Identification of a DR1 beta-chain determinant recognized in the mixed lymphocyte reaction. J Immunol 1988; 140:4019-23.
238. Merryman P, Gregersen PK, Lee S et al. Nucleotide sequence of a DRw10 beta chain cDNA clone. Identity of the third D region with that of the DRw53 allele of the beta 2 locus and as the probable site encoding a polymorphic MHC class II epitope. J Immunol 1988; 140:2447-52.
239. Coppin HL, Avoustin P, Fabron J et al. Evolution of the HLA-DR1 gene family. Structural and functional analysis of the new allele "DR-BON". J Immunol 1990; 144:984-9.
240. Gregersen PK, Todd JA, Erlich HA et al. Immunobiology of HLA. 1989; First domain sequence diversity of DR and DQ subregion alleles. p. 1027-31.
241. Guignier F, Mercier B, Roz P et al. A novel HLA-DRB1*01 allele (DRB1*0104). Tissue Antigens 1993; 42:42-4.
242. Bell JI, Denney D, Jr., Foster L et al. Allelic variation in the DR subregion of the human major histocompatibility complex. Proc Natl Acad Sci U S A 1987; 84:6234-8.
243. Gorski J, Mach B. Polymorphism of human Ia antigens: gene conversion between two DR beta loci results in a new HLA-D/DR specificity. Nature 1986; 322:67-70.
244. Gustafsson K, Wiman K, Emmoth E et al. Mutations and selection in the generation of class II histocompatibility antigen polymorphism. EMBO J 1984; 3:1655-61.
245. Horn GT, Bugawan TL, Long CM et al. Sequence analysis of HLA class II genes from insulin-dependent diabetic individuals. Hum Immunol 1988; 21:249-63.
246. Todd JA, Bell JI, McDevitt HO. HLA-DQ beta gene contributes to susceptibility and resistance to insulin-dependent diabetes mellitus. Nature 1987; 329:599-604.
247. Buyse I, Emonds MP, Bouillon R et al. Novel class II HLA-DRB4 and DPB1 alleles found in the Belgian population. Immunogenetics 1993; 38:380.
248. Eberle M, Baxter-Lowe LA. A silent mutation in HLA-DRB1*0301 can affect oligotyping. Tissue Antigens 1992; 40: 150-2.
249. Hurley CK, Gregersen PK, Gorski J et al. The DR3(w18), DQw4 haplotype differs from DR3(w17), DQw2 haplotypes at multiple class II loci. Hum Immunol 1989; 25:37-50.
250. Ellis JM, Steiner N, Wang J et al. Diversity and evolution of the DRB1*03 family: Description of DRB1*03022, *0307, *0308. Tissue Antigens 1997; 49:41-5.
251. Apple RJ, Erlich HA. Two new HLA DRB1 alleles found in African Americans: implications for balancing selection at positions 57 and 86. Tissue Antigens 1992; 40:69-74.
252. Anholts JD, Verduyn W, Parlevliet A et al. Irregular polymerase chain reaction-

sequence-specific oligonucleotide hybridization patterns reveal seven new HLA-DRB1 alleles related to DR2, DR3, DR6, DR8, and DR11. Implications for sequence-specific priming. Hum Immunol 1995; 42:15-22.
253. Asu U, Taylor M, Dunn D et al. A new DRB1 allele: DRB1*03 new. Hum Immunol 1994; 40:36.
254. Fenske BA, Lemieux J, Hoar D et al. A novel DRB1*0306 allele identified by PCR-RFLP. Hum Immunol 1996; 46: 55-7.
255. Dufossé F, Guignier F, Cracco P et al. A novel HLA-DRB1 allele (DRB1*0309). [In Press] Tissue Antigens 1997.
256. Martinez-Quiles N, Martin-Villa JM, Matinez-Laso J et al. Description of two new DRB1 (DRB1*0310) and DRB3 (DRB3*01012) alleles found in a Spanish infant. [In Press] Tissue Antigens 1997.
257. Curtsinger JM, Hilden JM, Cairns JS et al. Evolutionary and genetic implications of sequence variation in two nonallelic HLA-DR beta-chain cDNA sequences. Proc Natl Acad Sci U S A 1987; 84: 209-13.
258. Spies T, Sorrentino R, Boss JM et al. Structural organization of the DR subregion of the human major histocompatibility complex. Proc Natl Acad Sci U S A 1985; 82:5165-9.
259. Gregersen PK, Shen M, Song QL et al. Molecular diversity of HLA-DR4 haplotypes. Proc Natl Acad Sci U S A 1986; 83:2642-6.
260. Thonnard J, Gervais T, Heusterpreute M et al. A new silent mutation at codon 35 in exon 2 yielding DRB1*04012 allele. Tissue Antigens 1997;49 Part 1:274-6.
261. Gregersen PK, Goyert SM, Song QL et al. Microheterogeneity of HLA-DR4 haplotypes: DNA sequence analysis of LD "KT2" and LD "TAS" haplotypes. Hum Immunol 1987; 19:287-92.
262. Cairns JS, Curtsinger JM, Dahl CA et al. Sequence polymorphism of HLA DR beta 1 alleles relating to T-cell-recognized determinants. Nature 1985; 317:166-8.
263. Morales P, Martinez-Laso J, Martin-Villa JM et al. High frequency of the HLA-DRB1*0405-(Dw15)-DQw8 haplotype in Spaniards and its relationship to diabetes susceptibility. Hum Immunol 1991; 32:170-5.
264. Moribe T, Kaneshige T, Hirakata et al. Identification of a DRB1*0405 variant (DRB1*04052) using the PCR-RFLP method. Tissue Antigens 1996; 47:450-3.
265. Lang B, Navarrete C, LoGalbo PR et al. Further DNA sequence microheterogeneity of the HLA-DR4/Dw13 haplotype group: importance of amino acid position 86 of the DR beta 1 chain for T-cell recognition. Hum Immunol 1990; 27: 378-89.
266. Lanchbury JS, Hall MA, Welsh KI et al. Sequence analysis of HLA-DR4B1 subtypes: additional first domain variability is detected by oligonucleotide hybridization and nucleotide sequencing. Hum Immunol 1990; 27:136-44.
267. Lanchbury JS, Jaeger EE, Welsh KI et al. Nucleotide sequence of a novel HLA-DRB4B1 allele, DRB1*0409. Immunogenetics 1991; 33:210-2.
268. Gao X, Veale A, Serjeantson SW. HLA class II diversity in Australian aborigines: unusual HLA-DRB1 alleles. Immunogenetics 1992; 36:333-7.
269. Petersdorf EW, Smith AG, Mickelson EM et al. Ten HLA-DR4 alleles defined by sequence polymorphisms within the DRB1 first domain. Immunogenetics 1991; 33:267-75.
270. Petersdorf EW, Smith AG, Martin PJ et al. HLA-DRB1 first domain sequence for a novel DR4 allele designated DRB1*0413. Tissue Antigens 1992; 40:267-8.
271. Pile KD, Willcox N, Bell JI et al. A novel HLA-DR4 allele (DRB1*0414) in a patient with myasthenia gravis. Tissue Antigens 1992; 40:264-6.
272. Tiercy JM, Gebührer L, Betuel H et al. A new HLA-DR4 allele with a DR11 alpha-helix sequence. Tissue Antigens 1993; 41:97-101.
273. Middleton D, Hughes DJ, Trainor F et al. An HLA-DRB1*04 first domain sequence (DRB1*0416) which differs from HLA-DRB1*0401 at codon 59. Tissue Antigens 1994; 43:44-6.
274. Zhang S, Fernandez-Vina M, Falco M et al. A novel HLA-DRB1 allele (DRB1*0417) in South American Indians. Immunogenetics 1993; 38:463.
275. Mehra NK, Bouwens AG, Naipal A et al.

Asian Indian HLA-DR2-, DR4-, and DR52-related DR-DQ genotypes analyzed by polymerase chain reaction based on nonradioactive oligonucleotide typing. Unique haplotypes and a novel DR4 subtype. Hum Immunol 1994; 39:202-10.
276. Smith AG, Petersdorf EW, Mickelson E et al. HLA-DRB1 first domain sequences of two new DR11 alleles and one novel DR4 allele. Tissue Antigens 1993; 42: 533-5.
277. Cassidy S, Lester S, Humphreys I et al. A new HLA-DRB1*04 allele: DRB1*0420. Tissue Antigens 1995; 45:353-5.
278. Keller E, Yao Z, Volgger A et al. A novel variant of DR4 (DRB1*0421) identified in a patient with polychondritis. Immunogenetics 1995; 41:171.
279. Gebührer L, Adami N, Javaux F et al. Sequence of a new HLA-DR4 allele with an unusual residue at position 88 that does not seem to affect T-cell allo recognition. Hum Immunol 1996; 51:60-2.
280. Guethlein LA, Bias WB, Schmeckpeper BJ. Re-evaluation of DRB1*0702: evidence for only one allele, DRB1*0701, encoding the beta chain of the HLA-DR7 antigen. Tissue Antigens 1994; 43:124-8.
281. Young JA, Wilkinson D, Bodmer WF et al. Sequence and evolution of HLA-DR7- and -DRw53-associated beta-chain genes. Proc Natl Acad Sci U S A 1987; 84: 4929-33.
282. Karr RW, Gregersen PK, Obata F et al. Analysis of DR beta and DQ beta chain cDNA clones from a DR7 haplotype. J Immunol 1986; 137:2886-90.
283. Gregersen PK, Moriuchi T, Karr RW et al. Polymorphism of HLA-DR beta chains in DR4, -7, and -9 haplotypes: implications for the mechanisms of allelic variation. Proc Natl Acad Sci U S A 1986; 83:9149-53.
284. Jonsson AK, Andersson L, Rask L. A cellular and functional split in the DRw8 haplotype is due to a single amino acid replacement (DR beta ser 57-asp 57). Immunogenetics 1989; 29:308-16.
285. Gorski J. The HLA-DRw8 lineage was generated by a deletion in the DR B region followed by first domain diversification. J Immunol 1989; 142:4041-5.
286. Watanabe Y, Tokunaga K, Matsuki K et al. Direct sequencing of a HLA-DRB gene by polymerase chain reaction: sequence variation in DRw8 specificity. Jinrui Idengaku Zasshi 1990; 35:151-7.
287. Abe A, Ito I, Ohkubo M et al. Two distinct subtypes of the HLA-DRw12 haplotypes in the Japanese population detected by nucleotide sequence analysis and oligonucleotide genotyping. Immunogenetics 1989; 30:422-6.
288. O'Brien RM, Cram DS, Russ GR et al. Nucleotide sequences of the HLA-DRw12 and DRw8 B1 chains from an Australian aborigine. Hum Immunol 1992; 34: 147-51.
289. Hurley CK, Lee KW, Mickelson E et al. DRw8 microvariation: a new DRB1 allele identified in association with DQw7 in American blacks. Hum Immunol 1991; 31:109-13.
290. Eberle M, Baxter-Lowe LA. Molecular analysis of HLA-DRB1*08/12 alleles. Identification of two additional alleles. Hum Immunol 1992; 34:24-30.
291. Titus-Trachtenberg EA, Rickards O, De Stefano GF et al. Analysis of HLA class II haplotypes in the Cayapa Indians of Ecuador: a novel DRB1 allele reveals evidence for convergent evolution and balancing selection at position 86. Am J Hum Genet 1994; 55:160-7.
292. Loeffler D, Woelpl A, Eiermann TH. Nucleotide sequence of a novel HLA-DRB1 allele, DRB1*0806. Immunogenetics 1995; 41:56.
293. Benmamar D, Martinez-Laso J, Varela P et al. Evolutionary relationships of HLA-DR8 alleles and description of a new subtype (DRB1*0806) in the Algerian population. Hum Immunol 1993; 36:172-8.
294. Smith AG, Mickelson EM, McKinney S et al. Analysis of HLA-DRB1 alleles among 23 Brazilian families reveals a new DR8 allele. Tissue Antigens 1996, in press.
295. Kashiwase K, Tokunaga K, Lin L et al. A new HLA-DR8 subtype showing unusual serological reaction and the confirmatory sequence of DRB1*0809. Tissue Antigens 1995; 46:340-2.
296. She JX, Zhang LP, Scornik J et al. Nucleotide sequence of a novel HLA-DRB1 allele, DRB1*0810 [corrected] [published erratum appears in Immunogenetics 1994; 39:379]. Immunogenetics 1994; 39:78.

297. Williams TM, Wu J, Foutz T et al. A new DRB1 allele (DRB1*0811) identified in Native Americans. Immunogenetics 1994; 40:314.
298. Versluis LF, Savelkoul PH, van der Zwan AW et al. Identification of the new HLA-DRB1*0812 allele detected by sequenced based typing. Immunogenetics 1996; 44:84.
299. Smith AG, Nelson JL, Regen L et al. Six new DR52-associated DRB1 alleles, three DR8, two DR11, and one DR6 reflect a variety of mechanismms which generate polymorphism in the MHC. Tissue Antigens 1996; 48:118-26.
300. Trejaut J, Greville W, Duncan N et al. A novel allele (DRB1*0815) defined in an Australian Aborigine. [In Press] Tissue Antigens 1997.
301. Naruse TK, Ando R, Nose Y et al. HLA-DRB4 genotyping by PCR-RFLP: diversity in the association between HLA-DRB4 and DRB1 alleles. Tissue Antigens 1997; 49:152-9.
302. Tieber VL, Abruzzini LF, Didier DK et al. Complete characterization and sequence of an HLA class II DR beta chain cDNA from the DR5 haplotype. J Biol Chem 1986; 261:2738-42.
303. Lee KW, Johnson AH, Tang T et al. DRw11 haplotypes: continuum of DRB1 diversity augmented by unique DQ/DRw52 associations [published erratum appears in Hum Immunol 1992; 34:75]. Hum Immunol 1991; 32: 150-5.
304. Murru MR, Costa GR, Muntoni F et al. A new allelic variant of HLA-DRB1*1101 (DRB1*11013) segregating in a Sardinian family. Tissue Antigens 1996; 48:604-6.
305. Steimle V, Hinkkanen A, Schlesier M et al. A novel HLA-DR beta I sequence from the DRw11 haplotype. Immunogenetics 1988; 28:208-10.
306. Numez-Roldan A, Gregersen PK, Winchester RJ et al. Analysis of class II genes from a DR5, DQW haplotype: Implications for haplotype evolution. Human Immunology 1991; 32:150-5.
307. Apple RJ, Bugawan TL, Griffith R et al. A new DRB1 allele and a novel DR4 haplotype found in a Filipino family. Tissue Antigens 1993; 41:51-4.
308. Bannai M, Tokunaga K, Lin L et al. A new HLA-DR11 DRB1 allele found in a Korean. Hum Immunol 1994; 39:230-2.
309. Lin YN, Ren EC, Chan SH. A new DR11 allele in Singaporean Chinese. Tissue Antigens 1993; 41:204-5.
310. Middleton D, Hughes DJ, Williams F et al. A new DRB1 allele DRB1*1107—a combination of DRB1*11 and DRB1*03. Tissue Antigens 1993; 42:160-3.
311. Williams F, Hughes DJ, Middleton D. A new HLA-DRB1*11 allele (DRB1*1109) differing at codons 32, 34 and 37. Tissue Antigens 1994; 44:63-4.
312. Eberle M, Szmania S, Baxter-Lowe LA. Molecular evolution of HLA: A continuum of diversity. J Immunol 1993; 150:175.
313. Smith AG, Safirman C, Kelso C et al. Two new DR52-associated alleles, DRB1*1111 and *1312, identified by PCR/SSOP and confirmed by DNA sequencing. Tissue Antigens 1994; 44:52-6.
314. Rosenberg SM, Wollenzien TF, Johnson MM et al. A description of a new DR allele, DRB1*1113. Tissue Antigens 1995; 45:125-8.
315. Heron SD, McKeen ME, Cizman BB et al. Identification of HLA-DRB1*1114 by oligonucleotide typing and DNA sequencing. Immunogenetics 1995; 42: 436-7.
316. Robbins F, Tang T, Yao H et al. Direct sequencing of SSP-PCR-amplified cDNA to identify new alleles in the DR52-associated DRB1 group: identification of DRB1*1115, DRB1*1117 and DRB1*1319. Tissue Antigens 1995; 45: 302-8.
317. Fischer GF, Fae I, Petrasek M et al. An HLA-DR11 variant (HLA-DRB1*1115) segregating in a family of Turkish origin. Tissue Antigens 1995; 45:143-4.
318. Thonnard J, Blaimond B, Heusterspreut M et al. A new HLA-DRB1*1116 allele sharing DR13 and DR11 sequence motifs. Tissue Antigens 1995; 46:124-7.
319. Nielsen J, Zhang G, Spalding T et al. Molecular cloning and automated sequencing of a new HLA-DRB1 allele within the DRB1*14 family. Hum Immunol 1995; 44-1:52.
320. Heine U, Mason JM, Begovich AB et al. Two novel DRB1 alleles, DRB1*1118 and DRB1*1119, detected by PCR-SSOP and confirmed by DNA sequencing. Tissue Antigens 1995; 46:68-70.
321. Cizman BB, Kearns DJ, McKeen ME et

al. New DRB1*1120 allele; another example of the transition between the DR11 and DR13 families of alleles. Tissue Antigens 1996; 48:52-4.
322. Verduyn W, Anholts JDH, Versluis LF et al. Six newly identified HLA-DRB alleles: DRB1*1121, *1419, *1420, *1421, DRB3*0203 and DR5*0103. Tissue Antigens 1996; 48:80-6.
323. Adami N, Jeannet M, Tiercy J. Sequence of a new HLA-DR11 allele with a DR4-specific first hypervariable region. Immunogenetics 1995; 42:448-9.
324. Schranz P, Seelig R, Seidl C et al. Nucleotide sequence of a new HLA-DRB1(*)11 allele (DRB1(*)1124). Immunogenetics 1996; 43:242-3.
325. Perrier P, Reveillere C, Schuhmacher A. A new DRB1 allele (DRB1*1125) sharing DR11 and DR8 sequence motifs. Tissue Antigens 1997; 49:84-7.
326. Knipper AJ, Enczmann J, Schuch B et al. A novel HLA-DRB1*11 allele (DRB1*1127). Tissue Antigens 1997; 49:414-6.
327. Navarrete C, Seki T, Miranda A et al. DNA sequence analysis of the HLA-DRw12 allele. Hum Immunol 1989; 25:51-8.
328. Behar E, Lin X, Grumet FC et al. A new DRB1*1202 allele (DRB1*12022) found in association with DQA1*0102 and DQB1*0602 in two black narcoleptic subjects. Immunogenetics 1995; 41:52.
329. Rodriguez SG, Crevling CL, Steiner N et al. Identification of a new allele, DRB1*1204, during routine PCR-SSOP typing of National Marrow Donor Program volunteers. Tissue Antigens 1996; 48:221-3.
330. Tiercy JM, Gorski J, Betuel H et al. DNA typing of DRw6 subtypes: correlation with DRB1 and DRB3 allelic sequences by hybridization with oligonucleotide probes. Hum Immunol 1989; 24:1-14.
331. Noreen HJ, Santamaria P, Davidson ML et al. Serology, restriction fragment length polymorphism, and sequence analysis of a unique HLA class II antigen, DR5x6. Hum Immunol 1991; 30: 168-73.
332. Corell A, Martin-Villa JM, Varela P et al. Exon 2 DNA sequence of the HLA-DRw13b allele obtained from genomes of five different individuals [published erratum appears in Mol Immunol 1990; 27:471]. Mol Immunol 1990; 27:313-6.
333. Lee KW, Johnson AH, Hurley CK. Two divergent routes of evolution gave rise to the DRw13 haplotypes. J Immunol 1990; 145:3119-25.
334. Tiercy JM, Jeannet M, Mach B. A new HLA-DRB1 allele within the DRw52 supertypic specificity (DRw13-DwHAG): sequencing and direct identification by oligonucleotide typing. Eur J Immunol 1990; 20:237-41.
335. Petersdorf EW, Griffith RL, Erlich HA et al. Unique sequences for two HLA-DRB1 genes expressed on distinct DRw6 haplotypes. Immunogenetics 1990; 32: 96-103.
336. Tiercy JM, Gebührer L, Freidel C et al. Additional complexity within the HLA-D region: sequence analysis of two new DRw13-DQw7 haplotypes. Hum Immunol 1991; 32:95-101.
337. Petersdorf EW, Smith AG, Haase AM et al. Polymorphism of HLA-DRw52-associated DRB1 genes as defined by sequence-specific oligonucleotide probe hybridization and sequencing. Tissue Antigens 1991; 38:169-77.
338. Kaneshige T, Hashimoto M, Matsumoto Y et al. Serologic and nucleotide sequencing analyses of a novel DR52-associated DRB1 allele with the DR 'NJ25' specificity, designated DRB1*1307. Hum Immunol 1994; 41:151-9.
339. Lee KW. DR6 in Koreans. DR11 frequently acts as a recipient gene to create DR13 alleles. Hum Immunol 1993; 37: 229-36.
340. Horne C, Goodfellow PJ, McDonald HL et al. A new HLA-DRB1 allele formed by an intraexonic interallelic crossover. Tissue Antigens 1993; 42:141-3.
341. Yunis JJ, Kineke E, Yunis EJ. Characterization of a new DRB1 allele, DRB1*1309, by PCR-SSOP and sequencing. Tissue Antigens 1994; 43:54-7.
342. Dufossé F, Cracco P, Becuwe D et al. A novel HLA DR52-associated DRB1 allele (DRB1*1311). Tissue Antigens 1994; 43:271-3.
343. Blasczyk R, van Lessen A, Schwella N et al. A novel HLA-DR13 allele (DRB1*1314) identified by single-strand confor-

mation polymorphism analysis and confirmed by direct sequencing. Hum Immunol 1995; 43:309-12.
344. Dinauer DM, Glumm R, Baxter-Lowe LA. DRB1*1316: evolutionary and functional implications of a novel polymorphism at codon 86. Hum Immunol 1996; 45:37-41.
345. Cizman BB, Heron SD, McKeen ME et al. Identification of a DRB1 allele (DRB1*1316) with aspartate at position 86: Evolutionary considerations and functional implications. Tissue Antigens 1996; 47:153-4.
346. Rosenberg SM, Wollenzien TF, Robbins FM et al. Yet another novel HLA-DRB1 allele (DRB1*1317) and its misidentification by PCR-SSP. Tissue Antigens 1995; 46:128-30.
347. Dormoy A, Delbosc A, Galy-Floc'h M et al. A novel DRB1*13 allele (DRB1*1318) with a short DRB1*08 sequence. Immunogenetics 1996; 43:240-1.
348. Hashemi S, Couture C, Buyse I et al. Identification of a new DRB1*13 allele (DRB1*1320) and a novel DRB1*15 allele (DRB1*15012) with a silent mutation affecting oligotyping. Tissue Antigens 1996; 47:147-9.
349. Poli F, Bianchi P, Crespiatico L et al. Identification of a new DRB1 allele (DRB1*1325) by PCR-SSP and DNA sequencing. Tissue Antigens 1996; 48: 714-6.
350. Voorter CEM, de Bruyn-Geraets D, Verduyn W et al. Identification of a new HLA-DRB1*13 allele (DRB1*1326) with a short DRB1*16 sequence. Tissue Antigens 1997; 49:88-91.
351. Schaffer M, Olerup O. A novel DRB1*13 allele (DRB1*1327) on a DR17, DQ2 haplotype with a DRB1*0301 sequence motif in the second hyperpolymorphic region. Tissue Antigens 1997; 49:186-8.
352. Gorski J. First domain sequence of the HLA-DRB1 chain from two HLA-DRw14 homozygous typing cell lines: TEM (Dw9) and AMALA (Dw16). Hum Immunol 1989; 24:145-9.
353. Obata F, Abe A, Ohkubo M et al. Sequence analysis and oligonucleotide genotyping of HLA-DR"JX6", a DR "blank" haplotype found in the Japanese population. Hum Immunol 1990; 27: 269-84.
354. McClure GR, Ruberti G, Fathman CG et al. DRB1*LY10—a new DRB1 allele and its haplotypic association. Immunogenetics 1990; 32:214-7.
355. Gorski J, Radka SF, Masewicz S et al. Mapping of distinct serologic and T cell recognition epitopes on an HLA-DR beta-chain. J Immunol 1990; 145:2020-4.
356. Obata F, Ito I, Ito K et al. Sequence analysis and HLA-DR genotyping of a novel HLA-DRw14 allele. Immunogenetics 1990; 32:313-20.
357. Dong RP, Kimura A, Sasazuki T. Sequence analysis of three novel DRw14-DRB1 alleles. Immunogenetics 1992; 36:130-3.
358. Laforet M, Urlacher A, Falkenrodt A et al. A new DR14 allele (DRB1*1411) containing a short DR11 sequence and its haplotypic association. Hum Immunol 1993; 36:179-85.
359. Hashimoto M, Kaneshige T, Kinoshita T et al. A new DR14-related DRB1 allele, DRB1*1412, which differs from DRB1 *1403 only at codon 86. Tissue Antigens 1994; 43:133-5.
360. Pando M, Theiler G, Melano R et al. A new HLA-DR6 allele (DRB1*1413) found in a tribe of Brazilian Indians. Immunogenetics 1994; 39:377
361. Lester S, Cassidy S, Humphreys I et al. Evolution in HLA-DRB1 and major histocompatibility complex class II haplotypes of Australian aborigines. Definition of a new DRB1 allele and distribution of DRB1 gene frequencies. Hum Immunol 1995; 42:154-60.
362. Fogdell A, Olerup O. A novel DRB1 allele (DRB1*1415) formed by interallelic crossing over between the DRB1*1404 and the DRB1*0802 or 0804 alleles. Tissue Antigens 1994; 43:327-9.
363. Hashemi S, Aye MT, Zeibadawi A et al. A novel HLA-DRB1*14 allele (DRB1* 1417). Tissue Antigens 1994; 44:189-92.
364. Adami N, Aubert V, Jeannet M et al. Sequencing of a new HLA-DR14 allele (DRB1*1422). Immunogenetics 1996; 43:248-9.
365. Lee BS, Rust NA, McMichael AJ et al. HLA-DR2 subtypes form an additional

supertypic family of DR beta alleles. Proc Natl Acad Sci U S A 1987; 84:4591-5.
366. Lock CB, So AK, Welsh KI et al. MHC class II sequences of an HLA-DR2 narcoleptic. Immunogenetics 1988; 27:449-55.
367. Wu S, Saunders TL, Bach FH. Polymorphism of human Ia antigens generated by reciprocal intergenic exchange between two DR beta loci. Nature 1986; 324: 676-9.
368. Wu S, Yabe T, Madden M et al. cDNA cloning and sequencing reveals that the electrophoretically constant DRβ2 molecules, as well as the variable β1 molecules, from HLA-DR2 subtypes have different amnio acid sequences including a hypervariable region for a functionally important epitope. J Immunol 1987; 138:2953-9.
369. Demopulos JT, Hodge TW, Wooten V et al. A novel DRB1 allele in DR2-positive American blacks. Hum Immunol 1991; 30:41-4.
370. Fan LA, Smith AG, Chandanayingyong D et al. DRB1*1504 (DR2Dai): a new DR2 allele identified in the Dai minority population of southwest China. Tissue Antigens 1994; 44:326-8.
371. Fei H, Lu Y, Lin B et al. The nucleotide sequence of a new HLA DR15(2) allele in Chinese. Chin Microbiol Immunol 1995; 15:45-8.
372. Shinno K, Tsuboyama K, Mine H et al. Nucleotide sequence of a New DRB1*15 variant, 1505, in a Japanese family. Tissue Antigens 1995; 46:411-3.
373. van den Berg-Loonen EM, Rani R, Singal D et al. A new DRB1*15 allele (DRB1 *1506) identified by sequence based typing. Tissue Antigens 1997; 49:189-91.
374. White JM, Baxter-Lowe LA. Sequence of DRB1*1601. Tissue Antigens 1997; 49: 192-3.
375. Liu CP, Bach FH, Wu SK. Molecular studies of a rare DR2/LD-5a/DQw3 HLA class II haplotype. Multiple genetic mechanisms in the generation of polymorphic HLA class II genes [published erratum appears in J Immunol 1990; 144:1544]. J Immunol 1988; 140: 3631-9.
376. Trejaut J, Bhatia K, Greville WD et al. HLA-DR2 haplotypic diversity in four populations of Southeast Asia and Northern China, and five Melanesian populations using PCR-RFLP for DRB1, DRB5, DQB1 and DQA1. Eur J Immunogenetics 1996; 23: 437-49.
377. Rosenlicht JW, Hartung K, Deicher H et al. A novel HLA-DRB1-DR2 allele associated with HLA mistyping. Immunogenetics 1993; 37:479.
378. Laforet M, Urlacher A, Tongio MM. A new HLA DR16 allele (DRB1*1604) with a short DR8 sequence. Tissue Antigens 1994; 43:257-60.
379. Bettinotti MP, McNicholas A, Keller E et al. DRB1*1605: a new DR2-DRB1 allele found in a German family. Immunogenetics 1994; 39:300.
380. Anholts JDH, Bouwens AGM, Verduyn W et al. Sequence of HLA-DRB1*1606 is incorrect. Hum Immunol 1996; 46:65-6.
381. Israel S, Smith AG, Miller K et al. Two new DR2 alleles; DRB1*1607 identified in a Jewish Ashkenazi family and DRB1*15022 found in a single caucasian donor. Tissue Antigens 1997; 49:173-5.
382. Gorski J. HLA-DR beta-chain polymorphism. Second domain polymorphism reflects evolutionary relatedness of alleles and may explain public serologic epitopes. J Immunol 1989; 143:329-33.
383. Long EO, Wake CT, Gorski J et al. Complete sequence of an HLA-DR beta chain deduced from a cDNA clone and identification of multiple non-allelic DR beta chain genes. EMBO J 1983; 2: 389-94.
384. Didier DK, Schiffenbauer J, Shuman S et al. Characterization of two distinct DR beta chain alleles at the beta III locus of the DR5 haplotype: beta III alleles are highly conserved. J Immunol 1986; 137: 2627-31.
385. Gorski J, Irle C, Mickelson EM et al. Correlation of structure with T cell responses of the three members of the HLA-DRw52 allelic series. J Exp Med 1989; 170:1027-32.
386. Sutton VR, Knowles RW. An aberrant DRB4 null gene transcript is found that could encode a novel HLA-DR beta chain. Immunogenetics 1990; 31:112-7.
387. Andersson G, Larhammar D, Widmark E et al. Class II genes of the human major histocompatibility complex. Organization and evolutionary relationship of the DR beta genes [published erratum

appears in J Biol Chem 1988; 263: 8551]. J Biol Chem 1987; 262: 8748-58.
388. De Canck I, Demant C, Mersch G et al. Characterisation of a new DRB4 allele (DRB4*0104). Tissue Antigens 1996; 48:213-6.
389. Voorter CEM, Emonds M, van den Berg-Loonen EM. Identification of a new DRB4 allele (DRB4*0105) by sequence based typing. [In Press] Tissue Antigens 1997.
390. Poli F, Bianchi P, Crespiatico L et al. Characterisation of a new HLA-DRB5 allele (DRB5*0105) by PCR-SSP and direct sequencing. Tissue Antigens 1996; 47:338-40.
391. Freeman SM, Saunders TL, Madden M et al. Comparison of DRβ1 alleles from diabetic and normal individuals. Hum Immunol 1987; 19:1-6.
392. Grooms A, Dunckley H, Gao X et al. DRB5*HK: a new HLA-DRB5 allele in Cantonese. Tissue Antigens 1992; 40: 210-1.
393. Corell A, Martin Villa JM, Morales P et al. Exon-2 nucleotide sequences, polymorphism and haplotype distribution of a new HLA-DRB gene: HLA-DRB sigma. Mol Immunol 1991; 28:533-43.
394. Figueroa F, O'hUigin C, Inoki H et al. Primate DRB6 pseudogenes: clue to the evolutionary origin of the HLA-DR2 haplotype. Immunogenetics 1991; 34: 324-37.
395. Corell A, Morales P, Varela P et al. Allelic diversity at the primate major histocompatibility complex DRB6 locus. Immunogenetics 1992; 36:404-5.
396. Larhammar D, Servenius B, Rask L et al. Characterization of an HLA DR beta pseudogene. Proc Natl Acad Sci U S A 1985; 82:1475-9.
397. Yasunaga S, Kimura A, Hamaguchi K et al. Different contribution of HLA-DR and -DQ genes in susceptibility and resistance to Insulin-dependant Diabetes Mellitus (IDDM). Tissue Antigens 1996; 47:37-48.
398. Horn GT, Bugawan TL, Long CM et al. Allelic sequence variation of the HLA-DQ loci: relationship to serology and to insulin-dependent diabetes susceptibility. Proc Natl Acad Sci U S A 1988; 85: 6012-6.
399. Auffray C, Lillie JW, Arnot D et al. Isotypic and allotypic variation of human class II histocompatibility antigen alpha-chain genes. Nature 1984; 308:327-33.
400. Fogdell A, Olerup O. The DQA1*0104 allele is carried by DRB1*1001- and DRB1*1401-positive haplotypes in Caucasians, Africans and Orientals. Tissue Antigens 1994; 44:19-24.
401. Lee KW, Johnson AH, Hurley CK. New DQw1 diversity identified within DRw12 and DRw14 haplotypes. Tissue Antigens 1991; 38:231-4.
402. Chang HC, Moriuchi T, Silver J. The heavy chain of human B-cell alloantigen HLA-DS has a variable N-terminal region and a constant immunoglobulin-like region. Nature 1983; 305:813-5.
403. Auffray C, Korman AJ, Roux Dosseto M et al. cDNA clone for the heavy chain of the human B cell alloantigen DC1: strong sequence homology to the HLA-DR heavy chain. Proc Natl Acad Sci U S A 1982; 79:6337-41.
404. Jonsson AK, Hyldig Nielsen JJ, Servenius B et al. Class II genes of the human major histocompatibility complex. Comparisons of the DQ and DX alpha and beta genes. J Biol Chem 1987; 262: 8767-77.
405. Bell JI, Todd JA, McDevitt HO. The molecular basis of HLA-disease association. Adv Hum Genet 1989; 18:1-41.
406. Moriuchi J, Moriuchi T, Silver J. Nucleotide sequence of an HLA-DQ alpha chain derived from a DRw9 cell line: genetic and evolutionary implications. Proc Natl Acad Sci U S A 1985; 82:3420-4.
407. Jonsson AK, Andersson L, Rask L. Complete sequences of DQA1 and DQB1 cDNA clones corresponding to the DQw4 specificities. Immunogenetics 1989; 30:232-4.
408. Hurley CK, Gregersen P, Steiner N et al. Polymorphism of the HLA-D region in American blacks. A DR3 haplotype generated by recombination. J Immunol 1988; 140:885-92.
409. Schenning L, Larhammar D, Bill P et al. Both alpha and beta chains of HLA-DC class II histocompatibility antigens display extensive polymorphism in their amino-terminal domains. EMBO J 1984; 3:447-52.

410. Zimmerman PA, Phadke PM, Lee A et al. Migration of a novel DQA1* allele (DQA1*0502) from African origin to North and South America. Hum Immunol 1995; 42:233-40.
411. Hall MA, Lanchbury JS, Lee JS et al. HLA-DQ2 second-domain polymorphisms may explain increased trans-associated risk in celiac disease and dermatitis herpetiformis. Hum Immunol 1993; 38:284-92.
412. Boss JM, Strominger JL. Cloning and sequence analysis of the human major histocompatibility complex gene DC-3 beta. Proc Natl Acad Sci U S A 1984; 81:5199-203.
413. Trachtenberg EA, Keyeux G, Bernal J et al. Results of Expedicion Humana. II. Analysis of HLA class II alleles in three African American populations from Colombia using the PCR/SSOP: Identification of a novel DQB*02 (*0203) allele. Tissue Antigens 1996; 48:192-8.
414. Olerup O, Aldener-Cannava A, Fogdell-Hahn A et al. DQB1*0202 and the new DQB1*0203 allele: A fourth pair of DQB1 alleles only differing at coding 57. Tissue Antigens 1997; 49:271-3.
415. Michelsen B, Lernmark A. Molecular cloning of a polymorphic DNA endonuclease fragment associates insulin-dependent diabetes mellitus with HLA-DQ. J Clin Invest 1987; 79:1144-52.
416. Larhammar D, Hyldig-Nielsen JJ, Servenius B et al. Exon-intron organization and complete nucleotide sequence of a human major histocompatibility antigen DC beta gene. Proc Natl Acad Sci U S A 1983; 80:7313-7.
417. Briata P, Radka SF, Sartoris S et al. Alternative splicing of HLA-DQB transcripts and secretion of HLA-DQ beta-chain proteins: allelic polymorphism in splicing and polyadenylation sites. Proc Natl Acad Sci U S A 1989; 86:1003-7.
418. Giorda R, Turco E, Trucco M. Full length beta chain cDNAs of DQw9 and DQw8 molecules encode proteins that differ only at amino acid 57. Immunogenetics 1991; 33:404-8.
419. Tautz C, Zwollo P, Marsh DG et al. Sequence of a novel HLA-DQB1 allele. Immunogenetics 1992; 35:421-4.
420. Fenske TS, Baxter-Lowe LA. Characterization of a novel DQB1 allele associated with HLA-DQw3: implications for oligotyping. Hum Immunol 1992; 33:224-7.
421. Cucca F, Frau F, Lampis R et al. HLA-DQB1*0305 and -DQB1*0304 alleles among Sardinians. Evolutionary and practical implications for oligotyping. Hum Immunol 1994; 40:143-9.
422. Cucca F, Muntoni F, Lampis R et al. A novel HLA-DQB1 allele: evidence for gene conversion event promoted by chi-like sequence at DQB1 locus. Tissue Antigens 1993; 41:263-6.
423. Saito S, Ota S, Hashizume K et al. A new HLA-DQB1*0306 allele sharing DQB1 *03032 and DQB1*04 sequences. Tissue Antigens 1996; 48:580-5.
424. Thye T, Muntau B, Stelma FE, Horstmann RD. Novel allele DQB1*0307 in a West African family. [In Press] Tissue Antigens 1997.
425. Lee BS, Bell JI, Rust NA et al. Structural and functional variability among DQ beta alleles of DR2 subtypes. Immunogenetics 1987; 26:85-91.
426. Wu SK, Lu D, Madden M et al. Full-length DQ beta cDNA sequences of HLA-DR2/DQw1 subtypes: genetic interactions between two DQ beta loci generate human class II HLA diversity. Hum Immunol 1990; 27:305-22.
427. Scharf SJ, Freidmann A, Steinman L et al. Specific HLA-DQB and HLA-DRB1 alleles confer susceptibility to pemphigus vulgaris [published erratum appears in Proc Natl Acad Sci U S A 1989; 86:10023]. Proc Natl Acad Sci U S A 1989; 86:6215-9.
428. Bugawan TL, Erlich HA. Rapid typing of HLA-DQB1 DNA polymorphism using nonradioactive oligonucleotide probes and amplified DNA. Immunogenetics 1991; 33:163-70.
429. Tsukamoto K, Yasunami M, Kimura A et al. DQw1 beta gene from HLA-DR2-Dw12 consists of six exons and expresses multiple DQw1 beta polypeptides through alternative splicing. Immunogenetics 1987; 25:343-6.
430. Schranz P, Nessler G, Schindera F et al. Nucleotide sequence of the corrected DQB1*06011 allele. Tissue Antigens 1996; 48:139-40.
431. Singal DP, Qiu X, Sood SK. Molecular

analysis of novel HLA-DR2.DQwl haplotypes in Asian Indians. Tissue Antigens 1992; 40:104-7.
432. Turco E, Care A, Compagnone Post P et al. Allelic forms of the alpha- and beta-chain genes encoding DQw1-positive heterodimers. Immunogenetics 1987; 26:282-90.
433. Fronek Z, Timmerman LA, McDevitt HO. A rare HLA DQB allele sequenced from patients with systemic lupus erythematosus. Hum Immunol 1991; 30: 77-84.
434. Meyer CG, Spauke D. DQB1*MDvR-I: a synonymous mutation at DQB1 codon 57 (DQB1*06052). Tissue Antigens 1994; 43:314-5.
435. Meyer CG, Gallin M, Erttmann K et al. DQB1*WA1—a new DQB1 allele identified in West Africa. Tissue Antigens 1992; 39:147-9.
436. Aldener A, Olerup O. Characterization of a novel DQB1 (DQB1*0609) allele by PCR amplification with sequence-specific primers (PCR-SSP) and nucleotide sequencing. Tissue Antigens 1993; 42: 536-8.
437. Mersch G, Semana G, De Canck I et al. Characterization of a new DQB1 allele (DQB1*0610) which differs from DQB1 *0602 at the highly polymorphic 57-codon. Tissue Antigens 1996; 48:217-20.
438. Williams TM, Bassinger S, Moehlenkamp C et al. Strategy for distinguishing a new DQB1 allele (DQB1*0611) from the closely related DQB1*0602 allele via sequence specific PCR or direct DNA sequencing. Tissue Antigens 1996; 48: 143-7.
439. Vilches C, Garcia-Pacheco J, de Pablo R et al. Complete coding region of the HLA-DQB1*0612 allele, obtained by RT-PCR. Tissue Antigens 1996; 48:589-92.
440. Rozemuller EH, Bouwens AG, van Oort E et al. Sequencing-based typing reveals new insight in HLA-DPA1 polymorphism. Tissue Antigens 1995; 45:57-62.
441. Gustafsson K, Widmark E, Jonsson AK et al. Class II genes of the human major histocompatibility complex. Evolution of the DP region as deduced from nucleotide sequences of the four genes. J Biol Chem 1987; 262:8778-86.
442. Trowsdale J, Young JA, Kelly AP et al. Structure, sequence and polymorphism in the HLA-D region. Immunol Rev 1985; 85:5-43.
443. Lawrance SK, Das HK, Pan J et al. The genomic organisation and nucleotide sequence of the HLA-SB(DP) alpha gene. Nucleic Acids Res 1985; 13:7515-28.
444. Bugawan TL, Horn GT, Long CM et al. Analysis of HLA-DP allelic sequence polymorphism using the in vitro enzymatic DNA amplification of DP-alpha and DP-beta loci. J Immunol 1988; 141:4024-30.
445. Okada K, Prentice HL, Boss JM et al. SB subregion of the human major histocompatibility complex: gene organization, allelic polymorphism and expression in transformed cells. EMBO J 1985; 4: 739-48.
446. May J, Kretschmer C, Schnittger L et al. DPA1*0105, a novel DPA1-variant in a negroid population. Tissue Antigens 1996; 48:593-4.
447. Meyer CG, May J, Spauke D et al. DPA1*02012: a DPA1*0201-related Mhc class II allele in west Africa. Immunogenetics 1994; 40:309
448. Guethlein LA, Bias WB, Schmeckpeper BJ. New DP sequences: three DPA1 and one DPB1. Tissue Antigens 1993; 41: 269-72.
449. Harada H, Kimura A, Dong RP et al. Sequencing and population analysis of four novel HLA-DPA1 alleles. Hum Immunol 1992; 35:173-8.
450. Muntau B, Thye T, Pirmez C, Horstmann RD. A novel DPA1 allele (*0203) composed of known epitopes. [In Press] Tissue Antigens 1997.
451. Lee JS, Sartoris S, Briata P et al. Sequence polymorphism of HLA-DP beta chains. Immunogenetics 1989; 29:346-9.
452. Korioth F, Hartung K, Deicher H et al. A new HLA-DPB1 allele from a patient with systemic lupus erythematosus. Tissue Antigens 1992; 39:216-9.
453. Meyer CG, Schnittger L. A silent mutation in HLA-DPB1*0101 and its evolutionary implications. Hum Immunol 1993; 38:123-6.
454. Kappes DJ, Arnot D, Okada K et al. Structure and polymorphism of the HLA class II SB light chain genes. EMBO J 1984; 3:2985-93.

455. Roux Dosseto M, Auffray C, Lillie JW et al. Genetic mapping of a human class II antigen beta-chain cDNA clone to the SB region of the HLA complex. Proc Natl Acad Sci U S A 1983; 80:6036-40.
456. Schranz P, Renz M, Wojtzyk I et al. Nucleotide sequence of a new HLA-DPB1 allele, DPB1*02013. Immunogenetics 1996; 44:159-60.
457. Kelly A, Trowsdale J. Complete nucleotide sequence of a functional HLA-DP beta gene and the region between the DP beta 1 and DP alpha 1 genes: comparison of the 5' ends of HLA class II genes. Nucleic Acids Res 1985; 13:1607-21.
458. Gustafsson K, Emmoth E, Widmark E et al. Isolation of a cDNA clone coding for an SB beta-chain. Nature 1984; 309: 76-8.
459. Gorski J, Rollini P, Long E et al. Molecular organization of the HLA-SB region of the human major histocompatibility complex and evidence for two SB beta-chain genes. Proc Natl Acad Sci U S A 1984; 81:3934-8.
460. Lair B, Alber C, Yu WY et al. A newly characterized HLA-DP beta-chain allele. Evidence for DP beta heterogeneity within the DPw4 specificity. J Immunol 1988; 141:1353-7.
461. Moonsamy PV, Aldrich CL, Petersdorf EW et al. Seven new DPB1 alleles and their population distribution. Tissue Antigens 1994; 43:249-52.
462. Bugawan TL, Angelini G, Larrick J et al. A combination of a particular HLA-DP beta allele and an HLA-DQ heterodimer confers susceptibility to coeliac disease. Nature 1989; 339:470-3.
463. Begovich AB, Bugawan TL, Nepom BS et al. A specific HLA-DP beta allele is associated with pauciarticular juvenile rheumatoid arthritis but not adult rheumatoid arthritis. Proc Natl Acad Sci U S A 1989; 86:9489-93.
464. Madsen HO, Ryder LP, Fugger L et al. New DPB1 alleles. Tissue Antigens 1992; 39:102-3.
465. Savage DA, Middleton D, Trainor F et al. Frequency of HLA-DPB1 alleles, including a novel DPB1 sequence, in the Northern Ireland population. Hum Immunol 1992; 33:235-42.
466. de Koster HS, Kenter MJ, D'Amaro J et al. Positive correlation between oligonucleotide typing and T-cell recognition of HLA-DP molecules. Immunogenetics 1991; 34:12-22.
467. Hessner MJ, Baxter-Lowe LA. Characterization of novel HLA-DPB1 alleles by oligotyping and nucleotide sequencing. Tissue Antigens 1992; 40:261-3.
468. Dekker JW, Croft L, Easteal S. Nucleotide sequence of a novel HLA-DPB1 allele. Immunogenetics 1992; 36:341-3.
469. Moonsamy PV, Suraj VC, Bugawan TL et al. Genetic diversity within the HLA class II region: ten new DPB1 alleles and their population distribution. Tissue Antigens 1992; 40:153-7.
470. Gao X, Veale A, Serjeantson S. AB1: a novel HLA-DPB1 allele found in one third of an Australian population. Immunogenetics 1992; 36:64-6.
471. Eiermann TH, Uhl S, Fakler J et al. A novel HLA-DPB1 sequence, DPB1*2301. Tissue Antigens 1992; 40:108-10.
472. Meyer CG, Schnittger L, Gallin M et al. DPB1*WA2 and DPB1*WA3—novel West African HLA DPB1 alleles closely related to the allele DPB1*0101 common in negroid populations. Tissue Antigens 1992; 39:144-6.
473. Meyer CG, Spauke D, Schnittger L. MHC class II DPB1*26012: a novel DPB1 sequence and its presumed origin. Tissue Antigens 1994; 43:324-6.
474. Easteal S, Croft L. Two new HLA-DPB1 alleles from Java, Indonesia [published erratum appears in Immunogenetics 1994; 39:160]. Immunogenetics 1993; 37:478
475. Easteal S, Grooms A, Croft L. A second new HLA-DPB1 allele from Santa Cruz Island, Solomon Islands. Immunogenetics 1993; 38:79.
476. Ogawa K, Itho H, Nakajyo S et al. A novel HLA-DPB1 allele, DPB1*3601 (DPB1*KT). Tissue Antigens 1994; 44: 134-6.
477. Mitsunaga S, Kuwata S, Tokunaga K et al. Family study on HLA-DPB1 polymorphism: linkage analysis with HLA-DR/DQ and two "new" alleles. Hum Immunol 1992; 34:203-11.
478. Meyer CG, Schnittger L, Begovich AB et al. DPB1*WA4—an additional HLA class

II allele identified in west Africa. Tissue Antigens 1992; 40:98-9.
479. Mizuki N, Ohno S, Sugimura K et al. Identification of a new HLA-DPB1 allele detected by PCR-RFLP and its nucleotide sequence determination by direct sequencing after PCR amplification. Tissue Antigens 1993; 41:259-62.
480. Easteal S, Croft L. A new HLA-DPB1 allele from the Santa Cruz Islands, Solomon Islands. Immunogenetics 1993; 38:78.
481. de Vries N, Meijerink JP, Tijssen H et al. A novel HLA-DPB1 allele (DPB1 *4501) in a Dutch Caucasian healthy control. Tissue Antigens 1993; 41:255-8.
482. Rani R, Fernandez-Vina MA, Zhang S et al. HLA-DPB1 alleles in a population from north India and description of a new variant (DPB1*5601). Tissue Antigens 1995; 45:264-9.
483. Koshizaka T, Taguchi M, Onishi H et al. A new HLA-DPB1 allele, DPB1*SUT (DPB1*4701). Tissue Antigens 1994; 43:50-3.
484. Mitsunaga S, Shinno K, Maruya E et al. Nucleotide sequence of a novel DPB1 allele, DPB1*4701. Hum Immunol 1993; 37:198-200.
485. Kaneshige T, Kinoshita T, Hashimoto M et al. Direct sequencing of a novel DPB1 allele (DPB1*5101) of the heterozygote from the membrane of reverse dot blot analysis. Tissue Antigens 1994; 44:204-7.
486. Argyris EG, Gibson CF, Cizman B et al. Identification of a new HLA-DPB1 allele (DPB1*5101) by oligotyping and nucleotide sequencing. Immunogenetics 1994; 40:164.
487. Schnittger L, Aldrich C, Spauke D et al. DPB1*5101—a novel DPB1*0402-related allele in west Africa affects DPB1 genotyping. Tissue Antigens 1994; 44:59-62.
488. Mersch G, Mytilineos J, De Canck I et al. Characterization of a new DPB1 allele (DPB1*5701) isolated from a Caucasian individual. Tissue Antigens 1995; 46:208-12.
489. Versluis LF, Daly LN, Degli-Eposti MA et al. Identification of the novel HLA-DPB1*5801 allele detected by sequenced based typing. Immunogenetics 1995; 41:173.
490. Naughton MJ, Limm TM, Ashdown ML et al. DPB1 locus PCR-RFLP typing of the fourth Asia-Oceania histocompatibility workshop cell panel reveals a novel DPB1 allele. Eur J Immunogenetics 1994; 21:351-64.
491. Noble JA, Cavalli AS, Erlich HA. DPB1 *5901: A novel HLA-DPB1 allele from a caucasian IDDM family. Tissue Antigens 1996; 47:159-62.
492. Noreen H, Steiner L, Davidson M et al. Six new DPB1 alleles identified in a study of 1,302 unrelated bone marrow donor-recipient pairs. Tissue Antigens 1997; 49:512-6.
493. Zimmermann PA, Steiner LL, Titanji VPK et al. Three new DPB1 alleles identified in a Bantu-speaking population in central Cameroon. Tissue Antigens 1996; 47:293-9.
494. Steiner LL, McCurdy DK, Cavalli A et al. Two new DPB1 alleles identified in a study of the genetics of susceptibility to pauciarticular juvenile rheumatoid arthritis. Tissue Antigens 1997; 49 Part 1:262-6.
495. Versluis LF, Phillipe M, van den Zwan A et al. Identification of a new HLA-DPB1*6501 allele in a Caucasian individual. Immunogenetics 1996; 44:483-4.
496. Schnittger L, May J, Kretschmer C et al. DPB1*BR—an MHC class II DPB1 allele (DPB1*6601) of negroid origin. Immunogenetics 1996; 44:405-6.
497. Meyer CG, May J, Simon C et al. DPB1 *TF, a novel HLA class II DPB1 allele identified in a Turkish family. Tissue Antigens 1996; 48:231-2.
498. Cresswell P, Androlewicz MJ, Ortmann B. Assembly and transport of class I MHC-peptide complexes. Ciba Found Symp 1994; 187:150-69.
499. Saper MA, Bjorkman PJ, Wiley DC. Refined structure of the human histocompatibility antigen HLA-A2 at 2.6 Å resolution. J Mol Biol 1991; 219:277-319.
500. Hughes AL, Nei M. Pattern of nucleotide substitution at major histocompatibility complex class I loci reveals overdominant selection. Nature 1988; 335:167-70.
501. Hughes AL, Nei M. Maintenance of MHC polymorphism. Nature 1992; 355:402-3.

502. Hughes AL, Nei M. Evolutionary relationships of the classes of major histocompatibility complex genes. Immunogenetics 1993; 37:337-46.
503. Hughes AL, Nei M. Models of host-parasite interaction and MHC polymorphism. Genetics 1992; 132: 863-4.
504. Wakeland EK, Boehme S, She JX. The generation and maintenance of MHC class II gene polymorphism in rodents. Immunol Rev 1990; 113:207-26.
505. Okada K, Boss JM, Prentice H et al. Gene organization of DC and DX subregions of the human major histocompatibility complex. Proc Natl Acad Sci U S A 1985; 82:3410-4.
506. Lawlor DA, Zemmour J, Ennis PD et al. Evolution of class-I MHC genes and proteins: from natural selection to thymic selection. Annu Rev Immunol 1990; 8:23-63.
507. Riley EM, Olerup O, Bennett S et al. MHC and malaria: the relationship between HLA class II alleles and immune responses to Plasmodium falciparum. Int Immunol 1992; 4:1055-63.
508. Hill AV. Genetic susceptibility to malaria and other infectious diseases: from the MHC to the whole genome. Parasitology 1996; 112 Suppl:s75-84.
509. Riley EM. The role of MHC- and non-MHC-associated genes in determining the human immune response to malaria antigens. Parasitology 1996; 112 Suppl:s39-51.
510. Klein J. Origin of major histocompatibility complex polymorphism: the trans-species hypothesis. Hum Immunol 1987; 19:155-62.
511. Ciccone E, Colonna M, Viale O et al. Susceptibility or resistance to lysis by alloreactive natural killer cells is governed by a gene in the human major histocompatibility complex between BF and HLA-B [published erratum appears in Proc Natl Acad Sci USA 1991; 88: 5477]. Proc Natl Acad Sci USA 1990; 87:9794-7.
512. Grossberger D, Hein W, Marcuz A. Class I major histocompatibility complex cDNA clones from sheep thymus: alternative splicing could make a long cytoplasmic tail. Immunogenetics 1990; 32:77-87.
513. Salter-Cid L, Flajnik MF. Evolution and developmental regulation of the major histocompatibility complex. Crit Rev Immunol 1995; 15:31-75.
514. Bjorkman PJ, Parham P. Structure, function, and diversity of class I major histocompatibility complex molecules. Annu Rev Biochem 1990; 59:253-88.
515. Geraghty DE, Koller BH, Hansen JA et al. The HLA class I gene family includes at least six genes and twelve pseudogenes and gene fragments. J Immunol 1992; 149:1934-46.
516. Houlihan JM, Biro PA, Fergar Payne A et al. Evidence for the expression of non-HLA-A,-B,-C class I genes in the human fetal liver. J Immunol 1992; 149:668-75.
517. Koller BH, Geraghty DE, DeMars R et al. Chromosomal organization of the human major histocompatibility complex class I gene family [published erratum appears in J Exp Med 1989; 169:1517]. J Exp Med 1989; 169:469-80.
518. el Kahloun A, Vernet C, Jouanolle AM et al. A continuous restriction map from HLA-E to HLA-F. Structural comparison between different HLA-A haplotypes. Immunogenetics 1992; 35:183-9.
519. Shawar SM, Vyas JM, Rodgers JR et al. Antigen presentation by major histocompatibility complex class I-B molecules. Annu Rev Immunol 1994; 12:839-80.
520. Bahram S, Bresnahan M, Geraghty DE et al. A second lineage of mammalian major histocompatibility complex class I genes. Proc Natl Acad Sci U S A 1994; 91:6259-63.
521. Geraghty DE, Wei XH, Orr HT et al. Human leukocyte antigen F (HLA-F). An expressed HLA gene composed of a class I coding sequence linked to a novel transcribed repetitive element. J Exp Med 1990; 171:1-18.
522. Koller BH, Geraghty DE, Shimizu Y et al. HLA-E. A novel HLA class I gene expressed in resting T lymphocytes. J Immunol 1988; 141:897-904.
523. Ulbrecht M, Kellermann J, Johnson JP et al. Impaired intracellular transport and cell surface expression of nonpolymorphic HLA-E: evidence for inefficient peptide binding. J Exp Med 1992; 176: 1083-90.
524. Bahram S, Arnold D, Bresnahan M et al. Two putative subunits of a peptide pump

encoded in the human major histocompatibility complex class II region. Proc Natl Acad Sci U S A 1991; 88: 10094-8.
525. Bahram S, Mizuki N, Inoko H et al. Nucleotide sequence of the human MHC class I MICA gene. Immunogenetics 1996; 44:80-1.
526. Bahram S, Spies T. Nucleotide sequence of a human MHC class I MICB cDNA. Immunogenetics 1996; 43:230-3.
527. Malissen M, Malissen B, Jordan BR. Exon/intron organization and complete nucleotide sequence of an HLA gene. Proc Natl Acad Sci U S A 1982; 79:893-7.
528. Fodil N, Laloux L, Wanner V et al. Allelic repertoire of the human MHC class I MICA gene. Immunogenetics 1996; 44:351-7.
529. Pham Dinh D, Jones EP, Pitiot G et al. Physical mapping of the human and mouse MOG gene at the distal end of the MHC class Ib region. Immunogenetics 1995; 42:386-91.
530. Pham Dinh D, Mattei MG, Nussbaum JL et al. Myelin/oligodendrocyte glycoprotein is a member of a subset of the immunoglobulin superfamily encoded within the major histocompatibility complex. Proc Natl Acad Sci U S A 1993; 90:7990-4.
531. Steinman L. Connections between the immune system and the nervous system. Proc Natl Acad Sci USA 1993; 90:7912-4.
532. Gardinier MV, Amiguet P, Linington C et al. Myelin/oligodendrocyte glycoprotein is a unique member of the immunoglobulin superfamily. J Neurosci Res 1992; 33:177-87.
533. Roth MP, Malfroy L, Offer C et al. The human myelin oligodendrocyte glycoprotein (MOG) gene: complete nucleotide sequence and structural characterization. Genomics 1995; 28:241-50.
534. Guillemot F, Billault A, Auffray C. Physical linkage of a guanine nucleotide-binding protein-related gene to the chicken major histocompatibility complex. Proc Natl Acad Sci U S A 1989; 86:4594-8.
535. Kaufman J, Salomonsen J, Skjodt K. B-G cDNA clones have multiple small repeats and hybridize to both chicken MHC regions. Immunogenetics 1989; 30:440-51.
536. Kaufman J, Salomonsen J. B-G: we know what it is, but what does it do? Immunol Today 1992; 13:1-3.
537. Kaufman J, Skjodt K, Salomonsen J. The B-G multigene family of the chicken major histocompatibility complex. Crit Rev Immunol 1991; 11:113-43.
538. Vernet C, Ribouchon MT, Chimini G et al. Structure and evolution of a member of a new subfamily of GTP-binding proteins mapping to the human MHC class I region. Mamm Genome 1994; 5:100-5.
539. Guillaudeux T, Mattei MG, Depetris D et al. In situ hybridization localizes the human OTF3 to chromosome 6p21.3—>p22 and OTF3L to 12p13. Cytogenet Cell Genet 1993; 63:212-4.
540. Crouau Roy B, Amadou C, Bouissou C et al. Localization of the OTF3 gene within the human MHC class I region by physical and meiotic mapping. Genomics 1994; 21:241-3.
541. Wei H, Fan WF, Xu H et al. Genes in one megabase of the HLA class I region. Proc Natl Acad Sci USA 1993; 90: 11870-4.
542. Chu TW, Capossela A, Coleman R et al. Cloning of a new "finger" protein gene (ZNF173) within the class I region of the human MHC. Genomics 1995; 29: 229-39.
543. el Kahloun A, Chauvel B, Mauvieux V et al. Localization of seven new genes around the HLA-A locus. Hum Mol Genet 1993; 2:55-60.
544. Goei VL, Parimoo S, Capossela A et al. Isolation of novel non-HLA gene fragments from the hemochromatosis region (6p21.3) by cDNA hybridization selection. Am J Hum Genet 1994; 54:244-51.
545. Chien YH, Davis MM. How alpha beta T-cell receptors 'see' peptide/MHC complexes. Immunol Today 1993; 14: 597-602.
546. David-Watine B, Israel A, Kourilsky P. The regulation and expression of MHC class I genes. Immunol Today 1990; 11:286-92.
547. Ting JP, Baldwin AS. Regulation of MHC gene expression. Curr Opin Immunol 1993; 5:8-16.
548. Tatake RJ, Zeff RA. Regulated expression of the major histocompatibility complex class I genes. Proc Soc Exp Biol Med 1993; 203:405-17.

549. Benoist C, Mathis D. Regulation of major histocompatibility complex class-II genes: X, Y and other letters of the alphabet. Annu Rev Immunol 1990; 8: 681-715.
550. Glimcher LH, Kara CJ. Sequences and factors: a guide to MHC class-II transcription. Annu Rev Immunol 1992; 10:13-49.
551. Kara CJ, Liou HC, Ivashkiv LB et al. A cDNA for a human cyclic AMP response element-binding protein which is distinct from CREB and expressed preferentially in brain. Mol Cell Biol 1990; 10:1347-57.
552. Dey A, Thornton AM, Lonergan M et al. Occupancy of upstream regulatory sites in vivo coincides with major histocompatibility complex class I gene expression in mouse tissues. Mol Cell Biol 1992; 12:3590-9.
553. Miyazaki J, Appella E, Ozato K. Negative regulation of the major histocompatibility class I gene in undifferentiated embryonal carcinoma cells. Proc Natl Acad Sci U S A 1986; 83:9537-41.
554. Flanagan JR, Murata M, Burke PA et al. Negative regulation of the major histocompatibility complex class I promoter in embryonal carcinoma cells. Proc Natl Acad Sci U S A 1991; 88:3145-9.
555. Ehrlich R, Maguire JE, Singer DS. Identification of negative and positive regulatory elements associated with a class I major histocompatibility complex gene. Mol Cell Biol 1988; 8:695-703.
556. Katoh S, Ozawa K, Kondoh S et al. Identification of sequences responsible for positive and negative regulation by E1A in the promoter of H-2K^{bm1} class I MHC gene. EMBO J 1990; 9:127-35.
557. Nagata T, Segars JH, Levi BZ et al. Retinoic acid-dependent transactivation of major histocompatibility complex class I promoters by the nuclear hormone receptor H-2RIIBP in undifferentiated embryonal carcinoma cells. Proc Natl Acad Sci U S A 1992; 89:937-41.
558. Marks MS, Hallenbeck PL, Nagata T et al. H-2RIIBP (RXR beta) heterodimerization provides a mechanism for combinatorial diversity in the regulation of retinoic acid and thyroid hormone responsive genes. EMBO J 1992; 11: 1419-35.
559. Hamada K, Gleason SL, Levi BZ et al. H-2RIIBP, a member of the nuclear hormone receptor superfamily that binds to both the regulatory element of major histocompatibility class I genes and the estrogen response element. Proc Natl Acad Sci U S A 1989; 86:8289-93.
560. Sugita K, Miyazaki J, Appella E et al. Interferons increase transcription of a major histocompatibility class I gene via a 5' interferon consensus sequence. Mol Cell Biol 1987; 7:2625-30.
561. Korber B, Hood L, Stroynowski I. Regulation of murine class I genes by interferons is controlled by regions located both 5' and 3' to the transcription initiation site. Proc Natl Acad Sci U S A 1987; 84:3380-4.
562. Bikoff EK, Jaffe L, Ribaudo RK et al. MHC class I surface expression in embryo-derived cell lines inducible with peptide or interferon. Nature 1991; 354:235-8.
563. Trowsdale J, Hanson I, Mockridge I et al. Sequences encoded in the class II region of the MHC related to the 'ABC' superfamily of transporters. Nature 1990; 348:741-4.
564. Goldberg AL, Rock KL. Proteolysis, proteasomes and antigen presentation. Nature 1992; 357:375-9.
565. Wan YJ, Orrison BM, Lieberman R et al. Induction of major histocompatibility class I antigens by interferons in undifferentiated F9 cells. J Cell Physiol 1987; 130:276-83.
566. Hanson I, Ragoussis J, Trowsdale J. Organization of the human HLA-class-II region. Int J Cancer Suppl 1991; 6:18-9.
567. Hanson IM, Poustka A, Trowsdale J. New genes in the class II region of the human major histocompatibility complex. Genomics 1991; 10:417-24.
568. Howard JC. Supply and transport of peptides presented by class I MHC molecules. Curr Opin Immunol 1995; 7: 69-76.
569. Klein D, Ono H, O'hUigin C et al. Extensive MHC variability in cichlid fishes of Lake Malawi. Nature 1993; 364:330-4.
570. Trowsdale J. "Both man & bird & beast": comparative organization of MHC genes. Immunogenetics 1995; 41:1-17.
571. Stern LJ, Brown JH, Jardetzky TS et al.

Crystal structure of the human class II MHC protein HLA-DR1 complexed with an influenza virus peptide. Nature 1994; 368:215-21.
572. Campbell RD, Trowsdale J. Map of the human MHC. Immunol Today 1993; 14:349-52.
573. Boss JM, Mengler R, Okada K et al. Sequence analysis of the human major histocompatibility gene SX alpha. Mol Cell Biol 1985; 5:2677-83.
574. Servenius B, Gustafsson K, Widmark E et al. Molecular map of the human HLA-SB (HLA-DP) region and sequence of an SB alpha (DP alpha) pseudogene. EMBO J 1984; 3:3209-14.
575. Young JA, Trowsdale J. A processed pseudogene in an intron of the HLA-DP beta 1 chain gene is a member of the ribosomal protein L32 gene family. Nucleic Acids Res 1985; 13:8883-91.
576. Young JA, Trowsdale J. The HLA-DNA (DZA) gene is correctly expressed as a 1.1 kb mature mRNA transcript. Immunogenetics 1990; 31:386-8.
577. Karlsson L, Peterson PA. The alpha chain gene of H-2O has an unexpected location in the major histocompatibility complex. J Exp Med 1992; 176:477-83.
578. Karlsson L, Surh CD, Sprent J et al. A novel class II MHC molecule with unusual tissue distribution. Nature 1991; 351:485-8.
579. Trowsdale J, Kelly A. The human HLA class II alpha chain gene DZ alpha is distinct from genes in the DP, DQ and DR subregions. EMBO J 1985; 4:2231-7.
580. Kelly AP, Monaco JJ, Cho SG et al. A new human HLA class II-related locus, DM. Nature 1991; 353:571-3.
581. Shaman J, von Scheven E, Morris P et al. Analysis of HLA-DMB mutants and -DMB genomic structure. Immunogenetics 1995; 41:117-24.
582. Radley E, Alderton RP, Kelly A et al. Genomic organization of HLA-DMA and HLA-DMB. Comparison of the gene organization of all six class II families in the human major histocompatibility complex. J Biol Chem 1994; 269:18834-8.
583. Carrington M, Yeager M, Mann D. Characterization of HLA-DMB polymorphism. Immunogenetics 1993; 38:446-9.
584. Sanderson F, Powis SH, Kelly AP et al. Limited polymorphism in HLA-DM does not involve the peptide binding groove. Immunogenetics 1994; 39:56-8.
585. Kern I, Steimle V, Siegrist CA et al. The two novel MHC class II transactivators RFX5 and CIITA both control expression of HLA-DM genes. Int Immunol 1995; 7:1295-9.
586. Chang CH, Flavell RA. Class II transactivator regulates the expression of multiple genes involved in antigen presentation. J Exp Med 1995; 181:765-7.
587. Kropshofer H, Hämmerling GJ, Vogt AB. How HLA-DM edits the MHC class II peptide repertoire: survival of the fittest? Immunol Today 1997; 18:77-82.
588. Cho S, Attaya M, Brown MG et al. A cluster of transcribed sequences between the Pb and Ob genes of the murine major histocompatibility complex. Proc Natl Acad Sci U S A 1991; 88:5197-201.
589. Hermel E, Yuan J, Monaco JJ. Characterization of polymorphism within the H2-M MHC class II loci. Immunogenetics 1995; 42:136-42.
590. Walter W, Loos M, Maeurer MJ. H2-M polymorphism in mice susceptible to collagen-induced arthritis involves the peptide binding groove. Immunogenetics 1996; 44:19-26.
591. Hermel E, Monaco JJ. RT1.DMa and RT1.DMb: the rat homologues of H2-DMa and H2-DMb. Immunogenetics 1995; 42:446-7.
592. Beck S, Hanson I, Kelly A et al. A homologue of the Drosophila female sterile homeotic (fsh) gene in the class II region of the human MHC. DNA Seq 1992; 2:203-10.
593. Salter-Cid L, Du Pasquier L, Flajnik M. RING3 is linked to the Xenopus major histocompatibility complex. Immunogenetics 1996; 44:397-9.
594. Beck S, Kelly A, Radley E et al. DNA sequence analysis of 66 kb of the human MHC class II region encoding a cluster of genes for antigen processing. J Mol Biol 1992; 228:433-41.
595. Glynne R, Powis SH, Beck S et al. A proteasome-related gene between the two ABC transporter loci in the class II region of the human MHC. Nature 1991; 353:357-60.
596. Monaco JJ. Genes in the MHC that may

affect antigen processing. Curr Opin Immunol 1992; 4:70-3.
597. Martinez CK, Monaco JJ. Post-translational processing of a major histocompatibility complex-encoded proteasome subunit, LMP-2. Mol Immunol 1993; 30:1177-83.
598. Kelly A, Powis SH, Glynne R et al. Second proteasome-related gene in the human MHC class II region. Nature 1991; 353:667-8.
599. Glynne R, Kerr LA, Mockridge I et al. The major histocompatibility complex-encoded proteasome component LMP7: alternative first exons and post-translational processing. Eur J Immunol 1993; 23:860-6.
600. Powis SH, Tonks S, Mockridge I et al. Alleles and haplotypes of the MHC-encoded ABC transporters TAP1 and TAP2 [published erratum appears in Immunogenetics 1993; 37: 480]. Immunogenetics 1993; 37:373-80.
601. Powis SH, Mockridge I, Kelly A et al. Polymorphism in a second ABC transporter gene located within the class II region of the human major histocompatibility complex. Proc Natl Acad Sci U S A 1992; 89:1463-7.
602. Belich MP, Glynne RJ, Senger G et al. Proteasome components with reciprocal expression to that of the MHC-encoded LMP proteins. Curr Biol 1994; 4:769-76.
603. Carrington M, Colonna M, Spies T et al. Haplotypic variation of the transporter associated with antigen processing (TAP) genes and their extension of HLA class II region haplotypes. Immunogenetics 1993; 37:266-73.
604. Cerundolo V, Kelly A, Elliott T et al. Genes encoded in the major histocompatibility complex affecting the generation of peptides for TAP transport [published erratum appears in Eur J Immunol 1995; 25:1485]. Eur J Immunol 1995; 25:554-62.
605. Kelly A, Powis SH, Kerr LA et al. Assembly and function of the two ABC transporter proteins encoded in the human major histocompatibility complex. Nature 1992; 355:641-4.
606. Belich MP, Trowsdale J. Proteasome and class I antigen processing and presentation. Mol Biol Rep 1995; 21:53-6.
607. Martinez CK, Monaco JJ. Homology of proteasome subunits to a major histocompatibility complex-linked LMP gene. Nature 1991; 353:664-7.
608. Zhou P, Zanelli E, Smart M et al. Genomic organization and tissue expression of mouse proteasome gene Lmp-2. Genomics 1993; 16:664-8.
609. Zanelli E, Zhou P, Cao H et al. Genetic polymorphism of the mouse major histocompatibility complex-associated proteasome subunit Lmp7. Immunogenetics 1995; 41:251-4.
610. Spies T, Bresnahan M, Bahram S et al. A gene in the human major histocompatibility complex class II region controlling the class I antigen presentation pathway. Nature 1990; 348: 744-7.
611. Monaco JJ, Cho S, Attaya M. Transport protein genes in the murine MHC: possible implications for antigen processing. Science 1990; 250:1723-6.
612. Androlewicz MJ, Cresswell P. How selective is the transporter associated with antigen processing? Immunity 1996; 5:1-5.
613. Momburg F, Roelse J, Hammerling GJ et al. Peptide size selection by the major histocompatibility complex-encoded peptide transporter. J Exp Med 1994; 179: 1613-23.
614. Momburg F, Roelse J, Howard JC et al. Selectivity of MHC-encoded peptide transporters from human, mouse and rat. Nature 1994; 367:648-51.
615. Attaya M, Jameson S, Martinez CK et al. Ham-2 corrects the class I antigen-processing defect in RMA-S cells. Nature 1992; 355:647-9.
616. Fruh K, Gossen M, Wang K et al. Displacement of housekeeping proteasome subunits by MHC-encoded LMPs: a newly discovered mechanism for modulating the multicatalytic proteinase complex. EMBO J 1994; 13:3236-44.
617. Akiyama K, Yokota K, Kagawa S et al. cDNA cloning and interferon gamma down-regulation of proteasomal subunits X and Y. Science 1994; 265:1231-4.
618. Daar AS, Fuggle SV, Fabre JW et al. The detailed distribution of MHC Class II antigens in normal human organs. Transplantation 1984; 38:293-8.
619. Seidl C, Saraiya C, Osterweil Z et al.

Genetic complexity of regulatory mutants defective for HLA class II gene expression. J Immunol 1992; 148:1576-84.
620. Sültmann H, Mayer WE, Figueroa F et al. Zebrafish Mhc class II alpha chain-encoding genes: polymorphism, expression, and function. Immunogenetics 1993; 38:408-20.
621. Sültmann H, Mayer WE, Figueroa F et al. Organization of Mhc class II B genes in the zebrafish (Brachydanio rerio). Genomics 1994; 23:1-14.
622. Brown AM, Wright KL, Ting JPY. Human major histocompatibility complex class II-associated invariant chain gene promoter. Functional analysis and in vivo protein/DNA interactions of constitutive and IFN-gamma-induced expression. J Biol Chem 1993; 268:26328-33.
623. Guardiola J, Maffei A. Control of MHC class II gene expression in autoimmune, infectious, and neoplastic diseases. Crit Rev Immunol 1993; 13:247-68.
624. Sloan JH, Hasegawa SL, Boss JM. Single base pair substitutions within the HLA-DRA gene promoter separate the functions of the X1 and X2 boxes. J Immunol 1992; 148:2591-9.
625. Reith W, Ucla C, Barras E et al. RFX1, a transactivator of hepatitis B virus enhancer I, belongs to a novel family of homodimeric and heterodimeric DNA-binding proteins. Mol Cell Biol 1994; 14:1230-44.
626. van Huijsduijnen RH, Li XY, Black D et al. Co-evolution from yeast to mouse: cDNA cloning of the two NF-Y (CP-1/CBF) subunits. EMBO J 1990; 9:3119-27.
627. Hasegawa SL, Boss JM. Two B-cell factors bind the HLA-DRA X box region and recognize different subsets of HLA class II promoters. Nucleic Acids Res 1991; 19:6269-76.
628. Moreno CS, Emery P, West JE et al. Purified X2 binding protein (X2BP) cooperatively binds the class II MHC X box in the presence of purified RFX, the X box factor deficient in the bare lymphocyte syndrome. J Immunol 1995; 155: 4313-21.
629. Mach B, Steimle V, Martinez-Soria E et al. Regulation of MHC class II genes: Lessons from a Disease. Ann Rev Immunol 1996; 14:301-31.
630. Steimle V, Siegrist CA, Mottet A et al. Regulation of MHC class II expression by interferon-gamma mediated by the transactivator gene CIITA. Science 1994; 265:106-9.
631. Steimle V, Mach B. Complementation cloning of mammalian transcriptional regulators: the example of MHC class II gene regulators. Curr Opin Genet Dev 1995; 5:646-51.
632. Mach B, Steimle V, Reith W. MHC class II-deficient combined immunodeficiency: a disease of gene regulation. Immunol Rev 1994; 138:207-21.
633. Riley JL, Westerheide SD, Price JA et al. Activation of class II MHC genes requires both the X box region and the class II transactivator (CIITA). Immunity 1995; 2:533-43.
634. Chang CH, Fontes JD, Peterlin M et al. Class II transactivator (CIITA) is sufficient for the inducible expression of major histocompatibility complex class II genes. J Exp Med 1994; 180:1367-74.
635. Lennon A, Ottone C, Rigaud G et al. Isolation of a B-cell-specific promotor for the human class II transactivator. Immunogenetics 1997; 45:266-73.
636. Martinez-Soria E, Siegrist CA, Mach B. Highly efficient peptide binding and T cell activation by MHC class II molecules of CIITA-transfected cells. Int Immunol 1996; 8:543-9.
637. Sims TN, Elliott JF, Ramassar V et al. Mouse class II transactivator: cDNA sequence and amino acid comparison with the human class II transactivator. Immunogenetics 1997; 45:220-2.
638. Nepom GT, Erlich H. MHC class-II molecules and autoimmunity. Annu Rev Immunol 1991; 9:493-525.
639. Andersen LC, Beaty JS, Nettles JW et al. Allelic polymorphism in transcriptional regulatory regions of HLA-DQB genes. J Exp Med 1991; 173:181-92.
640. Woolfrey AE, Andersen LC, Shewey L et al. Analysis of differential HLA-DQB expression in autologous B cell lines. J Leukoc Biol 1993; 53:697-706.
641. Louis P, Vincent R, Cavadore P et al. Differential transcriptional activities of HLA-DR genes in the various haplotypes. J Immunol 1994; 153:5059-67.
642. Vincent R, Louis P, Gongora C et al.

Quantitative analysis of the expression of the HLA-DRB genes at the transcriptional level by competitive polymerase chain reaction. J Immunol 1996; 156: 603-10.
643. Symington FW, Levine F, Braun M et al. Differential Ia antigen expression by autologous human erythroid and B lymphoblastoid cell lines. J Immunol 1985; 135:1026-32.
644. Lee JS. Regulation of HLA class II gene expression. In:Dupont B, ed. Immunology of HLA, Vol II. New York: Springer-Verlag, 1989:49-61.
645. Morzycka-Wroblewska E, Harwood JI, Smith JR et al. Structure and evolution of the promoter regions of the DQA genes. Immunogenetics 1993; 37:364-72.
646. Dorn A, Benoist C, Mathis D. New B-lymphocyte-specific enhancer-binding protein. Mol Cell Biol 1989; 9:312-20.
647. Morzycka-Wroblewska E, Munshi A, Ostermayer M et al. Differential expression of HLA-DQA1 alleles associated with promoter polymorphisms. Immunogenetics 1997; 45:163-70.
648. Newell WR, Trowsdale J, Beck S. MHCDB—database of the human MHC. Immunogenetics 1994; 40:109-15.
649. Globerman H, Amor M, Parker KL et al. Nonsense mutation causing steroid 21-hydroxylase deficiency. J Clin Invest 1988; 82:139-44.
650. Higashi Y, Tanae A, Inoue H et al. Evidence for frequent gene conversion in the steroid 21-hydroxylase P-450(C21) gene: implications for steroid 21-hydroxylase deficiency. Am J Hum Genet 1988; 42:17-25.
651. Kawaguchi H, O'hUigin C, Klein J. In: Klein J, Klein D, eds.Molecular Evolution of the Major Histocompatibility Complex. Berlin, Heidelberg: Springer-Verlag; 1991:357-81.
652. Carroll MC, Campbell RD, Porter RR. Mapping of steroid 21-hydroxylase genes adjacent to complement component C4 genes in HLA, the major histocompatibility complex in man. Proc Natl Acad Sci USA 1985; 82:521-5.
653. Spies T, Morton CC, Nedospasov SA et al. Genes for the tumor necrosis factors alpha and beta are linked to the human major histocompatibility complex. Proc Natl Acad Sci U S A 1986; 83:8699-702.
654. Higashi Y, Yoshioka H, Yamane M et al. Complete nucleotide sequence of two steroid 21-hydroxylase genes tandemly arranged in human chromosome: a pseudogene and a genuine gene. Proc Natl Acad Sci U S A 1986; 83:2841-5.
655. Higashi Y, Tanae A, Inoue H et al. Aberrant splicing and missense mutations cause steroid 21-hydroxylase [P-450 (C21)] deficiency in humans: possible gene conversion products. Proc Natl Acad Sci U S A 1988; 85:7486-90.
656. Sottrup-Jensen L, Stepanik TM, Kristensen T et al. Common evolutionary origin of alpha 2-macroglobulin and complement components C3 and C4. Proc Natl Acad Sci U S A 1985; 82:9-13.
657. Carroll MC, Alper CA. Polymorphism and molecular genetics of human C4. Br Med Bull 1987; 43:50-65.
658. Prentice HL, Schneider PM, Strominger JL. C4B gene polymorphism detected in a human cosmid clone. Immunogenetics 1986; 23:274-6.
659. Yu CY, Belt KT, Giles CM et al. Structural basis of the polymorphism of human complement components C4A and C4B: gene size, reactivity and antigenicity. EMBO J 1986; 5:2873-81.
660. So AK, Fielder AH, Warner CA et al. DNA polymorphism of major histocompatibility complex class II and class III genes in systemic lupus erythematosus. Tissue Antigens 1990; 35:144-7.
661. Raum D, Glass D, Carpenter CB et al. Mapping of the structural gene for the second component of complement with respect to the human major histocompatibility complex. Am J Hum Genet 1979; 31:35-41.
662. Dunham I, Sargent CA, Trowsdale J et al. Molecular mapping of the human major histocompatibility complex by pulsed-field gel electrophoresis. Proc Natl Acad Sci U S A 1987; 84:7237-41.
663. Campbell RD, Porter RR. Molecular cloning and characterization of the gene coding for human complement protein factor B. Proc Natl Acad Sci U S A 1983; 80:4464-8.
664. Ruddle NH. Activation of human poly-

morphonuclear neutrophil functions by interferon-gamma and tumor necrosis factors. J Immunol 1986; 136: 2335-6.
665. Kehrl JH, Alvarez Mon M, Delsing GA et al. Lymphotoxin is an important T cell-derived growth factor for human B cells. Science 1987; 238:1144-6.
666. Levi-Strauss M, Carroll MC, Steinmetz M et al. A previously undetected MHC gene with an unusual periodic structure. Science 1988; 240:201-4.
667. Speiser PW, White PC. Structure of the human RD gene: a highly conserved gene in the class III region of the major histocompatibility complex. DNA 1989; 8:745-51.
668. Harrison GS, Drabkin HA, Kao FT et al. Chromosomal location of human genes encoding major heat-shock protein HSP70. Somat Cell Mol Genet 1987; 13:119-30.
669. Sargent CA, Dunham I, Trowsdale J et al. Human major histocompatibility complex contains genes for the major heat shock protein HSP70. Proc Natl Acad Sci U S A 1989; 86:1968-72.
670. Moseley WS, Watson ML, Kingsmore SF et al. CD1 defines conserved linkage group border between human chromosomes 1 and mouse chromosomes 1 and 3. Immunogenetics 1989; 30:378-82.
671. Yu CY, Wu LC, Buluwela L et al. Cosmid cloning and walking to map human CD1 leukocyte differentiation antigen genes. Methods Enzymol 1993; 217: 378-98.
672. Martin LH, Calabi F, Lefebvre FA et al. Structure and expression of the human thymocyte antigens CD1a, CD1b, and CD1c. Proc Natl Acad Sci U S A 1987; 84:9189-93.
673. Aida Y, Kohda C, Morooka A et al. Cloning of cDNAs and the molecular evolution of a bovine MHC class II DRA gene. Biochem Biophys Res Commun 1994; 204:195-202.
674. Beckman EM, Porcelli SA, Morita CT et al. Recognition of a lipid antigen by CD1-restricted alpha beta+ T cells. Nature 1994; 372:691-4.
675. Goodfellow PN, Jones EA, Van Heyningen V et al. The beta2-microglobulin gene is on chromosome 15 and not in the HL-A region. Nature 1975; 254: 267-9.
676. McAdam SN, Boyson JE, Liu X et al. Chimpanzee MHC class I A locus alleles are related to only one of the six families of human A locus alleles. J Immunol 1995; 154:6421-9.
677. Lawlor DA, Warren E, Taylor P et al. Gorilla class I major histocompatibility complex alleles: comparison to human and chimpanzee class I. J Exp Med 1991; 174:1491-509.
678. Lawlor DA, Warren E, Ward FE et al. Comparison of class I MHC alleles in humans and apes. Immunol Rev 1990; 113:147-85.
679. Miller MD, Yamamoto H, Hughes AL et al. Definition of an epitope and MHC class I molecule recognized by gag-specific cytotoxic T lumphocytes in SIV mac-infected rhesus monkeys. J Immunol 1991; 147:320-9.
680. Watkins DI, Letvin NL, Hughes AL et al. Molecular cloning of cDNA that encode MHC class I molecules from a New World primate (Saguinus oedipus). Natural selection acts at positions that may affect peptide presentation to T cells. J Immunol 1990; 144:1136-43.
681. Yuhki N, O'Brien SJ. DNA recombination and natural selection pressure sustain genetic sequence diversity of the feline MHC class I genes. J Exp Med 1990; 172:621-30.
682. Burnett RC, Geraghty DE. Structure and expression of a divergent canine class I gene. J Immunol 1995; 155:4278-85.
683. Ellis SA, Martin AJ, Holmes EC et al. At least four MHC class I genes are transcribed in the horse: phylogenetic analysis suggests an unusual evolutionary history for the MHC in this species. Eur J Immunogenet 1995; 22:249-60.
684. Frels WI, Bordallo C, Golding H et al. Expression of a class I MHC transgene: regulation by a tissue-specific negative regulatory DNA sequence element. New Biol 1990; 2:1024-33.
685. Tykocinski ML, Marche PN, Max EE et al. Rabbit class I MHC genes: cDNA clones define full-length transcripts of an expressed gene and a putative pseudogene. J Immunol 1984; 133: 2261-9.
686. Salgar SK, Sawai H, Kunz HW et al. Cloning and expression of the rat class I MHC gene RT1.Al. Immunogenetics 1994; 39:447

687. Duran LW, Horton RM, Birschbach CW et al. Structural relationships among the H-2 D-regions of murine MHC haplotypes. J Immunol 1989; 142:288-96.
688. Brown P, Spooner RL, Clark AJ. Cloning and characterization of a BoLA class I cDNA clone. Immunogenetics 1989; 29:58-60.
689. Wettstein PJ, Strausbauch M, Lamb T et al. Phylogeny of six Sciurus aberti subspecies based on nucleotide sequences of cytochrome b. Mol Phylogenet Evol 1995; 4:150-62.
690. Kroemer G, Zoorob R, Auffray C. Structure and expression of a chicken MHC class I gene. Immunogenetics 1990; 31:405-9.
691. Grossberger D, Parham P. Reptilian class I major histocompatibility complex genes reveal conserved elements in class I structure. Immunogenetics 1992; 36: 166-74.
692. Sammut B, Laurens V, Tournefier A. Isolation of MHC class I cDNAs from the axolotl Ambystoma mexicanum. Immunogenetics 1997; 45:285-94.
693. Flajnik MF, Kasahara M, Shum BP et al. A novel type of class I gene organization in vertebrates: a large family of non-MHC-linked class I genes is expressed at the RNA level in the amphibian Xenopus. EMBO J 1993; 12:4385-96.
694. Hashimoto K, Nakanishi T, Kurosawa Y. Isolation of carp genes encoding major histocompatibility complex antigens. Proc Natl Acad Sci U S A 1990; 87: 6863-7.
695. Eccles SJ, McMaster WR. DNA sequence analysis of a rat RT1 class II A beta gene. Immunogenetics 1985; 22:653-63.
696. Kenter M, Otting N, Anholts J et al. MHC-DRB diversity of the chimpanzee (Pan troglodytes). Immunogenetics 1992; 37:1-11.
697. Trtkova K, Mayer WE, O'hUigin C et al. MHC-DRB genes and the origin of New World monkeys. Mol Phylogenet Evol 1995; 4:408-19.
698. Zhu ZF, Vincek V, Figueroa F et al. Mhc-DRB genes of the pigtail macaque (Macaca nemestrina): implications for the evolution of human DRB genes. Mol Biol Evol 1991; 8:563-78.
699. Gaur LK, Nepom GT. Ancestral major histocompatibility complex DRB genes beget conserved patterns of localized polymorphisms. Proc Natl Acad Sci U S A 1996; 93:5380-3.
700. Figueroa F, O'hUigin C, Tichy H et al. The origin of the primate MHC-DRB genes and allelic lineages as deduced from the study of prosimians. J Immunol 1994; 152:4455-65.
701. Swarbrick PA, Schwaiger FW, Epplen JT et al. Cloning and sequencing of expressed DRB genes of the red deer (Cervus elaphus) MHC. Immunogenetics 1995; 42:1-9.
702. Gustafsson K, Andersson L. Structure and polymorphism of horse MHC class II DRB genes: convergent evolution in the antigen binding site. Immunogenetics 1994; 39:355-8.
703. Vage DI, Olsaker I, Lingaas F et al. Isolation and sequence determination of porcine class II DRB alleles amplified by PCR. Anim Genet 1994; 25:73-5.
704. Mikko S, Andersson L. Low major histocompatibility complex class II diversity in European and North American moose. Proc Natl Acad Sci U S A 1995; 92: 4259-63.
705. Fraser DC, Craigmile S, Campbell JD et al. Functional expression of a cattle MHC class II DR-like antigen on mouse L cells. Immunogenetics 1996; 43:296-303.
706. Ballingall KT, Dutia BM, Hopkins J et al. Analysis of the fine specificities of sheep major histocompatibility complex class II-specific monoclonal antibodies using mouse L-cell transfectants. Anim Genet 1995; 26:79-84.
707. Zoorob R, Bernot A, Renoir DM et al. Chicken major histocompatibility complex class II B genes: analysis of interallelic and interlocus sequence variance. Eur J Immunol 1993; 23:1139-45.
708. Kobari F, Sato K, Shum BP et al. Exon-intron organization of Xenopus MHC class II beta chain genes. Immunogenetics 1995; 42:376-85.
709. Schneider S, Vincek V, Tichy H et al. MHC class II genes of a marsupial, the red-necked wallaby (Macropus rufogriseus): identification of new gene families. Mol Biol Evol 1991; 8:753-66.
710. Edwards SV, Grahn M, Potts WK. Dynamics of MHC evolution in birds and

crocodilians: amplification of class II genes with degenerate primers. Mol Ecol 1995; 4:719-29.
711. van Erp SH, Dixon B, Figueroa F et al. Identification and characterization of a novel class I gene in carp (Cyprinus carpio L.). Immunogenetics 1996; 44: 49-61.
712. Miller KM, Withler RE. Sequence analysis of a polymorphic MHC class II gene in Pacific salmon. Immunogenetics 1996; 43:337-51.
713. Bohme J, Andersson M, Andersson G et al. HLA-DR beta genes vary in number between different DR specificities, whereas the number of DQ beta genes is constant. J Immunol 1985; 135:2149-55.
714. Kawai J, Ando A, Sato T et al. Analysis of gene structure and antigen determinants of DR2 antigens using DR gene transfer into mouse L cells. J Immunol 1989; 142:312-7.
715. Kasahara M, Klein D, Vincek V et al. Comparative anatomy of the primate major histocompatibility complex DR subregion: evidence for combinations of DRB genes conserved across species. Genomics 1992; 14:340-9.
716. Schönbach C, Vincek V, Mayer WE et al. Multiplication of MHC-DRB5 loci in the orangutan: implications for the evolution of DRB haplotypes. Mamm Genome 1993; 4:159-70.
717. Grahovać B, Mayer WE, Vincek V et al. Major-histocompatibility-complex DRB genes of a New-World monkey, the cottontop tamarin (Saguinus oedipus). Mol Biol Evol 1992; 9:403-16.
718. Brändle U, Ono H, Vincek V et al. Trans-species evolution of MHC-DRB haplotype polymorphism in primates: organization of DRB genes in the chimpanzee. Immunogenetics 1992; 36:39-48.
719. Grahovać B, Schönbach C, Brändle U et al. Conservative evolution of the Mhc-DP region in anthropoid primates. Hum Immunol 1993; 37:75-84.
720. Gasser DL, Sternberg NL, Pierce JC et al. P1 and cosmid clones define the organization of 280 kb of the mouse H-2 complex containing the Cps-1 and Hsp70 loci. Immunogenetics 1994; 39:48-55.
721. Kawaguchi H, Klein J. Organization of C4 and CYP21 loci in gorilla and orangutan. Hum Immunol 1992; 33:153-62.
722. Seeger A, Mayer WE, Klein J. A complement factor B-like cDNA clone from the zebrafish (Brachydanio rerio). Mol Immunol 1996; 33:511-20.
723. Trtkova K, Kupfermann H, Grahovać B et al. MHC-DRB genes of platyrrhine primates. Immunogenetics 1993; 38:210-22.
724. Marché PN, Tykocinski ML, Max EE et al. Structure of a functional rabbit class I MHC gene: similarity to human class I genes. Immunogenetics 1985; 21:71-82.
725. Sittisombut N, Mordacq J, Knight KL. Rabbit MHC. II. Sequence analysis of the R-DP alpha- and beta-genes. J Immunol 1988; 140:3237-43.
726. LeGuern C, Marché PN, Kindt TJ. Molecular evidence for five distinct MHC class II alpha genes in the rabbit. Immunogenetics 1985; 22:141-8.
727. Rebière MC, Marché PN, Kindt TJ. A rabbit class I major histocompatibility complex gene with a T cell-specific expression pattern. J Immunol 1987; 139: 2066-74.
728. Chouchane L, Brown TJ, Kindt TJ. Structure and expression of a nonpolymorphic rabbit class II gene with homology to HLA-DOB. Immunogenetics 1993; 38: 64-6.
729. Yuhki N, Heidecker GF, O'Brien SJ. Characterization of MHC cDNA clones in the domestic cat. Diversity and evolution of class I genes. J Immunol 1989; 142:3676-82.
730. Yuhki N, O'Brien SJ. Exchanges of short polymorphic DNA segments predating speciation in feline major histocompatibility complex class I genes. J Mol Evol 1994; 39:22-33.
731. Sarmiento UM, Storb R. Nucleotide sequence of a dog class I cDNA clone. Immunogenetics 1990; 31:400-4.
732. Sarmiento UM, Sarmiento JI, Storb R. Allelic variation in the DR subregion of the canine major histocompatibility complex. Immunogenetics 1990; 32:13-9.
733. Sarmiento UM, Storb R. Nucleotide sequence of a dog DRB cDNA clone. Immunogenetics 1990; 31:396-9.
734. Wettstein PJ, Lager P, Jin L et al. Phylogeny of mitochondrial DNA clones in

tassel-eared squirrels Sciurus aberti. Mol Ecol 1994; 3:541-50.
735. McGuire KL, Duncan WR, Tucker PW. Structure of a class I gene from Syrian hamster. J Immunol 1986; 137:366-72.
736. Ellegren H, Hartman G, Johansson M et al. Major histocompatibility complex monomorphism and low levels of DNA fingerprinting variability in a reintroduced and rapidly expanding population of beavers. Proc Natl Acad Sci U S A 1993; 90:8150-3.
737. Lafuse WP. Molecular biology of murine MHC class II genes. Crit Rev Immunol 1991; 11:167-94.
738. Hanson IM, Trowsdale J. Colinearity of novel genes in the class II regions of the MHC in mouse and human. Immunogenetics 1991; 34:5-11.
739. Weiss E, Golden L, Zakut R et al. The DNA sequence of the H-2K(b) gene: evidence for gene conversion as a mechanism for the generation of polymorphism in histocompatibility antigens. EMBO J 1983; 2:453-62.
740. Kvist S, Roberts L, Dobberstein B. Mouse histocompatibility genes: structure and organisation of a K^d gene. EMBO J 1983; 2:245-54.
741. Horton RM, Hildebrand WH, Martinko JM et al. Structural analysis of H-$2K^f$ and H-$2K^{fm1}$ by using H-2K locus-specific sequences. J Immunol 1990; 145: 1782-7.
742. Watts S, Vogel JM, Harriman WD et al. DNA sequence analysis of the C3H H-$2K^k$ and H-$2D^k$ loci. Evolutionary relationships to H-2 genes from four other mouse strains. J Immunol 1987; 139: 3878-85.
743. Jaulin C, Perrin A, Abastado JP et al. Polymorphism in mouse and human class I H-2 and HLA genes is not the result of random independent point mutations. Immunogenetics 1985; 22: 453-70.
744. Morita T, Delarbre C, Kress M et al. An H-2K gene of the tw32 mutant at the T/t complex is a close parent of an H-$2K^q$ gene. Immunogenetics 1985; 21:367-83.
745. Nairn R, Nathenson SG, Coligan JE. Amino acid sequence of cyanogen bromide fragment CN-C (residues 24-98) of the mouse histocompatibility antigen H-$2D^d$. A comparison of the amino-terminal 100 residues of H-$2D^d$, D^b, K^d, and K^b reveals discrete areas of diversity. Biochemistry 1981; 20:4739-45.
746. Cai ZL, Pease LR. An intragenic recombinant class I gene: H-$2D^{dx}$. Immunogenetics 1991; 34:273-6.
747. Hildebrand WH, Horton RM, Pease LR et al. Nucleotide sequence analysis of H-$2D^f$ and the spontaneous in vivo H-$2D^{fm2}$ mutation. Mol Immunol 1992; 29:61-9.
748. Schepart BS, Takahashi H, Cozad KM et al. The nucleotide sequence and comparative analysis of the H-$2D^p$ class I H-2 gene. J Immunol 1986; 136:3489-95.
749. Lee DR, Rubocki RJ, Lie WR et al. The murine MHC class I genes, H-$2D^q$ and H-$2L^q$, are strikingly homologous to each other, H-$2L^d$, and two genes reported to encode tumor-specific antigens. J Exp Med 1988; 168:1719-39.
750. Cai ZL, Pease LR. Locus-specific cDNA cloning in the class I multigene family: structure of H-$2D^r$ and H-$2D^s$. Immunogenetics 1990; 32:456-9.
751. Hemmi S, Geliebter J, Zeff RA et al. Three spontaneous H-$2D^b$ mutants are generated by genetic micro-recombination (gene conversion) events. Impact on the H-2-restricted immune responsiveness. J Exp Med 1988; 168:2319-35.
752. Lalanne JL, Transy C, Guerin S et al. Expression of class I genes in the major histocompatibility complex: identification of eight distinct mRNAs in DBA/2 mouse liver. Cell 1985; 41:469-78.
753. Lalanne JL, Cochet M, Kummer AM et al. Different exon-intron organization at the 5' part of a mouse class I gene is used to generate a novel H-$2K^d$-related mRNA. Proc Natl Acad Sci U S A 1983; 80:7561-5.
754. Lalanne JL, Delarbre C, Gachelin G et al. A cDNA clone containing the entire coding sequence of a mouse H-$2K^d$ histocompatibility antigen. Nucleic Acids Res 1983; 11:1567-77.
755. Moore KW, Sher BT, Sun YH et al. DNA sequence of a gene encoding a BALB/c mouse L^d transplantation antigen. Science 1982; 215:679-82.
756. Rubocki RJ, Lee DR, Lie WR et al. Molecular evidence that the H-2D and H-2L genes arose by duplication. Differences between the evolution of the class

I genes in mice and humans. J Exp Med 1990; 171:2043-61.
757. Matsumura M, Fremont DH, Peterson PA et al. Emerging principles for the recognition of peptide antigens by MHC class I molecules. Science 1992; 257:927-34.
758. Landais D, Matthes H, Benoist C et al. A molecular basis for the Ia.2 and Ia.19 antigenic determinants. Proc Natl Acad Sci U S A 1985; 82:2930-4.
759. Benoist CO, Mathis DJ, Kanter MR et al. The murine Ia alpha chains, E alpha and A alpha, show a surprising degree of sequence homology. Proc Natl Acad Sci U S A 1983; 80:534-8.
760. Mathis DJ, Benoist CO, Williams VE 2d et al. The murine E alpha immune response gene. Cell 1983; 32:745-54.
761. Hyldig-Nielsen JJ, Schenning L, Hämmerling U et al. The complete nucleotide sequence of the I-E alpha d immune response gene. Nucleic Acids Res 1983; 11:5055-71.
762. Kasahara M, Stojković I, Mayer WE et al. The nucleotide sequence of the mouse H-2E alpha w28 gene. Immunogenetics 1986; 24:324-7.
763. She JX, Boehme SA, Wang TW et al. Amplification of major histocompatibility complex class II gene diversity by intraexonic recombination. Proc Natl Acad Sci U S A 1991; 88:453-7.
764. Holmdahl R, Karlsson M, Andersson ME et al. Localization of a critical restriction site on the I-A beta chain that determines susceptibility to collagen-induced arthritis in mice. Proc Natl Acad Sci U S A 1989; 86:9475-9.
765. Malissen M, Hunkapillar T and Hood LE. Nucleotide sequence of light chain gene of the mouse I-A subregion.Aβ^d. Science 1983; 221:750-4.
766. Choi E, McIntyre K, Germain RN et al. Murine I-A beta chain polymorphism: nucleotide sequences of three allelic I-A beta genes. Science 1983; 221:283-6.
767. Estess P, Begovich AB, Koo M et al. Sequence analysis and structure-function correlation of murine q, k, u, s, and f haplotype I-A-beta cDNA clones. Proc Natl Acad Aci USA 1986;83:3594-8.
768. Ayane M, Mengle Gaw L, McDevitt HO et al. E alpha u and E beta u chain association: where lies the anomaly? J Immunol 1986; 137:948-51.
769. Ogawa S, Nishimura H, Awaji M et al. Nucleotide sequence analysis of MHC class II genes in autoimmune disease-prone (NZB x NZW)F1 mice. Immunogenetics 1990; 32:63-7.
770. Widera G, Flavell RA. The nucleotide sequence of the murine I-E beta b immune response gene: evidence for gene conversion events in class II genes of the major histocompatibility complex. EMBO J 1984; 3:1221-5.
771. Padgett KA, Shreffler DC, Saha BK. Molecular mapping of murine I region recombinants. III. Crossing over at two discrete sites within the beta 1-beta 2 intron of the E beta gene. J Immunol 1991; 147:2764-70.
772. King LB, Sharma S, Corley RB. Complete coding region sequence of E beta k cDNA clones: lack of polymorphism in the NH2-terminus between E beta k and E beta b molecules. J Immunogenet 1988; 15:209-14.
773. Braunstein NS, Germain RN. The mouse E beta 2 gene: a class II MHC beta gene with limited intraspecies polymorphism and an unusual pattern of transcription. EMBO J 1986; 5:2469-76.
774. Begovich AB, Vu TH, Jones PP. Characterization of the molecular defects in the mouse E beta f and E beta q genes. Implications for the origin of MHC polymorphism J Immunol 1990; 144:1957-64.
775. Wei BY, Cao H, Pan S et al. Sequence analysis of MHC class II Eb cDNAs from H2r and H2p haplotypes. Immunogenetics 1996; 44:231-2.
776. Stroynowski I, Fischer-Lindahl K. Antigen presentation by non-classical class I molecules. Curr Opin Immunol 1994; 6:38-44.
777. Teitell M, Cheroutre H, Panwala C et al. Structure and function of H-2 T (Tla) region class I MHC molecules. Crit Rev Immunol 1994; 14:1-27.
778. Hedrick SM. Dawn of the hunt for non-classical MHC function. Cell 1992; 70:177-80.
779. Joyce S, Tabaczewski P, Angeletti RH et al. A nonpolymorphic major histocompatibility complex class Ib molecule

binds a large array of diverse self-peptides. J Exp Med 1994; 179:579-88.
780. Rodgers JR, Mehta V, Cook RG. Surface expression of beta 2-microglobulin-associated thymus-leukemia antigen is independent of TAP2. Eur J Immunol 1995; 25:1001-7.
781. Fischer-Lindahl K, Hermel E, Loveland BE et al. Maternally transmitted antigen of mice: a model transplantation antigen. Annu Rev Immunol 1991; 9:351-72.
782. Xin JH, Kvist S, Dobberstein B. Identification of an H-2K^d gene using a specific cDNA probe. EMBO J 1982; 1:467-71.
783. Cho SG, Attaya M, Monaco JJ. New class II-like genes in the murine MHC. Nature 1991; 353:573-6.
784. Newell WR, Trowsdale J, Beck S. MHCDB: database of the human MHC (release 2). Immunogenetics 1996; 45: 6-8.
785. Carter CA, Murphy G, Fabre JW et al. Physical mapping of the rat MHC class II genes shows a high level of interspecies conservation. Genomics 1994; 22:451-5.
786. Walter L, Heine L, Günther E. Sequence, expression, and mapping of a rat Mhc class Ib gene. Immunogenetics 1994; 39:351-4.
787. Howard JC. Restrictions on the use of antigenic peptides by the immune system. Proc Natl Acad Sci U S A 1993; 90:3777-9.
788. Colonna M, Bresnahan M, Bahram S et al. Allelic variants of the human putative peptide transporter involved in antigen processing. Proc Natl Acad Sci U S A 1992; 89:3932-6.
789. Powis SH, Trowsdale J. Human major histocompatibility complex genes. Behring Inst Mitt 1994; 17-25.
790. Heemels MT, Ploegh HL. Substrate specificity of allelic variants of the TAP peptide transporter. Immunity 1994; 1:775-84.
791. Heemels MT, Schumacher TN, Wonigeit K et al. Peptide translocation by variants of the transporter associated with antigen processing. Science 1993; 262: 2059-63.
792. Momburg F, Neefjes JJ, Hammerling GJ. Peptide selection by MHC-encoded TAP transporters. Curr Opin Immunol 1994; 6:32-7.
793. Momburg F, Armandola EA, Post M et al. Residues in TAP2 peptide transporters controlling substrate specificity. J Immunol 1996; 156:1756-63.
794. Walter L, Fischer K, Günther E. Physical mapping of the Ring1, Ring2, Ke6, Ke4, Rxrb, Col11a2, and RT1.Hb genes in the rat major histocompatibility complex. Immunogenetics 1996; 44:218-21.
795. Ennis PD, Jackson AP, Parham P. Molecular cloning of bovine class I MHC cDNA. J Immunol 1988; 141:642-51.
796. Bensaid A, Kaushal A, Baldwin CL et al. Identification of expressed bovine class I MHC genes at two loci and demonstration of physical linkage. Immunogenetics 1991; 33:247-54.
797. Barbis DP, Maher JK, Stanek J et al. Horse cDNA clones encoding two MHC class I genes. Immunogenetics 1994; 40:163.
798. Cameron PU, Tabarias HA, Pulendran B et al. Conservation of the central MHC genome: PFGE mapping and RFLP analysis of complement, HSP70, and TNF genes in the goat. Immunogenetics 1990; 31:253-64.
799. Wright H, Ballingall KT, Redmond J. The DY sub-region of the sheep MHC contains an A/B gene pair. Immunogenetics 1994; 40:230-4.
800. Skow LC, Snaples SN, Davis SK et al. Localization of bovine lymphocyte antigen (BoLA) DYA and class I loci to different regions of chromosome 23. Mamm Genome 1996; 7:388-9.
801. Skow LC, Nall CA. A second polymorphism in exon 2 of the BoLA-DYA gene. Anim Genet 1996; 27:216-7.
802. Stone RT, Muggli-Cockett NE. BoLA-DIB: species distribution, linkage with DOB, and northern analysis. Anim Genet 1993; 24:41-5.
803. Willison K, Kelly A, Dudley K et al. The human homologue of the mouse t-complex gene, TCP1, is located on chromosome 6 but is not near the HLA region. EMBO J 1987; 6:1967-74.
804. Russell GC, Oliver RA, Sawhney SMS. Cloning, transfection, and DNA sequence of a second gene from the BoLA-A11 haplotype. Immunogenetics 1996; 44: 315-8.
805. Ennis PD, Jackson AP, Parham P. Mo-

lecular cloning of bovine class I MHC cDNA. J Immunol 1988; 141:642-51.

806. Niimi M, Nakai Y, Aida Y. Nucleotide sequences and the molecular evolution of the DMA and DMB genes of the bovine major histocompatibility complex. Biochem Biophys Res Commun 1997; 217:522-8.

807. Chardonnens X, Du Pasquier L. Induction of skin allograft tolerance during metamorphosis of the toad Xenopus laevis: a possible model for studying generation of self tolerance to histocompatibility antigens. Eur J Immunol 1973; 3:569-73.

808. Flajnik MF, Kaufman JF, Riegert P et al. Identification of class I major histocompatibility complex encoded molecules in the amphibian Xenopus. Immunogenetics 1984; 20:433-42.

809. Kaufman JF, Flajnik MF, Du Pasquier L et al. Xenopus MHC class II molecules. I. Identification and structural characterization. J Immunol 1985; 134:3248-57.

810. Shum BP, Avila D, Du Pasquier L et al. Isolation of a classical MHC class I cDNA from an amphibian. Evidence for only one class I locus in the Xenopus MHC. J Immunol 1993; 151:5376-86.

811. Sato K, Flajnik MF, Du Pasquier L et al. Evolution of the MHC: isolation of class II beta-chain cDNA clones from the amphibian Xenopus laevis. J Immunol 1993; 150:2831-43.

812. Salter-Cid L, Kasahara M, Flajnik MF. Hsp70 genes are linked to the Xenopus major histocompatibility complex. Immunogenetics 1994; 39:1-7.

813. Kato Y, Salter-Cid L, Flajnik MF et al. Isolation of the Xenopus complement factor B complementary DNA and linkage of the gene to the frog MHC. J Immunol 1994; 153:4546-54.

814. Plachy J, Pink JR, Hala K. Biology of the chicken MHC (B complex). Crit Rev Immunol 1992; 12:47-79.

815. Guillemot F, Billault A, Pourquie O et al. A molecular map of the chicken major histocompatibility complex: the class II beta genes are closely linked to the class I genes and the nucleolar organizer. EMBO J 1988; 7:2775-85.

816. Pharr GT, Bacon LD, Dodgson JB. Analysis of B-L beta-chain gene expression in two chicken cDNA libraries. Immunogenetics 1993; 37:381-5.

817. Kaufman J, Andersen R, Avila D et al. Different features of the MHC class I heterodimer have evolved at different rates. Chicken B-F and beta 2-microglobulin sequences reveal invariant surface residues. J Immunol 1992; 148:1532-46.

818. Koch C. A genetic polymorphism of the complement component factor B in chickens not linked to the major histocompatibility complex (MHC). Immunogenetics 1986; 23:364-7.

819. Miller MM, Goto RM, Taylor RL Jr et al. Assignment of Rfp-Y to the chicken major histocompatibility complex/NOR microchromosome and evidence for high-frequency recombination associated with the nucleolar organizer region. Proc Natl Acad Sci U S A 1996; 93:3958-62.

820. Miller MM, Goto R, Bernot A et al. Two Mhc class I and two Mhc class II genes map to the chicken Rfp-Y system outside the B complex. Proc Natl Acad Sci USA 1994; 91:4397-401.

821. Chen Y, Lillehoj HS, Hsu C et al. Functional characterization of a chicken major histocompatibility commplex class II B gene promoter. Immunogenetics 1997; 45:242-8.

822. Mayer WE, Williams NS, O'hUigin C et al. Class I major histocompatibility complex genes of the red-necked Wallaby, Macropus rufogriseus. Mol Phylogenet Evol 1993; 2:23-30.

823. Hashimoto K, Nakanishi T, Kurosawa Y. Identification of a shark sequence resembling the major histocompatibility complex class I alpha 3 domain. Proc Natl Acad Sci USA 1992; 89:2209-12.

824. Bartl S, Weissman IL. Isolation and characterization of major histocompatibility complex class IIB genes from the nurse shark. Proc Natl Acad Sci U S A 1994; 91:262-6.

825. Kasahara M, McKinney EC, Flajnik MF et al. The evolutionary origin of the major histocompatibility complex: polymorphism of class II alpha chain genes in the cartilaginous fish. Eur J Immunol 1993; 23:2160-5.

826. Ono H, O'hUigin C, Vincek V et al. New beta chain-encoding Mhc class II genes

in the carp. Immunogenetics 1993; 38:146-9.

827. Okamura K, Nakanishi T, Kurosawa Y et al. Expansion of genes that encode MHC class I molecules in cyprinid fishes. J Immunol 1993; 151:188-200.

828. Grimholt U, Hordvik I, Fosse VM et al. Molecular cloning of major histocompatibility complex class I cDNAs from Atlantic salmon (Salmo salar). Immunogenetics 1993; 37:469-73.

829. Juul-Madsen HR, Glamann J, Madsen HO et al. MHC class II beta-chain expression in the rainbow trout. Scand J Immunol 1992; 35:687-94.

830. Takeuchi H, Figueroa F, O'hUigin C et al. Cloning and characterization of class I Mhc genes of the zebrafish, Brachydanio rerio. Immunogenetics 1995; 42:77-84.

831. Ono H, O'hUigin C, Vincek V et al. Exon-intron organization of fish major histocompatibility complex class II B genes. Immunogenetics 1993; 38:223-34.

832. Ono H, Klein D, Vincek V et al. Major histocompatibility complex class II genes of zebrafish. Proc Natl Acad Sci U S A 1992; 89:11886-90.

833. Sato A, Figueroa F, O'hUigin C et al. Identification of major histocompatibility complex genes in the guppy, Poecilia reticulata. Immunogenetics 1996; 43: 38-49.

834. Betz UA, Mayer WE, Klein J. Major histocompatibility complex class I genes of the coelacanth Latimeria chalumnae. Proc Natl Acad Sci USA 1994; 91: 11065-9.

835. Brenner S, Elgar G, Sandford R et al. Characterization of the pufferfish (Fugu) genome as a compact model vertebrate genome. Nature 1993; 366:265-8.

CHAPTER 3

The Structure

MHC CLASS I

In our context the most important part is the peptide-binding groove. It is made up of the α1 and α2 domains. Amino acids $1\alpha_1$ to $48\alpha_1$, and $94\alpha_2$ to $135\alpha_2$ form a β-pleated sheet which makes up the floor of the groove[1,2] (see Fig. 3.1). The remaining parts of both domains are in α-helical conformation and form the rims of the groove. The peptide, usually but not always nine AA long, lies more or less extended between the two α-helical rims; both N and C termini are tightly fixed in the edges of the groove.[3] Clusters of conserved residues form hydrogen bonds with either of the termini. For the peptide N-terminus, these are Tyr7, Tyr59, Tyr71, Trp167, and Tyr159; for the C-terminus, Tyr84, Thr143, Lys146 and Trp147 form these bonds.[2] Most of the peptide-binding affinity is brought about by these forces, at least for those peptides of eight to ten AA, whose termini are then buried within the binding site.[3] Some longer ligands, however, are loose at one end so that they protrude over the groove's ends.[4] Other long peptides have their termini fixed in the groove but have their middle part bulged out to accommodate the extra length.[5] The specificity of interactions between peptide and the groove comes about by many contacts between peptide side chains and MHC residues. These contacts, apart from contributing to the binding forces, are responsible for the allele-specific binding characteristics of class I molecules.[6,7] The most prominent contacts of this kind are produced by pockets within the binding cleft. Specificity and location of these pockets vary considerably between different MHC alleles; thus, MHC sequence polymorphism directly affects peptide binding specificity. For example, A*0201 binds peptides with a large aliphatic side chain (Leu, Ile, or Met) at position 2, and a smaller aliphatic side chain (Leu or Val) at the C-terminus, which is mostly P9.[8] In contrast, A*0101 prefers peptides with an acidic residue at position 3 (Asp or Glu) and strictly a Tyr at the C-terminus.[9,10] These side chains are 'anchored' in the corresponding pockets of the groove. In addition to these prominent contact sites, other peptide side chains make contacts with groove residues contributing to binding specificity; the sum of these interactions then produces the allele-specific peptide specificity or 'peptide motif' of each MHC allelic product. In several cases, where crystals consisting of an MHC I molecule associated with a single peptide have been analyzed, the anchor-pocket interactions and the other peptide-groove contacts are exactly known, e.g., for HLA-A2 with five different peptides, for H-2K^b in three cases, for HLA-B53 in two cases, and for D^b, HLA-Aw68, and HLA-B35 for one peptide each.[7,11-14] Since the overall structure of MHC class I molecules is conserved even if one considers molecules from distant species, such as mouse and man, it is possible to predict anchor pocket interaction even for MHC-peptide combinations where crystals have not been analyzed.[15,16,17] Moreover, the determined[18,7,19] or predicted[15,17] nature of pockets nicely explains the peptide motifs determined by sequencing peptides eluted from MHC molecules. For example, the P2 pocket of HLA-A*0201 is lined by Tyr7, Phe9, Met45, Glu63, Lys66, Val67 and Tyr99.[6] The P2 pocket of B*2705 differs in several residues; most influential is Glu45, which lends a negative charge to the pocket. Thus, the P2 pocket of B*2705 prefers a positive charge (Arg) at P2 of the peptide. The pocket usually harboring the P2 side chain is also called the B-pocket, indicating that it is the second pocket in the groove. The first pocket then is called A, the third, however, D followed by C, E and F. The F pocket is usually identical to the P9 pocket. An exception to these connections is, e.g., the H2-M3 molecule which has the A pocket blocked.[20] Similarly, the conformation of ligands in HLA-B35 molecules is different from the standard.[21] Tables 3.1 to 3.18 list the MHC residues shown to be lining one of the pockets in crystals, or predicted to be possibly involved in pocket lining. This information is combined with the determined anchor specificity or the preferred residue at the respective peptide position—pocket A for position 1, pocket B for P2, pocket C for P6, pocket D for P3, pocket E for P7 and pocket F for the C-terminal peptide position. Thus, these tables can be used to predict pocket specificities in a limited manner—e.g., the C-terminal anchor of the B*0702 motif is a Leu or Phe; since all the B*0705 residues predicted to be possibly involved in the F pocket are identical, the C-terminal anchor of B*0705 is most likely also a Leu or Phe. However, if an MHC molecule binds peptides in a nonstandard way, such as H2-M3, such comparisons are more complex. On the other hand, the differences in pockets responsible for pocket specificity can be easily looked up—for example, the F-pocket of B*2705 tolerates positive anchor side chains, whereas B*2702, lacking one negative charge (Asn77 instead of Asp77) does not allow Arg, His or Lys at P9. The remaining domains of the class I molecule, α3, the transmembrane and the cytoplasmic tail as well as the light chain, β2-microglobulin, do not directly contribute to peptide specificity. However, T cells can distinguish between class I molecules associated with diverse allelic forms of β2-microglobulin. This is due either to recognition of a conformational difference, or possibly due to an indirect influence of β2-microglobulin on the peptide or peptides bound.[22,23] The α3 region of MHC I is important as a conserved contact region for the CD8 molecule of the T cell and thus contributes to the T cell target interaction in an antigen-nonspecific way.[24]

Once a T cell receptor has found its matching combination of MHC molecule and peptide, it binds in a manner that has only recently been elucidated by X-ray crystallography of TCR/peptide/MHC complexes for two antigens, an HTLV-1 peptide on HLA-A2,[26] and a self peptide on H-2K^b.[27] The size of the TCR and the MHC/peptide complex is roughly similar. The two chains of the T cell receptor, each immunoglobulin-like, sit diagonally on the top of the peptide groove. The CDR loops of the α chain attach to the 'lower left' of the MHC surface, the β chain CDRs to the 'upper right', based on the orientation, the MHC groove is usually depicted. The CDR3 loops of both TCR α and β chains are located next to each other on top of the center of the peptide. CDR1α spans the part from the peptide's N-terminus to its middle, CDR1β covers the C-terminal end of the peptide. Both CDR2 loops are over the MHC part of the complex, CDR2α over the α2 domain α-helix, and CDR2β over the α1 domain α-helix. Most of the peptide is buried within the groove; however, there are still direct contacts between peptide and TCR. For the case of the HTLV-1 peptide (LLFGYPVYV), these are L1, L2, and from G4 to Y8. The most prominent interaction between peptide and TCR is at Y5, which is bound in a deep pocket at the center of the TCR. Thus, although L2, whose side chain is anchored in the P2 pocket of the MHC molecule, is also touched by the TCR, the most intensive interaction between peptide and TCR is at a nonanchor residue. Intimate interactions occur at P6, V7, and Y8, whereas V9, the C-terminal anchor of the peptide, is not in direct contact with the TCR. Thus, the TCR touches both the MHC as well as the peptide surface. The overall contact area is similar to that of antibody-antigen interaction (around 1000Å^2). Most of the TCR-peptide contact is made up by the most diverse loop, CDR3β. The surface area shared between TCR and peptide is about half of that shared between TCR and the MHC-part of the complex.

MHC CLASS II

The overall three-dimensional structure of class II molecules is remarkably similar to that of class I, although the sequence homology is only limited.[2,11,28-31] The peptide-binding groove is formed by the α1 and β1 domains such that class IIα corresponds to class I α1, and class II β1 to class I α2 (Fig. 3.2). The groove is made up from a β-pleated sheet and two α-helices, very similar to the class I structure. The most striking difference between the two MHC classes is the length of peptides bound, and this is explained by rather small structural differences.[2] The termini of class II bound peptide are not fixed by conserved hydrogen bonds in the edge of the groove; the peptide's termini rather extend out of the groove. Instead, 15 hydrogen bonds between the main chain of the influenza hemagglutinin peptide and the DR1 groove are distributed along the binding site. These hydrogen bonds, which are again conserved, are probably responsible for most of the binding forces between peptide and MHC molecule. In addition, these bonds distributed over the groove-contained stretch of the peptide constrain its conformation to an extended one not allowing much bulging. The missing concentration of hydrogen bonds in the edge of the groove as well as some smaller MHC-II-residues and other changes within the groove's edges as compared to class I, allow the peptides to extend out of the site. A nine amino acid stretch of the bound peptide, usually approximately in its center, is fixed in the groove by the hydrogen bonds and is positioned by anchor-pocket interaction, much as in class I molecules. For the Flu-HA peptide/DR1 crystal, five of the nine peptide side chains are buried within complementary pockets;[30] the specificity of these pockets is rather degenerate, as compared to class I pockets. The most specific pocket is the one harboring the Tyr side chain at relative position 1 of the peptide (the entire peptide sequence is PKYVKQNTLKLAT; for motif description, the first anchor residue is defined at relative position 1).[32] Among the DR molecules, this pocket is influenced by β-chain polymorphism such that two principal specificities occur: if β86 is a Gly, as in DR1, pocket 1 has a preference for the bulky aromatic residues Phe, Tyr, and Trp, whereas aliphatic residues are also possible. If β86 is a Val, having a bigger side chain than the hydrogen atom of Gly, and therefore occupying more space in the pocket, the bulky residues are not allowed any more, and the pocket changes its preference towards the smaller aliphatic residues.[32] The other pockets of DR1 are rather degenerate, as revealed by peptide binding studies as well as by analysis of natural ligands, the most specific being P6 with a preference for small residues, especially Gly and Ala (see Chapter 4). For H2-E^k, crystal studies revealed anchoring of side chains at relative positions 1, 4, 6 and 9.[11] The P1 anchor is very similar to the corresponding one in the homologous human DR molecules, and is influenced in a similar way by the occupation of β86. The P9 anchor is remarkably specific for basic residues Arg and Lys, nicely explained by a negative countercharge within the peptide pocket, Glu β9. Thus again, spacing and specificity of pockets determine the peptide specificity of MHC class II molecules also. The residues of DRB and H2-E β chains likely to contribute to pockets are listed in Tables 3.19 - 3.23 and 3.24 -3.28, respectively; for the other polymorphic class II chains, the three-dimensional structure is not established, so that similar predictions cannot be made with some certainty. The DRA and Eα chains are only marginally polymorphic and are therefore not listed in this way.

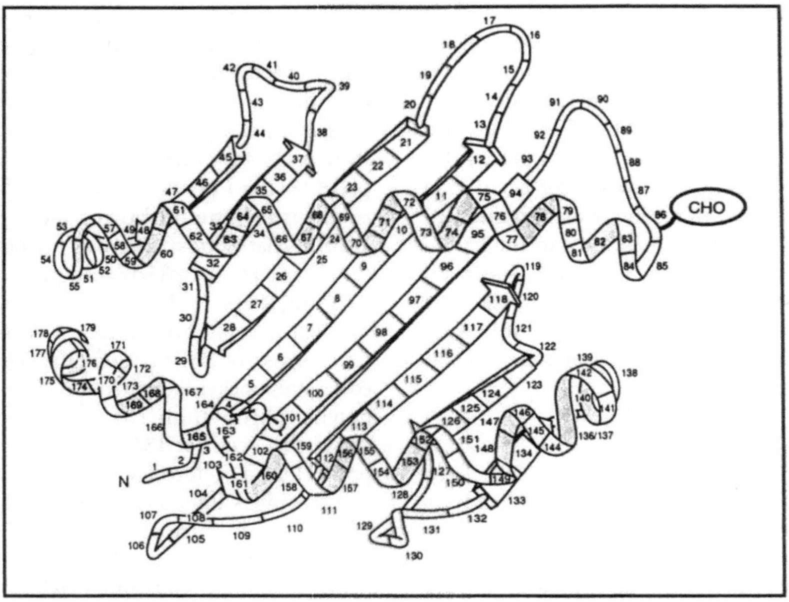

Fig. 3.1. MHC class I peptide binding groove. Reprinted from Parham P. Eur J Immunogenet 1992; 19:347-59 with permission from: Bjorkman PJ, Saper MA, Samraoui B et al. Nature 1987; 329:506-12 and Bjorkman PJ, Saper MA, Samraoui B et al. Nature 1987; 329:512-8. © 1987 Macmillan Magazines Limited.

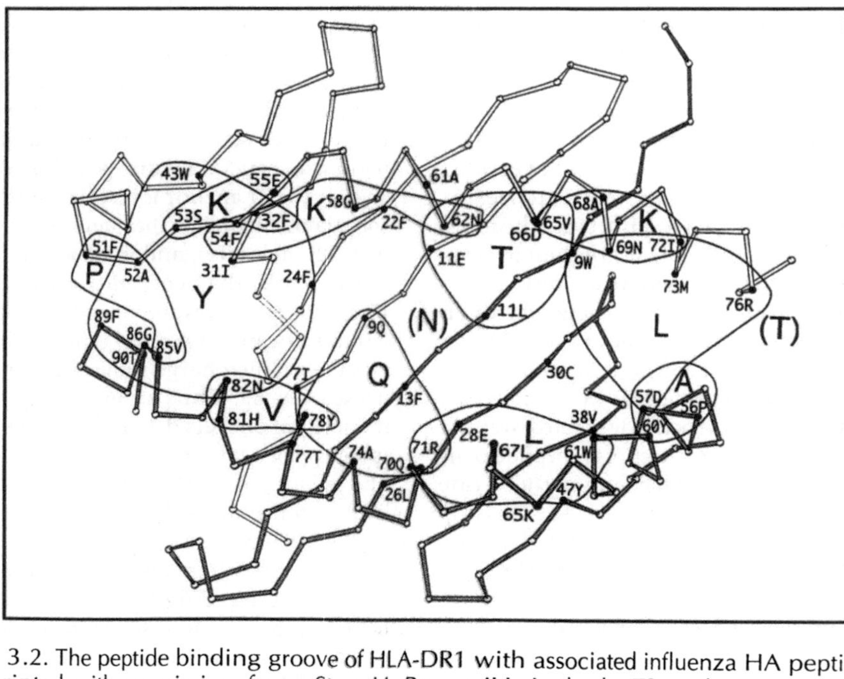

Fig. 3.2. The peptide binding groove of HLA-DR1 with associated influenza HA peptide. Reprinted with permission from: Stern LJ, Brown JH, Jardetzky TS et al. Nature 1994; 368:215-21 ©1994 Macmillan Magazines Limited.

Table 3.1. Pocket for peptide position 1 (Pocket A)

Chelvanayagam 1996[17]	5	7	33	59	62	63	66	99	159	163	167	171	Anchors/
Saper et al 1991[25]	5	7		59		63	66	99	159	163	167	171	preferred
Matsumura et al 1992[16]	5	7		59		63		99	159			171	residues
*A*0101*	M	Y	F	Y	Q	E	N	Y	Y	R	G	Y	
*A*0102*	M	Y	F	Y	Q	E	N	Y	Y	R	G	Y	
*A*0201*	M	Y	F	Y	G	E	K	Y	Y	T	W	Y	(I,L,F,K,M,Y,V)
*A*0202*	M	Y	F	Y	G	E	K	Y	Y	T	W	Y	(A,F,G,V,I)
*A*0203*	M	Y	F	Y	G	E	K	Y	Y	T	W	Y	
*A*0204*	M	Y	F	Y	G	E	K	Y	Y	T	W	Y	
*A*0205*	M	Y	F	Y	G	E	K	Y	Y	T	W	Y	(F,V,Y,A)
*A*0206*	M	Y	F	Y	G	E	K	Y	Y	T	W	Y	
*A*0207*	M	Y	F	Y	G	E	K	C	Y	T	W	Y	
*A*0208*	M	Y	F	Y	G	E	N	Y	Y	T	W	Y	
*A*0209*	M	Y	F	Y	G	E	K	Y	Y	T	W	Y	
*A*0210*	M	Y	F	Y	G	E	K	F	Y	T	W	Y	
*A*0211*	M	Y	F	Y	G	E	K	Y	Y	T	W	Y	
*A*0212*	M	Y	F	Y	G	E	K	Y	Y	T	W	Y	
*A*0213*	M	Y	F	Y	G	E	K	Y	Y	T	W	Y	
*A*0214*	M	Y	F	Y	G	E	K	Y	Y	T	W	Y	(F,Y,V,A)
*A*0215N*	M	Y	F	Y	G	E	K	C	Y	T	W	Y	
*A*0216*	M	Y	F	Y	G	E	K	Y	Y	E	W	Y	
*A*0217*	M	Y	F	Y	G	E	K	F	Y	T	W	Y	
*A*0218*	M	Y	F	Y	G	E	K	C	Y	T	W	Y	
*A*0219*	M	Y	F	Y	G	E	K	Y	Y	T	G	Y	
*A*0220*	M	Y	F	Y	G	E	N	Y	Y	T	W	Y	
*A*0221*	M	Y	F	Y	G	E	K	Y	Y	T	W	Y	
*A*0222*	M	Y	F	Y	G	E	K	Y	Y	T	W	Y	
*A*0301*	M	Y	F	Y	Q	E	N	Y	Y	T	W	Y	
*A*0302*	M	Y	F	Y	Q	E	N	Y	Y	T	W	Y	
*A*0303N*	M	Y	F	Y	Q	E	N	Y	Y	T	W	Y	
*A*1101*	M	Y	F	Y	Q	E	N	Y	Y	R	W	Y	(A)
*A*1102*	M	Y	F	Y	Q	E	N	Y	Y	R	W	Y	
*A*1103*	M	Y	F	Y	Q	E	N	Y	Y	R	W	Y	
*A*1104*	M	Y	F	Y	Q	E	N	Y	Y	T	W	Y	
*A*2301*	M	Y	F	Y	E	E	K	F	Y	T	G	Y	
*A*2402*	M	Y	F	Y	E	E	K	F	Y	T	G	Y	
*A*2403*	M	Y	F	Y	E	E	K	F	Y	T	W	Y	
*A*2404*	M	Y	F	Y	E	E	K	F	Y	T	G	Y	
*A*2405*	M	Y	F	Y	E	E	K	F	Y	T	G	Y	
*A*2406*	M	Y	F	Y	E	E	K	F	Y	T	G	Y	
*A*2407*	M	Y	F	Y	E	E	K	F	Y	T	G	Y	
*A*2408*	M	Y	F	Y	G	E	K	F	Y	T	G	Y	
*A*2409N*	M	Y	F	Y	E	E	K	F	Y	T	G	Y	
*A*2410*	M	Y	F	Y	E	E	K	F	Y	R	W	Y	
*A*2413*	M	Y	F	Y	E	E	K	F	Y	T	G	Y	
*A*2414*	M	Y	F	Y	E	E	K	Y	Y	T	G	Y	
*A*2501*	M	Y	F	Y	R	N	N	Y	Y	R	W	Y	
*A*2502*	M	Y	F	Y	R	N	N	Y	Y	R	W	Y	
*A*2601*	M	Y	F	Y	R	N	N	Y	Y	R	W	Y	
*A*2602*	M	Y	F	Y	R	N	N	Y	Y	R	W	Y	
*A*2603*	M	Y	F	Y	R	N	N	Y	Y	R	W	Y	
*A*2604*	M	Y	F	Y	R	N	N	Y	Y	L	W	Y	
*A*2605*	M	Y	F	Y	R	N	N	Y	Y	R	W	Y	
*A*2606*	M	Y	F	Y	R	N	N	Y	Y	R	W	Y	
*A*2607*	M	Y	F	Y	G	E	K	Y	Y	R	W	Y	
*A*2608*	M	Y	F	Y	R	N	N	Y	Y	R	W	Y	
*A*2901*	M	Y	F	Y	L	Q	N	Y	Y	T	W	Y	
*A*2902*	M	Y	F	Y	L	Q	N	Y	Y	T	W	Y	
*A*2903*	M	Y	F	Y	L	Q	N	Y	Y	T	G	Y	
*A*3001*	M	Y	F	Y	Q	E	N	Y	Y	T	W	Y	
*A*3002*	M	Y	F	Y	Q	E	N	Y	Y	T	W	Y	

Table 3.1. (con't)

Chelvanayagam 1996[17]	5	7	33	59	62	63	66	99	159	163	167	171	Anchors/
Saper et al 1991[25]	5	7		59		63	66	99	159	163	167	171	preferred
Matsumura et al 1992[16]	5	7		59		63		99	159			171	residues
*A*3003*	M	Y	F	Y	Q	E	N	Y	Y	T	W	Y	
*A*3004*	M	Y	F	Y	Q	E	N	Y	Y	T	W	Y	
*A*3005*	M	Y	F	Y	R	E	N	Y	Y	T	W	Y	
*A*31012*	M	Y	F	Y	Q	E	N	Y	Y	T	W	Y	(K,R)
*A*3201*	M	Y	F	Y	Q	E	N	Y	Y	T	W	Y	
*A*3202*	M	Y	F	Y	Q	E	N	Y	Y	T	W	Y	
*A*3301*	M	Y	F	Y	R	N	N	Y	Y	T	W	H	
*A*3302*	M	Y	F	Y	R	N	N	Y	Y	T	W	Y	(D,E,M)
*A*3303*	M	Y	F	Y	R	N	N	Y	Y	T	W	Y	
*A*3401*	M	Y	F	Y	R	N	K	Y	Y	T	W	Y	
*A*3402*	M	Y	F	Y	R	N	N	Y	Y	T	W	Y	
*A*3601*	M	Y	F	Y	Q	E	N	Y	Y	T	W	Y	
*A*4301*	M	Y	F	Y	L	Q	N	Y	Y	R	W	Y	
*A*6601*	M	Y	F	Y	R	N	N	Y	Y	R	W	Y	
*A*6602*	M	Y	F	Y	R	N	N	Y	Y	E	W	Y	
*A*6603*	M	Y	F	Y	R	N	N	Y	Y	E	W	Y	
*A*68011*	M	Y	F	Y	R	N	N	Y	Y	T	W	Y	D,E
*A*68012*	M	Y	F	Y	R	N	N	Y	Y	T	W	Y	
*A*6802*	M	Y	F	Y	R	N	N	Y	Y	T	W	Y	
*A*6803*	M	Y	F	Y	R	N	N	Y	Y	T	W	Y	
*A*6901*	M	Y	F	Y	R	N	N	Y	Y	T	W	Y	(E)
*A*7401*	M	Y	F	Y	Q	E	N	Y	Y	T	W	Y	
*A*7402*	M	Y	F	Y	Q	E	N	Y	Y	T	W	Y	
*A*7403*	M	Y	F	Y	Q	E	N	Y	Y	T	W	Y	
*A*8001*	M	Y	F	Y	E	E	N	Y	Y	E	G	Y	

HLA class I pockets actually shown[25,16] or predicted[17] to be participating in pocket structure at least in some allelic products. Capital letters designate 'preferred AA', amino acids that are less frequently found are shown in brackets. (.) indicate unavailability of information. This applies also to Tables 3.2 - 3.19.

Table 3.2. Pocket for peptide position 1 (Pocket A)

Chevalnayagam 1996[17]	5	7	33	59	62	63	66	99	159	163	167	171	Anchors/
Saper et al 1991[25]	5	7		59		63	66	99	159	163	167	171	preferred
Matsumura et al 1992[16]	5	7		59		63		99	159			171	residues
*B*0702*	M	Y	F	Y	R	N	I	Y	Y	E	W	Y	(A,R)
*B*0703*	M	Y	F	Y	R	N	I	Y	Y	E	W	Y	(A,R)
*B*0704*	M	Y	F	Y	R	N	I	Y	Y	E	W	Y	
*B*0705*	M	Y	F	Y	R	N	I	Y	Y	E	W	Y	(A,R)
*B*0706*	M	Y	F	Y	R	N	I	Y	Y	E	W	Y	
*B*0707*	M	Y	F	Y	R	N	I	Y	Y	E	W	Y	
*B*0801*	M	Y	F	Y	R	N	I	Y	Y	T	W	Y	
*B*0802*	M	Y	F	Y	R	N	I	Y	Y	T	W	Y	
*B*0803*	.	.	F	Y	R	N	I	Y	Y	T	W	Y	
*B*1301*	M	Y	F	Y	R	E	I	Y	Y	E	W	Y	
*B*1302*	M	Y	F	Y	R	E	I	Y	Y	E	W	Y	
*B*1303*	M	Y	F	Y	R	E	I	Y	Y	L	W	Y	
*B*1401*	M	Y	F	Y	R	N	I	Y	Y	T	W	H	
*B*1402*	M	Y	F	Y	R	N	I	Y	Y	T	W	H	
*B*1501*	M	Y	F	Y	R	E	I	Y	Y	L	W	Y	(I)
*B*1502*	M	Y	F	Y	R	N	I	Y	Y	L	W	Y	
*B*1503*	M	Y	F	Y	R	E	I	Y	Y	L	W	Y	
*B*1504*	M	Y	F	Y	R	E	I	Y	Y	L	W	Y	
*B*1505*	M	Y	F	Y	R	E	I	Y	Y	L	W	Y	
*B*1506*	M	Y	F	Y	R	E	I	F	Y	L	W	Y	
*B*1507*	M	Y	F	Y	R	E	I	Y	Y	L	W	Y	

Table 3.2. (con't)

Chevalnayagam 1996[17]	5	7	33	59	62	63	66	99	159	163	167	171	Anchors/
Saper et al 1991[25]	5	7		59		63	66	99	159	163	167	171	preferred
Matsumura et al 1992[16]	5	7		59		63		99	159			171	residues
*B*1508*	M	Y	F	Y	R	N	I	Y	Y	L	W	Y	
*B*1509*	M	Y	F	Y	R	N	I	Y	Y	L	W	Y	
*B*1510*	M	Y	F	Y	R	N	I	Y	Y	L	W	Y	
*B*1511*	M	Y	F	Y	R	N	I	Y	Y	L	W	Y	
*B*1512*	M	Y	F	Y	R	E	I	Y	Y	L	G	Y	
*B*1513*	M	Y	F	Y	R	N	I	Y	Y	L	W	Y	
*B*1514*	M	Y	F	Y	R	E	I	Y	Y	L	S	Y	
*B*1515*	M	Y	F	Y	R	N	I	Y	Y	L	W	Y	
*B*1516*	M	Y	F	Y	R	E	N	Y	Y	L	W	Y	
*B*1517*	M	Y	F	Y	R	E	N	Y	Y	L	W	Y	
*B*1518*	M	Y	F	Y	R	N	I	Y	Y	L	W	Y	
*B*1519*	M	Y	F	Y	R	E	I	Y	Y	L	G	Y	
*B*1520*	M	Y	F	Y	R	E	I	Y	Y	L	W	Y	
*B*1521*	M	Y	F	Y	R	N	I	Y	Y	L	W	Y	
*B*1522*	M	Y	F	Y	R	N	I	Y	Y	L	W	Y	
*B*1523*	M	Y	F	Y	R	N	I	Y	Y	L	W	Y	
*B*1524*	M	Y	F	Y	R	E	I	Y	Y	L	W	Y	
*B*1525*	M	Y	F	Y	R	E	I	Y	Y	L	W	Y	
*B*1526N*	M	Y	F	Y	R	E	I	/	Y	L	W	Y	
*B*1527*	.	Y	F	Y	R	E	I	F	Y	L	W	Y	
*B*1528*	M	Y	F	Y	R	E	I	Y	Y	L	W	Y	
*B*1529*	M	Y	F	Y	R	N	I	Y	Y	L	W	Y	
*B*1530*	.	Y	F	Y	R	E	I	Y	Y	L	W	Y	
*B*1531*	.	Y	F	Y	R	N	I	Y	Y	L	W	Y	
*B*1532*	M	Y	F	Y	R	E	I	S	Y	L	W	Y	
*B*1533*	M	Y	F	Y	R	E	I	Y	Y	L	W	Y	
*B*1534*	M	Y	F	Y	R	E	I	Y	Y	L	W	Y	
*B*1535*	M	Y	F	Y	R	E	I	Y	Y	L	W	Y	
*B*1537*	M	Y	F	Y	R	N	I	Y	Y	L	W	H	
*B*1801*	M	Y	F	Y	R	N	I	Y	Y	T	W	H	
*B*1802*	M	Y	F	Y	R	N	I	Y	Y	T	W	H	
*B*1803*	M	Y	F	Y	R	N	I	Y	Y	T	W	H	
*B*1805*	M	Y	F	Y	R	N	I	Y	Y	T	W	H	
*B*2701*	M	Y	F	Y	R	E	I	Y	Y	E	W	Y	
*B*2702*	M	Y	F	Y	R	E	I	Y	Y	E	W	Y	(K)
*B*2703*	M	Y	F	H	R	E	I	Y	Y	E	W	Y	
*B*2704*	M	Y	F	Y	R	E	I	Y	Y	E	W	Y	
*B*27052*	M	Y	F	Y	R	E	I	Y	Y	E	W	Y	(A,G,K,R)
*B*27053*	.	.	F	Y	R	E	I	Y	Y	E	W	.	
*B*2706*	M	Y	F	Y	R	E	I	Y	Y	E	W	Y	
*B*2707*	M	Y	F	Y	R	E	I	Y	Y	E	W	Y	
*B*2708*	M	Y	F	Y	R	E	I	Y	Y	E	W	Y	
*B*2709*	M	Y	F	Y	R	E	I	Y	Y	E	W	Y	
*B*2710*	M	Y	F	Y	R	E	I	Y	Y	E	W	Y	
*B*3501*	M	Y	F	Y	R	N	I	Y	Y	L	W	Y	(M)
*B*3502*	M	Y	F	Y	R	N	I	Y	Y	L	W	Y	
*B*3503*	M	Y	F	Y	R	N	I	Y	Y	L	W	Y	(A)
*B*3504*	M	Y	F	Y	R	N	I	Y	Y	L	W	Y	
*B*3505*	M	Y	F	Y	R	N	I	Y	Y	L	W	Y	
*B*3506*	M	Y	F	Y	R	N	I	Y	Y	L	W	Y	
*B*3507*	M	Y	F	Y	R	N	I	Y	Y	L	W	Y	
*B*3508*	M	Y	F	Y	R	N	I	Y	Y	L	W	Y	
*B*35091*	M	Y	F	Y	R	N	I	Y	Y	L	W	Y	
*B*35092*	M	Y	F	Y	R	N	I	Y	Y	L	W	Y	
*B*3510*	M	Y	F	Y	R	E	I	Y	Y	L	W	Y	
*B*3511*	M	Y	F	Y	R	N	I	Y	Y	L	W	Y	
*B*3512*	M	Y	F	Y	R	N	I	Y	Y	L	W	Y	
*B*3513*	M	Y	F	Y	R	E	I	Y	Y	L	W	Y	
*B*3515*	M	Y	F	Y	R	N	I	Y	Y	E	W	Y	

Table 3.2. (con't)

Chevalnayagam 1996[17]	5	7	33	59	62	63	66	99	159	163	167	171	Anchors/
Saper et al 1991[25]	5	7		59		63	66	99	159	163	167	171	preferred
Matsumura et al 1992[16]	5	7		59		63		99	159			171	residues
*B*3516*	M	Y	F	Y	R	E	I	Y	Y	L	W	Y	
*B*3517*	M	Y	F	Y	R	N	I	Y	Y	L	W	Y	
*B*3518*	M	Y	F	Y	R	N	I	Y	Y	L	W	Y	
*B*3519*	M	Y	F	Y	R	N	I	Y	Y	L	W	Y	
*B*3520*	M	Y	F	Y	R	N	I	Y	Y	L	W	Y	
*B*3521*	M	Y	F	Y	R	N	I	Y	Y	L	W	H	
*B*3701*	M	Y	F	Y	R	E	I	S	Y	T	W	Y	(K,Q)
*B*3702*	M	Y	F	Y	R	E	I	Y	Y	E	W	Y	
*B*3801*	M	Y	F	Y	R	N	I	Y	Y	T	W	Y	(I)
*B*3802*	M	Y	F	Y	R	N	I	Y	Y	T	W	Y	
*B*39011*	M	Y	F	Y	R	N	I	Y	Y	T	W	Y	
*B*39013*	M	Y	F	Y	R	N	I	Y	Y	T	W	Y	
*B*39021*	M	Y	F	Y	R	E	I	Y	Y	T	W	Y	(K,A)
*B*39022*	M	Y	F	Y	R	E	I	Y	Y	T	W	Y	
*B*3903*	M	Y	F	Y	R	N	I	Y	Y	T	W	Y	
*B*3904*	M	Y	F	Y	R	N	I	Y	Y	T	W	Y	
*B*3905*	M	Y	F	Y	R	N	I	Y	Y	T	W	Y	
*B*39061*	M	Y	F	Y	R	N	I	Y	Y	T	W	Y	
*B*39062*	M	Y	F	Y	R	N	I	Y	Y	T	W	Y	
*B*3907*	.	.	.	Y	R	N	I	Y	Y	T	W	Y	
*B*3908*	M	Y	F	Y	R	E	I	Y	Y	T	W	Y	
*B*3909*	M	Y	F	Y	R	N	I	S	Y	T	W	Y	
*B*3910*	M	Y	F	Y	R	N	I	Y	Y	T	W	Y	
*B*3911*	.	.	F	Y	R	N	I	Y	Y	T	W	Y	
*B*3912*	M	Y	F	Y	R	N	I	Y	Y	T	W	Y	
*B*40011*	M	Y	F	Y	R	E	I	Y	Y	E	W	Y	
*B*40012*	M	Y	F	Y	R	E	I	Y	Y	E	W	Y	
*B*4002*	M	Y	F	Y	R	E	I	Y	Y	E	W	Y	
*B*4003*	M	Y	F	Y	R	E	I	Y	Y	E	W	Y	
*B*4004*	M	Y	F	Y	R	E	I	Y	Y	E	W	Y	
*B*4005*	M	Y	F	Y	R	E	I	Y	Y	L	W	Y	
*B*4006*	M	Y	F	Y	R	E	I	Y	Y	E	W	Y	(G,R)
*B*4007*	M	Y	F	Y	R	E	I	Y	Y	E	W	Y	
*B*4008*	M	Y	F	Y	R	N	I	Y	Y	E	W	Y	
*B*4009*	M	Y	F	Y	R	E	I	Y	Y	E	W	Y	
*B*4101*	M	Y	F	Y	R	E	I	Y	Y	T	W	Y	
*B*4102*	M	Y	F	Y	R	E	I	Y	Y	T	W	Y	
*B*4201*	M	Y	F	Y	R	N	I	Y	Y	T	W	Y	
*B*4402*	M	Y	F	Y	R	E	I	Y	Y	L	S	Y	(A,S,D)
*B*44031*	M	Y	F	Y	R	E	I	Y	Y	L	S	Y	(A,S)
*B*44032*	M	Y	F	Y	R	E	I	Y	Y	L	S	Y	
*B*4404*	M	Y	F	Y	R	E	I	Y	Y	T	S	Y	
*B*4405*	M	Y	F	Y	R	E	I	Y	Y	L	S	Y	
*B*4406*	M	Y	F	Y	R	N	I	Y	Y	L	S	Y	
*B*4407*	M	Y	F	Y	R	E	I	Y	Y	L	S	Y	
*B*4408*	M	Y	F	Y	R	E	I	Y	Y	L	S	Y	
*B*4410*	M	Y	F	Y	R	E	I	F	Y	L	S	Y	
*B*4501*	M	Y	F	Y	R	E	I	Y	Y	L	S	Y	
*B*4601*	M	Y	F	Y	R	E	K	Y	Y	L	W	Y	
*B*4701*	M	Y	F	Y	R	E	I	F	Y	E	W	Y	
*B*4702*	M	Y	F	Y	R	E	I	F	Y	T	W	Y	
*B*4801*	M	Y	F	Y	R	E	I	Y	Y	E	W	Y	
*B*4802*	M	Y	F	Y	R	E	I	Y	Y	L	W	Y	
*B*4803*	M	Y	F	Y	R	E	I	Y	Y	E	W	Y	
*B*4901*	M	Y	F	Y	R	E	I	Y	Y	L	W	Y	
*B*5001*	M	Y	F	Y	R	E	I	Y	Y	L	W	Y	
*B*51011*	M	Y	F	Y	R	N	I	Y	Y	L	W	H	(I,L,V,Y,D)
*B*51012*	M	Y	F	Y	R	N	I	Y	Y	L	W	H	
*B*51021*	M	Y	F	Y	R	N	I	Y	Y	L	W	Y	
*B*51022*	M	Y	F	Y	R	N	I	Y	Y	L	W	Y	

Table 3.2. (con't)

Chevalnayagam 1996[17]	5	7	33	59	62	63	66	99	159	163	167	171	Anchors/
Saper et al 1991[25]	5	7		59		63	66	99	159	163	167	171	preferred
Matsumura et al 1992[16]	5	7		59		63		99	159			171	residues
*B*5103*	M	Y	F	Y	R	N	I	Y	Y	L	G	H	(T,V,D)
*B*5104*	M	Y	F	Y	R	N	I	Y	Y	L	W	H	
*B*5105*	M	Y	F	Y	R	N	I	Y	Y	L	W	Y	
*B*5106*	M	Y	F	Y	R	N	I	Y	Y	L	W	H	
*B*5107*	M	Y	F	Y	R	N	I	Y	Y	L	W	H	
*B*5108*	.	.	F	Y	R	N	I	Y	Y	L	W	H	
*B*52011*	M	Y	F	Y	R	E	I	Y	Y	L	W	H	(V,L,I)
*B*52012*	M	Y	F	Y	R	E	I	Y	Y	L	W	H	
*B*5301*	M	Y	F	Y	R	N	I	Y	Y	L	W	Y	(S,Y,F,M)
*B*5401*	M	Y	F	Y	R	N	I	Y	Y	T	W	Y	(M,F)
*B*5501*	M	Y	F	Y	R	N	I	Y	Y	T	W	Y	(A)
*B*5502*	M	Y	F	Y	R	N	I	Y	Y	T	W	Y	(A)
*B*5503*	M	Y	F	Y	R	N	I	Y	Y	T	W	Y	
*B*5504*	M	Y	F	Y	R	N	I	Y	Y	T	W	Y	
*B*5505*	M	Y	F	Y	R	N	I	Y	Y	T	W	Y	
*B*5601*	M	Y	F	Y	R	N	I	Y	Y	L	W	Y	(A)
*B*5602*	M	Y	F	Y	R	N	I	Y	Y	L	W	Y	
*B*5603*	M	Y	F	Y	R	N	I	Y	Y	L	W	Y	
*B*5701*	M	Y	F	Y	G	E	N	Y	Y	L	W	Y	
*B*5702*	M	Y	F	Y	G	E	N	Y	Y	L	W	Y	
*B*5703*	M	Y	F	Y	G	E	N	Y	Y	L	W	Y	
*B*5704*	M	Y	F	Y	G	E	N	Y	Y	L	W	Y	
*B*5801*	M	Y	F	Y	G	E	N	Y	Y	L	W	Y	(K,R,I)
*B*5802*	M	Y	F	Y	G	E	N	Y	Y	L	W	Y	
*B*5901*	M	Y	F	Y	R	N	I	Y	Y	T	W	Y	
*B*67011*	M	Y	F	Y	R	N	I	Y	Y	T	W	Y	(A)
*B*67012*	M	Y	F	Y	R	N	I	Y	Y	T	W	Y	
*B*7301*	M	Y	F	Y	R	N	I	Y	Y	E	W	H	N
*B*7801*	M	Y	F	Y	R	N	I	Y	Y	L	W	H	
*B*78021*	M	Y	F	Y	R	N	I	Y	Y	L	W	H	
*B*78022*	M	Y	F	Y	R	N	I	Y	Y	L	W	H	
*B*8101*	M	Y	F	Y	R	N	I	Y	Y	E	W	Y	
*B*8201*	M	Y	F	Y	R	N	I	F	Y	L	S	Y	

Table 3.3 Pocket for peptide position 1 (Pocket A)

Chelvanayagam 1996[16]	5	7	33	59	62	63	66	99	159	163	167	171	Anchors/preferred residues
Saper et al 1991[25]	5	7		59		63	66	99	159	163	167	171	
Matsumura et al 1992[17]	5	7		59		63		99	159			171	
*Cw*0102*	M	Y	F	Y	R	E	K	C	Y	T	W	Y	
*Cw*0103*	M	Y	F	Y	R	E	K	C	Y	T	W	Y	
*Cw*02021*	M	Y	F	Y	R	E	K	Y	Y	E	W	Y	
*Cw*02022*	M	Y	F	Y	R	E	K	Y	Y	E	W	Y	
*Cw*02023*	M	Y	F	Y	R	E	K	Y	Y	E	W	Y	
*Cw*0302*	M	Y	F	Y	R	E	K	Y	Y	L	W	Y	
*Cw*0303*	M	Y	F	Y	R	E	K	Y	Y	L	W	Y	
*Cw*0304*	M	Y	F	Y	R	E	K	Y	Y	L	W	Y	
*Cw*0401*	M	Y	F	Y	R	E	K	F	Y	T	W	Y	
*Cw*0402*	M	Y	F	Y	R	E	K	F	Y	T	W	Y	
*Cw*0403*	M	Y	F	Y	R	E	K	F	Y	T	W	Y	
*Cw*0501*	M	Y	F	Y	R	E	K	Y	Y	T	W	Y	
*Cw*0602*	M	Y	F	Y	R	E	K	Y	Y	T	W	Y	(I, F, K, Y)
*Cw*0701*	M	Y	F	Y	R	E	N	Y	Y	T	W	Y	
*Cw*0702*	M	Y	F	Y	R	E	K	S	Y	T	W	Y	
*Cw*0703*	M	Y	F	Y	R	E	K	S	Y	T	W	Y	
*Cw*0704*	M	Y	F	Y	R	E	K	Y	Y	L	W	Y	
*Cw*0705*	M	Y	F	Y	R	E	K	Y	Y	T	W	Y	
*Cw*0706*	M	Y	F	Y	R	E	N	Y	Y	T	W	Y	
*Cw*0707*	M	Y	F	Y	R	E	N	Y	Y	T	W	Y	

Cw*0801	M	Y	F	Y	R	E	K	Y	Y	T	W	Y
Cw*0802	M	Y	F	Y	R	E	K	Y	Y	T	W	Y
Cw*0803	M	Y	F	Y	R	E	K	Y	Y	T	W	Y
Cw*12021	M	Y	F	Y	R	E	K	Y	Y	T	W	Y
Cw*12022	M	Y	F	Y	R	E	K	Y	Y	T	W	Y
Cw*1203	M	Y	F	Y	R	E	K	Y	Y	T	W	Y
Cw*1204	M	Y	F	Y	R	E	K	Y	Y	T	W	Y
Cw*1301	M	Y	F	Y	R	E	K	Y	Y	T	W	Y
Cw*1402	M	Y	F	Y	R	E	K	F	Y	T	W	Y
Cw*1403	M	Y	F	Y	R	E	K	F	Y	T	W	Y
Cw*1502	M	Y	F	Y	R	E	N	Y	Y	T	W	Y
Cw*1503	M	Y	F	Y	R	E	N	Y	Y	T	W	Y
Cw*1504	M	Y	F	Y	R	E	N	Y	Y	T	W	Y
Cw*15051	M	Y	F	Y	R	E	N	Y	Y	T	W	Y
Cw*15052	M	Y	F	Y	R	E	N	Y	Y	T	W	Y
Cw*1601	M	Y	F	Y	R	E	K	Y	Y	T	W	Y
Cw*1602	M	Y	F	Y	R	E	K	Y	Y	T	W	Y
Cw*1701	M	Y	F	Y	R	E	K	Y	Y	E	W	Y
Cw*1702	M	Y	F	Y	R	E	K	Y	Y	E	W	Y
Cw*1801	M	Y	F	Y	R	E	K	F	Y	T	W	Y
Cw*1802	M	Y	F	Y	R	E	K	F	Y	T	W	Y

Table 3.4. Pocket for peptide position 2 (Pocket B)

Chelvanayagam 1996[17]	7	9	24	25	26	34	35	36	45	62	63	66	67	70	99	159	163	167	Anchors/preferred residues
Saper et al. 1991[25]	7	9	24	25		34			45		63	66	67	70	99				
Matsumura et al. 1992[16]	7	9	24			34			45		63		67	70	99				
*A*0101*	Y	F	A	V	G	V	R	F	M	Q	E	N	M	H	Y	Y	R	G	S,T, (L)
*A*0102*	Y	S	A	V	G	V	R	F	M	Q	E	N	M	H	Y	Y	R	G	
*A*0201*	Y	F	A	V	G	V	R	F	M	G	E	K	V	H	Y	Y	T	W	L,M
*A*0202*	Y	F	A	V	G	V	R	F	M	G	E	K	V	H	Y	Y	T	W	L,(A)
*A*0203*	Y	F	A	V	G	V	R	F	M	G	E	K	V	H	Y	Y	T	W	
*A*0204*	Y	F	A	V	G	V	R	F	M	G	E	K	V	H	Y	Y	T	W	L
*A*0205*	Y	Y	A	V	G	V	R	F	M	G	E	K	V	H	Y	Y	T	W	V,L,I,M,(Q)
*A*0206*	Y	Y	A	V	G	V	R	F	M	G	E	K	V	H	Y	Y	T	W	V,Q
*A*0207*	Y	F	A	V	G	V	R	F	M	G	E	K	V	H	C	Y	T	W	L
*A*0208*	Y	Y	A	V	G	V	R	F	M	G	E	N	V	H	Y	Y	T	W	
*A*0209*	Y	F	A	V	G	V	R	F	M	G	E	K	V	H	Y	Y	T	W	
*A*0210*	Y	Y	A	V	G	V	R	F	M	G	E	K	V	H	F	Y	T	W	
*A*0211*	Y	F	A	V	G	V	R	F	M	G	E	K	V	H	Y	Y	T	W	
*A*0212*	Y	F	A	V	G	V	R	F	M	G	E	K	V	H	Y	Y	T	W	
*A*0213*	Y	F	A	V	G	V	R	F	M	G	E	K	V	H	Y	Y	T	W	
*A*0214*	Y	Y	A	V	G	V	R	F	M	G	E	K	V	H	Y	Y	T	W	V,Q,L,(A)
*A*0215N*	Y	F	A	V	G	V	R	F	M	G	E	K	V	H	C	Y	T	W	
*A*0216*	Y	F	A	V	G	V	R	F	M	G	E	K	V	H	Y	Y	E	W	
*A*0217*	Y	F	A	V	G	V	R	F	M	G	E	K	V	H	F	Y	T	W	
*A*0218*	Y	F	A	V	G	V	R	F	M	G	E	K	V	H	C	Y	T	W	
*A*0219*	Y	F	A	V	G	V	R	F	M	G	E	K	V	H	Y	Y	T	G	
*A*0220*	Y	F	A	V	G	V	R	F	M	G	E	N	V	H	Y	Y	T	W	
*A*0221*	Y	Y	A	V	G	V	R	F	M	G	E	K	V	H	Y	Y	T	W	
*A*0222*	Y	F	A	V	G	V	R	F	M	G	E	K	V	H	Y	Y	T	W	
*A*0301*	Y	F	A	V	G	V	R	F	M	Q	E	N	V	Q	Y	Y	T	W	L,V, M
*A*0302*	Y	F	A	V	G	V	R	F	M	Q	E	N	V	Q	Y	Y	T	W	
*A*0303N*	Y	F	A	V	G	V	R	F	M	Q	E	N	V	Q	Y	Y	T	W	
*A*1101*	Y	Y	A	V	G	V	R	F	M	Q	E	N	V	Q	Y	Y	R	W	V,I,F,Y,(T)
*A*1102*	Y	Y	A	V	G	V	R	F	M	Q	E	N	V	Q	Y	Y	R	W	
*A*1103*	Y	Y	A	V	G	V	R	F	M	Q	E	N	V	Q	Y	Y	R	W	
*A*1104*	Y	Y	A	V	G	V	R	F	M	Q	E	N	V	Q	Y	Y	T	W	
*A*2301*	Y	S	A	V	G	V	R	F	M	E	E	K	V	H	F	Y	T	G	

*A*2402*	Y	S	A	V	G	V	R	F	M	E	E	K	V	H	F	Y	T	G	Y
*A*2403*	Y	S	A	V	G	V	R	F	M	E	E	K	V	H	F	Y	T	W	
*A*2404*	Y	S	A	V	G	V	R	F	M	E	E	K	V	H	F	Y	T	G	
*A*2405*	Y	S	A	V	G	V	R	F	M	E	E	K	V	H	F	Y	T	G	
*A*2406*	Y	S	A	V	G	V	R	F	M	E	E	K	V	H	F	Y	T	G	
*A*2407*	Y	S	A	V	G	V	R	F	M	E	E	K	V	Q	F	Y	T	G	
*A*2408*	Y	S	A	V	G	V	R	F	M	G	E	K	V	H	F	Y	T	G	
*A*2409N*	Y	S	A	V	G	V	R	F	M	E	E	K	V	H	F	Y	T	G	
*A*2410*	Y	S	A	V	G	V	R	F	M	E	E	K	V	H	F	Y	R	W	
*A*2413*	Y	S	A	V	G	V	R	F	M	E	E	K	V	H	F	Y	T	G	
*A*2414*	Y	S	A	V	G	V	R	F	M	E	E	K	V	H	Y	Y	T	G	
*A*2501*	Y	Y	A	V	G	V	R	F	M	R	N	N	V	H	Y	Y	R	W	
*A*2502*	Y	Y	A	V	G	V	R	F	M	R	N	N	V	Q	Y	Y	R	W	
*A*2601*	Y	Y	A	V	G	V	R	F	M	R	N	N	V	H	Y	Y	R	W	
*A*2602*	Y	Y	A	V	G	V	R	F	M	R	N	N	V	H	Y	Y	R	W	
*A*2603*	Y	Y	A	V	G	V	R	F	M	R	N	N	V	H	Y	Y	R	W	
*A*2604*	Y	Y	A	V	G	V	R	F	M	R	N	N	V	H	Y	Y	L	W	
*A*2605*	Y	Y	A	V	G	V	R	F	M	R	N	N	V	H	Y	Y	R	W	
*A*2606*	Y	Y	A	V	G	V	R	F	M	R	N	N	V	H	Y	Y	R	W	
*A*2607*	Y	Y	A	V	G	V	R	F	M	G	E	K	V	H	Y	Y	R	W	
*A*2608*	Y	Y	A	V	G	V	R	F	M	R	N	N	V	H	Y	Y	R	W	
*A*2901*	Y	T	A	V	G	V	R	F	M	L	Q	N	V	Q	Y	Y	T	W	
*A*2902*	Y	T	A	V	G	V	R	F	M	L	Q	N	V	Q	Y	Y	T	W	E,(M)
*A*2903*	Y	T	A	V	G	V	R	F	M	L	Q	N	V	Q	Y	Y	T	G	
*A*3001*	Y	S	A	V	G	V	R	F	M	Q	E	N	V	Q	Y	Y	T	W	
*A*3002*	Y	S	A	V	G	V	R	F	M	Q	E	N	V	H	Y	Y	T	W	
*A*3003*	Y	S	A	V	G	V	R	F	M	Q	E	N	V	H	Y	Y	T	W	
*A*3004*	Y	S	A	V	G	V	R	F	M	Q	E	N	V	H	Y	Y	T	W	
*A*3005*	Y	S	A	V	G	V	R	F	M	R	E	N	V	H	Y	Y	T	W	
*A*31012*	Y	T	A	V	G	V	R	F	M	Q	E	N	V	H	Y	Y	T	W	L,V,Y,F,(T,Q)
*A*3201*	Y	F	A	V	G	V	R	F	M	Q	E	N	V	H	Y	Y	T	W	
*A*3202*	Y	F	A	V	G	V	R	F	M	Q	E	N	V	H	Y	Y	T	W	
*A*3301*	Y	T	A	V	G	V	R	F	M	R	N	N	V	H	Y	Y	T	W	
*A*3302*	Y	T	A	V	G	V	R	F	M	R	N	N	V	H	Y	Y	T	W	A,I,L,F,Y,V,(T)
*A*3303*	Y	T	A	V	G	V	R	F	M	R	N	N	V	H	Y	Y	T	W	
*A*3401*	Y	Y	A	V	G	V	R	F	M	R	N	K	V	Q	Y	Y	T	W	

Table 3.4. (con't)

Chelvanayagam 1996[17]	7	9	24	25	26	34	35	36	45	62	63	66	67	70	99	159	163	167	Anchors/preferred residues
Saper et al. 1991[25]	7	9	24	25		34			45		63	66	67	70	99				
Matsumura et al. 1992[16]	7	9	24			34			45		63		67	70	99				
*A*3402*	Y	Y	A	V	G	V	R	F	M	R	N	N	V	Q	Y	Y	T	W	
*A*3601*	Y	F	A	V	G	V	R	F	M	Q	E	N	M	H	Y	Y	T	W	
*A*4301*	Y	Y	A	V	G	V	R	F	M	L	Q	N	V	H	Y	Y	R	W	
*A*6601*	Y	Y	A	V	G	V	R	F	M	R	N	N	V	Q	Y	Y	R	W	
*A*6602*	Y	Y	A	V	G	V	R	F	M	R	N	N	V	Q	Y	Y	E	W	
*A*6603*	Y	Y	A	V	G	V	R	F	M	R	N	N	V	H	Y	Y	E	W	
*A*68011*	Y	Y	A	V	G	V	R	F	M	R	N	N	V	Q	Y	Y	T	W	V,T
*A*68012*	Y	Y	A	V	G	V	R	F	M	R	N	N	V	Q	Y	Y	T	W	
*A*6802*	Y	Y	A	V	G	V	R	F	M	R	N	N	V	Q	Y	Y	T	W	
*A*6803*	Y	Y	A	V	G	V	R	F	M	R	N	N	V	H	Y	Y	T	W	
*A*6901*	Y	Y	A	V	G	V	R	F	M	R	N	N	V	Q	Y	Y	T	W	V,T,A
*A*7401*	Y	F	A	V	G	V	R	F	M	Q	E	N	V	H	Y	Y	T	W	
*A*7402*	Y	F	A	V	G	V	R	F	M	Q	E	N	V	H	Y	Y	T	W	
*A*7403*	Y	F	A	V	G	V	R	F	M	Q	E	N	V	H	Y	Y	T	W	
*A*8001*	Y	F	A	V	G	V	Q	F	M	E	E	N	V	H	Y	Y	E	G	

Table 3.5. Pocket for peptide position 2 (Pocket B)

Chelvanayagam 1996[17]	7	9	24	25	26	34	35	36	45	62	63	66	67	70	99	159	163	167	Anchors/preferred residues
Saper et al 1991[25]	7	9	24	25		34			45		63	66	67	70	99				
Matsumura et al 1992[16]	7	9	24			34			45		63		67	70	99				
*B*0702*	Y	Y	S	V	G	V	R	F	E	R	N	I	Y	Q	Y	Y	E	W	P,(V)
*B*0703*	Y	Y	S	V	G	V	R	F	E	R	N	I	Y	N	Y	Y	E	W	P,(N,D)
*B*0704*	Y	Y	S	V	G	V	R	F	E	R	N	I	Y	Q	Y	Y	E	W	
*B*0705*	Y	Y	S	V	G	V	R	F	E	R	N	I	Y	Q	Y	Y	E	W	P
*B*0706*	Y	Y	S	V	G	V	R	F	E	R	N	I	Y	Q	Y	Y	E	W	
*B*0707*	Y	Y	S	V	G	V	R	F	E	R	N	I	Y	Q	Y	Y	E	W	
*B*0801*	Y	D	S	V	G	V	R	F	E	R	N	I	F	N	Y	Y	T	W	
*B*0802*	Y	D	S	V	G	V	R	F	E	R	N	I	F	N	Y	Y	T	W	
*B*0803*	.	D	S	V	G	V	R	F	E	R	N	I	F	N	Y	Y	T	W	
*B*1301*	Y	Y	T	V	G	V	R	F	M	R	E	I	S	N	Y	Y	E	W	
*B*1302*	Y	Y	T	V	G	V	R	F	M	R	E	I	S	N	Y	Y	E	W	

*B*1303*	Y	Y	T	V	G	V	R	F	M	R	E	I	S	N	Y	Y	L	W	
*B*1401*	Y	Y	S	V	G	V	R	F	E	R	N	I	C	N	Y	Y	T	W	R,K
*B*1402*	Y	Y	S	V	G	V	R	F	E	R	N	I	C	N	Y	Y	T	W	
*B*1501*	Y	Y	A	V	G	V	R	F	M	R	E	I	S	N	Y	Y	L	W	Q,L,(M,V)
*B*1502*	Y	Y	A	V	G	V	R	F	M	R	N	I	S	N	Y	Y	L	W	
*B*1503*	Y	Y	S	V	G	V	R	F	E	R	E	I	S	N	Y	Y	L	W	
*B*1504*	Y	Y	A	V	G	V	R	F	M	R	E	I	S	N	Y	Y	L	W	
*B*1505*	Y	Y	A	V	G	V	R	F	M	R	E	I	S	N	Y	Y	L	W	
*B*1506*	Y	Y	A	V	G	V	R	F	M	R	E	I	S	N	F	Y	L	W	
*B*1507*	Y	Y	A	V	G	V	R	F	M	R	E	I	S	N	Y	Y	L	W	
*B*1508*	Y	Y	A	V	G	V	R	F	M	R	N	I	F	N	Y	Y	L	W	
*B*1509*	Y	Y	S	V	G	V	R	F	E	R	N	I	C	N	Y	Y	L	W	
*B*1510*	Y	Y	S	V	G	V	R	F	E	R	N	I	C	N	Y	Y	L	W	
*B*1511*	Y	Y	A	V	G	V	R	F	M	R	N	I	Y	N	Y	Y	L	W	
*B*1512*	Y	Y	A	V	G	V	R	F	M	R	E	I	S	N	Y	Y	L	G	
*B*1513*	Y	Y	A	V	G	V	R	F	M	R	N	I	S	N	Y	Y	L	W	
*B*1514*	Y	Y	A	V	G	V	R	F	M	R	E	I	S	N	Y	Y	L	S	
*B*1515*	Y	Y	A	V	G	V	R	F	M	R	N	I	S	N	Y	Y	L	W	
*B*1516*	Y	Y	A	V	G	V	R	F	M	R	E	N	M	S	Y	Y	L	W	
*B*1517*	Y	Y	A	V	G	V	R	F	M	R	E	N	M	S	Y	Y	L	W	
*B*1518*	Y	Y	S	V	G	V	R	F	E	R	N	I	C	N	Y	Y	L	W	
*B*1519*	Y	Y	A	V	G	V	R	F	M	R	E	I	S	N	Y	Y	L	G	
*B*1520*	Y	Y	A	V	G	V	R	F	M	R	E	I	S	N	Y	Y	L	W	
*B*1521*	Y	Y	A	V	G	V	R	F	M	R	N	I	C	N	Y	Y	L	W	
*B*1522*	Y	Y	A	V	G	V	R	F	T	R	N	I	F	N	Y	Y	L	W	
*B*1523*	Y	Y	S	V	G	V	R	F	E	R	N	I	C	N	Y	Y	L	W	
*B*1524*	Y	Y	A	V	G	V	R	F	M	R	E	I	S	N	Y	Y	L	W	
*B*1525*	Y	Y	A	V	G	V	R	F	M	R	E	I	S	N	Y	Y	L	W	
*B*1526N*	Y	Y	A	V	G	V	R	F	M	R	E	I	S	N	/	Y	L	W	
*B*1527*	Y	Y	A	V	G	V	R	F	M	R	E	I	S	N	F	Y	L	W	
*B*1528*	Y	Y	A	V	G	V	R	F	M	R	E	I	S	N	Y	Y	L	W	
*B*1529*	Y	Y	S	V	G	V	R	F	E	R	N	I	F	N	Y	Y	L	W	
*B*1530*	Y	Y	A	V	G	V	R	F	M	R	E	I	S	N	Y	Y	L	W	
*B*1531*	Y	Y	A	V	G	V	R	F	M	R	N	I	S	N	Y	Y	L	W	
*B*1532*	Y	Y	A	V	G	V	R	F	M	R	E	I	S	N	S	Y	L	W	
*B*1533*	Y	Y	A	V	G	V	R	F	M	R	E	I	S	N	Y	Y	L	W	

Table 3.5. (con't)

Chelvanayagam 1996[17]	7	9	24	25	26	34	35	36	45	62	63	66	67	70	99	159	163	167	Anchors/preferred residues
Saper et al 1991[25]	7	9	24	25		34			45		63	66	67	70	99				
Matsumura et al 1992[16]	7	9	24			34			45		63		67	70	99				
*B*1534*	Y	Y	A	V	G	V	R	F	M	R	E	I	S	N	Y	Y	L	W	
*B*1535*	Y	Y	A	V	G	V	R	F	M	R	E	I	S	N	Y	Y	L	W	
*B*1537*	Y	Y	S	V	G	V	R	F	E	R	N	I	C	N	Y	Y	L	W	
*B*1801*	Y	H	S	V	G	V	R	F	T	R	N	I	S	N	Y	Y	T	W	
*B*1802*	Y	H	S	V	G	V	R	F	T	R	N	I	S	N	Y	Y	T	W	
*B*1803*	Y	H	S	V	G	V	R	F	T	R	N	I	S	N	Y	Y	T	W	
*B*1805*	Y	H	S	V	G	V	R	F	T	R	N	I	S	N	Y	Y	T	W	
*B*2701*	Y	H	T	V	G	V	R	F	E	R	E	I	C	K	Y	Y	E	W	
*B*2702*	Y	H	T	V	G	V	R	F	E	R	E	I	C	K	Y	Y	E	W	R
*B*2703*	Y	H	T	V	G	V	R	F	E	R	E	I	C	K	Y	Y	E	W	
*B*2704*	Y	H	T	V	G	V	R	F	E	R	E	I	C	K	Y	Y	E	W	
*B*27052*	Y	H	T	V	G	V	R	F	E	R	E	I	C	K	Y	Y	E	W	R
*B*27053*	.	.	.	.	.	V	R	F	E	R	E	I	C	K	Y	Y	E	W	
*B*2706*	Y	H	T	V	G	V	R	F	E	R	E	I	C	K	Y	Y	E	W	
*B*2707*	Y	H	T	V	G	V	R	F	E	R	E	I	C	K	Y	Y	E	W	
*B*2708*	Y	H	T	V	G	V	R	F	E	R	E	I	C	K	Y	Y	E	W	
*B*2709*	Y	H	T	V	G	V	R	F	E	R	E	I	C	K	Y	Y	E	W	
*B*2710*	Y	H	T	V	G	V	R	F	E	R	E	I	C	K	Y	Y	E	W	
*B*3501*	Y	Y	A	V	G	V	R	F	T	R	N	I	F	N	Y	Y	L	W	P,(A,V,Y,R,D)
*B*3502*	Y	Y	A	V	G	V	R	F	T	R	N	I	F	N	Y	Y	L	W	
*B*3503*	Y	Y	A	V	G	V	R	F	T	R	N	I	F	N	Y	Y	L	W	P,(M,I,L,F,V)
*B*3504*	Y	Y	A	V	G	V	R	F	T	R	N	I	F	N	Y	Y	L	W	
*B*3505*	Y	Y	A	V	G	V	R	F	T	R	N	I	F	N	Y	Y	L	W	
*B*3506*	Y	Y	A	V	G	V	R	F	T	R	N	I	F	N	Y	Y	L	W	
*B*3507*	Y	Y	A	V	G	V	R	F	T	R	N	I	F	N	Y	Y	L	W	
*B*3508*	Y	Y	A	V	G	V	R	F	T	R	N	I	F	N	Y	Y	L	W	
*B*35091*	Y	Y	A	V	G	V	R	F	T	R	N	I	F	N	Y	Y	L	W	
*B*35092*	Y	Y	A	V	G	V	R	F	T	R	N	I	F	N	Y	Y	L	W	
*B*3510*	Y	Y	A	V	G	V	R	F	T	R	E	I	F	N	Y	Y	L	W	
*B*3511*	Y	Y	A	V	G	V	R	F	T	R	N	I	F	N	Y	Y	L	W	
*B*3512*	Y	Y	A	V	G	V	R	F	T	R	N	I	F	N	Y	Y	L	W	
*B*3513*	Y	Y	A	V	G	V	R	F	T	R	E	I	F	N	Y	Y	L	W	
*B*3515*	Y	Y	A	V	G	V	R	F	T	R	N	I	F	N	Y	Y	E	W	
*B*3516*	Y	Y	A	V	G	V	R	F	T	R	E	I	F	N	Y	Y	L	W	
*B*3517*	Y	Y	A	V	G	V	R	F	T	R	N	I	F	N	Y	Y	L	W	
*B*3518*	Y	Y	A	V	G	V	R	F	T	R	N	I	F	N	Y	Y	L	W	
*B*3519*	Y	Y	A	V	G	V	R	F	K	R	N	I	F	N	Y	Y	L	W	

*B*3520*	Y	Y	A	V	G	V	R	F	T	R	N	I	S	N	Y	Y	L	W	
*B*3521*	Y	Y	A	V	G	V	R	F	T	R	N	I	F	N	Y	Y	L	W	
*B*3701*	Y	H	S	V	G	V	R	F	T	R	E	I	S	N	S	Y	T	W	D,E, (H,P,G,S,L)
*B*3702*	Y	H	S	V	G	V	R	F	T	R	E	I	S	N	Y	Y	E	W	
*B*3801*	Y	Y	S	V	G	V	R	F	E	R	N	I	C	N	Y	Y	T	W	H,(F,P,W,Y)
*B*3802*	Y	Y	S	V	G	V	R	F	E	R	N	I	C	N	Y	Y	T	W	
*B*39011*	Y	Y	S	V	G	V	R	F	E	R	N	I	C	N	Y	Y	T	W	R,H
*B*39013*	Y	Y	S	V	G	V	R	F	E	R	N	I	C	N	Y	Y	T	W	
*B*39021*	Y	Y	S	V	G	V	R	F	E	R	E	I	S	N	Y	Y	T	W	K,Q
*B*39022*	Y	Y	S	V	G	V	R	F	E	R	E	I	S	N	Y	Y	T	W	
*B*3903*	Y	Y	S	V	G	V	R	F	E	R	N	I	C	N	Y	Y	T	W	
*B*3904*	Y	Y	S	V	G	V	R	F	E	R	N	I	C	N	Y	Y	T	W	
*B*3905*	Y	Y	S	V	G	V	R	F	E	R	N	I	C	N	Y	Y	T	W	
*B*39061*	Y	Y	S	V	G	V	R	F	E	R	N	I	C	N	Y	Y	T	W	
*B*39062*	Y	Y	S	V	G	V	R	F	E	R	N	I	C	N	Y	Y	T	W	
*B*3907*	.	.	.	.	.	.	.	F	E	R	N	I	C	N	Y	Y	T	W	
*B*3908*	Y	Y	S	V	G	V	R	F	E	R	E	I	S	N	Y	Y	T	W	
*B*3909*	Y	Y	S	V	G	V	R	F	E	R	N	I	C	N	S	Y	T	W	
*B*3910*	Y	Y	S	V	G	V	R	F	E	R	N	I	Y	N	Y	Y	T	W	
*B*3911*	.	Y	S	V	G	V	R	F	E	R	N	I	C	N	Y	Y	T	W	
*B*3912*	Y	D	S	V	G	V	R	F	E	R	N	I	C	N	Y	Y	T	W	
*B*40011*	Y	H	T	V	G	V	R	F	K	R	E	I	S	N	Y	Y	E	W	
*B*40012*	Y	H	T	V	G	V	R	F	K	R	E	I	S	N	Y	Y	E	W	E
*B*4002*	Y	H	T	V	G	V	R	F	K	R	E	I	S	N	Y	Y	E	W	
*B*4003*	Y	H	T	V	G	V	R	F	K	R	E	I	S	N	Y	Y	E	W	
*B*4004*	Y	H	T	V	G	V	R	F	K	R	E	I	S	N	Y	Y	E	W	
*B*4005*	Y	H	T	V	G	V	R	F	K	R	E	I	S	N	Y	Y	L	W	
*B*4006*	Y	H	T	V	G	V	R	F	K	R	E	I	S	N	Y	Y	E	W	E,(P)
*B*4007*	Y	H	T	V	G	V	R	F	K	R	E	I	F	N	Y	Y	E	W	
*B*4008*	Y	H	T	V	G	V	R	F	K	R	N	I	F	N	Y	Y	E	W	
*B*4009*	Y	H	T	V	G	V	R	F	K	R	E	I	S	N	Y	Y	E	W	
*B*4101*	Y	H	T	V	G	V	R	F	K	R	E	I	S	N	Y	Y	T	W	
*B*4102*	Y	H	T	V	G	V	R	F	K	R	E	I	S	N	Y	Y	T	W	
*B*4201*	Y	Y	S	V	G	V	R	F	E	R	N	I	Y	Q	Y	Y	T	W	
*B*4402*	Y	Y	T	V	G	V	R	F	K	R	E	I	S	N	Y	Y	L	S	E,(M,I,L,D,N)
*B*44031*	Y	Y	T	V	G	V	R	F	K	R	E	I	S	N	Y	Y	L	S	E,(M,I,L,V,D,N)
*B*44032*	Y	Y	T	V	G	V	R	F	K	R	E	I	S	N	Y	Y	L	S	
*B*4404*	Y	Y	T	V	G	V	R	F	K	R	E	I	S	N	Y	Y	T	S	
*B*4405*	Y	Y	T	V	G	V	R	F	K	R	E	I	S	N	Y	Y	L	S	
*B*4406*	Y	Y	A	V	G	V	R	F	T	R	N	I	F	N	Y	Y	L	S	
*B*4407*	Y	Y	T	V	G	V	R	F	K	R	E	I	S	N	Y	Y	L	S	
*B*4408*	Y	Y	T	V	G	V	R	F	M	R	E	I	S	N	Y	Y	L	S	

Table 3.5. (con't)

Chelvanayagam 1996[17]	7	9	24	25	26	34	35	36	45	62	63	66	67	70	99	159	163	167	Anchors/preferred residues
Saper et al 1991[25]	7	9	24	25		34			45		63	66	67	70	99				
Matsumura et al 1992[16]	7	9	24			34			45		63		67	70	99				
*B*4410*	Y	Y	T	V	G	V	R	F	K	R	E	I	S	N	F	Y	L	S	
*B*4501*	Y	H	T	V	G	V	R	F	K	R	E	I	S	N	Y	Y	L	S	
*B*4601*	Y	Y	A	V	G	V	R	F	M	R	E	K	Y	Q	Y	Y	L	W	M,(I)
*B*4701*	Y	Y	T	V	G	V	R	F	K	R	E	I	S	N	F	Y	E	W	
*B*4702*	Y	Y	T	V	G	V	R	F	K	R	E	I	S	N	F	Y	T	W	
*B*4801*	Y	Y	S	V	G	V	R	F	E	R	E	I	S	N	Y	Y	E	W	
*B*4802*	Y	Y	S	V	G	V	R	F	E	R	E	I	S	N	Y	Y	L	W	
*B*4803*	Y	Y	S	V	G	V	R	F	E	R	E	I	S	N	Y	Y	E	W	
*B*4901*	Y	H	T	V	G	V	R	F	K	R	E	I	S	N	Y	Y	L	W	
*B*5001*	Y	H	T	V	G	V	R	F	K	R	E	I	S	N	Y	Y	L	W	
*B*51011*	Y	Y	A	V	G	V	R	F	T	R	N	I	F	N	Y	Y	L	W	A,P,G,(W,F)
*B*51012*	Y	Y	A	V	G	V	R	F	T	R	N	I	F	N	Y	Y	L	W	
*B*51021*	Y	Y	A	V	G	V	R	F	T	R	N	I	F	N	Y	Y	L	W	P,A,G
*B*51022*	Y	Y	A	V	G	V	R	F	T	R	N	I	F	N	Y	Y	L	W	
*B*5103*	Y	Y	A	V	G	V	R	F	T	R	N	I	F	N	Y	Y	L	G	P,A,G,(W,F)
*B*5104*	Y	Y	A	V	G	V	R	F	T	R	N	I	F	N	Y	Y	L	W	
*B*5105*	Y	Y	A	V	G	V	R	F	T	R	N	I	F	N	Y	Y	L	W	
*B*5106*	Y	Y	A	V	G	V	R	F	T	R	N	I	F	N	Y	Y	L	W	
*B*5107*	Y	Y	A	V	G	V	R	F	T	R	N	I	S	N	Y	Y	L	W	
*B*5108*	.	.	A	V	G	V	R	F	T	R	N	I	F	N	Y	Y	L	W	
*B*52011*	Y	Y	A	V	G	V	R	F	T	R	E	I	S	N	Y	Y	L	W	Q,(M,F,P)
*B*52012*	Y	Y	A	V	G	V	R	F	T	R	E	I	S	N	Y	Y	L	W	
*B*5301*	Y	Y	A	V	G	V	R	F	T	R	N	I	F	N	Y	Y	L	W	P
*B*5401*	Y	Y	A	V	G	V	R	F	G	R	N	I	Y	Q	Y	Y	T	W	P
*B*5501*	Y	Y	A	V	G	V	R	F	E	R	N	I	Y	Q	Y	Y	T	W	P
*B*5502*	Y	Y	A	V	G	V	R	F	E	R	N	I	Y	Q	Y	Y	T	W	P
*B*5503*	Y	Y	A	V	G	V	R	F	E	R	N	I	Y	Q	Y	Y	T	W	
*B*5504*	Y	Y	A	V	G	V	R	F	E	R	N	I	Y	Q	Y	Y	T	W	
*B*5505*	Y	Y	A	V	G	V	R	F	E	R	N	I	Y	Q	Y	Y	T	W	
*B*5601*	Y	Y	A	V	G	V	R	F	E	R	N	I	Y	Q	Y	Y	L	W	P
*B*5602*	Y	Y	A	V	G	V	R	F	E	R	N	I	Y	Q	Y	Y	L	W	
*B*5603*	Y	Y	A	V	G	V	R	F	E	R	N	I	Y	Q	Y	Y	L	W	
*B*5701*	Y	Y	A	V	G	V	R	F	M	G	E	N	M	S	Y	Y	L	W	
*B*5702*	Y	Y	A	V	G	V	R	F	M	G	E	N	M	S	Y	Y	L	W	
*B*5703*	Y	Y	A	V	G	V	R	F	M	G	E	N	M	S	Y	Y	L	W	

*B*5704*	Y	Y	A	V	G	V	R	F	M	G	E	N	M	S	Y	Y	L	W	
*B*5801*	Y	Y	A	V	G	V	R	F	T	G	E	N	M	S	Y	Y	L	W	A,S,T,(G)
*B*5802*	Y	Y	A	V	G	V	R	F	T	G	E	N	M	S	Y	Y	L	W	
*B*5901*	Y	Y	A	V	G	V	R	F	E	R	N	I	F	N	Y	Y	T	W	
*B*67011*	Y	Y	S	V	G	V	R	F	E	R	N	I	Y	Q	Y	Y	T	W	P
*B*67012*	Y	Y	S	V	G	V	R	F	E	R	N	I	Y	Q	Y	Y	T	W	
*B*7301*	Y	H	T	V	G	V	R	F	E	R	N	I	C	K	Y	Y	E	W	R
*B*7801*	Y	Y	A	V	G	V	R	F	T	R	N	I	F	N	Y	Y	L	W	P,A,G
*B*78021*	Y	Y	A	V	G	V	R	F	T	R	N	I	F	N	Y	Y	L	W	
*B*78022*	Y	Y	A	V	G	V	R	F	T	R	N	I	F	N	Y	Y	L	W	
*B*8101*	Y	Y	S	V	G	V	R	F	E	R	N	I	Y	Q	Y	Y	E	W	
*B*8201*	Y	Y	S	V	G	V	R	F	E	R	N	I	Y	Q	F	Y	L	S	

Table 3.6. Pocket for peptide position 2 (Pocket B)

Chelvanayagam 1996[17]	7	9	24	25	26	34	35	36	45	62	63	66	67	70	99	159	163	167	Anchors/preferred residues
Saper et al 1991[25]	7	9	24	25		34			45		63	66	67	70	99				
Matsumura et al 1992[16]	7	9	24			34			45		63		67	70	99				
*Cw*0102*	Y	F	S	V	G	V	R	F	G	R	E	K	Y	Q	C	Y	T	W	A, L
*Cw*0103*	Y	F	S	V	G	V	R	F	G	R	E	K	Y	Q	C	Y	T	W	
*Cw*02021*	Y	Y	A	V	G	V	R	F	G	R	E	K	Y	Q	Y	Y	E	W	
*Cw*02022*	Y	Y	A	V	G	V	R	F	G	R	E	K	Y	Q	Y	Y	E	W	
*Cw*02023*	Y	Y	A	V	G	V	R	F	G	R	E	K	Y	Q	Y	Y	E	W	
*Cw*0302*	Y	Y	A	V	G	V	R	F	G	R	E	K	Y	Q	Y	Y	L	W	
*Cw*0303*	Y	Y	A	V	G	V	R	F	G	R	E	K	Y	Q	Y	Y	L	W	
*Cw*0304*	Y	Y	A	V	G	V	R	F	G	R	E	K	Y	Q	Y	Y	L	W	A
*Cw*0401*	Y	S	A	V	G	V	R	F	G	R	E	K	Y	Q	F	Y	T	W	Y,P,F
*Cw*0402*	Y	S	A	V	G	V	R	F	G	R	E	K	Y	Q	F	Y	T	W	
*Cw*0403*	Y	Y	A	V	G	V	R	F	G	R	E	K	Y	Q	F	Y	T	W	
*Cw*0501*	Y	Y	A	V	G	V	Q	F	G	R	E	K	Y	Q	Y	Y	T	W	
*Cw*0602*	Y	D	S	V	G	V	R	F	G	R	E	K	Y	Q	Y	Y	T	W	(P,R)
*Cw*0701*	Y	D	S	V	G	V	R	F	G	R	E	N	Y	Q	Y	Y	T	W	Y,P,(R,D)
*Cw*0702*	Y	D	S	V	G	V	R	F	G	R	E	K	Y	Q	S	Y	T	W	
*Cw*0703*	Y	D	S	V	G	V	R	F	G	R	E	K	Y	Q	S	Y	L	W	
*Cw*0704*	Y	D	S	V	G	V	R	F	G	R	E	K	Y	Q	Y	Y	T	W	
*Cw*0705*	Y	D	S	V	G	V	R	F	G	R	E	K	Y	Q	Y	Y	T	W	

Table 3.6. (con't)

Chelvanayagam 1996[17]	7	9	24	25	26	34	35	36	45	62	63	66	67	70	99	159	163	167	Anchors/preferred residues
Saper et al 1991[25]	7	9	24	25		34			45		63	66	67	70	99				
Matsumura et al 1992[16]	7	9	24			34			45		63		67	70	99				
*Cw*0706*	Y	D	S	V	G	V	R	F	G	R	E	N	Y	Q	Y	Y	T	W	
*Cw*0707*	Y	D	S	V	G	V	R	F	G	R	E	N	Y	Q	Y	Y	T	W	
*Cw*0801*	Y	Y	A	V	G	V	Q	F	G	R	E	K	Y	Q	Y	Y	T	W	
*Cw*0802*	Y	Y	A	V	G	V	Q	F	G	R	E	K	Y	Q	Y	Y	T	W	
*Cw*0803*	Y	Y	A	V	G	V	Q	F	G	R	E	K	Y	Q	Y	Y	T	W	
*Cw*12021*	Y	Y	A	V	G	V	R	F	G	R	E	K	Y	Q	Y	Y	T	W	
*Cw*12022*	Y	Y	A	V	G	V	R	F	G	R	E	K	Y	Q	Y	Y	T	W	
*Cw*1203*	Y	Y	A	V	G	V	R	F	G	R	E	K	Y	Q	Y	Y	T	W	
*Cw*1204*	Y	Y	A	V	G	V	R	F	G	R	E	K	Y	Q	Y	Y	T	W	
*Cw*1301*	Y	Y	A	V	G	V	R	F	G	R	E	K	Y	Q	Y	Y	T	W	
*Cw*1402*	Y	S	A	V	G	V	R	F	G	R	E	K	Y	Q	F	Y	T	W	
*Cw*1403*	Y	S	A	V	G	V	R	F	G	R	E	K	Y	Q	F	Y	T	W	
*Cw*1502*	Y	Y	A	V	G	V	R	F	G	R	E	N	Y	Q	Y	Y	T	W	
*Cw*1503*	Y	Y	A	V	G	V	R	F	G	R	E	N	Y	Q	Y	Y	T	W	
*Cw*1504*	Y	Y	A	V	G	V	R	F	G	R	E	N	Y	Q	Y	Y	T	W	
*Cw*15051*	Y	Y	A	V	G	V	R	F	G	R	E	N	Y	Q	Y	Y	T	W	
*Cw*15052*	Y	Y	A	V	G	V	R	F	G	R	E	N	Y	Q	Y	Y	T	W	
*Cw*1601*	Y	Y	A	V	G	V	R	F	G	R	E	K	Y	Q	Y	Y	T	W	
*Cw*1602*	Y	Y	A	V	G	V	R	F	G	R	E	K	Y	Q	Y	Y	T	W	
*Cw*1701*	Y	Y	A	V	G	V	R	F	G	R	E	K	Y	Q	Y	Y	E	W	
*Cw*1702*	Y	Y	A	V	G	V	R	F	G	R	E	K	Y	Q	Y	Y	E	W	
*Cw*1801*	Y	D	S	V	G	V	R	F	G	R	E	K	Y	Q	F	Y	T	W	
*Cw*1802*	Y	D	S	V	G	V	R	F	G	R	E	K	Y	Q	F	Y	T	W	

Table 3.7. Pocket for peptide position 3 (Pocket D)

Chelvanayagam 1996[17]	7	9	62	66	70	97	99		114	152	155	156	159		163	Anchors/preferred residues
Saper et al 1991[25]							99	113	114		155	156	159	160		
Matsumura et al 1992[16]							99		114			156	159	160		
*A*0101*	Y	F	Q	N	H	I	Y	Y	R	A	Q	R	Y	L	R	D,E
*A*0102*	Y	S	Q	N	H	I	Y	Y	R	A	Q	R	Y	L	R	
*A*0201*	Y	F	G	K	H	R	Y	Y	H	V	Q	L	Y	L	T	(A,Y,F,P,M,S,R)
*A*0202*	Y	F	G	K	H	R	Y	Y	H	V	Q	W	Y	L	T	(F,A)
*A*0203*	Y	F	G	K	H	R	Y	Y	H	E	Q	W	Y	L	T	

*A*0204*	Y	F	G	K	H	M	Y	Y	H	V	Q	L	Y	L	T	
*A*0205*	Y	Y	G	K	H	R	Y	Y	H	V	Q	W	Y	L	T	(I,M,Y,P,F)
*A*0206*	Y	Y	G	K	H	R	Y	Y	H	V	Q	L	Y	L	T	I,L
*A*0207*	Y	F	G	K	H	R	C	Y	H	V	Q	L	Y	L	T	D,P
*A*0208*	Y	Y	G	N	H	R	Y	Y	H	V	Q	W	Y	L	T	
*A*0209*	Y	F	G	K	H	R	Y	Y	H	V	Q	L	Y	L	T	
*A*0210*	Y	Y	G	K	H	R	F	Y	H	V	Q	L	Y	L	T	
*A*0211*	Y	F	G	K	H	R	Y	Y	H	V	Q	L	Y	L	T	
*A*0212*	Y	F	G	K	H	R	Y	Y	H	V	Q	Q	Y	L	T	
*A*0213*	Y	F	G	K	H	R	Y	Y	H	E	Q	Q	Y	L	T	
*A*0214*	Y	Y	G	K	H	R	Y	Y	H	V	Q	L	Y	L	T	(I,L,M,D,Y,P)
*A*0215N*	Y	F	G	K	H	R	C	Y	H	V	Q	L	Y	L	T	
*A*0216*	Y	F	G	K	H	R	Y	Y	H	V	Q	L	Y	L	E	
*A*0217*	Y	F	G	K	H	M	F	Y	H	V	Q	L	Y	L	T	
*A*0218*	Y	F	G	K	H	R	C	Y	H	V	Q	L	Y	L	T	
*A*0219*	Y	F	G	K	H	R	Y	Y	H	V	Q	Q	Y	L	T	
*A*0220*	Y	F	G	N	H	R	Y	Y	H	V	Q	L	Y	L	T	
*A*0221*	Y	Y	G	K	H	R	Y	Y	H	V	Q	L	Y	L	T	
*A*0222*	Y	F	G	K	H	R	Y	Y	H	V	Q	W	Y	L	T	
*A*0301*	Y	F	Q	N	Q	I	Y	Y	R	E	Q	L	Y	L	T	Y,F
*A*0302*	Y	F	Q	N	Q	I	Y	Y	R	V	Q	Q	Y	L	T	
*A*0303N*	Y	F	Q	N	Q	I	Y	Y	R	E	Q	L	Y	L	T	
*A*1101*	Y	Y	Q	N	Q	I	Y	Y	R	A	Q	Q	Y	L	R	M,L,F,Y,I,A,(N,D,E,Q)
*A*1102*	Y	Y	Q	N	Q	I	Y	Y	R	A	Q	Q	Y	L	R	
*A*1103*	Y	Y	Q	N	Q	I	Y	Y	R	E	Q	Q	Y	L	R	
*A*1104*	Y	Y	Q	N	Q	I	Y	Y	R	A	Q	Q	Y	L	T	
*A*2301*	Y	S	E	K	H	M	F	Y	H	V	Q	L	Y	L	T	
*A*2402*	Y	S	E	K	H	M	F	Y	H	V	Q	Q	Y	L	T	
*A*2403*	Y	S	E	K	H	M	F	Y	H	V	Q	Q	Y	L	T	
*A*2404*	Y	S	E	K	H	M	F	Y	H	V	Q	Q	Y	L	T	
*A*2405*	Y	S	E	K	H	M	F	Y	H	V	Q	Q	Y	L	T	
*A*2406*	Y	S	E	K	H	M	F	Y	H	V	Q	W	Y	L	T	
*A*2407*	Y	S	E	K	Q	M	F	Y	H	V	Q	Q	Y	L	T	
*A*2408*	Y	S	G	K	H	M	F	Y	H	V	Q	Q	Y	L	T	
*A*2409N*	Y	S	E	K	H	M	F	Y	H	V	Q	Q	Y	L	T	
*A*2410*	Y	S	E	K	H	M	F	Y	H	V	Q	Q	Y	L	R	
*A*2413*	Y	S	E	K	H	M	F	Y	H	V	Q	L	Y	L	T	
*A*2414*	Y	S	E	K	H	R	Y	Y	H	V	Q	L	Y	L	T	
*A*2501*	Y	Y	R	N	H	R	Y	Y	Q	E	Q	W	Y	L	R	
*A*2502*	Y	Y	R	N	Q	R	Y	Y	Q	E	Q	W	Y	L	R	
*A*2601*	Y	Y	R	N	H	R	Y	Y	Q	E	Q	W	Y	L	R	
*A*2602*	Y	Y	R	N	H	R	Y	Y	Q	E	Q	W	Y	L	R	

Table 3.7. (con't)

Chelvanayagam 1996[17]	7	9	62	66	70	97	99		114	152	155	156	159		163	Anchors/preferred residues
Saper et al 1991[25]							99	113	114		155	156	159	160		
Matsumura et al 1992[16]							99		114			156	159	160		
*A*2603*	Y	Y	R	N	H	R	Y	Y	Q	E	Q	W	Y	L	R	
*A*2604*	Y	Y	R	N	H	R	Y	Y	Q	E	Q	W	Y	L	L	
*A*2605*	Y	Y	R	N	H	R	Y	Y	Q	E	Q	W	Y	L	R	
*A*2606*	Y	Y	R	N	H	R	Y	Y	Q	E	Q	W	Y	L	R	
*A*2607*	Y	Y	G	K	H	R	Y	Y	Q	E	Q	W	Y	L	R	
*A*2608*	Y	Y	R	N	H	R	Y	Y	Q	E	Q	Q	Y	L	R	
*A*2901*	Y	T	L	N	Q	M	Y	Y	R	V	Q	L	Y	L	T	
*A*2902*	Y	T	L	N	Q	M	Y	Y	R	V	Q	L	Y	L	T	F,(V,I,A,K,L)
*A*2903*	Y	T	L	N	Q	M	Y	Y	R	V	Q	L	Y	L	T	
*A*3001*	Y	S	Q	N	Q	I	Y	Y	E	W	Q	L	Y	L	T	
*A*3002*	Y	S	Q	N	H	I	Y	Y	E	R	Q	L	Y	L	T	
*A*3003*	Y	S	Q	N	H	I	Y	Y	E	R	Q	L	Y	L	T	
*A*3004*	Y	S	Q	N	H	I	Y	Y	E	V	Q	W	Y	L	T	
*A*3005*	Y	S	R	N	H	I	Y	Y	E	V	Q	W	Y	L	T	
*A*31012*	Y	T	Q	N	H	M	Y	Y	Q	V	Q	L	Y	L	T	F,L,Y,W,(K,N)
*A*3201*	Y	F	Q	N	H	M	Y	Y	Q	V	Q	L	Y	L	T	
*A*3202*	Y	F	Q	N	H	M	Y	Y	Q	V	Q	Q	Y	L	T	
*A*3301*	Y	T	R	N	H	M	Y	Y	Q	V	Q	L	Y	L	T	
*A*3302*	Y	T	R	N	H	M	Y	Y	Q	V	Q	L	Y	L	T	(L,K,Q,W,E,N)
*A*3303*	Y	T	R	N	H	M	Y	Y	Q	V	Q	L	Y	L	T	
*A*3401*	Y	Y	R	K	Q	R	Y	Y	Q	E	Q	W	Y	L	T	
*A*3402*	Y	Y	R	N	Q	I	Y	Y	R	E	Q	L	Y	L	T	
*A*3601*	Y	F	Q	N	H	I	Y	Y	R	A	Q	R	Y	L	T	
*A*4301*	Y	Y	L	N	H	R	Y	Y	Q	E	Q	W	Y	L	R	
*A*6601*	Y	Y	R	N	Q	R	Y	Y	Q	E	Q	W	Y	L	R	
*A*6602*	Y	Y	R	N	Q	R	Y	Y	Q	E	Q	W	Y	L	E	
*A*6603*	Y	Y	R	N	H	R	Y	Y	Q	E	Q	W	Y	L	E	

Table 3.8. Pocket for peptide position 3 (Pocket D)

Chelvanayagam 1996[17]	7	9	62	66	70	97	99		114	152	155	156	159		163	Anchors/preferred residues
Saper et al 1992[25]							99	113	114		155	156	159	160		
Matsumura et al 1992[16]							99		114			156	159	160		
*B*0702*	Y	Y	R	I	Q	S	Y	H	D	E	Q	R	Y	L	E	(R,K,N,H,F,M,Q,L,Y)
*B*0703*	Y	Y	R	I	N	S	Y	H	D	E	Q	R	Y	L	E	R,(A,T,Q,M,F,H)
*B*0704*	Y	Y	R	I	Q	S	Y	H	D	E	Q	D	Y	L	E	
*B*0705*	Y	Y	R	I	Q	S	Y	H	N	E	Q	R	Y	L	E	(A,L,M,Q,Y,S,I,F,K,N,E,T,W)
*B*0706*	Y	Y	R	I	Q	S	Y	H	N	E	Q	R	Y	L	E	
*B*0707*	Y	Y	R	I	Q	R	Y	H	D	E	Q	R	Y	L	E	
*B*0801*	Y	D	R	I	N	S	Y	H	N	V	Q	D	Y	L	T	
*B*0802*	Y	D	R	I	N	S	Y	H	N	V	Q	D	Y	L	T	
*B*0803*	.	D	R	I	N	S	Y	H	N	V	Q	D	Y	L	T	
*B*1301*	Y	Y	R	I	N	R	Y	H	N	V	Q	L	Y	L	E	
*B*1302*	Y	Y	R	I	N	T	Y	H	N	V	Q	L	Y	L	E	
*B*1303*	Y	Y	R	I	N	T	Y	H	N	V	Q	L	Y	L	L	
*B*1401*	Y	Y	R	I	N	W	Y	Y	N	E	Q	L	Y	L	T	
*B*1402*	Y	Y	R	I	N	W	Y	Y	N	E	Q	L	Y	L	T	
*B*1501*	Y	Y	R	I	N	R	Y	H	D	E	Q	W	Y	L	L	(K,A,N,F,P,Y,H,R)
*B*1502*	Y	Y	R	I	N	R	Y	Y	D	E	Q	L	Y	L	L	
*B*1503*	Y	Y	R	I	N	R	Y	H	D	E	Q	L	Y	L	L	
*B*1504*	Y	Y	R	I	N	T	Y	H	D	E	Q	W	Y	L	L	
*B*1505*	Y	Y	R	I	N	R	Y	H	D	V	Q	L	Y	L	L	
*B*1506*	Y	Y	R	I	N	R	F	Y	D	E	Q	L	Y	L	L	
*B*1507*	Y	Y	R	I	N	S	Y	H	D	E	Q	W	Y	L	L	
*B*1508*	Y	Y	R	I	N	R	Y	H	D	E	Q	W	Y	L	L	
*B*1509*	Y	Y	R	I	N	R	Y	H	N	E	Q	L	Y	L	L	
*B*1510*	Y	Y	R	I	N	R	Y	H	D	E	Q	L	Y	L	L	
*B*1511*	Y	Y	R	I	N	R	Y	H	D	E	Q	W	Y	L	L	

Table 3.8. (con't)

Chelvanayagam 1996[17]	7	9	62	66	70	97	99		114	152	155	156	159		163	Anchors/preferred residues
Saper et al 1992[25]							99	113	114		155	156	159	160		
Matsumura et al 1992[16]							99		114			156	159	160		
*B*1512*	Y	Y	R	I	N	R	Y	H	D	E	Q	W	Y	L	L	
*B*1513*	Y	Y	R	N	S	R	Y	H	D	E	Q	L	Y	L	L	
*B*1517*	Y	Y	R	N	S	R	Y	Y	H	E	Q	L	Y	L	L	
*B*1518*	Y	Y	R	I	N	R	Y	H	D	E	Q	L	Y	L	L	
*B*1519*	Y	Y	R	I	N	R	Y	H	D	E	Q	W	Y	L	L	
*B*1520*	Y	Y	R	I	N	R	Y	H	D	V	Q	L	Y	L	L	
*B*1521*	Y	Y	R	I	N	R	Y	Y	D	E	Q	L	Y	L	L	
*B*1522*	Y	Y	R	I	N	R	Y	H	D	E	Q	W	Y	L	L	
*B*1523*	Y	Y	R	I	N	R	Y	H	D	E	Q	L	Y	L	L	
*B*1524*	Y	Y	R	I	N	R	Y	H	D	E	Q	W	Y	L	L	
*B*1525*	Y	Y	R	I	N	R	Y	Y	D	E	Q	L	Y	L	L	
*B*1526N*	Y	Y	R	I	N	R	/	H	D	E	Q	W	Y	L	L	
*B*1527*	Y	Y	R	I	N	R	F	H	D	E	Q	W	Y	L	L	
*B*1528*	Y	Y	R	I	N	R	Y	H	D	E	Q	W	Y	L	L	
*B*1529*	Y	Y	R	I	N	R	Y	H	D	E	Q	L	Y	L	L	
*B*1530*	Y	Y	R	I	N	R	Y	H	N	E	Q	W	Y	L	L	
*B*1531*	Y	Y	R	I	N	R	Y	Y	D	V	Q	L	Y	L	L	
*B*1532*	Y	Y	R	I	N	R	S	H	D	E	Q	W	Y	L	L	
*B*1533*	Y	Y	R	I	N	R	Y	H	D	E	Q	W	Y	L	L	
*B*1534*	Y	Y	R	I	N	R	Y	H	D	E	Q	W	Y	L	L	
*B*1535*	Y	Y	R	I	N	T	Y	H	D	E	Q	W	Y	L	L	
*B*1537*	Y	Y	R	I	N	R	Y	H	D	E	Q	L	Y	L	L	
*B*1801*	Y	H	R	I	N	R	Y	H	D	V	Q	L	Y	L	T	
*B*1802*	Y	H	R	I	N	N	Y	H	D	V	Q	L	Y	L	T	
*B*1803*	Y	H	R	I	N	R	Y	H	D	V	Q	L	Y	L	T	
*B*1805*	Y	H	R	I	N	R	Y	H	D	V	Q	L	Y	L	T	
*B*2701*	Y	H	R	I	K	N	Y	Y	H	V	Q	L	Y	L	E	
*B*2702*	Y	H	R	I	K	N	Y	Y	H	V	Q	L	Y	L	E	
*B*2704*	Y	H	R	I	K	N	Y	Y	H	E	Q	L	Y	L	E	
*B*27052*	Y	H	R	I	K	N	Y	Y	H	V	Q	L	Y	L	E	(L,I,F)
*B*27053*	.	.	R	I	K	N	Y	Y	H	V	Q	L	Y	L	E	
*B*2706*	Y	H	R	I	K	N	Y	Y	D	E	Q	L	Y	L	E	
*B*2707*	Y	H	R	I	K	S	Y	H	N	V	Q	L	Y	L	E	

*B*2708*	Y	H	R	I	K	N	Y	Y	H	V	Q	L	Y	L	E	
*B*2709*	Y	H	R	I	K	N	Y	Y	H	V	Q	L	Y	L	E	
*B*2710*	Y	H	R	I	K	N	Y	Y	H	E	Q	L	Y	L	E	
*B*3501*	Y	Y	R	I	N	R	Y	H	D	V	Q	L	Y	L	L	(I,L,F,V,M,E,T,Y,N)
*B*3502*	Y	Y	R	I	N	R	Y	H	N	V	Q	L	Y	L	L	
*B*3503*	Y	Y	R	I	N	R	Y	H	D	V	Q	L	Y	L	L	(E,G,N,D,K,H)
*B*3504*	Y	Y	R	I	N	R	Y	H	N	V	Q	L	Y	L	L	
*B*3505*	Y	Y	R	I	N	S	Y	H	D	V	Q	L	Y	L	L	
*B*3506*	Y	Y	R	I	N	R	Y	H	N	V	Q	L	Y	L	L	
*B*3507*	Y	Y	R	I	N	R	Y	H	D	V	Q	L	Y	L	L	
*B*3508*	Y	Y	R	I	N	R	Y	H	D	V	Q	R	Y	L	L	
*B*35091*	Y	Y	R	I	N	R	Y	H	N	V	Q	L	Y	L	L	
*B*35092*	Y	Y	R	I	N	R	Y	H	N	V	Q	L	Y	L	L	
*B*3510*	Y	Y	R	I	N	R	Y	H	D	V	Q	L	Y	L	L	
*B*3511*	Y	Y	R	I	N	R	Y	H	D	E	Q	L	Y	L	L	
*B*3512*	Y	Y	R	I	N	R	Y	H	N	V	Q	L	Y	L	L	
*B*3513*	Y	Y	R	I	N	R	Y	H	D	V	Q	L	Y	L	L	
*B*3515*	Y	Y	R	I	N	R	Y	H	D	V	Q	L	Y	L	E	
*B*3516*	Y	Y	R	I	N	S	Y	H	D	V	Q	L	Y	L	L	
*B*3517*	Y	Y	R	I	N	S	Y	H	D	V	Q	L	Y	L	L	
*B*3518*	Y	Y	R	I	N	R	Y	H	N	V	Q	R	Y	L	L	
*B*3519*	Y	Y	R	I	N	R	Y	H	D	V	Q	L	Y	L	L	
*B*3520*	Y	Y	R	I	N	R	Y	H	D	V	Q	L	Y	L	L	
*B*3521*	Y	Y	R	I	N	R	Y	H	D	E	Q	L	Y	L	L	
*B*3701*	Y	H	R	I	N	R	S	Y	N	V	Q	D	Y	L	T	
*B*3702*	Y	H	R	I	N	N	Y	Y	H	V	Q	L	Y	L	E	
*B*3801*	Y	Y	R	I	N	R	Y	H	N	V	Q	L	Y	L	T	D,E,(I,A,S,N,M,V)
*B*3802*	Y	Y	R	I	N	R	Y	H	N	V	Q	L	Y	L	T	
*B*39011*	Y	Y	R	I	N	R	Y	H	N	V	Q	L	Y	L	T	(A,D,I,L,F,V,M,S,T,Y)
*B*39013*	Y	Y	R	I	N	R	Y	H	N	V	Q	L	Y	L	T	
*B*39021*	Y	Y	R	I	N	R	Y	H	N	V	Q	L	Y	L	T	(A,I,F,V,N,L,T,Y,E,H,S)
*B*39022*	Y	Y	R	I	N	R	Y	H	N	V	Q	L	Y	L	T	
*B*3903*	Y	Y	R	I	N	S	Y	H	N	V	Q	L	Y	L	T	
*B*3904*	Y	Y	R	I	N	R	Y	H	N	V	Q	L	Y	L	T	
*B*3905*	Y	Y	R	I	N	R	Y	H	N	V	Q	L	Y	L	T	
*B*39061*	Y	Y	R	I	N	T	Y	H	N	V	Q	L	Y	L	T	
*B*39062*	Y	Y	R	I	N	T	Y	H	N	V	Q	L	Y	L	T	
*B*3907*	.	.	R	I	N	R	Y	H	D	V	Q	L	Y	L	T	

Table 3.8. (con't)

Chelvanayagam 1996[17]	7	9	62	66	70	97	99		114	152	155	156	159		163	Anchors/preferred residues
Saper et al 1992[25]							99	113	114		155	156	159	160		
Matsumura et al 1992[16]							99		114			156	159	160		
*B*3908*	Y	Y	R	I	N	R	Y	H	N	V	Q	R	Y	L	T	
*B*3909*	Y	Y	R	I	N	R	S	H	N	V	Q	L	Y	L	T	
*B*3910*	Y	Y	R	I	N	R	Y	H	N	V	Q	L	Y	L	T	
*B*3911*	.	Y	R	I	N	R	Y	H	N	V	Q	R	Y	L	T	
*B*3912*	Y	D	R	I	N	R	Y	H	N	V	Q	L	Y	L	T	
*B*40011*	Y	H	R	I	N	R	Y	H	N	V	Q	L	Y	L	E	
*B*40012*	Y	H	R	I	N	R	Y	H	N	V	Q	L	Y	L	E	(A,V,I,L,M,F,S,D,N)
*B*4002*	Y	H	R	I	N	S	Y	H	N	V	Q	L	Y	L	E	
*B*4003*	Y	H	R	I	N	S	Y	H	D	V	Q	L	Y	L	E	
*B*4004*	Y	H	R	I	N	R	Y	H	N	V	Q	L	Y	L	E	
*B*4005*	Y	H	R	I	N	S	Y	H	N	E	Q	L	Y	L	L	
*B*4006*	Y	H	R	I	N	T	Y	H	N	V	Q	L	Y	L	E	F,I,L,V,Y,W,(M,T)
*B*4007*	Y	H	R	I	N	R	Y	H	N	V	Q	L	Y	L	E	
*B*4008*	Y	H	R	I	N	S	Y	H	N	V	Q	L	Y	L	E	
*B*4009*	Y	H	R	I	N	S	Y	Y	D	V	Q	L	Y	L	E	
*B*4101*	Y	H	R	I	N	R	Y	H	N	V	Q	D	Y	L	T	
*B*4102*	Y	H	R	I	N	S	Y	H	N	V	Q	D	Y	L	T	
*B*4201*	Y	Y	R	I	Q	S	Y	H	N	V	Q	D	Y	L	T	
*B*4402*	Y	Y	R	I	N	R	Y	Y	D	V	Q	D	Y	L	L	(I,P,R,K)
*B*44031*	Y	Y	R	I	N	R	Y	Y	D	V	Q	L	Y	L	L	(I,V,K)
*B*44032*	Y	Y	R	I	N	R	Y	Y	D	V	Q	L	Y	L	L	
*B*4404*	Y	Y	R	I	N	R	Y	Y	D	V	Q	R	Y	L	T	
*B*4405*	Y	Y	R	I	N	R	Y	Y	D	V	Q	D	Y	L	L	
*B*4406*	Y	Y	R	I	N	R	Y	Y	D	V	Q	D	Y	L	L	
*B*4407*	Y	Y	R	I	N	R	Y	Y	D	V	Q	L	Y	L	L	
*B*4408*	Y	Y	R	I	N	R	Y	Y	D	V	Q	D	Y	L	L	
*B*4410*	Y	Y	R	I	N	R	F	H	N	V	Q	L	Y	L	L	
*B*4501*	Y	H	R	I	N	R	Y	Y	N	V	Q	D	Y	L	L	
*B*4601*	Y	Y	R	K	Q	R	Y	H	D	E	Q	W	Y	L	L	K,R,N,(I,P,F)
*B*4701*	Y	Y	R	I	N	R	F	Y	H	V	Q	L	Y	L	E	
*B*4702*	Y	Y	R	I	N	R	F	Y	H	V	Q	L	Y	L	T	
*B*4801*	Y	Y	R	I	N	S	Y	H	N	V	Q	L	Y	L	E	
*B*4802*	Y	Y	R	I	N	R	Y	H	D	V	Q	L	Y	L	L	
*B*4803*	Y	Y	R	I	N	R	Y	H	N	V	Q	L	Y	L	E	

*B*4901*	Y	H	R	I	N	R	Y	Y	N	E	Q	L	Y	L	L	
*B*5001*	Y	H	R	I	N	R	Y	Y	N	E	Q	L	Y	L	L	
*B*51011*	Y	Y	R	I	N	T	Y	H	N	E	Q	L	Y	L	L	(I,L,M,F,W,Y,V,E,H,D,R,N)
*B*51012*	Y	Y	R	I	N	T	Y	H	N	E	Q	L	Y	L	L	
*B*51021*	Y	Y	R	I	N	T	Y	H	N	E	Q	L	Y	L	L	Y,(F,V,L,I)
*B*51022*	Y	Y	R	I	N	T	Y	H	N	E	Q	L	Y	L	L	
*B*5103*	Y	Y	R	I	N	T	Y	H	N	E	Q	L	Y	L	L	Y(F,D,L)
*B*5104*	Y	Y	R	I	N	R	Y	H	N	E	Q	L	Y	L	L	
*B*5105*	Y	Y	R	I	N	T	Y	H	N	V	Q	R	Y	L	L	
*B*5106*	Y	Y	R	I	N	R	Y	H	N	E	Q	L	Y	L	L	
*B*5107*	Y	Y	R	I	N	T	Y	H	N	E	Q	L	Y	L	L	
*B*5108*	.	.	R	I	N	T	Y	H	N	V	Q	D	Y	L	L	
*B*52011*	Y	Y	R	I	N	T	Y	H	N	E	Q	L	Y	L	L	F,Y,W,(I,L,P,D,K)
*B*52012*	Y	Y	R	I	N	T	Y	H	N	E	Q	L	Y	L	L	
*B*5301*	Y	Y	R	I	N	R	Y	H	D	V	Q	L	Y	L	L	(F,K,N,Q)
*B*5401*	Y	Y	R	I	Q	T	Y	H	N	V	Q	L	Y	L	T	(F,M,R,Y,N,K,L,Q)
*B*5501*	Y	Y	R	I	Q	T	Y	H	N	E	Q	L	Y	L	T	(R,M,Y,K,N,F,L)
*B*5502*	Y	Y	R	I	Q	T	Y	H	N	V	Q	L	Y	L	T	(R,M,Y,F,H,K,L,Q)
*B*5503*	Y	Y	R	I	Q	T	Y	H	N	E	Q	L	Y	L	T	
*B*5504*	Y	Y	R	I	Q	S	Y	H	N	V	Q	L	Y	L	T	
*B*5505*	Y	Y	R	I	Q	T	Y	H	N	E	Q	L	Y	L	T	
*B*5601*	Y	Y	R	I	Q	T	Y	H	N	V	Q	L	Y	L	L	Y,(N,R,F,Q,K,H,L,M)
*B*5602*	Y	Y	R	I	Q	R	Y	H	N	V	Q	L	Y	L	L	
*B*5603*	Y	Y	R	I	Q	R	Y	H	D	E	Q	W	Y	L	L	
*B*5701*	Y	Y	G	N	S	V	Y	H	D	V	Q	L	Y	L	L	
*B*5702*	Y	Y	G	N	S	V	Y	H	N	V	Q	R	Y	L	L	
*B*5703*	Y	Y	G	N	S	V	Y	H	N	V	Q	L	Y	L	L	
*B*5704*	Y	Y	G	N	S	V	Y	Y	D	V	Q	R	Y	L	L	
*B*5801*	Y	Y	G	N	S	R	Y	H	D	V	Q	L	Y	L	L	(G,T,I,L,V,F,Y,N,Q)
*B*5802*	Y	Y	G	N	S	W	Y	H	D	V	Q	L	Y	L	L	
*B*5901*	Y	Y	R	I	N	T	Y	H	N	V	Q	L	Y	L	T	
*B*67011*	Y	Y	R	I	Q	R	Y	H	N	V	Q	L	Y	L	T	(F,M,Y,I,A,L,E,N,T,Q,D,G)
*B*67012*	Y	Y	R	I	Q	R	Y	H	N	V	Q	L	Y	L	T	
*B*7301*	Y	H	R	I	K	T	Y	Y	N	V	Q	L	Y	L	E	N,L,F,V,A,I,M,Y,H,T,D,W,K,(S)
*B*7801*	Y	Y	R	I	N	T	Y	H	N	E	Q	L	Y	L	L	(Y,D,W)
*B*78021*	Y	Y	R	I	N	T	Y	H	N	E	Q	L	Y	L	L	
*B*78022*	Y	Y	R	I	N	T	Y	H	N	E	Q	L	Y	L	L	
*B*8101*	Y	Y	R	I	Q	S	Y	H	N	V	Q	L	Y	L	E	
*B*8201*	Y	Y	R	I	Q	R	F	H	N	V	Q	D	Y	L	L	

Table 3.9. Pocket for peptide position 3 (Pocket D)

Chelvanayagam 1996[17]	7	9	62	66	70	97	99		114	152	155	156	159		163	Anchors/preferred residues
Saper et al 1991[25]							99	113	114		155	156	159	160		
Matsumura et al 1992[16]							99		114			156	159	160		
*Cw*0102*	Y	F	R	K	Q	W	C	Y	D	E	Q	R	Y	L	T	(P, Q)
*Cw*0103*	Y	F	R	K	Q	W	C	Y	N	E	Q	R	Y	L	T	
*Cw*02021*	Y	Y	R	K	Q	R	Y	Y	D	E	Q	W	Y	L	E	
*Cw*02022*	Y	Y	R	K	Q	R	Y	Y	D	E	Q	W	Y	L	E	
*Cw*02023*	Y	Y	R	K	Q	R	Y	Y	D	E	Q	W	Y	L	E	
*Cw*0302*	Y	Y	R	K	Q	R	Y	Y	D	E	Q	L	Y	L	L	
*Cw*0303*	Y	Y	R	K	Q	R	Y	Y	D	E	Q	L	Y	L	L	
*Cw*0304*	Y	Y	R	K	Q	R	Y	Y	D	E	Q	L	Y	L	L	V,I,Y,P,M,(F,N)
*Cw*0401*	Y	S	R	K	Q	R	F	Y	N	E	Q	R	Y	L	T	(D,H)
*Cw*0402*	Y	S	R	K	Q	R	F	Y	N	E	E	R	Y	L	T	
*Cw*0403*	Y	Y	R	K	Q	R	F	Y	N	E	Q	R	Y	L	T	
*Cw*0501*	Y	Y	R	K	Q	R	Y	Y	N	E	Q	R	Y	L	T	
*Cw*0602*	Y	D	R	K	Q	W	Y	Y	D	E	Q	W	Y	L	T	(P,I,G,F,Y,K,N,A)
*Cw*0701*	Y	D	R	N	Q	R	Y	Y	D	A	Q	L	Y	L	T	
*Cw*0702*	Y	D	R	K	Q	R	S	Y	D	A	Q	L	Y	L	T	(P,G,A)
*Cw*0703*	Y	D	R	K	Q	R	S	Y	D	A	Q	L	Y	L	L	
*Cw*0704*	Y	D	R	K	Q	R	Y	Y	D	A	Q	D	Y	L	T	
*Cw*0705*	Y	D	R	K	Q	N	Y	Y	D	A	Q	L	Y	L	T	
*Cw*0706*	Y	D	R	N	Q	R	Y	Y	D	A	Q	L	Y	L	T	
*Cw*0707*	Y	D	R	N	Q	R	Y	Y	D	A	Q	L	Y	L	T	
*Cw*0801*	Y	Y	R	K	Q	R	Y	Y	N	T	Q	L	Y	L	T	
*Cw*0802*	Y	Y	R	K	Q	R	Y	Y	N	E	Q	R	Y	L	T	
*Cw*0803*	Y	Y	R	K	Q	R	Y	Y	N	T	Q	L	Y	L	T	
*Cw*12021*	Y	Y	R	K	Q	R	Y	Y	D	E	Q	W	Y	L	T	
*Cw*12022*	Y	Y	R	K	Q	R	Y	Y	D	E	Q	W	Y	L	T	
*Cw*1203*	Y	Y	R	K	Q	W	Y	Y	D	E	Q	W	Y	L	T	
*Cw*1204*	Y	Y	R	K	Q	W	Y	Y	D	E	Q	W	Y	L	T	
*Cw*1301*	Y	Y	R	K	Q	R	Y	Y	D	E	Q	W	Y	L	T	
*Cw*1402*	Y	S	R	K	Q	W	F	Y	D	E	Q	R	Y	L	T	
*Cw*1403*	Y	S	R	K	Q	W	F	Y	D	E	Q	R	Y	L	T	
*Cw*1502*	Y	Y	R	N	Q	R	Y	H	D	E	Q	L	Y	L	T	
*Cw*1503*	Y	Y	R	N	Q	R	Y	H	D	E	Q	L	Y	L	T	
*Cw*1504*	Y	Y	R	N	Q	R	Y	Y	D	E	Q	L	Y	L	T	

*Cw*15051*	Y	Y	R	N	Q	R	Y	H	D	E	Q	L	Y	L	T
*Cw*15052*	Y	Y	R	N	Q	R	Y	H	D	E	Q	L	Y	L	T
*Cw*1601*	Y	Y	R	K	Q	W	Y	Y	D	A	Q	Q	Y	L	T
*Cw*1602*	Y	Y	R	K	Q	W	Y	Y	D	A	Q	Q	Y	L	T
*Cw*1701*	Y	Y	R	K	Q	R	Y	Y	N	E	Q	L	Y	L	E
*Cw*1702*	Y	Y	R	K	Q	R	Y	Y	N	E	Q	L	Y	L	E
*Cw*1801*	Y	D	R	K	Q	R	F	Y	N	E	Q	R	Y	L	T
*Cw*1802*	Y	D	R	K	Q	R	F	Y	N	E	Q	R	Y	L	T

Table 3.10. Pocket for peptide position 6 (Pocket C)

Chelvanayagam 1996[17]	7	9	22	24	66	69	70	73	74	97	99	114	116	133	147	152	155	156	Anchors/preferred residues
Saper et al. 1991[25]		9					70	73	74	97									
Matsumura et al. 1992[16]		9	22				70		74	97	99	114	116						
*A*0101*	Y	F	F	A	N	A	H	T	D	I	Y	R	D	W	W	A	Q	R	
*A*0102*	Y	S	F	A	N	A	H	T	D	I	Y	R	D	W	W	A	Q	R	
*A*0201*	Y	F	F	A	K	A	H	T	H	R	Y	H	Y	W	W	V	Q	L	V,(I,L,T)
*A*0202*	Y	F	F	A	K	A	H	T	H	R	Y	H	Y	W	W	V	Q	W	(I,L,V,T)
*A*0203*	Y	F	F	A	K	A	H	T	H	R	Y	H	Y	W	W	E	Q	W	
*A*0204*	Y	F	F	A	K	A	H	T	H	M	Y	H	Y	W	W	V	Q	L	(L,I)
*A*0205*	Y	Y	F	A	K	A	H	T	H	R	Y	H	Y	W	W	V	Q	W	I,V,L,A,(T)
*A*0206*	Y	Y	F	A	K	A	H	T	H	R	Y	H	Y	W	W	V	Q	L	(L)
*A*0207*	Y	F	F	A	K	A	H	T	H	R	C	H	Y	W	W	V	Q	L	(I)
*A*0208*	Y	Y	F	A	N	A	H	T	H	R	Y	H	Y	W	W	V	Q	W	
*A*0209*	Y	F	F	A	K	A	H	T	H	R	Y	H	Y	W	W	V	Q	L	
*A*0210*	Y	Y	F	A	K	A	H	T	H	R	F	H	Y	W	W	V	Q	L	
*A*0211*	Y	F	F	A	K	A	H	I	D	R	Y	H	Y	W	W	V	Q	L	
*A*0212*	Y	F	F	A	K	A	H	T	H	R	Y	H	Y	W	W	V	Q	Q	
*A*0213*	Y	F	F	A	K	A	H	T	H	R	Y	H	Y	W	W	E	Q	Q	
*A*0214*	Y	Y	F	A	K	A	H	T	H	R	Y	H	Y	W	W	V	Q	L	I,L,V,F,(K,N)
*A*0215N*	Y	F	F	A	K	A	H	T	H	R	C	H	Y	W	W	V	Q	L	
*A*0216*	Y	F	F	A	K	A	H	T	H	R	Y	H	Y	W	W	V	Q	L	

Table 3.10. (con't)

	7	9	22	24	66	69	70	73	74	97	99	114	116	133	147	152	155	156	Anchors/preferred residues
Chelvanayagam 1996[17]	7	9	22	24	66	69	70	73	74	97	99	114	116	133	147	152	155	156	
Saper et al 1991[25]		9					70	73	74	97									
Matsumura et al 1992[16]		9	22				70		74	97	99	114	116						
*A*0217*	Y	F	F	A	K	A	H	T	H	M	F	H	Y	W	W	V	Q	L	
*A*0218*	Y	F	F	A	K	A	H	T	H	R	C	H	Y	W	W	V	Q	L	
*A*0219*	Y	F	F	A	K	A	H	T	H	R	Y	H	Y	W	W	V	Q	Q	
*A*0220*	Y	F	F	A	N	A	H	T	H	R	Y	H	Y	W	W	V	Q	L	
*A*0221*	Y	Y	F	A	K	A	H	T	H	R	Y	H	Y	W	W	V	Q	L	
*A*0222*	Y	F	F	A	K	A	H	T	H	R	Y	H	Y	W	W	V	Q	W	
*A*0301*	Y	F	F	A	N	A	Q	T	D	I	Y	R	D	W	W	E	Q	L	
*A*0302*	Y	F	F	A	N	A	Q	T	D	I	Y	R	D	W	W	V	Q	Q	
*A*0303N*	Y	F	F	A	N	A	Q	T	D	I	Y	R	D	W	W	E	Q	L	
*A*1101*	Y	Y	F	A	N	A	Q	T	D	I	Y	R	D	W	W	A	Q	Q	(I,V,M)
*A*1102*	Y	Y	F	A	N	A	Q	T	D	I	Y	R	D	W	W	A	Q	Q	
*A*1103*	Y	Y	F	A	N	A	Q	T	D	I	Y	R	D	W	W	E	Q	Q	
*A*1104*	Y	Y	F	A	N	A	Q	T	D	I	Y	R	D	W	W	A	Q	Q	
*A*2301*	Y	S	F	A	K	A	H	T	D	M	F	H	Y	W	W	V	Q	L	
*A*2402*	Y	S	F	A	K	A	H	T	D	M	F	H	Y	W	W	V	Q	Q	
*A*2403*	Y	S	F	A	K	A	H	T	D	M	F	H	Y	W	W	V	Q	Q	
*A*2404*	Y	S	F	A	K	A	H	T	D	M	F	H	Y	W	W	V	Q	Q	
*A*2405*	Y	S	F	A	K	A	H	T	D	M	F	H	Y	W	W	V	Q	Q	
*A*2406*	Y	S	F	A	K	A	H	T	D	M	F	H	Y	W	W	V	Q	W	
*A*2407*	Y	S	F	A	K	A	Q	T	D	M	F	H	Y	W	W	V	Q	Q	
*A*2408*	Y	S	F	A	K	A	H	T	D	M	F	H	Y	W	W	V	Q	Q	
*A*2409N*	Y	S	F	A	K	A	H	T	D	M	F	H	Y	W	W	V	Q	Q	
*A*2410*	Y	S	F	A	K	A	H	T	D	M	F	H	Y	W	W	V	Q	Q	
*A*2413*	Y	S	F	A	K	A	H	T	D	M	F	H	Y	W	W	V	Q	L	
*A*2414*	Y	S	F	A	K	A	H	T	D	R	Y	H	Y	W	W	V	Q	L	
*A*2501*	Y	Y	F	A	N	A	H	T	D	R	Y	Q	D	W	W	E	Q	W	
*A*2502*	Y	Y	F	A	N	A	Q	T	D	R	Y	Q	D	W	W	E	Q	W	
*A*2601*	Y	Y	F	A	N	A	H	T	D	R	Y	Q	D	W	W	E	Q	W	
*A*2602*	Y	Y	F	A	N	A	H	T	D	R	Y	Q	N	W	W	E	Q	W	
*A*2603*	Y	Y	F	A	N	A	H	T	H	R	Y	Q	D	W	W	E	Q	W	
*A*2604*	Y	Y	F	A	N	A	H	T	D	R	Y	Q	D	W	W	E	Q	W	
*A*2605*	Y	Y	F	A	N	A	H	T	D	R	Y	Q	D	W	W	E	Q	W	
*A*2606*	Y		F	A	N	A	H	T	H	R	Y	Q	D	W	W	E	Q	W	
*A*2607*	Y	Y	F	A	K	A	H	T	D	R	Y	Q	D	W	W	E	Q	W	
*A*2608*	Y	Y	F	A	N	A	H	T	D	R	Y	Q	D	W	W	E	Q	Q	
*A*2901*	Y	T	F	A	N	A	Q	T	D	M	Y	R	D	W	W	V	Q	L	

*A*2902*	Y	T	F	A	N	A	Q	T	D	M	Y	R	D	W	W	V	Q	L	
*A*2903*	Y	T	F	A	N	A	Q	T	D	M	Y	R	D	W	W	V	Q	L	
*A*3001*	Y	S	F	A	N	A	Q	T	D	I	Y	E	H	W	W	W	Q	L	
*A*3002*	Y	S	F	A	N	A	H	T	D	I	Y	E	H	W	W	R	Q	L	
*A*3003*	Y	S	F	A	N	A	H	T	D	I	Y	E	H	W	W	R	Q	L	
*A*3004*	Y	S	F	A	N	A	H	T	D	I	Y	E	H	W	W	V	Q	W	
*A*3005*	Y	S	F	A	N	A	H	T	D	I	Y	E	H	W	W	V	Q	W	
*A*31012*	Y	T	F	A	N	A	H	I	D	M	Y	Q	D	W	W	V	Q	L	L,F,V,I,(T,N,D,E,R)
*A*3201*	Y	F	F	A	N	A	H	T	D	M	Y	Q	D	W	W	V	Q	L	
*A*3202*	Y	F	F	A	N	A	H	T	D	M	Y	Q	D	W	W	V	Q	Q	
*A*3301*	Y	T	F	A	N	A	H	I	D	M	Y	Q	D	W	W	V	Q	L	
*A*3302*	Y	T	F	A	N	A	H	I	D	M	Y	Q	D	W	W	V	Q	L	(I,L,F,R,D,H,Y)
*A*3303*	Y	T	F	A	N	A	H	I	D	M	Y	Q	D	W	W	V	Q	L	
*A*3401*	Y	Y	F	A	K	A	Q	T	D	R	Y	Q	D	W	W	E	Q	W	
*A*3402*	Y	Y	F	A	N	A	Q	T	D	I	Y	R	D	W	W	E	Q	L	
*A*3601*	Y	F	F	A	N	A	H	T	D	I	Y	R	D	W	W	A	Q	R	
*A*4301*	Y	Y	F	A	N	A	H	T	D	R	Y	Q	D	W	W	E	Q	W	
*A*6601*	Y	Y	F	A	N	A	Q	T	D	R	Y	Q	D	W	W	E	Q	W	
*A*6602*	Y	Y	F	A	N	A	Q	T	D	R	Y	Q	D	W	W	E	Q	W	
*A*6603*	Y	Y	F	A	N	A	H	T	D	R	Y	Q	D	W	W	E	Q	W	
*A*68011*	Y	Y	F	A	N	A	Q	T	D	M	Y	R	D	W	W	V	Q	W	
*A*68012*	Y	Y	F	A	N	A	Q	T	D	M	Y	R	D	W	W	V	Q	W	
*A*6802*	Y	Y	F	A	N	A	Q	T	D	R	Y	H	Y	W	W	V	Q	W	
*A*6803*	Y	Y	F	A	N	A	H	T	D	M	Y	R	D	W	W	V	Q	W	
*A*6901*	Y	Y	F	A	N	A	Q	T	D	R	Y	H	Y	W	W	V	Q	L	I,F,L,(V)
*A*7401*	Y	F	F	A	N	A	H	T	D	M	Y	Q	D	W	W	V	Q	L	
*A*7402*	Y	F	F	A	N	A	H	T	D	M	Y	Q	D	W	W	V	Q	L	
*A*7403*	Y	F	F	A	N	A	H	T	D	M	Y	Q	D	W	W	V	Q	L	
*A*8001*	Y	F	F	A	N	A	H	T	N	I	Y	R	D	W	W	R	Q	L	

Table 3.11. Pocket for peptide position 6 (Pocket C)

	7	9	22	24	66	69	70	73	74	97	99	114	116	133	147	152	155	156	Anchors/preferred residues
Chelvanayagam 1996[17]	7	9	22	24	66	69	70	73	74	97	99	114	116	133	147	152	155	156	
Saper et al 1991[25]		9					70	73	74	97									
Matsumura et al 1992[16]		9	22				70		74	97	99	114	116						
*B*0702*	Y	Y	F	S	I	A	Q	T	D	S	Y	D	Y	W	W	E	Q	R	(R,T)
*B*0703*	Y	Y	F	S	I	T	N	T	D	S	Y	D	Y	W	W	E	Q	R	(R,D)
*B*0704*	Y	Y	F	S	I	A	Q	T	D	S	Y	D	Y	W	W	E	Q	D	
*B*0705*	Y	Y	F	S	I	A	Q	T	D	S	Y	N	Y	W	W	E	Q	R	
*B*0706*	Y	Y	F	S	I	A	Q	T	D	S	Y	N	Y	W	W	E	Q	R	
*B*0707*	Y	Y	F	S	I	A	Q	T	D	R	Y	D	Y	W	W	E	Q	R	
*B*0801*	Y	D	F	S	I	T	N	T	D	S	Y	N	Y	W	W	V	Q	D	
*B*0802*	Y	D	F	S	I	T	N	T	D	S	Y	N	Y	W	W	V	Q	D	
*B*0803*	.	D	F	S	I	T	N	T	Y	S	Y	N	Y	W	W	V	Q	D	
*B*1301*	Y	Y	F	T	I	T	N	T	Y	R	Y	N	L	W	W	V	Q	L	
*B*1302*	Y	Y	F	T	I	T	N	T	Y	T	Y	N	L	W	W	V	Q	L	
*B*1303*	Y	Y	F	T	I	T	N	T	Y	T	Y	N	L	W	W	V	Q	L	
*B*1401*	Y	Y	F	S	I	T	N	T	D	W	Y	N	F	W	W	E	Q	L	
*B*1402*	Y	Y	F	S	I	T	N	T	D	W	Y	N	F	W	W	E	Q	L	
*B*1501*	Y	Y	F	A	I	T	N	T	Y	R	Y	D	S	W	W	E	Q	W	(V,T,G,I)
*B*1502*	Y	Y	F	A	I	T	N	T	Y	R	Y	D	S	W	W	E	Q	L	
*B*1503*	Y	Y	F	S	I	T	N	T	Y	R	Y	D	S	W	W	E	Q	L	
*B*1504*	Y	Y	F	A	I	T	N	T	Y	T	Y	D	S	W	W	E	Q	W	
*B*1505*	Y	Y	F	A	I	T	N	T	Y	R	Y	D	S	W	W	V	Q	L	
*B*1506*	Y	Y	F	A	I	T	N	T	Y	R	F	D	S	W	W	E	Q	L	
*B*1507*	Y	Y	F	A	I	T	N	T	Y	S	Y	D	S	W	W	E	Q	W	
*B*1508*	Y	Y	F	A	I	T	N	T	Y	R	Y	D	S	W	W	E	Q	W	
*B*1509*	Y	Y	F	S	I	T	N	T	Y	R	Y	N	Y	W	W	E	Q	L	
*B*1510*	Y	Y	F	S	I	T	N	T	Y	R	Y	D	Y	W	W	E	Q	L	
*B*1511*	Y	Y	F	A	I	T	N	T	Y	R	Y	D	S	W	W	E	Q	W	
*B*1512*	Y	Y	F	A	I	T	N	T	Y	R	Y	D	S	W	W	E	Q	W	
*B*1513*	Y	Y	F	A	I	T	N	T	Y	R	Y	D	S	W	W	E	Q	L	
*B*1514*	Y	Y	F	A	I	T	N	T	Y	R	Y	D	S	W	W	E	Q	W	
*B*1515*	Y	Y	F	A	I	T	N	T	Y	R	Y	D	S	W	W	E	Q	W	
*B*1516*	Y	Y	F	A	N	A	S	T	Y	R	Y	D	S	W	W	E	Q	L	
*B*1517*	Y	Y	F	A	N	A	S	T	Y	R	Y	H	D	W	W	E	Q	L	
*B*1518*	Y	Y	F	S	I	T	N	T	Y	R	Y	D	S	W	W	E	Q	L	

B*1519	Y	Y	F	A	I	T	N	T	Y	R	Y	D	S	W	W	E	Q	W	
B*1520	Y	Y	F	A	I	T	N	T	Y	R	Y	D	S	W	W	V	Q	L	
B*1521	Y	Y	F	A	I	T	N	T	Y	R	Y	D	S	W	W	E	Q	L	
B*1522	Y	Y	F	A	I	T	N	T	Y	R	Y	D	S	W	W	E	Q	W	
B*1523	Y	Y	F	S	I	T	N	T	Y	R	Y	D	S	W	W	E	Q	L	
B*1524	Y	Y	F	A	I	T	N	T	Y	R	Y	D	S	W	W	E	Q	W	
B*1525	Y	Y	F	A	I	T	N	T	Y	R	Y	D	S	W	W	E	Q	L	
B*1526N	Y	Y	F	A	I	T	N	T	Y	R	/	D	S	W	W	E	Q	W	
B*1527	Y	Y	F	A	I	T	N	T	Y	R	F	D	S	W	W	E	Q	W	
B*1528	Y	Y	F	A	I	T	N	T	Y	R	Y	D	S	W	W	E	Q	W	
B*1529	Y	Y	F	S	I	T	N	T	Y	R	Y	D	S	W	W	E	Q	L	
B*1530	Y	Y	F	A	I	T	N	T	Y	R	Y	N	Y	W	W	E	Q	W	
B*1531	Y	Y	F	A	I	T	N	T	Y	R	Y	D	S	W	W	V	Q	L	
B*1532	Y	Y	F	A	I	T	N	T	Y	R	S	D	S	W	W	E	Q	W	
B*1533	Y	Y	F	A	I	T	N	T	Y	R	Y	D	S	W	W	E	Q	W	
B*1534	Y	Y	F	A	I	T	N	T	Y	R	Y	D	S	W	W	E	Q	W	
B*1535	Y	Y	F	A	I	T	N	T	Y	T	Y	D	S	W	W	E	Q	W	
B*1537	Y	Y	F	S	I	T	N	T	Y	R	Y	D	Y	W	W	E	Q	L	
B*1801	Y	H	F	S	I	T	N	T	Y	R	Y	D	S	W	W	V	Q	L	
B*1802	Y	H	F	S	I	T	N	T	Y	N	Y	D	S	W	W	V	Q	L	
B*1803	Y	H	F	S	I	T	N	T	D	R	Y	D	S	W	W	V	Q	L	
B*1805	Y	H	F	S	I	T	N	T	Y	R	Y	D	S	W	W	V	Q	L	
B*2701	Y	H	F	T	I	A	K	T	Y	N	Y	H	D	W	W	V	Q	L	
B*2702	Y	H	F	T	I	A	K	T	D	N	Y	H	D	W	W	V	Q	L	(I,V,Y,R,D,H,E,Q)
B*2703	Y	H	F	T	I	A	K	T	D	N	Y	H	D	W	W	V	Q	L	
B*2704	Y	H	F	T	I	A	K	T	D	N	Y	H	D	W	W	E	Q	L	
B*27052	Y	H	F	T	I	A	K	T	D	N	Y	H	D	W	W	V	Q	L	(I,A,N,Q,D,V,K)
B*27053	.	.	.	.	I	A	K	T	D	N	Y	H	D	W	W	V	Q	L	
B*2706	Y	H	F	T	I	A	K	T	D	N	Y	D	Y	W	W	E	Q	L	
B*2707	Y	H	F	T	I	A	K	T	D	S	Y	N	Y	W	W	V	Q	L	
B*2708	Y	H	F	T	I	A	K	T	D	N	Y	H	D	W	W	V	Q	L	
B*2709	Y	H	F	T	I	A	K	T	D	N	Y	H	H	W	W	V	Q	L	
B*2710	Y	H	F	T	I	A	K	T	D	N	Y	H	D	W	W	E	Q	L	
B*3501	Y	Y	F	A	I	T	N	T	Y	R	Y	D	S	W	W	V	Q	L	(I,Q,K,V,L,M)
B*3502	Y	Y	F	A	I	T	N	T	Y	R	Y	N	Y	W	W	V	Q	L	
B*3503	Y	Y	F	A	I	T	N	T	Y	R	Y	D	F	W	W	V	Q	L	(Y,T,N)

Table 3.11. (con't)

	7	9	22	24	66	69	70	73	74	97	99	114	116	133	147	152	155	156	Anchors/preferred residues
Chelvanayagam 1996[17]	7	9	22	24	66	69	70	73	74	97	99	114	116	133	147	152	155	156	
Saper et al. 1991[25]		9					70	73	74	97									
Matsumura et al. 1992[16]		9	22				70		74	97	99	114	116						
*B*3504*	Y	Y	F	A	I	T	N	T	Y	R	Y	N	Y	W	W	V	Q	L	
*B*3505*	Y	Y	F	A	I	T	N	T	Y	S	Y	D	S	W	W	V	Q	L	
*B*3506*	Y	Y	F	A	I	T	N	T	Y	R	Y	N	F	W	W	V	Q	L	
*B*3507*	Y	Y	F	A	I	T	N	T	Y	R	Y	D	S	W	W	V	Q	L	
*B*3508*	Y	Y	F	A	I	T	N	T	Y	R	Y	D	S	W	W	V	Q	R	
*B*35091*	Y	Y	F	A	I	T	N	T	Y	R	Y	N	Y	W	W	V	Q	L	
*B*35092*	Y	Y	F	A	I	T	N	T	Y	R	Y	N	Y	W	W	V	Q	L	
*B*3510*	Y	Y	F	A	I	T	N	T	Y	R	Y	D	S	W	W	V	Q	L	
*B*3511*	Y	Y	F	A	I	T	N	T	Y	R	Y	D	S	W	W	E	Q	L	
*B*3512*	Y	Y	F	A	I	T	N	T	Y	R	Y	N	Y	W	W	V	Q	L	
*B*3513*	Y	Y	F	A	I	T	N	T	Y	R	Y	D	F	W	W	V	Q	L	
*B*3515*	Y	Y	F	A	I	T	N	T	Y	R	Y	D	S	W	W	V	Q	L	
*B*3516*	Y	Y	F	A	I	T	N	T	Y	S	Y	D	S	W	W	V	Q	L	
*B*3517*	Y	Y	F	A	I	T	N	T	Y	S	Y	D	S	W	W	V	Q	L	
*B*3518*	Y	Y	F	A	I	T	N	T	Y	R	Y	N	Y	W	W	V	Q	R	
*B*3519*	Y	Y	F	A	I	T	N	T	Y	R	Y	D	S	W	W	V	Q	L	
*B*3520*	Y	Y	F	A	I	T	N	T	Y	R	Y	D	S	W	W	V	Q	L	
*B*3521*	Y	Y	F	A	I	T	N	T	Y	R	Y	D	S	W	W	E	Q	L	
*B*3701*	Y	H	F	S	I	T	N	T	Y	R	S	N	F	W	W	V	Q	D	
*B*3702*	Y	H	F	S	I	T	N	T	Y	N	Y	H	D	W	W	V	Q	L	
*B*3801*	Y	Y	F	S	I	T	N	T	Y	R	Y	N	F	W	W	V	Q	L	(V,I,T,K,R,N,H)
*B*3802*	Y	Y	F	S	I	T	N	T	Y	R	Y	N	F	W	W	V	Q	L	
*B*39011*	Y	Y	F	S	I	T	N	T	D	R	Y	N	F	W	W	V	Q	L	I,V,L,(N)
*B*39013*	Y	Y	F	S	I	T	N	T	D	R	Y	N	F	W	W	V	Q	L	
*B*39021*	Y	Y	F	S	I	T	N	T	D	R	Y	N	F	W	W	V	Q	L	(V,Y,T,H,F,I,M,P,R)
*B*39022*	Y	Y	F	S	I	T	N	T	D	R	Y	N	F	W	W	V	Q	L	
*B*3903*	Y	Y	F	S	I	T	N	T	D	S	Y	N	F	W	W	V	Q	L	
*B*3904*	Y	Y	F	S	I	T	N	T	D	R	Y	N	F	W	W	V	Q	L	
*B*3905*	Y	Y	F	S	I	T	N	T	Y	R	Y	N	F	W	W	V	Q	L	
*B*39061*	Y	Y	F	S	I	T	N	T	D	T	Y	N	F	W	W	V	Q	L	
*B*39062*	Y	Y	F	S	I	T	N	T	D	T	Y	N	F	W	W	V	Q	L	
*B*3907*	.	.	.	.	I	T	N	T	Y	R	Y	D	S	W	W	V	Q	L	
*B*3908*	Y	Y	F	S	I	T	N	T	Y	R	Y	N	F	W	W	V	Q	R	
*B*3909*	Y	Y	F	S	I	T	N	T	D	R	S	N	F	W	W	V	Q	L	
*B*3910*	Y	Y	F	S	I	T	N	T	D	R	Y	N	F	W	W	V	Q	L	

*B*3911*	.	Y	F	S	I	T	N	T	Y	R	Y	N	F	W	W	V	Q	R	
*B*3912*	Y	D	F	S	I	T	N	T	D	R	Y	N	F	W	W	V	Q	L	
*B*40011*	Y	H	F	T	I	T	N	T	Y	R	Y	N	Y	W	L	V	Q	L	
*B*40012*	Y	H	F	T	I	T	N	T	Y	R	Y	N	Y	W	L	V	Q	L	(K,N,P,V,I,D,R,Q)
*B*4002*	Y	H	F	T	I	T	N	T	Y	S	Y	N	Y	W	W	V	Q	L	
*B*4003*	Y	H	F	T	I	T	N	T	Y	S	Y	D	S	W	W	V	Q	L	
*B*4004*	Y	H	F	T	I	T	N	T	Y	R	Y	N	Y	W	W	V	Q	L	
*B*4005*	Y	H	F	T	I	T	N	T	Y	S	Y	N	Y	W	W	E	Q	L	
*B*4006*	Y	H	F	T	I	T	N	T	Y	T	Y	N	Y	W	W	V	Q	L	I,(N)
*B*4007*	Y	H	F	T	I	T	N	T	Y	R	Y	N	Y	W	L	V	Q	L	
*B*4008*	Y	H	F	T	I	T	N	T	Y	S	Y	N	Y	W	W	V	Q	L	
*B*4009*	Y	H	F	T	I	T	N	T	Y	S	Y	D	Y	W	W	V	Q	L	
*B*4101*	Y	H	F	T	I	T	N	T	Y	R	Y	N	Y	W	W	V	Q	D	
*B*4102*	Y	H	F	T	I	T	N	T	Y	S	Y	N	Y	W	W	V	Q	D	
*B*4201*	Y	Y	F	S	I	A	Q	T	D	S	Y	N	Y	W	W	V	Q	D	
*B*4402*	Y	Y	F	T	I	T	N	T	Y	R	Y	D	D	W	W	V	Q	D	
*B*44031*	Y	Y	F	T	I	T	N	T	Y	R	Y	D	D	W	W	V	Q	L	
*B*44032*	Y	Y	F	T	I	T	N	T	Y	R	Y	D	D	W	W	V	Q	L	
*B*4404*	Y	Y	F	T	I	T	N	T	Y	R	Y	D	D	W	W	V	Q	R	
*B*4405*	Y	Y	F	T	I	T	N	T	Y	R	Y	D	Y	W	W	V	Q	D	
*B*4406*	Y	Y	F	A	I	T	N	T	Y	R	Y	D	D	W	W	V	Q	D	
*B*4407*	Y	Y	F	T	I	T	N	T	Y	R	Y	D	D	W	W	V	Q	L	
*B*4408*	Y	Y	F	T	I	T	N	T	Y	R	Y	D	D	W	W	V	Q	D	
*B*4410*	Y	Y	F	T	I	T	N	T	Y	R	F	N	L	W	W	V	Q	L	
*B*4501*	Y	H	F	T	I	T	N	T	Y	R	Y	N	L	W	W	V	Q	D	
*B*4601*	Y	Y	F	A	K	R	Q	T	D	R	Y	D	S	W	W	E	Q	W	S,(A)
*B*4701*	Y	Y	F	T	I	T	N	T	Y	R	F	H	D	W	W	V	Q	L	
*B*4702*	Y	Y	F	T	I	T	N	T	Y	R	F	H	D	W	W	V	Q	L	
*B*4801*	Y	Y	F	S	I	T	N	T	Y	S	Y	N	Y	W	L	V	Q	L	
*B*4802*	Y	Y	F	S	I	T	N	T	Y	R	Y	D	S	W	W	V	Q	L	
*B*4803*	Y	Y	F	S	I	T	N	T	Y	R	Y	N	Y	W	L	V	Q	L	
*B*4901*	Y	H	F	T	I	T	N	T	Y	R	Y	N	L	W	W	E	Q	L	
*B*5001*	Y	H	F	T	I	T	N	T	Y	R	Y	N	L	W	W	E	Q	L	
*B*51011*	Y	Y	F	A	I	T	N	T	Y	T	Y	N	Y	W	W	E	Q	L	(N,I,L,K,Q)
*B*51012*	Y	Y	F	A	I	T	N	T	Y	T	Y	N	Y	W	W	E	Q	L	
*B*51021*	Y	Y	F	A	I	T	N	T	Y	T	Y	N	Y	W	W	E	Q	L	(I,N,Q,T)
*B*51022*	Y	Y	F	A	I	T	N	T	Y	T	Y	N	Y	W	W	E	Q	L	
*B*5103*	Y	Y	F	A	I	T	N	T	Y	T	Y	N	Y	W	W	E	Q	L	(I,K,T)
*B*5104*	Y	Y	F	A	I	T	N	T	Y	R	Y	N	Y	W	W	E	Q	L	

Table 3.11 (con't)

Chelvanayagam 1996[17]	7	9	22	24	66	69	70	73	74	97	99	114	116	133	147	152	155	156	Anchors/preferred residues
Saper et al. 1991[25]		9					70	73	74	97									
Matsumura et al. 1992[16]		9	22				70		74	97	99	114	116						
*B*5105*	Y	Y	F	A	I	T	N	T	Y	T	Y	N	Y	W	W	V	Q	R	
*B*5106*	Y	Y	F	A	I	T	N	T	Y	R	Y	N	Y	W	W	E	Q	L	
*B*5107*	Y	Y	F	A	I	T	N	T	Y	T	Y	N	Y	W	W	E	Q	L	
*B*5108*	.	.	F	A	I	T	N	T	Y	T	Y	N	Y	W	W	V	Q	D	
*B*52011*	Y	Y	F	A	I	T	N	T	Y	T	Y	N	Y	W	W	E	Q	L	(K,N,L,T,S)
*B*52012*	Y	Y	F	A	I	T	N	T	Y	T	Y	N	Y	W	W	E	Q	L	
*B*5301*	Y	Y	F	A	I	T	N	T	Y	R	Y	D	S	W	W	V	Q	L	(Y)
*B*5401*	Y	Y	F	A	I	A	Q	T	D	T	Y	N	L	W	W	V	Q	L	
*B*5501*	Y	Y	F	A	I	A	Q	T	D	T	Y	N	L	W	W	E	Q	L	(F,G)
*B*5502*	Y	Y	F	A	I	A	Q	T	D	T	Y	N	L	W	W	V	Q	L	
*B*5503*	Y	Y	F	A	I	A	Q	T	D	T	Y	N	L	W	W	E	Q	L	
*B*5504*	Y	Y	F	A	I	A	Q	T	D	S	Y	N	Y	W	W	V	Q	L	
*B*5505*	Y	Y	F	A	I	A	Q	T	D	T	Y	N	L	W	W	E	Q	L	
*B*5601*	Y	Y	F	A	I	A	Q	T	D	T	Y	N	L	W	W	V	Q	L	
*B*5602*	Y	Y	F	A	I	A	Q	T	D	R	Y	N	L	W	W	V	Q	L	
*B*5603*	Y	Y	F	A	I	A	Q	T	D	R	Y	D	S	W	W	E	Q	W	
*B*5701*	Y	Y	F	A	N	A	S	T	Y	V	Y	D	S	W	W	V	Q	L	
*B*5702*	Y	Y	F	A	N	A	S	T	Y	V	Y	N	Y	W	W	V	Q	R	
*B*5703*	Y	Y	F	A	N	A	S	T	Y	V	Y	N	Y	W	W	V	Q	L	
*B*5704*	Y	Y	F	A	N	A	S	T	Y	V	Y	D	D	W	W	V	Q	R	
*B*5801*	Y	Y	F	A	N	A	S	T	Y	R	Y	D	S	W	W	V	Q	L	(I,V,L,F)
*B*5802*	Y	Y	F	A	N	A	S	T	Y	W	Y	D	S	W	W	V	Q	L	
*B*5901*	Y	Y	F	A	I	T	N	T	Y	T	Y	N	L	W	W	V	Q	L	
*B*67011*	Y	Y	F	S	I	A	Q	T	D	R	Y	N	F	W	W	V	Q	L	M
*B*67012*	Y	Y	F	S	I	A	Q	T	D	R	Y	N	F	W	W	V	Q	L	
*B*7301*	Y	H	F	T	I	A	K	T	D	T	Y	N	F	W	W	V	Q	L	D
*B*7801*	Y	Y	F	A	I	T	N	T	D	T	Y	N	Y	W	W	E	Q	L	I,L,F,V
*B*78021*	Y	Y	F	A	I	T	N	T	Y	T	Y	N	Y	W	W	E	Q	L	
*B*78022*	Y	Y	F	A	I	T	N	T	Y	T	Y	N	Y	W	W	E	Q	L	
*B*8101*	Y	Y	F	S	I	A	Q	T	D	S	Y	N	Y	W	L	V	Q	L	
*B*8201*	Y	Y	F	S	I	A	Q	T	D	R	F	N	L	W	W	V	Q	D	

Table 3.12. Pocket for peptide position 6 (Pocket C)

Chelvanayagam 1996[17]	7	9	22	24	66	69	70	73	74	97	99	114	116	133	147	152	155	156	Anchors/preferred residues
Saper et al 1991[25]		9					70	73	74	97									
Matsumura et al 1992[16]			22				70		74	97	99	114	116						
*Cw*0102*	Y	F	F	S	K	R	Q	T	D	W	C	D	Y	W	W	E	Q	R	V,I,K,(H)
*Cw*0103*	Y	F	F	S	K	R	Q	T	D	W	C	N	F	W	W	E	Q	R	
*Cw*02021*	Y	Y	F	A	K	R	Q	T	D	R	Y	D	S	W	W	E	Q	W	
*Cw*02022*	Y	Y	F	A	K	R	Q	T	D	R	Y	D	S	W	W	E	Q	W	
*Cw*02023*	Y	Y	F	A	K	R	Q	T	D	R	Y	D	S	W	W	E	Q	W	
*Cw*0302*	Y	Y	F	A	K	R	Q	T	D	R	Y	D	S	W	W	E	Q	L	
*Cw*0303*	Y	Y	F	A	K	R	Q	T	D	R	Y	D	Y	W	W	E	Q	L	
*Cw*0304*	Y	Y	F	A	K	R	Q	T	D	R	Y	D	Y	W	W	E	Q	L	(G,Y)
*Cw*0401*	Y	S	F	A	K	R	Q	A	D	R	F	N	F	W	W	E	Q	R	V,I,L
*Cw*0403*	Y	Y	F	A	K	R	Q	A	D	R	F	N	F	W	W	E	Q	R	
*Cw*0402*	Y	S	F	A	K	R	Q	A	D	R	F	N	F	W	W	E	E	R	
*Cw*0501*	Y	Y	F	A	K	R	Q	T	D	R	Y	N	F	W	W	E	Q	R	
*Cw*0602*	Y	D	F	S	K	R	Q	A	D	W	Y	D	S	W	W	E	Q	W	V,I,L,(A,T,S)
*Cw*0701*	Y	D	F	S	N	R	Q	A	D	R	Y	D	S	W	L	A	Q	L	
*Cw*0702*	Y	D	F	S	K	R	Q	A	D	R	S	D	S	W	L	A	Q	L	V,I,L,M,(A,R)
*Cw*0703*	Y	D	F	S	K	R	Q	A	D	R	S	D	S	W	W	A	Q	L	
*Cw*0704*	Y	D	F	S	K	R	Q	A	D	R	Y	D	F	W	L	A	Q	D	
*Cw*0705*	Y	D	F	S	K	R	Q	A	D	N	Y	D	S	W	L	A	Q	L	
*Cw*0706*	Y	D	F	S	N	R	Q	A	D	R	Y	D	S	W	L	A	Q	L	
*Cw*0707*	Y	D	F	S	N	R	Q	A	D	R	Y	D	S	W	L	A	Q	L	
*Cw*0801*	Y	Y	F	A	K	R	Q	T	D	R	Y	N	F	W	W	T	Q	L	
*Cw*0802*	Y	Y	F	A	K	R	Q	T	D	R	Y	N	F	W	W	E	Q	R	
*Cw*0803*	Y	Y	F	A	K	R	Q	T	D	R	Y	N	F	W	W	T	Q	L	
*Cw*12021*	Y	Y	F	A	K	R	Q	A	D	R	Y	D	S	W	W	E	Q	W	
*Cw*12022*	Y	Y	F	A	K	R	Q	A	D	R	Y	D	S	W	W	E	Q	W	
*Cw*1203*	Y	Y	F	A	K	R	Q	A	D	W	Y	D	S	W	W	E	Q	W	
*Cw*1204*	Y	Y	F	A	K	R	Q	A	D	W	Y	D	S	W	W	E	Q	W	
*Cw*1301*	Y	Y	F	A	K	R	Q	A	D	R	Y	D	S	W	W	E	Q	W	
*Cw*1402*	Y	S	F	A	K	R	Q	T	D	W	F	D	S	W	W	E	Q	R	
*Cw*1403*	Y	S	F	A	K	R	Q	T	D	W	F	D	S	W	W	E	Q	R	
*Cw*1502*	Y	Y	F	A	N	R	Q	T	D	R	Y	D	L	W	W	E	Q	L	
*Cw*1503*	Y	Y	F	A	N	R	Q	A	D	R	Y	D	L	W	W	E	Q	L	

Table 3.12. (con't)

Chelvanayagam 1996[17]	7	9	22	24	66	69	70	73	74	97	99	114	116	133	147	152	155	156	Anchors/preferred residues
Saper et al 1991[25]		9					70	73	74	97									
Matsumura et al 1992[16]			22				70		74	97	99	114	116						
*Cw*1504*	Y	Y	F	A	N	R	Q	T	D	R	Y	D	S	W	W	E	Q	L	
*Cw*15051*	Y	Y	F	A	N	R	Q	T	D	R	Y	D	F	W	W	E	Q	L	
*Cw*15052*	Y	Y	F	A	N	R	Q	T	D	R	Y	D	F	W	W	E	Q	L	
*Cw*1601*	Y	Y	F	A	K	R	Q	T	D	W	Y	D	S	W	W	A	Q	Q	
*Cw*1602*	Y	Y	F	A	K	R	Q	T	D	W	Y	D	S	W	W	A	Q	Q	
*Cw*1701*	Y	Y	F	A	K	R	Q	A	D	R	Y	N	F	W	L	E	Q	L	
*Cw*1702*	Y	Y	F	A	K	R	Q	A	D	R	Y	N	F	W	L	E	Q	L	
*Cw*1801*	Y	D	F	S	K	R	Q	A	D	R	F	N	F	W	W	E	Q	R	
*Cw*1802*	Y	D	F	S	K	R	Q	A	D	R	F	N	F	W	W	E	Q	R	

Table 3.13. Pocket for peptide position 7 (Pocket E)

Chelvanayagam 1996[17]	73	77	97	114	116	133	146	147	150	152	155	156	Anchors/preferred residues
Saper et al 1991[25]			97	114				147		152		156	
Matsumura et al 1992[16]			97	114	116			147		152		156	
*A*0101*	T	N	I	R	D	W	K	W	V	A	Q	R	L
*A*0102*	T	N	I	R	D	W	K	W	V	A	Q	R	
*A*0201*	T	D	R	H	Y	W	K	W	A	V	Q	L	(A,Y,H)
*A*0202*	T	D	R	H	Y	W	K	W	A	V	Q	W	(H,Q)
*A*0203*	T	D	R	H	Y	W	K	W	A	E	Q	W	
*A*0204*	T	D	M	H	Y	W	K	W	A	V	Q	L	
*A*0205*	T	D	R	H	Y	W	K	W	A	V	Q	W	(Q,H,V)
*A*0206*	T	D	R	H	Y	W	K	W	A	V	Q	L	
*A*0207*	T	D	R	H	Y	W	K	W	A	V	Q	L	
*A*0208*	T	D	R	H	Y	W	K	W	A	V	Q	W	
*A*0209*	T	D	R	H	Y	W	K	W	A	V	Q	L	
*A*0210*	T	D	R	H	Y	W	K	W	A	V	Q	L	
*A*0211*	I	D	R	H	Y	W	K	W	A	V	Q	L	
*A*0212*	T	D	R	H	Y	W	K	W	A	V	Q	Q	
*A*0213*	T	D	R	H	Y	W	K	W	A	E	Q	Q	

A*0214	T	D	R	H	Y	W	K	W	A	V	Q	L	
A*0215N	T	D	R	H	Y	W	K	W	A	V	Q	L	
A*0216	T	D	R	H	Y	W	K	W	A	V	Q	L	
A*0217	T	D	M	H	Y	W	K	W	A	V	Q	L	
A*0218	T	D	R	H	Y	W	K	W	A	V	Q	L	
A*0219	T	D	R	H	Y	W	K	W	A	V	Q	Q	
A*0220	T	D	R	H	Y	W	K	W	A	V	Q	L	
A*0221	T	D	R	H	Y	W	K	W	A	V	Q	L	
A*0222	T	D	R	H	Y	W	K	W	A	V	Q	W	
A*0301	T	D	I	R	D	W	K	W	A	E	Q	L	
A*0302	T	D	I	R	D	W	K	W	A	V	Q	Q	
A*0303N	T	D	I	R	D	W	K	W	A	E	Q	L	
A*1101	T	D	I	R	D	W	K	W	A	A	Q	Q	L,I,Y,V,F
A*1102	T	D	I	R	D	W	K	W	A	A	Q	Q	
A*1103	T	D	I	R	D	W	K	W	A	E	Q	Q	
A*1104	T	D	I	R	D	W	K	W	A	A	Q	Q	
A*2301	T	N	M	H	Y	W	K	W	A	V	Q	L	
A*2402	T	N	M	H	Y	W	K	W	A	V	Q	Q	
A*2403	T	N	M	H	Y	W	K	W	A	V	Q	Q	
A*2404	T	N	M	H	Y	W	K	W	A	V	Q	Q	
A*2405	T	N	M	H	Y	W	K	W	A	V	Q	Q	
A*2406	T	N	M	H	Y	W	K	W	A	V	Q	W	
A*2407	T	N	M	H	Y	W	K	W	A	V	Q	Q	
A*2408	T	N	M	H	Y	W	K	W	A	V	Q	Q	
A*2409N	T	N	M	H	Y	W	K	W	A	V	Q	Q	
A*2410	T	N	M	H	Y	W	K	W	A	V	Q	Q	
A*2413	T	N	M	H	Y	W	K	W	A	V	Q	L	
A*2414	T	N	R	H	Y	W	K	W	A	V	Q	L	
A*2501	T	S	R	Q	D	W	K	W	A	E	Q	W	
A*2502	T	S	R	Q	D	W	K	W	A	E	Q	W	
A*2601	T	N	R	Q	D	W	K	W	A	E	Q	W	
A*2602	T	N	R	Q	N	W	K	W	A	E	Q	W	
A*2603	T	D	R	Q	D	W	K	W	A	E	Q	W	
A*2604	T	N	R	Q	D	W	K	W	A	E	Q	W	
A*2605	T	N	R	Q	D	W	K	W	A	E	Q	W	

Table 3.13. (con't)

Chelvanayagam 1996[17]	73	77	97	114	116	133	146	147	150	152	155	156	Anchors/preferred residues
Saper et al 1991[25]			97	114				147		152		156	
Matsumura et al 1992[16]			97	114	116			147		152		156	
*A*2606*	T	D	R	Q	D	W	K	W	A	E	Q	W	
*A*2607*	T	N	R	Q	D	W	K	W	A	E	Q	W	
*A*2608*	T	N	R	Q	D	W	K	W	A	E	Q	Q	
*A*2901*	T	N	M	R	D	W	K	W	A	V	Q	L	
*A*2902*	T	N	M	R	D	W	K	W	A	V	Q	L	(Y)
*A*2903*	T	N	M	R	D	W	K	W	A	V	Q	L	
*A*3001*	T	D	I	E	H	W	K	W	A	W	Q	L	
*A*3002*	T	N	I	E	H	W	K	W	A	R	Q	L	
*A*3003*	T	N	I	E	H	W	K	W	A	R	Q	L	
*A*3004*	T	N	I	E	H	W	K	W	A	V	Q	W	
*A*3005*	T	N	I	E	H	W	K	W	A	V	Q	W	
*A*31012*	I	D	M	Q	D	W	K	W	A	V	Q	L	(N,V,R,F,T,H,L,Y)
*A*3201*	T	S	M	Q	D	W	K	W	A	V	Q	L	
*A*3202*	T	S	M	Q	D	W	K	W	A	V	Q	Q	
*A*3301*	I	D	M	Q	D	W	K	W	A	V	Q	L	
*A*3302*	I	D	M	Q	D	W	K	W	A	V	Q	L	(H,Y,V,T,S)
*A*3303*	I	D	M	Q	D	W	K	W	A	V	Q	L	
*A*3401*	T	D	R	Q	D	W	K	W	A	E	Q	W	
*A*3402*	T	D	I	R	D	W	K	W	A	E	Q	L	
*A*3601*	T	N	I	R	D	W	K	W	V	A	Q	R	
*A*4301*	T	N	R	Q	D	W	K	W	A	E	Q	W	
*A*6601*	T	D	R	Q	D	W	K	W	A	E	Q	W	
*A*6602*	T	D	R	Q	D	W	K	W	A	E	Q	W	
*A*6603*	T	D	R	Q	D	W	K	W	A	E	Q	W	
*A*68011*	T	D	M	R	D	W	K	W	A	V	Q	W	
*A*68012*	T	D	M	R	D	W	K	W	A	V	Q	W	
*A*6802*	T	D	R	H	Y	W	K	W	A	V	Q	W	
*A*6803*	T	D	M	R	D	W	K	W	A	V	Q	W	
*A*6901*	T	D	R	H	Y	W	K	W	A	V	Q	L	
*A*7401*	T	D	M	Q	D	W	K	W	A	V	Q	L	
*A*7402*	T	D	M	Q	D	W	K	W	A	V	Q	L	
*A*7403*	T	D	M	Q	D	W	K	W	A	V	Q	L	
*A*8001*	T	N	I	R	D	W	K	W	A	R	Q	L	

Table 3.14. Pocket for peptide position 7 (Pocket E)

	73	77	97	114	116	133	146	147	150	152	155	156	Anchors/preferred residues
Chelvanayagam 1996[17]	73	77	97	114	116	133	146	147	150	152	155	156	Anchors/preferred residues
Saper et al 1991[25]			97	114				147		152		156	
Matsumura et al 1992[16]			97	114	116			147		152		156	
*B*0702*	T	S	S	D	Y	W	K	W	A	E	Q	R	(Y,L)
*B*0703*	T	S	S	D	Y	W	K	W	A	E	Q	R	
*B*0704*	T	S	S	D	Y	W	K	W	A	E	Q	D	
*B*0705*	T	S	S	N	Y	W	K	W	A	E	Q	R	
*B*0706*	T	S	S	N	Y	W	K	W	A	E	Q	R	
*B*0707*	T	S	R	D	Y	W	K	W	A	E	Q	R	
*B*0801*	T	S	S	N	Y	W	K	W	A	V	Q	D	
*B*0802*	T	N	S	N	Y	W	K	W	A	V	Q	D	
*B*0803*	T	N	S	N	Y	W	K	W	A	V	Q	D	
*B*1301*	T	N	R	N	L	W	K	W	A	V	Q	L	
*B*1302*	T	N	T	N	L	W	K	W	A	V	Q	L	
*B*1303*	T	N	T	N	L	W	K	W	A	V	Q	L	
*B*1401*	T	S	W	N	F	W	K	W	A	E	Q	L	
*B*1402*	T	S	W	N	F	W	K	W	A	E	Q	L	
*B*1501*	T	S	R	D	S	W	K	W	A	E	Q	W	(M,V,L,T,I)
*B*1502*	T	S	R	D	S	W	K	W	A	E	Q	L	
*B*1503*	T	S	R	D	S	W	K	W	A	E	Q	L	
*B*1504*	T	S	T	D	S	W	K	W	A	E	Q	W	
*B*1505*	T	S	R	D	S	W	K	W	A	V	Q	L	
*B*1506*	T	S	R	D	S	W	K	W	A	E	Q	L	
*B*1507*	T	S	S	D	S	W	K	W	A	E	Q	W	
*B*1508*	T	S	R	D	S	W	K	W	A	E	Q	W	
*B*1509*	T	S	R	N	Y	W	K	W	A	E	Q	L	
*B*1510*	T	S	R	D	Y	W	K	W	A	E	Q	L	
*B*1511*	T	S	R	D	S	W	K	W	A	E	Q	W	
*B*1512*	T	S	R	D	S	W	K	W	A	E	Q	W	
*B*1513*	T	N	R	D	S	W	K	W	A	E	Q	L	
*B*1514*	T	S	R	D	S	W	K	W	A	E	Q	W	
*B*1515*	T	S	R	D	S	W	K	W	A	E	Q	W	
*B*1516*	T	N	R	D	S	W	K	W	A	E	Q	L	
*B*1517*	T	N	R	H	D	W	K	W	A	E	Q	L	
*B*1518*	T	S	R	D	S	W	K	W	A	E	Q	L	
*B*1519*	T	S	R	D	S	W	K	W	A	E	Q	W	

Table 3.14. (con't)

Chelvanayagam 1996[17] Saper et al 1991[25] Matsumura et al 1992[16]	73	77	97 97 97	114 114 114	116 116	133	146	147 147 147	150	152 152 152	155	156 156 156	Anchors/preferred residues
*B*1520*	T	S	R	D	S	W	K	W	A	V	Q	L	
*B*1521*	T	S	R	D	S	W	K	W	A	E	Q	L	
*B*1522*	T	S	R	D	S	W	K	W	A	E	Q	W	
*B*1523*	T	N	R	D	S	W	K	W	A	E	Q	L	
*B*1524*	T	N	R	D	S	W	K	W	A	E	Q	W	
*B*1525*	T	S	R	D	S	W	K	W	A	E	Q	L	
*B*1526N*	T	S	R	D	S	W	K	W	A	E	Q	W	
*B*1527*	T	S	R	D	S	W	K	W	A	E	Q	W	
*B*1528*	T	S	R	D	S	W	K	W	A	E	Q	W	
*B*1529*	T	S	R	D	S	W	K	W	A	E	Q	L	
*B*1530*	T	S	R	N	Y	W	K	W	A	E	Q	W	
*B*1531*	T	S	R	D	S	W	K	W	A	V	Q	L	
*B*1532*	T	S	R	D	S	W	K	W	A	E	Q	W	
*B*1533*	T	S	R	D	S	W	K	W	A	E	Q	W	
*B*1534*	T	S	R	D	S	W	K	W	A	E	Q	W	
*B*1535*	T	S	T	D	S	W	K	W	A	E	Q	W	
*B*1537*	T	S	R	D	Y	W	K	W	A	E	Q	L	
*B*1801*	T	S	R	D	S	W	K	W	A	V	Q	L	
*B*1802*	T	S	N	D	S	W	K	W	A	V	Q	L	
*B*1803*	T	S	R	D	S	W	K	W	A	V	Q	L	
*B*1805*	T	S	R	D	S	W	K	W	A	V	Q	L	
*B*2701*	T	N	N	H	D	W	K	W	A	V	Q	L	
*B*2702*	T	N	N	H	D	W	K	W	A	V	Q	L	(Y,L,V,T,F)
*B*2703*	T	D	N	H	D	W	K	W	A	V	Q	L	
*B*2704*	T	S	N	H	D	W	K	W	A	E	Q	L	
*B*27052*	T	D	N	H	D	W	K	W	A	V	Q	L	(I,T,Y,M,L,W,N,V,P)
*B*27053*	T	D	N	H	D	W	K	W	A	V	Q	L	
*B*2706*	T	S	N	D	Y	W	K	W	A	E	Q	L	
*B*2707*	T	D	S	N	Y	W	K	W	A	V	Q	L	
*B*2708*	T	S	N	H	D	W	K	W	A	V	Q	L	
*B*2709*	T	D	N	H	H	W	K	W	A	V	Q	L	
*B*2710*	T	D	N	H	D	W	K	W	A	E	Q	L	
*B*3501*	T	S	R	D	S	W	K	W	A	V	Q	L	(V,N,E,Q,T,K)
*B*3502*	T	S	R	N	Y	W	K	W	A	V	Q	L	

*B*3503*	T	S	R	D	F	W	K	W	A	V	Q	L	
*B*3504*	T	S	R	N	Y	W	K	W	A	V	Q	L	
*B*3505*	T	S	S	D	S	W	K	W	A	V	Q	L	
*B*3506*	T	S	R	N	F	W	K	W	A	V	Q	L	
*B*3507*	T	S	R	D	S	W	K	W	A	V	Q	L	
*B*3508*	T	S	R	D	S	W	K	W	A	V	Q	R	
*B*35091*	T	S	R	N	Y	W	K	W	A	V	Q	L	
*B*35092*	T	S	R	N	Y	W	K	W	A	V	Q	L	
*B*3510*	T	S	R	D	S	W	K	W	A	V	Q	L	
*B*3511*	T	S	R	D	S	W	K	W	A	E	Q	L	
*B*3512*	T	S	R	N	Y	W	K	W	A	V	Q	L	
*B*3513*	T	S	R	D	F	W	K	W	A	V	Q	L	
*B*3515*	T	S	R	D	S	W	K	W	A	V	Q	L	
*B*3516*	T	S	S	D	S	W	K	W	A	V	Q	L	
*B*3517*	T	S	S	D	S	W	K	W	A	V	Q	L	
*B*3518*	T	S	R	N	Y	W	K	W	A	V	Q	R	
*B*3519*	T	S	R	D	S	W	K	W	A	V	Q	L	
*B*3520*	T	S	R	D	S	W	K	W	A	V	Q	L	
*B*3521*	T	S	R	D	S	W	K	W	A	E	Q	L	
*B*3701*	T	D	R	N	F	W	K	W	A	V	Q	D	(Q,K,Y,L)
*B*3702*	T	D	N	H	D	W	K	W	A	V	Q	L	
*B*3801*	T	N	R	N	F	W	K	W	A	V	Q	L	(Y,V,N)
*B*3802*	T	N	R	N	F	W	K	W	A	V	Q	L	
*B*39011*	T	S	R	N	F	W	K	W	A	V	Q	L	(N,Y,F)
*B*39013*	T	S	R	N	F	W	K	W	A	V	Q	L	
*B*39021*	T	S	R	N	F	W	K	W	A	V	Q	L	(V,L,T,Y,N,D,H)
*B*39022*	T	S	R	N	F	W	K	W	A	V	Q	L	
*B*3903*	T	S	S	N	F	W	K	W	A	V	Q	L	
*B*3904*	T	S	R	N	F	W	K	W	A	V	Q	L	
*B*3905*	T	S	R	N	F	W	K	W	A	V	Q	L	
*B*39061*	T	S	T	N	F	W	K	W	A	V	Q	L	
*B*39062*	T	S	T	N	F	W	K	W	A	V	Q	L	
*B*3907*	T	S	R	D	S	W	K	W	A	V	Q	L	
*B*3908*	T	S	R	N	F	W	K	W	A	V	Q	R	
*B*3909*	T	S	R	N	F	W	K	W	A	V	Q	L	

Table 3.14. (con't)

Chelvanayagam 1996[17]	73	77	97	114	116	133	146	147	150	152	155	156	Anchors/preferred residues
Saper et al 1991[25]			97	114				147		152		156	
Matsumura et al 1992[16]			97	114	116			147		152		156	
*B*3910*	T	S	R	N	F	W	K	W	A	V	Q	L	
*B*3911*	T	S	R	N	F	W	K	W	A	V	Q	R	
*B*3912*	T	S	R	N	F	W	K	W	A	V	Q	L	
*B*40011*	T	S	R	N	Y	W	K	L	A	V	Q	L	
*B*40012*	T	S	R	N	Y	W	K	L	A	V	Q	L	I,V,(L,Y,M)
*B*4002*	T	S	S	N	Y	W	K	W	A	V	Q	L	
*B*4003*	T	S	S	D	S	W	K	W	A	V	Q	L	
*B*4004*	T	S	R	N	Y	W	K	W	A	V	Q	L	
*B*4005*	T	S	S	N	Y	W	K	W	A	E	Q	L	
*B*4006*	T	S	T	N	Y	W	K	W	A	V	Q	L	(Y,V,L,W,I,T,R,D,Q,G)
*B*4007*	T	S	R	N	Y	W	K	L	A	V	Q	L	
*B*4008*	T	S	S	N	Y	W	K	W	A	V	Q	L	
*B*4009*	T	S	S	D	Y	W	K	W	A	V	Q	L	
*B*4101*	T	S	R	N	Y	W	K	W	A	V	Q	D	
*B*4102*	T	S	S	N	Y	W	K	W	A	V	Q	D	
*B*4201*	T	S	S	N	Y	W	K	W	A	V	Q	D	
*B*4402*	T	N	R	D	D	W	K	W	A	V	Q	D	
*B*44031*	T	N	R	D	D	W	K	W	A	V	Q	L	
*B*44032*	T	N	R	D	D	W	K	W	A	V	Q	L	
*B*4404*	T	N	R	D	D	W	K	W	A	V	Q	R	
*B*4405*	T	N	R	D	Y	W	K	W	A	V	Q	D	
*B*4406*	T	N	R	D	D	W	K	W	A	V	Q	D	
*B*4407*	T	N	R	D	D	W	K	W	A	V	Q	L	
*B*4408*	T	N	R	D	D	W	K	W	A	V	Q	D	
*B*4410*	T	N	R	N	L	W	K	W	A	V	Q	L	
*B*4501*	T	S	R	N	L	W	K	W	A	V	Q	D	
*B*4601*	T	S	R	D	S	W	K	W	A	E	Q	W	E,(G)
*B*4701*	T	D	R	H	D	W	K	W	A	V	Q	L	
*B*4702*	T	S	R	H	D	W	K	W	A	V	Q	L	
*B*4801*	T	S	S	N	Y	W	K	L	A	V	Q	L	
*B*4802*	T	S	R	D	S	W	K	W	A	V	Q	L	
*B*4803*	T	S	R	N	Y	W	K	L	A	V	Q	L	
*B*4901*	T	N	R	N	L	W	K	W	A	E	Q	L	
*B*5001*	T	S	R	N	L	W	K	W	A	E	Q	L	

*B*51011*	T	N	T	N	Y	W	K	W	A	E	Q	L	(K,Q,R,E)
*B*51012*	T	N	T	N	Y	W	K	W	A	E	Q	L	
*B*51021*	T	N	T	N	Y	W	K	W	A	E	Q	L	(R,E,Q,K)
*B*51022*	T	N	T	N	Y	W	K	W	A	E	Q	L	
*B*5103*	T	N	T	N	Y	W	K	W	A	E	Q	L	(V,M)
*B*5104*	T	N	R	N	Y	W	K	W	A	E	Q	L	
*B*5105*	T	N	T	N	Y	W	K	W	A	V	Q	R	
*B*5106*	T	N	R	N	Y	W	K	W	A	E	Q	L	
*B*5107*	T	N	T	N	Y	W	K	W	A	E	Q	L	
*B*5108*	T	N	T	N	Y	W	K	W	A	V	Q	D	
*B*52011*	T	N	T	N	Y	W	K	W	A	E	Q	L	(K,E,Q,Y)
*B*52012*	T	N	T	N	Y	W	K	W	A	E	Q	L	
*B*5301*	T	N	R	D	S	W	K	W	A	V	Q	L	
*B*5401*	T	S	T	N	L	W	K	W	A	V	Q	L	
*B*5501*	T	S	T	N	L	W	K	W	A	E	Q	L	(V)
*B*5502*	T	S	T	N	L	W	K	W	A	V	Q	L	(V)
*B*5503*	T	S	T	N	L	W	K	W	A	E	Q	L	
*B*5504*	T	S	S	N	Y	W	K	W	A	V	Q	L	
*B*5505*	T	S	T	N	L	W	K	W	A	E	Q	L	
*B*5601*	T	S	T	N	L	W	K	W	A	V	Q	L	(V)
*B*5602*	T	S	R	N	L	W	K	W	A	V	Q	L	
*B*5603*	T	S	R	D	S	W	K	W	A	E	Q	W	
*B*5701*	T	N	V	D	S	W	K	W	A	V	Q	L	
*B*5702*	T	N	V	N	Y	W	K	W	A	V	Q	R	
*B*5703*	T	N	V	N	Y	W	K	W	A	V	Q	L	
*B*5704*	T	N	V	D	D	W	K	W	A	V	Q	R	
*B*5801*	T	N	R	D	S	W	K	W	A	V	Q	L	(L,Y,M,N)
*B*5802*	T	N	W	D	S	W	K	W	A	V	Q	L	
*B*5901*	T	N	T	N	L	W	K	W	A	V	Q	L	
*B*67011*	T	S	R	N	F	W	K	W	A	V	Q	L	
*B*67012*	T	S	R	N	F	W	K	W	A	V	Q	L	
*B*7301*	T	G	T	N	F	W	K	W	A	V	Q	L	T,Y,(E)
*B*7801*	T	S	T	N	Y	W	K	W	A	E	Q	L	(A,V,N,K,Q,E)
*B*78021*	T	S	T	N	Y	W	K	W	A	E	Q	L	
*B*78022*	T	S	T	N	Y	W	K	W	A	E	Q	L	
*B*8101*	T	S	S	N	Y	W	K	L	A	V	Q	L	
*B*8201*	T	S	R	N	L	W	K	W	A	V	Q	D	

Table 3.15. Pocket for peptide position 7 (Pocket E)

Chelvanayagam 1996[17]	73	77	97	114	116	133	146	147	150	152	155	156	Anchors/preferred residues
Saper et al 1991[25]			97	114				147		152		156	
Matsumura et al 1992[16]			97	114	116			147		152		156	
*Cw*0102*	T	S	W	D	Y	W	K	W	A	E	Q	R	(F)
*Cw*0103*	T	S	W	N	F	W	K	W	A	E	Q	R	
*Cw*02021*	T	N	R	D	S	W	K	W	A	E	Q	W	
*Cw*02022*	T	N	R	D	S	W	K	W	A	E	Q	W	
*Cw*02023*	T	N	R	D	S	W	K	W	A	E	Q	W	
*Cw*0302*	T	S	R	D	S	W	K	W	A	E	Q	L	
*Cw*0303*	T	S	R	D	Y	W	K	W	A	E	Q	L	
*Cw*0304*	T	S	R	D	Y	W	K	W	A	E	Q	L	M,E,(R)
*Cw*0401*	A	N	R	N	F	W	K	W	A	E	Q	R	(A)
*Cw*0402*	A	N	R	N	F	W	K	W	A	E	E	R	
*Cw*0403*	A	N	R	N	F	W	K	W	A	E	Q	R	
*Cw*0501*	T	N	R	N	F	W	K	W	A	E	Q	R	
*Cw*0602*	A	N	W	D	S	W	K	W	A	E	Q	W	(R,K,Q,N)
*Cw*0701*	A	S	R	D	S	W	K	L	A	A	Q	L	
*Cw*0702*	A	S	R	D	S	W	K	L	A	A	Q	L	(Y,M,N,R,V,F,E)
*Cw*0703*	A	S	R	D	S	W	K	W	A	A	Q	L	
*Cw*0704*	A	S	R	D	F	W	K	L	A	A	Q	D	
*Cw*0705*	A	S	N	D	S	W	K	L	A	A	Q	L	
*Cw*0706*	A	S	R	D	S	W	K	L	A	A	Q	L	
*Cw*0707*	A	N	R	D	S	W	K	L	A	A	Q	L	
*Cw*0801*	T	S	R	N	F	W	K	W	A	T	Q	L	
*Cw*0802*	T	S	R	N	F	W	K	W	A	E	Q	R	
*Cw*0803*	T	S	R	N	F	W	K	W	A	T	Q	L	
*Cw*12021*	A	S	R	D	S	W	K	W	A	E	Q	W	
*Cw*12022*	A	S	R	D	S	W	K	W	A	E	Q	W	
*Cw*1203*	A	S	W	D	S	W	K	W	A	E	Q	W	
*Cw*1204*	A	N	W	D	S	W	K	W	A	E	Q	W	
*Cw*1301*	A	S	R	D	S	W	K	W	A	E	Q	W	
*Cw*1402*	T	S	W	D	S	W	K	W	A	E	Q	R	
*Cw*1403*	T	S	W	D	S	W	K	W	A	E	Q	R	
*Cw*1502*	T	N	R	D	L	W	K	W	A	E	Q	L	
*Cw*1503*	A	N	R	D	L	W	K	W	A	E	Q	L	

*Cw*1504*	T	N	R	D	S	W	K	W	A	E	Q	L
*Cw*15051*	T	N	R	D	F	W	K	W	A	E	Q	L
*Cw*15052*	T	N	R	D	F	W	K	W	A	E	Q	L
*Cw*1601*	T	S	W	D	S	W	K	W	A	A	Q	Q
*Cw*1602*	T	N	W	D	S	W	K	W	A	A	Q	Q
*Cw*1701*	A	N	R	N	F	W	K	L	A	E	Q	L
*Cw*1702*	A	N	R	N	F	W	K	L	A	E	Q	L
*Cw*1801*	A	N	R	N	F	W	K	W	A	E	Q	R
*Cw*1802*	A	N	R	N	F	W	K	W	A	E	Q	R

Table 3.16. Pocket for peptide C-terminus (Pocket F)

Chelvanayagam 1996[17]	70	73	74	76	77	80	81	84	95	96	97	114	116		123	124	142	143	146	147	Anchors/
Saper et al 1991[25]					77	80	81	84					116		123			143	146	147	preferred
Matsumura et al 1992[16]					77		81		95				116	118	123	124		143		147	residues
*A*0101*	H	T	D	A	N	T	L	Y	I	Q	I	R	D	Y	Y	I	I	T	K	W	Y
*A*0102*	H	T	D	A	N	T	L	Y	I	Q	I	R	D	Y	Y	I	I	T	K	W	
*A*0201*	H	T	H	V	D	T	L	Y	V	Q	R	H	Y	Y	Y	I	T	T	K	W	V,L
*A*0202*	H	T	H	V	D	T	L	Y	L	Q	R	H	Y	Y	Y	I	T	T	K	W	L,(V)
*A*0203*	H	T	H	V	D	T	L	Y	V	Q	R	H	Y	Y	Y	I	T	T	K	W	
*A*0204*	H	T	H	V	D	T	L	Y	V	Q	M	H	Y	Y	Y	I	T	T	K	W	L
*A*0205*	H	T	H	V	D	T	L	Y	L	Q	R	H	Y	Y	Y	I	T	T	K	W	L
*A*0206*	H	T	H	V	D	T	L	Y	V	Q	R	H	Y	Y	Y	I	T	T	K	W	V,L
*A*0207*	H	T	H	V	D	T	L	Y	V	Q	R	H	Y	Y	Y	I	T	T	K	W	L
*A*0208*	H	T	H	V	D	T	L	Y	L	Q	R	H	Y	Y	Y	I	T	T	K	W	
*A*0209*	H	T	H	V	D	T	L	Y	V	Q	R	H	Y	Y	Y	I	T	T	K	W	
*A*0210*	H	T	H	V	D	T	L	Y	V	Q	R	H	Y	Y	Y	I	T	T	K	W	
*A*0211*	H	I	D	V	D	T	L	Y	V	Q	R	H	Y	Y	Y	I	T	T	K	W	
*A*0212*	H	T	H	V	D	T	L	Y	V	Q	R	H	Y	Y	Y	I	T	T	K	W	
*A*0213*	H	T	H	V	D	T	L	Y	V	Q	R	H	Y	Y	Y	I	T	T	K	W	
*A*0214*	H	T	H	V	D	T	L	Y	L	Q	R	H	Y	Y	Y	I	T	T	K	W	L,(V,M)
*A*0215N*	H	T	H	V	D	T	L	Y	V	Q	R	H	Y	Y	Y	I	T	T	K	W	

Table 3.16. (con't)

	70	73	74	76	77	80	81	84	95	96	97	114	116		123	124	142	143	146	147	Anchors/
Chelvanayagam 1996[17]	70	73	74	76	77	80	81	84	95	96	97	114	116		123	124	142	143	146	147	Anchors/
Saper et al 1991[25]					77	80	81	84					116		123			143	146	147	preferred
Matsumura et al 1992[16]					77		81		95				116	118	123	124		143		147	residues
A*0216	H	T	H	V	D	T	L	Y	V	Q	R	H	Y	Y	Y	I	T	T	K	W	
A*0217	H	T	H	V	D	T	L	Y	L	Q	M	H	Y	Y	Y	I	T	T	K	W	
A*0218	H	T	H	V	D	T	L	Y	V	Q	R	H	Y	Y	Y	I	T	T	K	W	
A*0219	H	T	H	V	D	T	L	Y	V	Q	R	H	Y	Y	Y	I	I	T	K	W	
A*0220	H	T	H	V	D	T	L	Y	V	Q	R	H	Y	Y	Y	I	T	T	K	W	
A*0221	H	T	H	V	D	T	L	Y	V	Q	R	H	Y	Y	Y	I	T	T	K	W	
A*0222	H	T	H	V	D	T	L	Y	V	Q	R	H	Y	Y	Y	I	T	T	K	W	
A*0301	Q	T	D	V	D	T	L	Y	I	Q	I	R	D	Y	Y	I	I	T	K	W	K,Y,F
A*0302	Q	T	D	V	D	T	L	Y	I	Q	I	R	D	Y	Y	I	I	T	K	W	
A*0303N	Q	T	D	V	D	T	L	Y	I	Q	I	R	D	Y	Y	I	I	T	K	W	
A*1101	Q	T	D	V	D	T	L	Y	I	Q	I	R	D	Y	Y	I	I	T	K	W	K,(R)
A*1102	Q	T	D	V	D	T	L	Y	I	Q	I	R	D	Y	Y	I	I	T	K	W	
A*1103	Q	T	D	V	D	T	L	Y	I	Q	I	R	D	Y	Y	I	I	T	K	W	
A*1104	Q	T	D	V	D	T	L	Y	I	Q	I	R	D	Y	Y	I	I	T	K	W	
A*2301	H	T	D	E	N	I	A	Y	L	Q	M	H	Y	Y	Y	I	I	T	K	W	
A*2402	H	T	D	E	N	I	A	Y	L	Q	M	H	Y	Y	Y	I	I	T	K	W	
A*2403	H	T	D	E	N	I	A	Y	L	Q	M	H	Y	Y	Y	I	I	T	K	W	
A*2404	H	T	D	A	N	T	L	Y	L	Q	M	H	Y	Y	Y	I	I	T	K	W	
A*2405	H	T	D	E	N	I	A	Y	L	Q	M	H	Y	Y	Y	I	I	T	K	W	
A*2406	H	T	D	E	N	I	A	Y	L	Q	M	H	Y	Y	Y	I	I	T	K	W	
A*2407	Q	T	D	E	N	I	A	Y	L	Q	M	H	Y	Y	Y	I	I	T	K	W	
A*2408	H	T	D	E	N	I	A	Y	L	Q	M	H	Y	Y	Y	I	I	T	K	W	
A*2409N	H	T	D	E	N	I	A	Y	L	Q	M	H	Y	Y	Y	I	I	T	K	W	
A*2410	H	T	D	E	N	I	A	Y	L	Q	M	H	Y	Y	Y	I	I	T	K	W	
A*2413	H	T	D	E	N	I	A	Y	L	Q	M	H	Y	Y	Y	I	I	T	K	W	
A*2414	H	T	D	E	N	I	A	Y	R	Q	R	H	Y	Y	Y	I	I	T	K	W	
A*2501	H	T	D	E	S	I	A	Y	I	Q	R	Q	D	Y	Y	I	I	T	K	W	
A*2502	Q	T	D	E	S	I	A	Y	I	Q	R	Q	D	Y	Y	I	I	T	K	W	
A*2601	H	T	D	A	N	T	L	Y	I	Q	R	Q	D	Y	Y	I	I	T	K	W	
A*2602	H	T	D	A	N	T	L	Y	I	Q	R	Q	N	Y	Y	I	I	T	K	W	
A*2603	H	T	H	V	D	T	L	Y	I	Q	R	Q	D	Y	Y	I	I	T	K	W	
A*2604	H	T	D	A	N	T	L	Y	I	Q	R	Q	D	Y	Y	I	I	T	K	W	
A*2605	H	T	D	E	N	T	L	Y	I	Q	R	Q	D	Y	Y	I	I	T	K	W	
A*2606	H	T	H	V	D	T	L	Y	I	Q	R	Q	D	Y	Y	I	I	T	K	W	

*A*2607*	H	T	D	A	N	T	L	Y	I	Q	R	Q	D	Y	Y	I	I	T	K	W	
*A*2608*	H	T	D	A	N	T	L	Y	I	Q	R	Q	D	Y	Y	I	I	T	K	W	
*A*2901*	Q	T	D	A	N	T	L	Y	I	Q	M	R	D	Y	Y	I	I	T	K	W	
*A*2902*	Q	T	D	A	N	T	L	Y	I	Q	M	R	D	Y	Y	I	I	T	K	W	Y,(L)
*A*2903*	Q	T	D	A	N	T	L	Y	I	Q	M	R	D	Y	Y	I	I	T	K	W	
*A*3001*	Q	T	D	V	D	T	L	Y	I	Q	I	E	H	Y	Y	I	I	T	K	W	
*A*3002*	H	T	D	E	N	T	L	Y	I	Q	I	E	H	Y	Y	I	I	T	K	W	
*A*3003*	H	T	D	E	N	T	L	Y	I	Q	I	E	H	Y	Y	I	I	T	K	W	
*A*3004*	H	T	D	E	N	T	L	Y	I	Q	I	E	H	Y	Y	I	I	T	K	W	
*A*3005*	H	T	D	E	N	T	L	Y	I	Q	I	E	H	Y	Y	I	I	T	K	W	
*A*31012*	H	I	D	V	D	T	L	Y	I	Q	M	Q	D	Y	Y	I	I	T	K	W	R
*A*3201*	H	T	D	E	S	I	A	Y	I	Q	M	Q	D	Y	Y	I	I	T	K	W	
*A*3202*	H	T	D	E	S	I	A	Y	I	Q	M	Q	D	Y	Y	I	I	T	K	W	
*A*3301*	H	I	D	V	D	T	L	Y	I	Q	M	Q	D	Y	Y	I	I	T	K	W	
*A*3302*	H	I	D	V	D	T	L	Y	I	Q	M	Q	D	Y	Y	I	I	T	K	W	R
*A*3303*	H	I	D	V	D	T	L	Y	I	Q	M	Q	D	Y	Y	I	I	T	K	W	
*A*3401*	Q	T	D	V	D	T	L	Y	I	Q	R	Q	D	Y	Y	I	I	T	K	W	
*A*3402*	Q	T	D	V	D	T	L	Y	I	Q	I	R	D	Y	Y	I	I	T	K	W	
*A*3601*	H	T	D	A	N	T	L	Y	I	Q	I	R	D	Y	Y	I	I	T	K	W	
*A*4301*	H	T	D	A	N	T	L	Y	I	Q	R	Q	D	Y	Y	I	I	T	K	W	
*A*6601*	Q	T	D	V	D	T	L	Y	I	Q	R	Q	D	Y	Y	I	I	T	K	W	
*A*6602*	Q	T	D	V	D	T	L	Y	I	Q	R	Q	D	Y	Y	I	I	T	K	W	
*A*6603*	H	T	D	V	D	T	L	Y	I	Q	R	Q	D	Y	Y	I	I	T	K	W	
*A*68011*	Q	T	D	V	D	T	L	Y	I	Q	M	R	D	Y	Y	I	T	T	K	W	R,K
*A*68012*	Q	T	D	V	D	T	L	Y	I	Q	M	R	D	Y	Y	I	T	T	K	W	
*A*6802*	Q	T	D	V	D	T	L	Y	I	Q	R	H	Y	Y	Y	I	T	T	K	W	
*A*6803*	H	T	D	V	D	T	L	Y	I	Q	M	R	D	Y	Y	I	T	T	K	W	
*A*6901*	Q	T	D	V	D	T	L	Y	V	Q	R	H	Y	Y	Y	I	T	T	K	W	V,L,(M)
*A*7401*	H	T	D	V	D	T	L	Y	I	Q	M	Q	D	Y	Y	I	I	T	K	W	
*A*7402*	H	T	D	V	D	T	L	Y	I	Q	M	Q	D	Y	Y	I	I	T	K	W	
*A*7403*	H	T	D	V	D	T	L	Y	I	Q	M	Q	D	Y	Y	I	I	T	K	W	
*A*8001*	H	T	N	A	N	T	L	Y	I	Q	I	R	D	Y	Y	I	I	T	K	W	

Table 3.17 Pocket for peptide C-terminus (Pocket F)

Chelvanayagam 1996[17]	70	73	74	76	77	80	81	84	95	96	97	114	116	118	123	124	142	143	146	147	Anchors/preferred
Saper et al 1991[25]					77	80	81						116		123			143	146	147	residues
Matsumura et al 1992[16]					77		81		95				116	118	123	124		143		147	
B*0702	Q	T	D	E	S	N	L	Y	L	Q	S	D	Y	Y	Y	I	I	T	K	W	L
B*0703	N	T	D	E	S	N	L	Y	L	Q	S	D	Y	Y	Y	I	I	T	K	W	L
B*0704	Q	T	D	E	S	N	L	Y	L	Q	S	D	Y	Y	Y	I	I	T	K	W	
B*0705	Q	T	D	E	S	N	L	Y	L	Q	S	N	Y	Y	Y	I	I	T	K	W	L,(F)
B*0706	Q	T	D	E	S	N	L	Y	L	Q	S	N	Y	Y	Y	I	I	T	K	W	
B*0707	Q	T	D	E	S	N	L	Y	L	Q	R	D	Y	Y	Y	I	I	T	K	W	
B*0801	N	T	D	E	S	N	L	Y	L	Q	S	N	Y	Y	Y	I	I	T	K	W	
B*0802	N	T	D	E	N	T	A	Y	L	Q	S	N	Y	Y	Y	I	I	T	K	W	
B*0803	N	T	Y	E	N	I	A	Y	L	Q	S	N	Y	Y	Y	I	I	T	K	W	
B*1301	N	T	Y	E	N	T	A	Y	I	Q	R	N	L	Y	Y	I	I	T	K	W	
B*1302	N	T	Y	E	N	T	A	Y	W	Q	T	N	L	Y	Y	I	I	T	K	W	
B*1303	N	T	Y	E	N	T	A	Y	W	Q	T	N	L	Y	Y	I	I	T	K	W	
B*1401	N	T	D	E	S	N	L	Y	L	Q	W	N	F	Y	Y	I	I	T	K	W	
B*1402	N	T	D	E	S	N	L	Y	L	Q	W	N	F	Y	Y	I	I	T	K	W	
B*1501	N	T	Y	E	S	N	L	Y	L	Q	R	D	S	Y	Y	I	I	T	K	W	F,Y
B*1502	N	T	Y	E	S	N	L	Y	I	Q	R	D	S	Y	Y	I	I	T	K	W	
B*1503	N	T	Y	E	S	N	L	Y	L	Q	R	D	S	Y	Y	I	I	T	K	W	
B*1504	N	T	Y	E	S	N	L	Y	W	Q	T	D	S	Y	Y	I	I	T	K	W	
B*1505	N	T	Y	E	S	N	L	Y	L	Q	R	D	S	Y	Y	I	I	T	K	W	
B*1506	N	T	Y	E	S	N	L	Y	L	Q	R	D	S	Y	Y	I	I	T	K	W	
B*1507	N	T	Y	E	S	N	L	Y	L	Q	S	D	S	Y	Y	I	I	T	K	W	
B*1508	N	T	Y	E	S	N	L	Y	L	Q	R	D	S	Y	Y	I	I	T	K	W	
B*1509	N	T	Y	E	S	N	L	Y	L	Q	R	N	Y	Y	Y	I	I	T	K	W	
B*1510	N	T	Y	E	S	N	L	Y	L	Q	R	D	Y	Y	Y	I	I	T	K	W	
B*1511	N	T	Y	E	S	N	L	Y	L	Q	R	D	S	Y	Y	I	I	T	K	W	
B*1512	N	T	Y	E	S	N	L	Y	L	Q	R	D	S	Y	Y	I	I	T	K	W	
B*1513	N	T	Y	E	N	I	A	Y	I	Q	R	D	S	Y	Y	I	I	T	K	W	
B*1514	N	T	Y	E	S	N	L	Y	L	Q	R	D	S	Y	Y	I	I	T	K	W	
B*1515	N	T	Y	E	S	N	L	Y	L	Q	R	D	S	Y	Y	I	I	T	K	W	
B*1516	S	T	Y	E	N	I	A	Y	W	Q	R	D	S	Y	Y	I	I	T	K	W	
B*1517	S	T	Y	E	N	I	A	Y	L	Q	R	H	D	Y	Y	I	I	T	K	W	

B*1518	N	T	Y	E	S	N	L	Y	L	Q	R	D	S	Y	Y	I	I	T	K	W	
B*1519	N	T	Y	E	S	N	L	Y	L	Q	R	D	S	Y	Y	I	I	T	K	W	
B*1520	N	T	Y	E	S	N	L	Y	I	Q	R	D	S	Y	Y	I	I	T	K	W	
B*1521	N	T	Y	E	S	N	L	Y	I	Q	R	D	S	Y	Y	I	I	T	K	W	
B*1522	N	T	Y	E	S	N	L	Y	L	Q	R	D	S	Y	Y	I	I	T	K	W	
B*1523	N	T	Y	E	N	I	A	Y	L	Q	R	D	S	Y	Y	I	I	T	K	W	
B*1524	N	T	Y	E	N	I	A	Y	L	Q	R	D	S	Y	Y	I	I	T	K	W	
B*1525	N	T	Y	E	S	N	L	Y	I	Q	R	D	S	Y	Y	I	I	T	K	W	
B*1526N	N	T	Y	E	S	N	L	Y	L	Q	R	D	S	Y	Y	I	I	T	K	W	
B*1527	N	T	Y	E	S	N	L	Y	L	Q	R	D	S	Y	Y	I	I	T	K	W	
B*1528	N	T	Y	E	S	N	L	Y	L	Q	R	D	S	Y	Y	I	I	T	K	W	
B*1529	N	T	Y	E	S	N	L	Y	L	Q	R	D	S	Y	Y	I	I	T	K	W	
B*1530	N	T	Y	E	S	N	L	Y	L	Q	R	N	Y	Y	Y	I	I	T	K	W	
B*1531	N	T	Y	E	S	N	L	Y	L	Q	R	D	S	Y	Y	I	I	T	K	W	
B*1532	N	T	Y	E	S	N	L	Y	L	Q	R	D	S	Y	Y	I	I	T	K	W	
B*1533	N	T	Y	E	S	N	L	Y	L	Q	R	D	S	Y	Y	I	I	T	K	W	
B*1534	N	T	Y	E	S	N	L	Y	L	Q	R	D	S	Y	Y	I	I	T	K	W	
B*1535	N	T	Y	E	S	N	L	Y	L	Q	T	D	S	Y	Y	I	I	T	K	W	
B*1537	N	T	Y	E	S	N	L	Y	L	Q	R	D	Y	Y	Y	I	I	T	K	W	
B*1801	N	T	Y	E	S	N	L	Y	L	Q	R	D	S	Y	Y	I	I	T	K	W	
B*1802	N	T	Y	E	S	N	L	Y	L	Q	N	D	S	Y	Y	I	I	T	K	W	
B*1803	N	T	D	E	S	N	L	Y	L	Q	R	D	S	Y	Y	I	I	T	K	W	
B*1805	N	T	Y	E	S	N	L	Y	L	Q	R	D	S	Y	Y	I	I	T	K	W	
B*2701	K	T	Y	E	N	T	A	Y	L	Q	N	H	D	Y	Y	I	I	T	K	W	
B*2702	K	T	D	E	N	I	A	Y	L	Q	N	H	D	Y	Y	I	I	T	K	W	F,Y,I,L,W
B*2703	K	T	D	E	D	T	L	Y	L	Q	N	H	D	Y	Y	I	I	T	K	W	
B*2704	K	T	D	E	S	T	L	Y	L	Q	N	H	D	Y	Y	I	I	T	K	W	
B*27052	K	T	D	E	D	T	L	Y	L	Q	N	H	D	Y	Y	I	I	T	K	W	L,F,(Y,M,I,R,H,K)
B*27053	K	T	D	E	D	T	L	Y	L	Q	N	H	D	Y	Y	I	I	T	K	W	
B*2706	K	T	D	E	S	T	L	Y	L	Q	N	D	Y	Y	Y	I	I	T	K	W	
B*2707	K	T	D	E	D	T	L	Y	L	Q	S	N	Y	Y	Y	I	I	T	K	W	

Table 3.17. (con't)

	70	73	74	76	77	80	81	84	95	96	97	114	116	118	123	124	142	143	146	147	Anchors/preferred residues
Chelvanayagam 1996[17]	70	73	74	76	77	80	81	84	95	96	97	114	116	118	123	124	142	143	146	147	
Saper et al 1991[25]					77	80	81						116		123			143	146	147	
Matsumura et al 1992[16]					77		81		95				116	118	123	124		143		147	
B*2708	K	T	D	E	S	N	L	Y	L	Q	N	H	D	Y	Y	I	I	T	K	W	
B*2709	K	T	D	E	D	T	L	Y	L	Q	N	H	H	Y	Y	I	I	T	K	W	
B*2710	K	T	D	E	D	T	L	Y	L	Q	N	H	D	Y	Y	I	I	T	K	W	
B*3501	N	T	Y	E	S	N	L	Y	I	Q	R	D	S	Y	Y	I	I	T	K	W	Y,F,M,L,I
B*3502	N	T	Y	E	S	N	L	Y	I	Q	R	N	Y	Y	Y	I	I	T	K	W	
B*3503	N	T	Y	E	S	N	L	Y	I	Q	R	D	F	Y	Y	I	I	T	K	W	M,L,(F)
B*3504	N	T	Y	E	S	N	L	Y	I	Q	R	N	Y	Y	Y	I	I	T	K	W	
B*3505	N	T	Y	E	S	N	L	Y	L	Q	S	D	S	Y	Y	I	I	T	K	W	
B*3506	N	T	Y	E	S	N	L	Y	I	Q	R	N	F	Y	Y	I	I	T	K	W	
B*3507	N	T	Y	E	S	N	L	Y	I	Q	R	D	S	Y	Y	I	I	T	K	W	
B*3508	N	T	Y	E	S	N	L	Y	I	Q	R	D	S	Y	Y	I	I	T	K	W	
B*35091	N	T	Y	E	S	N	L	Y	I	Q	R	N	Y	Y	Y	I	I	T	K	W	
B*35092	N	T	Y	E	S	N	L	Y	I	Q	R	N	Y	Y	Y	I	I	T	K	W	
B*3510	N	T	Y	E	S	N	L	Y	I	Q	R	D	S	Y	Y	I	I	T	K	W	
B*3511	N	T	Y	E	S	N	L	Y	I	Q	R	D	S	Y	Y	I	I	T	K	W	
B*3512	N	T	Y	E	S	N	L	Y	I	Q	R	N	Y	Y	Y	I	I	T	K	W	
B*3513	N	T	Y	E	S	N	L	Y	I	Q	R	D	F	Y	Y	I	I	T	K	W	
B*3515	N	T	Y	E	S	N	L	Y	I	Q	R	D	S	Y	Y	I	I	T	K	W	
B*3516	N	T	Y	E	S	N	L	Y	I	Q	S	D	S	Y	Y	I	I	T	K	W	
B*3517	N	T	Y	E	S	N	L	Y	I	Q	S	D	S	Y	Y	I	I	T	K	W	
B*3518	N	T	Y	E	S	N	L	Y	I	Q	R	N	Y	Y	Y	I	I	T	K	W	
B*3519	N	T	Y	E	S	N	L	Y	I	Q	R	D	S	Y	Y	I	I	T	K	W	
B*3520	N	T	Y	E	S	N	L	Y	I	Q	R	D	S	Y	Y	I	I	T	K	W	
B*3521	N	T	Y	E	S	N	L	Y	I	Q	R	D	S	Y	Y	I	I	T	K	W	
B*3701	N	T	Y	E	D	T	L	Y	I	Q	R	N	F	Y	Y	I	I	T	K	W	I,L
B*3702	N	T	Y	E	D	T	L	Y	L	Q	N	H	D	Y	Y	I	I	T	K	W	
B*3801	N	T	Y	E	N	I	A	Y	L	Q	R	N	F	Y	Y	I	I	T	K	W	F,L,(I)
B*3802	N	T	Y	E	N	T	A	Y	L	Q	R	N	F	Y	Y	I	I	T	K	W	
B*39011	N	T	D	E	S	N	L	Y	L	Q	R	N	F	Y	Y	I	I	T	K	W	L,(V,I,M)
B*39013	N	T	D	E	S	N	L	Y	L	Q	R	N	F	Y	Y	I	I	T	K	W	
B*39021	N	T	D	E	S	N	L	Y	L	Q	R	N	F	Y	Y	I	I	T	K	W	L,(F,M)
B*39022	N	T	D	E	S	N	L	Y	L	Q	R	N	F	Y	Y	I	I	T	K	W	
B*3903	N	T	D	E	S	N	L	Y	L	Q	S	N	F	Y	Y	I	I	T	K	W	

B*3904	N	T	D	E	S	N	L	Y	L	Q	R	N	F	Y	Y	I	I	T	K	W	
B*3905	N	T	Y	E	S	N	L	Y	L	Q	R	N	F	Y	Y	I	I	T	K	W	
B*39061	N	T	D	E	S	N	L	Y	W	Q	T	N	F	Y	Y	I	I	T	K	W	
B*39062	N	T	D	E	S	N	L	Y	W	Q	T	N	F	Y	Y	I	I	T	K	W	
B*3907	N	T	Y	E	S	N	L	Y	L	Q	R	D	S	Y	Y	I	I	T	K	W	
B*3908	N	T	Y	E	S	N	L	Y	L	Q	R	N	F	Y	Y	I	I	T	K	W	
B*3909	N	T	D	E	S	N	L	Y	L	Q	R	N	F	Y	Y	I	I	T	K	W	
B*3910	N	T	D	E	S	N	L	Y	L	Q	R	N	F	Y	Y	I	I	T	K	W	
B*3911	N	T	Y	E	S	N	L	Y	L	Q	R	N	F	Y	Y	I	I	T	K	W	
B*3912	N	T	D	E	S	N	L	Y	L	Q	R	N	F	Y	Y	I	I	T	K	W	
B*40011	N	T	Y	E	S	N	L	Y	L	Q	R	N	Y	Y	Y	I	I	S	K	L	
B*40012	N	T	Y	E	S	N	L	Y	L	Q	R	N	Y	Y	Y	I	I	S	K	L	L
B*4002	N	T	Y	E	S	N	L	Y	L	Q	S	N	Y	Y	Y	I	I	T	K	W	
B*4003	N	T	Y	E	S	N	L	Y	L	Q	S	D	S	Y	Y	I	I	T	K	W	
B*4004	N	T	Y	E	S	N	L	Y	I	Q	R	N	Y	Y	Y	I	I	T	K	W	
B*4005	N	T	Y	E	S	N	L	Y	L	Q	S	N	Y	Y	Y	I	I	T	K	W	
B*4006	N	T	Y	E	S	N	L	Y	W	Q	T	N	Y	Y	Y	I	I	T	K	W	V,(A,P)
B*4007	N	T	Y	E	S	N	L	Y	L	Q	R	N	Y	Y	Y	I	I	S	K	L	
B*4008	N	T	Y	E	S	N	L	Y	L	Q	S	N	Y	Y	Y	I	I	T	K	W	
B*4009	N	T	Y	E	S	N	L	Y	L	Q	S	D	Y	Y	Y	I	I	T	K	W	
B*4101	N	T	Y	E	S	N	L	Y	W	Q	R	N	Y	Y	Y	I	I	T	K	W	
B*4102	N	T	Y	E	S	N	L	Y	L	Q	S	N	Y	Y	Y	I	I	T	K	W	
B*4201	Q	T	D	E	S	N	L	Y	L	Q	S	N	Y	Y	Y	I	I	T	K	W	
B*4402	N	T	Y	E	N	T	A	Y	I	Q	R	D	D	Y	Y	I	I	T	K	W	F,Y
B*44031	N	T	Y	E	N	T	A	Y	I	Q	R	D	D	Y	Y	I	I	T	K	W	F,Y
B*44032	N	T	Y	E	N	T	A	Y	I	Q	R	D	D	Y	Y	I	I	T	K	W	
B*4404	N	T	Y	E	N	T	A	Y	I	Q	R	D	D	Y	Y	I	I	T	K	W	
B*4405	N	T	Y	E	N	T	A	Y	I	Q	R	D	Y	Y	Y	I	I	T	K	W	
B*4406	N	T	Y	E	N	I	A	Y	I	Q	R	D	D	Y	Y	I	I	T	K	W	
B*4407	N	T	Y	E	N	T	A	Y	I	Q	R	D	D	Y	Y	I	I	T	K	W	
B*4408	N	T	Y	E	N	T	A	Y	I	Q	R	D	D	Y	Y	I	I	T	K	W	
B*4410	N	T	Y	E	N	T	A	Y	I	Q	R	N	L	Y	Y	I	I	T	K	W	
B*4501	N	T	Y	E	S	N	L	Y	W	Q	R	N	L	Y	Y	I	I	T	K	W	
B*4601	Q	T	D	V	S	N	L	Y	L	Q	R	D	S	Y	Y	I	I	T	K	W	F,Y
B*4701	N	T	Y	E	D	T	L	Y	L	Q	R	H	D	Y	Y	I	I	T	K	W	
B*4702	N	T	Y	E	S	N	L	Y	L	Q	R	H	D	Y	Y	I	I	T	K	W	
B*4801	N	T	Y	E	S	N	L	Y	L	Q	S	N	Y	Y	Y	I	I	S	K	L	
B*4802	N	T	Y	E	S	N	L	Y	I	Q	R	D	S	Y	Y	I	I	T	K	W	Y
B*4803	N	T	Y	E	S	N	L	Y	L	Q	R	N	Y	Y	Y	I	I	S	K	L	
B*4901	N	T	Y	E	N	I	A	Y	W	Q	R	N	L	Y	Y	I	I	T	K	W	
B*5001	N	T	Y	E	S	N	L	Y	W	Q	R	N	L	Y	Y	I	I	T	K	W	

Table 3.17. (con't)

Chelvanayagam 1996[17]	70	73	74	76	77	80	81	84	95	96	97	114	116	118	123	124	142	143	146	147	Anchors/preferred
Saper et al 1991[25]					77	80	81						116		123			143	146	147	residues
Matsumura et al 1992[16]					77		81		95				116	118	123	124		143		147	
B*51011	N	T	Y	E	N	I	A	Y	W	Q	T	N	Y	Y	Y	I	I	T	K	W	F,I,(W,M,V,L)
B*51012	N	T	Y	E	N	I	A	Y	W	Q	T	N	Y	Y	Y	I	I	T	K	W	
B*51021	N	T	Y	E	N	I	A	Y	W	Q	T	N	Y	Y	Y	I	I	T	K	W	I,V
B*51022	N	T	Y	E	N	I	A	Y	W	Q	T	N	Y	Y	Y	I	I	T	K	W	
B*5103	N	T	Y	E	N	I	A	Y	W	Q	T	N	Y	Y	Y	I	I	T	K	W	V,I,F
B*5104	N	T	Y	E	N	I	A	Y	I	Q	R	N	Y	Y	Y	I	I	T	K	W	
B*5105	N	T	Y	E	N	I	A	Y	W	Q	T	N	Y	Y	Y	I	I	T	K	W	
B*5106	N	T	Y	E	N	I	A	Y	L	Q	R	N	Y	Y	Y	I	I	T	K	W	
B*5107	N	T	Y	E	N	I	A	Y	W	Q	T	N	Y	Y	Y	I	I	T	K	W	
B*5108	N	T	Y	E	N	I	A	Y	W	Q	T	N	Y	Y	Y	I	I	T	K	W	
B*52011	N	T	Y	E	N	I	A	Y	W	Q	T	N	Y	Y	Y	I	I	T	K	W	I,V,(M,F)
B*52012	N	T	Y	E	N	I	A	Y	W	Q	T	N	Y	Y	Y	I	I	T	K	W	
B*5301	N	T	Y	E	N	I	A	Y	I	Q	R	D	S	Y	Y	I	I	T	K	W	
B*5401	Q	T	D	E	S	N	L	Y	W	Q	T	N	L	Y	Y	I	I	T	K	W	(A)
B*5501	Q	T	D	E	S	N	L	Y	W	Q	T	N	L	Y	Y	I	I	T	K	W	(A)
B*5502	Q	T	D	E	S	N	L	Y	W	Q	T	N	L	Y	Y	I	I	T	K	W	(A)
B*5503	Q	T	D	V	S	N	L	Y	W	Q	T	N	L	Y	Y	I	I	T	K	W	
B*5504	Q	T	D	E	S	N	L	Y	L	Q	S	N	Y	Y	Y	I	I	T	K	W	
B*5505	Q	T	D	E	S	N	L	Y	W	Q	T	N	L	Y	Y	I	I	T	K	W	
B*5601	Q	T	D	E	S	N	L	Y	W	Q	T	N	L	Y	Y	I	I	T	K	W	A,(L)
B*5602	Q	T	D	E	S	N	L	Y	L	Q	R	N	L	Y	Y	I	I	T	K	W	
B*5603	Q	T	D	E	S	N	L	Y	L	Q	R	D	S	Y	Y	I	I	T	K	W	
B*5701	S	T	Y	E	N	I	A	Y	I	Q	V	D	S	Y	Y	I	I	T	K	W	
B*5702	S	T	Y	E	N	I	A	Y	I	Q	V	N	Y	Y	Y	I	I	T	K	W	
B*5703	S	T	Y	E	N	I	A	Y	I	Q	V	N	Y	Y	Y	I	I	T	K	W	
B*5704	S	T	Y	E	N	I	A	Y	I	Q	V	D	D	Y	Y	I	I	T	K	W	
B*5801	S	T	Y	E	N	I	A	Y	I	Q	R	D	S	Y	Y	I	I	T	K	W	F,W,(Y)
B*5802	S	T	Y	E	N	I	A	Y	L	Q	W	D	S	Y	Y	I	I	T	K	W	
B*5901	N	T	Y	E	N	I	A	Y	W	Q	T	N	L	Y	Y	I	I	T	K	W	
B*67011	Q	T	D	E	S	N	L	Y	L	Q	R	N	F	Y	Y	I	I	T	K	W	(L)
B*67012	Q	T	D	E	S	N	L	Y	L	Q	R	N	F	Y	Y	I	I	T	K	W	
B*7301	K	T	D	V	G	N	L	Y	W	Q	T	N	F	Y	Y	I	I	T	K	W	P
B*7801	N	T	D	E	S	N	L	Y	W	Q	T	N	Y	Y	Y	I	I	T	K	W	A,(K,S)
B*78021	N	T	Y	E	S	N	L	Y	W	Q	T	N	Y	Y	Y	I	I	T	K	W	
B*78022	N	T	Y	E	S	N	L	Y	W	Q	T	N	Y	Y	Y	I	I	T	K	W	
B*8101	Q	T	D	E	S	N	L	Y	L	Q	S	N	Y	Y	Y	I	I	S	K	L	
B*8201	Q	T	D	E	S	N	L	Y	L	Q	R	N	L	Y	Y	I	I	T	K	W	

Table 3.18. Pocket for peptide C-terminus (Pocket F)

Chelvanayagam 1996[17]	70	73	74	76	77	80	81	84	95	96	97	114	116		123	124	142	143	146	147	Anchors/
Saper et al 1992[25]					77	80	81	84					116		123			143	146	147	preferred
Matsumura et al 1992[16]					77		81		95				116	118	123	124		143			residues
*Cw*0102*	Q	T	D	V	S	N	L	Y	L	Q	W	D	Y	Y	Y	I	I	T	K	W	L
*Cw*0103*	Q	T	D	V	S	N	L	Y	L	Q	W	N	F	Y	Y	I	I	T	K	W	
*Cw*02021*	Q	T	D	V	N	K	L	Y	L	Q	R	D	S	Y	Y	I	I	T	K	W	
*Cw*02022*	Q	T	D	V	N	K	L	Y	L	Q	R	D	S	Y	Y	I	I	T	K	W	
*Cw*02023*	Q	T	D	V	N	K	L	Y	L	Q	R	D	S	Y	Y	I	I	T	K	W	
*Cw*0302*	Q	T	D	V	S	N	L	Y	L	Q	R	D	S	Y	Y	I	I	T	K	W	
*Cw*0303*	Q	T	D	V	S	N	L	Y	I	Q	R	D	Y	Y	Y	I	I	T	K	W	
*Cw*0304*	Q	T	D	V	S	N	L	Y	I	Q	R	D	Y	Y	Y	I	I	T	K	W	L,M
*Cw*0401*	Q	A	D	V	N	K	L	Y	L	Q	R	N	F	Y	Y	I	I	T	K	W	L,F,M
*Cw*0402*	Q	A	D	V	N	K	L	Y	L	Q	R	N	F	Y	Y	I	I	T	K	W	
*Cw*0403*	Q	A	D	V	N	K	L	Y	L	Q	R	N	F	Y	Y	I	I	T	K	W	
*Cw*0501*	Q	T	D	V	N	K	L	Y	L	Q	R	N	F	Y	Y	I	I	T	K	W	
*Cw*0602*	Q	A	D	V	N	K	L	Y	L	Q	W	D	S	Y	Y	I	I	T	K	W	L,I,V,Y
*Cw*0701*	Q	A	D	V	S	N	L	Y	L	Q	R	D	S	Y	Y	I	I	T	K	L	
*Cw*0702*	Q	A	D	V	S	N	L	Y	L	Q	R	D	S	Y	Y	I	I	T	K	L	Y,F,L
*Cw*0703*	Q	A	D	V	S	N	L	Y	L	Q	R	D	S	Y	Y	I	I	T	K	W	
*Cw*0704*	Q	A	D	V	S	N	L	Y	F	Q	R	D	F	Y	Y	I	I	T	K	L	
*Cw*0705*	Q	A	D	V	S	N	L	Y	L	Q	N	D	S	Y	Y	I	I	T	K	L	
*Cw*0706*	Q	A	D	V	S	N	L	Y	L	Q	R	D	S	Y	Y	I	I	T	K	L	
*Cw*0707*	Q	A	D	V	N	K	L	Y	L	Q	R	D	S	Y	Y	I	I	T	K	L	
*Cw*0801*	Q	T	D	V	S	N	L	Y	L	Q	R	N	F	Y	Y	I	I	T	K	W	
*Cw*0802*	Q	T	D	V	S	N	L	Y	L	Q	R	N	F	Y	Y	I	I	T	K	W	
*Cw*0803*	Q	T	D	V	S	N	L	Y	L	Q	R	N	F	Y	Y	I	I	T	K	W	
*Cw*12021*	Q	A	D	V	S	N	L	Y	L	Q	R	D	S	Y	Y	I	I	T	K	W	
*Cw*12022*	Q	A	D	V	S	N	L	Y	L	Q	R	D	S	Y	Y	I	I	T	K	W	
*Cw*1203*	Q	A	D	V	S	N	L	Y	L	Q	W	D	S	Y	Y	I	I	T	K	W	
*Cw*1204*	Q	A	D	V	N	K	L	Y	L	Q	W	D	S	Y	Y	I	I	T	K	W	
*Cw*1301*	Q	A	D	V	S	N	L	Y	L	Q	R	D	S	Y	Y	I	I	T	K	W	

Table 3.18. (con't)

Chelvanayagam 1996[17]	70	73	74	76	77	80	81	84	95	96	97	114	116		123	124	142	143	146	147	Anchors/
Saper et al 1992[25]					77	80	81	84					116		123			143	146	147	preferred
Matsumura et al 1992[16]					77		81		95				116	118	123	124		143			residues
*Cw*1402*	Q	T	D	V	S	N	L	Y	L	Q	W	D	S	Y	Y	I	I	T	K	W	
*Cw*1403*	Q	T	D	V	S	N	L	Y	L	Q	W	D	S	Y	Y	I	I	T	K	W	
*Cw*1502*	Q	T	D	V	N	K	L	Y	I	Q	R	D	L	Y	Y	I	I	T	K	W	
*Cw*1503*	Q	A	D	V	N	K	L	Y	I	Q	R	D	L	Y	Y	I	I	T	K	W	
*Cw*1504*	Q	T	D	V	N	K	L	Y	I	Q	R	D	S	Y	Y	I	I	T	K	W	
*Cw*15051*	Q	T	D	V	N	K	L	Y	I	Q	R	D	F	Y	Y	I	I	T	K	W	
*Cw*15052*	Q	T	D	V	N	K	L	Y	I	Q	R	D	F	Y	Y	I	I	T	K	W	
*Cw*1601*	Q	T	D	V	S	N	L	Y	L	Q	W	D	S	Y	Y	I	I	T	K	W	
*Cw*1602*	Q	T	D	V	N	K	L	Y	L	Q	W	D	S	Y	Y	I	I	T	K	W	
*Cw*1701*	Q	A	D	V	N	K	L	Y	LI	Q	R	N	F	Y	Y	I	I	S	K	L	
*Cw*1702*	Q	A	D	V	N	K	L	Y	I	Q	R	N	F	Y	Y	I	I	S	K	L	
*Cw*1801*	Q	A	D	V	N	K	L	Y	L	Q	R	N	F	Y	Y	I	I	T	K	W	
*Cw*1802*	Q	A	D	V	N	K	L	Y	L	Q	R	N	F	Y	Y	I	I	T	K	W	

Table 3.19. HLA-DRB pocket for relative position P1

	β85	β86	β89	β90	Anchors/Preferred Residues
*DRB1*0101*	V	G	F	T	Y,V,L,F,I,A,M,W
*DRB1*01021*	A	V	F	T	I,L,V,M
*DRB1*01022*	A	V	F	T	
*DRB1*0103*	V	G	F	T	
*DRB1*0104*	V	V	.	.	
*DRB1*03011*	V	V	F	T	L,I,F,M,V
*DRB1*03012*	V	V	F	T	
*DRB1*03021*	V	G	F	T	
*DRB1*03022*	V	G	F	T	
*DRB1*0303*	V	V	F	T	
*DRB1*0304*	V	V	.	.	
*DRB1*0305*	V	G	F	T	
*DRB1*0306*	V	V	F	T	
*DRB1*0307*	V	V	F	T	
*DRB1*0308*	V	V	F	T	
*DRB1*0311*	V	V	F	T	
*DRB1*04011*	V	G	F	T	F,Y,W,I,L,V,M
*DRB1*04012*	V	G	F	T	
*DRB1*0402*	V	V	F	T	V,I,L,M
*DRB1*0403*	V	V	F	T	
*DRB1*0404*	V	V	F	T	V,I,L,M
*DRB1*04051*	V	G	F	T	F,Y,W,V,I,L,M
*DRB1*04052*	V	G	F	T	
*DRB1*0406*	V	V	F	T	
*DRB1*0407*	V	G	F	T	F,Y,W
*DRB1*0408*	V	G	.	.	
*DRB1*0409*	V	G	.	.	
*DRB1*0410*	V	V	F	T	
*DRB1*0411*	V	V	F	T	
*DRB1*0412*	V	V	F	T	
*DRB1*0413*	V	V	F	T	
*DRB1*0414*	V	G	.	.	
*DRB1*0415*	V	V	.	.	
*DRB1*0416*	V	G	.	.	
*DRB1*0417*	V	G	.	.	
*DRB1*0418*	V	V	F	T	
*DRB1*0419*	V	G	F	T	
*DRB1*0420*	V	G	.	.	
*DRB1*0421*	V	G	F	T	
*DRB1*0422*	V	V	F	T	
*DRB1*0423*	V	V	F	T	
*DRB1*0701*	V	G	F	T	
*DRB1*0801*	V	G	.	.	
*DRB1*08021*	V	G	F	T	
*DRB1*08022*	V	G	F	T	
*DRB1*08031*	V	G	F	T	
*DRB1*08032*	V	G	F	T	
*DRB1*08041*	V	V	F	T	
*DRB1*08042*	V	V	F	T	
*DRB1*0805*	V	G	.	.	
*DRB1*0806*	V	V	F	T	
*DRB1*0807*	V	G	F	T	
*DRB1*0808*	V	G	.	.	
*DRB1*0809*	V	G	.	.	
*DRB1*0810*	V	V	F	T	
*DRB1*0811*	V	.	.	.	
*DRB1*0812*	A	V	F	T	
*DRB1*0813*	V	G	.	.	
*DRB1*0814*	V	G	F	T	
*DRB1*0815*	V	G	F	T	

Table 3.19. (con't)

	β85	β86	β89	β90	Anchors/Preferred Residues
*DRB1*0816*	V	G	.	.	
*DRB1*09011*	V	G	F	T	W,Y,F,L
*DRB1*09012*	V	G	.	.	
*DRB1*1001*	V	G	F	T	
*DRB1*11011*	V	G	F	T	W,Y,F
*DRB1*11012*	V	G	F	T	
*DRB1*11013*	V	G	F	.	
*DRB1*1102*	V	V	F	T	
*DRB1*1103*	V	V	F	T	
*DRB1*11041*	V	V	F	T	I,L,V
*DRB1*11042*	V	V	F	T	
*DRB1*1105*	V	G	F	T	
*DRB1*1106*	A	V	F	T	
*DRB1*1107*	V	V	F	T	
*DRB1*11081*	V	G	F	T	
*DRB1*11082*	V	G	F	T	
*DRB1*1109*	V	G	F	T	
*DRB1*1110*	V	G	.	.	
*DRB1*1111*	V	G	F	T	
*DRB1*1112*	V	G	.	.	
*DRB1*1113*	V	V	F	T	
*DRB1*1114*	V	G	F	T	
*DRB1*1115*	V	G	F	T	
*DRB1*1116*	V	V	.	.	
*DRB1*1117*	V	V	F	T	
*DRB1*1118*	V	V	F	T	
*DRB1*1119*	V	G	F	T	
*DRB1*1120*	V	G	F	T	
*DRB1*1121*	A	V	.	.	
*DRB1*1122*	V	G	.	.	
*DRB1*1123*	V	G	.	.	
*DRB1*1124*	V	G	.	.	
*DRB1*1125*	V	V	F	T	
*DRB1*1126*	V	G	.	.	
*DRB1*1127*	V	G	.	.	
*DRB1*1129*	V	G	.	.	
*DRB1*1130*	V	G	F	T	
*DRB1*1201*	A	V	F	T	I,L,F,Y,V
*DRB1*12021*	A	V	.	.	
*DRB1*12022*	A	V	.	.	
*DRB1*12031*	V	V	F	T	
*DRB1*12032*	V	V	F	T	
*DRB1*1204*	A	V	.	.	
*DRB1*1205*	A	V	F	T	
*DRB1*1301*	V	V	F	T	I,L,V
*DRB1*1302*	V	G	F	T	V,F,Y,A,I
*DRB1*13031*	V	G	F	T	
*DRB1*13032*	V	G	F	T	
*DRB1*1304*	V	V	F	T	
*DRB1*1305*	V	G	F	T	
*DRB1*1306*	V	V	F	T	
*DRB1*1307*	V	G	F	T	
*DRB1*1308*	V	V	F	T	
*DRB1*1309*	V	V	F	T	
*DRB1*1310*	V	V	.	.	
*DRB1*1311*	V	V	F	T	
*DRB1*1312*	V	G	F	T	
*DRB1*1313*	V	G	F	T	
*DRB1*1314*	V	G	.	.	
*DRB1*1315*	V	V	.	.	
*DRB1*1316*	V	D	F	T	
*DRB1*1317*	V	V	F	T	
*DRB1*1318*	V	V	F	T	

Table 3.19. (con't)

	β85	β86	β89	β90	Anchors/Preferred Residues
*DRB1*1319*	V	V	F	T	
*DRB1*1320*	V	V	F	T	
*DRB1*1321*	V	G	F	T	
*DRB1*1322*	V	V	F	T	
*DRB1*1323*	V	G	F	T	
*DRB1*1324*	V	V	F	T	
*DRB1*1326*	V	G	.	.	
*DRB1*1327*	V	V	.	.	
*DRB1*1328*	V	V	F	T	
*DRB1*1329*	V	G	F	T	
*DRB1*1330*	V	G	F	T	
*DRB1*1401*	V	V	F	T	
*DRB1*1402*	V	G	F	T	
*DRB1*1403*	V	G	F	T	
*DRB1*1404*	V	V	F	T	
*DRB1*1405*	V	V	.	.	
*DRB1*1406*	V	V	F	T	
*DRB1*1407*	V	G	.	.	
*DRB1*1408*	V	V	F	T	
*DRB1*1409*	V	G	F	T	
*DRB1*1410*	V	V	F	T	
*DRB1*1411*	V	V	.	.	
*DRB1*1412*	V	V	.	.	
*DRB1*1413*	V	G	.	.	
*DRB1*1414*	V	G	F	T	
*DRB1*1415*	V	V	F	T	
*DRB1*1416*	V	V	.	.	
*DRB1*1417*	V	V	F	T	
*DRB1*1418*	V	V	F	T	
*DRB1*1419*	V	G	F	T	
*DRB1*1420*	V	V	.	.	
*DRB1*1421*	V	V	.	.	
*DRB1*1422*	V	G	F	T	
*DRB1*1423*	V	V	F	T	
*DRB1*1424*	V	G	F	T	
*DRB1*1425*	V	G	.	.	
*DRB1*1426*	V	V	F	T	
*DRB1*1427*	V	G	F	T	
*DRB1*1428*	A	V	.	.	
*DRB1*1429*	A	V	F	T	
*DRB1*15011*	V	V	F	T	L,V,I
*DRB1*15012*	V	V	F	T	
*DRB1*15021*	V	G	F	T	
*DRB1*15022*	V	G	.	.	
*DRB1*1503*	V	V	F	T	
*DRB1*1504*	V	V	.	.	
*DRB1*1505*	V	V	F	T	
*DRB1*1506*	V	V	.	.	
*DRB1*16011*	V	G	F	T	
*DRB1*16012*	V	G	F	T	
*DRB1*16021*	V	G	F	T	
*DRB1*16022*	V	G	.	.	
*DRB1*1603*	V	G	F	T	
*DRB1*1604*	V	G	.	.	
*DRB1*1605*	V	G	.	.	
*DRB1*1606*	V	G	.	.	
*DRB1*1608*	V	G	F	T	
*DRB3*01011*	V	G	F	T	
*DRB3*01013*	V	G	.	.	
*DRB3*0102*	V	G	.	.	
*DRB3*0201*	V	V	F	T	
*DRB3*0202*	V	G	F	T	Y,F,I,L
*DRB3*0203*	V	G	F	T	

Table 3.19. (con't)

	β85	β86	β89	β90	Anchors/Preferred Residues
*DRB3*0204*	V	V	F	T	
*DRB3*0205*	V	G	F	T	
*DRB3*0206*	V	G	.	.	
*DRB3*0301*	V	V	F	T	I,L,V
*DRB4*0101101*	V	V	F	T	
*DRB4*0102*	V	V	F	T	
*DRB4*0103101*	V	V	F	T	
*DRB4*0104*	V	V	F	T	
*DRB5*0101*	V	G	F	T	F,Y,L,M
*DRB5*0102*	V	G	F	T	
*DRB5*0103*	V	G	F	T	
*DRB5*0104*	V	G	F	T	
*DRB5*0105*	V	G	F	T	
*DRB5*0201*	A	V	F	T	
*DRB5*0202*	A	V	F	T	
*DRB5*0203*	V	G	F	T	
*DRB5*0204*	A	V	F	T	
*DRB6*0101*	V	F	.	.	
*DRB6*0201*	V	F	.	.	
*DRB6*0202*	V	F	.	.	

HLA class II pockets actually shown to be participating in pocket structure at least in some allelic products.[30] Capital letters designate preferred AA, amino acids that are less frequently found are shown in brackets. Unavailability of AA is indicated by a dot. This applies also to Tables 3.20 - 3.23.

Table 3.20. HLA-DRB pocket for relative position P4

	β13	β70	β71	β74	β78	Anchors/Preferred Residues
*DRB1*0101*	F	Q	R	A	Y	L,A,I,V,M,N,Q
*DRB1*01021*	F	Q	R	A	Y	A,L,M
*DRB1*01022*	F	Q	R	A	Y	
*DRB1*0103*	F	D	E	A	Y	
*DRB1*0104*	F	Q	R	A	Y	
*DRB1*03011*	S	Q	K	R	Y	D
*DRB1*03012*	S	Q	K	R	Y	
*DRB1*03021*	S	Q	K	R	Y	
*DRB1*03022*	S	Q	K	R	Y	
*DRB1*0303*	S	Q	K	R	Y	
*DRB1*0304*	S	Q	K	R	Y	
*DRB1*0305*	.	Q	K	R	Y	
*DRB1*0306*	S	Q	K	R	Y	
*DRB1*0307*	S	Q	K	R	Y	
*DRB1*0308*	S	Q	K	R	Y	
*DRB1*0311*	S	Q	K	Q	Y	
*DRB1*04011*	H	Q	K	A	Y	F,W,I,L,V,A,D,E, no R,K
*DRB1*04012*	H	Q	K	A	Y	
*DRB1*0402*	H	D	E	A	Y	Y,F,W,I,L,M,R,N, no D,E
*DRB1*0403*	H	Q	R	E	Y	
*DRB1*0404*	H	Q	R	A	Y	F,Y,W,I,L,V,M,A,D,E, no R,K
*DRB1*04051*	H	Q	R	A	Y	V,I,L,M,D,E
*DRB1*04052*	.	Q	R	A	Y	
*DRB1*0406*	H	Q	R	E	Y	
*DRB1*0407*	H	Q	R	E	Y	A,V,K
*DRB1*0408*	.	Q	R	A	Y	
*DRB1*0409*	.	Q	K	A	Y	
*DRB1*0410*	H	Q	R	A	Y	
*DRB1*0411*	H	Q	R	E	Y	
*DRB1*0412*	H	D	R	L	Y	
*DRB1*0413*	H	Q	K	A	Y	

Table 3.20. (con't)

	β13	β70	β71	β74	β78	Anchors/Preferred Residues
*DRB1*0414*	.	D	E	A	Y	
*DRB1*0415*	H	D	R	A	Y	
*DRB1*0416*	.	Q	K	A	Y	
*DRB1*0417*	.	Q	R	E	Y	
*DRB1*0418*	.	D	R	L	Y	
*DRB1*0419*	H	Q	R	A	Y	
*DRB1*0420*	.	Q	R	E	Y	
*DRB1*0421*	H	Q	K	A	Y	
*DRB1*0422*	H	Q	K	R	Y	
*DRB1*0423*	H	Q	R	A	Y	
*DRB1*0701*	Y	D	R	Q	V	
*DRB1*0801*	G	D	R	L	Y	
*DRB1*08021*	G	D	R	L	Y	
*DRB1*08022*	G	D	R	L	Y	
*DRB1*08031*	G	D	R	L	Y	
*DRB1*08032*	G	D	R	L	Y	
*DRB1*08041*	G	D	R	L	Y	
*DRB1*08042*	.	D	R	L	Y	
*DRB1*0805*	G	D	R	A	Y	
*DRB1*0806*	G	D	R	L	Y	
*DRB1*0807*	G	D	R	L	Y	
*DRB1*0808*	G	D	R	L	Y	
*DRB1*0809*	.	D	R	L	Y	
*DRB1*0810*	G	D	R	L	Y	
*DRB1*0811*	G	D	R	L	Y	
*DRB1*0812*	G	D	R	L	Y	
*DRB1*0813*	G	D	R	L	Y	
*DRB1*0814*	G	D	R	L	Y	
*DRB1*0815*	G	D	R	L	Y	
*DRB1*0816*	G	D	R	L	Y	
*DRB1*09011*	.	R	R	E	V	A,V,S,
*DRB1*09012*	F	R	R	E	V	
*DRB1*1001*	F	R	R	A	Y	
*DRB1*11011*	S	D	R	A	Y	M,L,V,A,F,Y
*DRB1*11012*	S	D	R	A	Y	
*DRB1*11013*	S	D	R	A	Y	
*DRB1*1102*	S	D	E	A	Y	
*DRB1*1103*	S	D	E	A	Y	
*DRB1*11041*	S	D	R	A	Y	L,V,M,A,F,Y
*DRB1*11042*	S	D	R	A	Y	
*DRB1*1105*	G	D	R	A	Y	
*DRB1*1106*	S	D	R	A	Y	
*DRB1*1107*	S	Q	K	R	Y	
*DRB1*11081*	S	D	R	A	Y	
*DRB1*11082*	S	D	R	A	Y	
*DRB1*1109*	.	D	R	A	Y	
*DRB1*1110*	.	D	R	A	Y	
*DRB1*1111*	S	D	E	A	Y	
*DRB1*1112*	.	D	R	A	Y	
*DRB1*1113*	S	R	R	A	Y	
*DRB1*1114*	S	D	E	A	Y	
*DRB1*1115*	S	D	R	A	Y	
*DRB1*1116*	S	D	E	A	Y	
*DRB1*1117*	S	R	R	E	Y	
*DRB1*1118*	S	D	R	A	Y	
*DRB1*1119*	S	D	R	A	Y	
*DRB1*1120*	S	D	E	A	Y	
*DRB1*1121*	S	D	E	A	Y	
*DRB1*1122*	H	D	R	A	Y	
*DRB1*1123*	S	D	R	L	Y	
*DRB1*1124*	S	D	R	L	Y	
*DRB1*1125*	S	D	R	L	Y	
*DRB1*1126*	S	Q	R	A	Y	

Table 3.20. (con't)

	β13	β70	β71	β74	β78	Anchors/Preferred Residues
*DRB1*1127*	S	D	R	A	Y	
*DRB1*1129*	S	D	R	A	Y	
*DRB1*1130*	S	D	R	A	Y	
*DRB1*1201*	G	D	R	A	Y	
*DRB1*12021*	G	D	R	A	Y	
*DRB1*12022*	G	D	R	A	Y	
*DRB1*12031*	G	D	R	A	Y	
*DRB1*12032*	G	D	R	A	Y	
*DRB1*1204*	G	D	R	A	Y	
*DRB1*1205*	G	D	R	A	Y	
*DRB1*1301*	S	D	E	A	Y	L,V,M,A,W,Y
*DRB1*1302*	S	D	E	A	Y	L,V,M,A,W,Y
*DRB1*13031*	S	D	K	A	Y	
*DRB1*13032*	S	D	K	A	Y	
*DRB1*1304*	S	D	E	A	Y	
*DRB1*1305*	S	D	R	A	Y	
*DRB1*1306*	.	D	R	A	Y	
*DRB1*1307*	S	D	R	A	Y	
*DRB1*1308*	S	D	E	A	Y	
*DRB1*1309*	S	Q	A	A	Y	
*DRB1*1310*	S	D	K	A	Y	
*DRB1*1311*	S	D	R	A	Y	
*DRB1*1312*	S	D	R	A	Y	
*DRB1*1313*	S	D	R	L	Y	
*DRB1*1314*	S	D	R	A	Y	
*DRB1*1315*	.	D	E	A	Y	
*DRB1*1316*	S	D	E	A	Y	
*DRB1*1317*	G	D	E	A	Y	
*DRB1*1318*	S	D	R	L	Y	
*DRB1*1319*	S	D	E	A	Y	
*DRB1*1320*	S	D	E	A	Y	
*DRB1*1321*	S	D	R	A	Y	
*DRB1*1322*	S	D	E	A	Y	
*DRB1*1323*	S	D	E	A	Y	
*DRB1*1324*	S	D	E	A	Y	
*DRB1*1326*	S	D	R	A	Y	
*DRB1*1327*	S	D	E	A	Y	
*DRB1*1328*	S	D	E	A	Y	
*DRB1*1329*	S	D	E	A	Y	
*DRB1*1330*	S	D	R	A	Y	
*DRB1*1401*	S	R	R	E	Y	
*DRB1*1402*	S	Q	R	A	Y	
*DRB1*1403*	S	D	R	L	Y	
*DRB1*1404*	G	R	R	E	Y	
*DRB1*1405*	S	R	R	E	Y	
*DRB1*1406*	S	Q	R	A	Y	
*DRB1*1407*	S	R	R	E	Y	
*DRB1*1408*	S	R	R	E	Y	
*DRB1*1409*	S	Q	R	A	Y	
*DRB1*1410*	H	R	R	E	Y	
*DRB1*1411*	G	R	R	E	Y	
*DRB1*1412*	S	D	R	L	Y	
*DRB1*1413*	S	Q	R	A	Y	
*DRB1*1414*	S	R	R	E	Y	
*DRB1*1415*	G	D	R	L	Y	
*DRB1*1416*	S	D	E	A	Y	
*DRB1*1417*	S	Q	R	A	Y	
*DRB1*1418*	.	R	R	E	Y	
*DRB1*1419*	S	Q	K	A	Y	
*DRB1*1420*	S	Q	R	A	Y	
*DRB1*1421*	S	Q	K	A	Y	
*DRB1*1422*	S	D	R	A	Y	
*DRB1*1423*	S	R	R	E	Y	

Table 3.20. (con't)

	β13	β70	β71	β74	β78	Anchors/Preferred Residues
*DRB1*1424*	S	Q	A	A	Y	
*DRB1*1425*	S	D	R	A	Y	
*DRB1*1426*	S	R	R	E	Y	
*DRB1*1427*	S	D	R	L	Y	
*DRB1*1428*	G	R	R	E	Y	
*DRB1*1429*	S	Q	R	A	Y	
*DRB1*15011*	R	Q	A	A	Y	F,Y,I
*DRB1*15012*	R	Q	A	A	Y	
*DRB1*15021*	R	Q	A	A	Y	
*DRB1*15022*	.	Q	A	A	Y	
*DRB1*1503*	R	Q	A	A	Y	
*DRB1*1504*	.	Q	A	A	Y	
*DRB1*1505*	R	Q	A	A	Y	
*DRB1*1506*	.	Q	A	A	Y	
*DRB1*16011*	R	D	R	A	Y	
*DRB1*16012*	R	D	R	A	Y	
*DRB1*16021*	R	D	R	A	Y	
*DRB1*16022*	R	D	R	A	Y	
*DRB1*1603*	R	D	R	A	Y	
*DRB1*1604*	R	D	R	L	Y	
*DRB1*1605*	.	D	R	A	Y	
*DRB1*1606*	R	D	R	A	Y	
*DRB1*1608*	R	D	R	A	Y	
*DRB3*01011*	S	Q	K	R	Y	
*DRB3*01013*	S	Q	K	R	Y	
*DRB3*0102*	S	Q	K	R	Y	
*DRB3*0201*	S	Q	K	Q	Y	
*DRB3*0202*	S	Q	K	Q	Y	N
*DRB3*0203*	S	Q	K	Q	Y	
*DRB3*0204*	S	Q	K	R	Y	
*DRB3*0205*	S	Q	K	Q	Y	
*DRB3*0206*	S	Q	K	Q	Y	
*DRB3*0301*	S	Q	K	Q	Y	N
*DRB4*0101101*	C	R	R	E	Y	
*DRB4*0102*	.	R	R	E	Y	
*DRB4*0103101*	C	R	R	E	Y	
*DRB4*0104*	C	R	R	E	Y	
*DRB4*0201N*	C	.	.	.	.	
*DRB5*0101*	Y	D	R	A	Y	Q,V,I,M
*DRB5*0102*	Y	D	R	A	Y	
*DRB5*0103*	Y	D	T	A	Y	
*DRB5*0104*	Y	D	R	L	Y	
*DRB5*0105*	Y	D	R	A	Y	
*DRB5*0201*	Y	Q	A	A	Y	
*DRB5*0202*	Y	Q	A	A	Y	
*DRB5*0203*	Y	Q	A	A	Y	
*DRB5*0204*	Y	Q	A	A	Y	
*DRB6*0101*	C	E	N	K	Y	
*DRB6*0201*	C	E	K	K	Y	
*DRB6*0202*	C	E	K	K	Y	

Table 3.21. HLA-DRB pocket for relative position P6

	β11	β13	Anchors/Preferred Residues
*DRB1*0101*	L	F	A,G,S,T,P
*DRB1*01021*	L	F	A,G,S,T,P
*DRB1*01022*	L	F	
*DRB1*0103*	L	F	
*DRB1*0104*	.	F	
*DRB1*03011*	S	S	K,R,E,Q,N
*DRB1*03012*	S	S	
*DRB1*03021*	S	S	
*DRB1*03022*	S	S	
*DRB1*0303*	S	S	
*DRB1*0304*	S	S	
*DRB1*0306*	S	S	
*DRB1*0307*	S	S	
*DRB1*0308*	S	S	
*DRB1*0311*	S	S	
*DRB1*04011*	V	H	N,S,T,Q,H,R
*DRB1*04012*	V	H	
*DRB1*0402*	V	H	N,Q,S,T,K
*DRB1*0403*	V	H	
*DRB1*0404*	V	H	N,T,S,Q,R
*DRB1*04051*	V	H	N,S,T,Q,K,D
*DRB1*0406*	V	H	
*DRB1*0407*	V	H	N,T,D,S
*DRB1*0410*	V	H	
*DRB1*0411*	V	H	
*DRB1*0412*	V	H	
*DRB1*0413*	.	H	
*DRB1*0415*	V	H	
*DRB1*0419*	.	H	
*DRB1*0421*	V	H	
*DRB1*0422*	V	H	
*DRB1*0423*	V	H	
*DRB1*0701*	G	Y	
*DRB1*0801*	S	G	
*DRB1*08021*	S	G	
*DRB1*08022*	S	G	
*DRB1*08031*	S	G	
*DRB1*08032*	S	G	
*DRB1*08041*	S	G	
*DRB1*0805*	S	G	
*DRB1*0806*	S	G	
*DRB1*0807*	.	G	
*DRB1*0808*	S	G	
*DRB1*0810*	S	G	
*DRB1*0811*	S	G	
*DRB1*0812*	S	G	
*DRB1*0813*	S	G	
*DRB1*0814*	S	G	
*DRB1*0815*	S	G	
*DRB1*0816*	S	G	
*DRB1*09012*	D	F	
*DRB1*1001*	V	F	
*DRB1*11011*	S	S	R,K,H
*DRB1*11012*	S	S	
*DRB1*11013*	S	S	
*DRB1*1102*	S	S	
*DRB1*1103*	S	S	
*DRB1*11041*	S	S	R,K,H
*DRB1*11042*	S	S	
*DRB1*1105*	S	G	

Table 3.21. (con't)

	β11	β13	Anchors/Preferred Residues
*DRB1*1106*	S	S	
*DRB1*1107*	S	S	
*DRB1*11081*	.	S	
*DRB1*11082*	.	S	
*DRB1*1111*	.	S	
*DRB1*1113*	S	S	
*DRB1*1114*	S	S	
*DRB1*1115*	S	S	
*DRB1*1116*	.	S	
*DRB1*1117*	S	S	
*DRB1*1118*	S	S	
*DRB1*1119*	S	S	
*DRB1*1120*	S	S	
*DRB1*1121*	S	S	
*DRB1*1122*	V	H	
*DRB1*1123*	.	S	
*DRB1*1124*	.	S	
*DRB1*1125*	S	S	
*DRB1*1126*	S	S	
*DRB1*1127*	S	S	
*DRB1*1129*	S	S	
*DRB1*1130*	L	S	
*DRB1*1201*	S	G	V,Y,F,I,N,A
*DRB1*12021*	S	G	
*DRB1*12022*	S	G	
*DRB1*12031*	S	G	
*DRB1*12032*	S	G	
*DRB1*1204*	S	G	
*DRB1*1205*	S	G	
*DRB1*1301*	S	S	R,K
*DRB1*1302*	S	S	R,K
*DRB1*13031*	S	S	
*DRB1*13032*	S	S	
*DRB1*1304*	S	S	
*DRB1*1305*	S	S	
*DRB1*1307*	S	S	
*DRB1*1308*	S	S	
*DRB1*1309*	S	S	
*DRB1*1310*	S	S	
*DRB1*1311*	S	S	
*DRB1*1312*	S	S	
*DRB1*1313*	S	S	
*DRB1*1314*	.	S	
*DRB1*1316*	S	S	
*DRB1*1317*	S	G	
*DRB1*1318*	S	S	
*DRB1*1319*	S	S	
*DRB1*1320*	S	S	
*DRB1*1321*	S	S	
*DRB1*1322*	S	S	
*DRB1*1323*	S	S	
*DRB1*1324*	S	S	
*DRB1*1326*	S	S	
*DRB1*1327*	.	S	
*DRB1*1328*	S	S	
*DRB1*1329*	S	S	
*DRB1*1330*	S	S	
*DRB1*1401*	S	S	
*DRB1*1402*	S	S	
*DRB1*1403*	S	S	
*DRB1*1404*	S	G	
*DRB1*1405*	S	S	

Table 3.21. (con't)

	β11	β13	Anchors/Preferred Residues
*DRB1*1406*	S	S	
*DRB1*1407*	S	S	
*DRB1*1408*	S	S	
*DRB1*1409*	S	S	
*DRB1*1410*	V	H	
*DRB1*1411*	S	G	
*DRB1*1412*	.	S	
*DRB1*1413*	S	S	
*DRB1*1414*	S	S	
*DRB1*1415*	S	G	
*DRB1*1416*	S	S	
*DRB1*1417*	S	S	
*DRB1*1419*	S	S	
*DRB1*1420*	S	S	
*DRB1*1421*	S	S	
*DRB1*1422*	S	S	
*DRB1*1423*	S	S	
*DRB1*1424*	.	S	
*DRB1*1425*	S	S	
*DRB1*1426*	S	S	
*DRB1*1427*	S	S	
*DRB1*1428*	S	G	
*DRB1*1429*	S	S	
*DRB1*15011*	P	R	
*DRB1*15012*	P	R	
*DRB1*15021*	P	R	
*DRB1*1503*	P	R	
*DRB1*1505*	P	R	
*DRB1*16011*	P	R	
*DRB1*16012*	P	R	
*DRB1*16021*	P	R	
*DRB1*16022*	.	R	
*DRB1*1603*	P	R	
*DRB1*1604*	P	R	
*DRB1*1606*	P	R	
*DRB1*1608*	P	R	
*DRB3*01011*	R	S	
*DRB3*01013*	R	S	
*DRB3*0102*	C	S	
*DRB3*0201*	L	S	
*DRB3*0202*	L	S	A,S,P,D,E
*DRB3*0203*	L	S	
*DRB3*0204*	L	S	
*DRB3*0205*	L	S	
*DRB3*0206*	L	S	
*DRB3*0301*	L	S	A,S,P,D,E
*DRB4*0101101*	A	C	
*DRB4*0103101*	A	C	
*DRB4*0104*	A	C	
*DRB4*0201N*	A	C	
*DRB5*0101*	D	Y	
*DRB5*0102*	D	Y	
*DRB5*0103*	D	Y	
*DRB5*0104*	D	Y	
*DRB5*0105*	D	Y	
*DRB5*0201*	D	Y	
*DRB5*0202*	D	Y	
*DRB5*0203*	D	Y	
*DRB5*0204*	D	Y	
*DRB6*0101*	.	C	
*DRB6*0201*	A	C	
*DRB6*0202*	.	C	

Table 3.22. HLA-DRB pocket for relative position P7

	β28	β47	β61	β67	β71	Anchors/Preferred Residues
*DRB1*0101*	E	Y	W	L	R	
*DRB1*01021*	E	Y	W	L	R	
*DRB1*01022*	E	Y	W	L	R	
*DRB1*0103*	E	Y	W	I	E	
*DRB1*0104*	E	Y	W	L	R	
*DRB1*03011*	D	F	W	L	K	
*DRB1*03012*	D	F	W	L	K	
*DRB1*03021*	E	Y	W	L	K	
*DRB1*03022*	E	Y	W	L	K	
*DRB1*0303*	E	Y	W	L	K	
*DRB1*0304*	D	F	W	L	K	
*DRB1*0305*	D	F	W	L	K	
*DRB1*0306*	D	Y	W	L	K	
*DRB1*0307*	D	F	W	L	K	
*DRB1*0308*	D	F	W	L	K	
*DRB1*0311*	D	F	W	L	K	
*DRB1*04011*	D	Y	W	L	K	polar, charged, aliphatic
*DRB1*04012*	D	Y	W	L	K	
*DRB1*0402*	D	Y	W	I	E	R,K,H,N,Q,P
*DRB1*0403*	D	Y	W	L	R	
*DRB1*0404*	D	Y	W	L	R	polar, charged, aliphatic
*DRB1*04051*	D	Y	W	L	R	polar, charged, aliphatic
*DRB1*04052*	D	Y	W	L	R	
*DRB1*0406*	D	Y	W	L	R	
*DRB1*0407*	D	Y	W	L	R	
*DRB1*0408*	D	Y	W	L	R	
*DRB1*0409*	D	Y	W	L	K	
*DRB1*0410*	D	Y	W	L	R	
*DRB1*0411*	D	Y	W	L	R	
*DRB1*0412*	D	Y	W	I	R	
*DRB1*0413*	D	Y	W	L	K	
*DRB1*0414*	D	Y	W	I	E	
*DRB1*0415*	D	Y	W	F	R	
*DRB1*0416*	D	Y	W	L	K	
*DRB1*0417*	D	Y	W	L	R	
*DRB1*0418*	D	Y	W	I	R	
*DRB1*0419*	D	Y	W	L	R	
*DRB1*0420*	D	Y	W	L	R	
*DRB1*0421*	D	Y	W	L	K	
*DRB1*0422*	D	Y	W	L	K	
*DRB1*0423*	D	Y	W	L	R	
*DRB1*0701*	E	Y	W	I	R	
*DRB1*0801*	D	Y	W	F	R	
*DRB1*08021*	D	Y	W	F	R	
*DRB1*08022*	D	Y	W	F	R	
*DRB1*08031*	D	Y	W	I	R	
*DRB1*08032*	D	Y	W	I	R	
*DRB1*08041*	D	Y	W	F	R	
*DRB1*08042*	D	Y	W	F	R	
*DRB1*0805*	D	Y	W	F	R	
*DRB1*0806*	D	Y	W	F	R	
*DRB1*0807*	D	Y	W	F	R	
*DRB1*0808*	D	Y	W	F	R	
*DRB1*0809*	D	Y	W	F	R	
*DRB1*0810*	D	Y	W	I	R	
*DRB1*0811*	D	Y	W	F	R	
*DRB1*0812*	D	Y	W	I	R	
*DRB1*0813*	D	Y	W	L	R	
*DRB1*0814*	D	Y	W	I	R	
*DRB1*0815*	D	Y	W	I	R	

Table 3.22. (con't)

	β28	β47	β61	β67	β71	Anchors/Preferred Residues
*DRB1*0816*	D	Y	W	F	R	
*DRB1*09011*	H	Y	W	F	R	
*DRB1*09012*	H	Y	W	F	R	
*DRB1*1001*	E	Y	W	L	R	
*DRB1*11011*	D	F	W	F	R	
*DRB1*11012*	D	F	W	F	R	
*DRB1*11013*	D	F	W	F	R	
*DRB1*1102*	D	F	W	I	E	
*DRB1*1103*	D	F	W	F	E	
*DRB1*11041*	D	F	W	F	R	
*DRB1*11042*	D	F	W	F	R	
*DRB1*1105*	D	F	W	F	R	
*DRB1*1106*	D	F	W	F	R	
*DRB1*1107*	D	F	W	L	K	
*DRB1*11082*	D	F	W	L	R	
*DRB1*1109*	D	F	W	F	R	
*DRB1*1110*	D	F	W	F	R	
*DRB1*1111*	D	F	W	F	E	
*DRB1*1112*	D	F	W	F	R	
*DRB1*1113*	D	F	W	L	R	
*DRB1*1114*	D	F	W	I	E	
*DRB1*1115*	D	F	W	F	R	
*DRB1*1116*	D	F	W	I	E	
*DRB1*1117*	D	Y	W	L	R	
*DRB1*1118*	D	F	W	I	R	
*DRB1*1119*	D	F	W	I	R	
*DRB1*1120*	D	F	W	I	E	
*DRB1*1121*	D	F	W	I	E	
*DRB1*1122*	D	F	W	F	R	
*DRB1*1123*	D	F	W	F	R	
*DRB1*1124*	D	F	W	F	R	
*DRB1*1125*	D	F	W	F	R	
*DRB1*1126*	D	F	W	L	R	
*DRB1*1127*	D	F	W	F	R	
*DRB1*1129*	D	F	W	F	R	
*DRB1*1130*	D	F	W	F	R	
*DRB1*1201*	E	F	W	I	R	
*DRB1*12021*	E	F	W	F	R	
*DRB1*12022*	E	F	W	F	R	
*DRB1*12031*	E	F	W	I	R	
*DRB1*12032*	E	F	W	I	R	
*DRB1*1204*	E	F	W	I	R	
*DRB1*1205*	E	F	W	I	R	
*DRB1*1301*	D	F	W	I	E	
*DRB1*1302*	D	F	W	I	E	
*DRB1*13031*	D	Y	W	I	K	
*DRB1*13032*	D	Y	W	I	K	
*DRB1*1304*	D	F	W	I	E	
*DRB1*1305*	D	F	W	F	R	
*DRB1*1306*	D	F	W	I	R	
*DRB1*1307*	D	Y	W	F	R	
*DRB1*1308*	D	Y	W	I	E	
*DRB1*1309*	D	F	W	I	A	
*DRB1*1310*	D	F	W	I	K	
*DRB1*1311*	D	F	W	F	R	
*DRB1*1312*	D	Y	W	I	R	
*DRB1*1313*	D	Y	W	I	R	
*DRB1*1314*	D	F	W	F	R	
*DRB1*1315*	E	F	W	I	E	
*DRB1*1316*	D	F	W	I	E	
*DRB1*1317*	D	F	W	I	E	
*DRB1*1318*	D	F	W	F	R	

Table 3.22. (con't)

	β28	β47	β61	β67	β71	Anchors/Preferred Residues
*DRB1*1319*	E	Y	W	I	E	
*DRB1*1320*	D	F	W	L	E	
*DRB1*1321*	D	F	W	F	R	
*DRB1*1322*	D	F	W	I	E	
*DRB1*1323*	D	F	W	I	E	
*DRB1*1324*	D	F	W	F	E	
*DRB1*1326*	E	Y	W	F	R	
*DRB1*1327*	D	F	W	I	E	
*DRB1*1328*	D	F	W	I	E	
*DRB1*1329*	D	F	W	L	E	
*DRB1*1330*	D	F	W	I	R	
*DRB1*1401*	D	Y	W	L	R	
*DRB1*1402*	E	Y	W	L	R	
*DRB1*1403*	E	Y	W	L	R	
*DRB1*1404*	D	Y	W	L	R	
*DRB1*1405*	D	Y	W	L	R	
*DRB1*1406*	E	Y	W	L	R	
*DRB1*1407*	D	Y	W	L	R	
*DRB1*1408*	D	Y	W	L	R	
*DRB1*1409*	D	Y	W	L	R	
*DRB1*1410*	D	Y	W	L	R	
*DRB1*1411*	D	Y	W	L	R	
*DRB1*1412*	E	Y	W	L	R	
*DRB1*1413*	E	Y	W	L	R	
*DRB1*1414*	D	Y	W	L	R	
*DRB1*1415*	D	Y	W	F	R	
*DRB1*1416*	D	Y	W	I	E	
*DRB1*1417*	D	F	W	L	R	
*DRB1*1418*	E	Y	W	L	R	
*DRB1*1419*	E	Y	W	L	K	
*DRB1*1420*	E	Y	W	L	R	
*DRB1*1421*	D	F	W	L	K	
*DRB1*1422*	D	Y	W	F	R	
*DRB1*1423*	D	Y	W	L	R	
*DRB1*1424*	E	Y	W	I	A	
*DRB1*1425*	D	Y	W	F	R	
*DRB1*1426*	D	Y	W	L	R	
*DRB1*1427*	E	Y	W	F	R	
*DRB1*1428*	D	Y	W	L	R	
*DRB1*1429*	E	Y	W	L	R	
*DRB1*15011*	D	F	W	I	A	I,L,V,M,F
*DRB1*15012*	D	F	W	I	A	
*DRB1*15021*	D	F	W	I	A	
*DRB1*15022*	D	F	W	I	A	
*DRB1*1503*	D	F	W	I	A	
*DRB1*1504*	D	F	W	F	A	
*DRB1*1505*	D	F	W	L	A	
*DRB1*1506*	D	F	W	I	A	
*DRB1*16011*	D	Y	W	F	R	
*DRB1*16012*	D	Y	W	F	R	
*DRB1*16021*	D	Y	W	L	R	
*DRB1*16022*	D	Y	W	L	R	
*DRB1*1603*	D	Y	W	F	R	
*DRB1*1604*	D	Y	W	F	R	
*DRB1*1605*	D	Y	W	I	R	
*DRB1*1606*	D	Y	W	I	R	
*DRB1*1608*	D	Y	W	F	R	
*DRB3*01011*	D	Y	W	L	K	
*DRB3*01013*	D	Y	W	L	K	
*DRB3*0102*	D	Y	W	L	K	
*DRB3*0201*	E	Y	W	L	K	
*DRB3*0202*	E	Y	W	L	K	

Table 3.22. (con't)

	β28	β47	β61	β67	β71	Anchors/Preferred Residues
*DRB3*0203*	E	Y	W	L	K	
*DRB3*0204*	E	Y	W	L	K	
*DRB3*0205*	E	Y	W	L	K	
*DRB3*0206*	E	Y	W	L	K	
*DRB3*0301*	E	Y	W	L	K	
*DRB4*0101101*	I	Y	W	L		
*DRB4*0102*	I	Y	W	L	R	
*DRB4*0103101*	I	Y	W	L		
*DRB4*0104*	I	Y	W	L	R	
*DRB4*0201N*	L	.	.	.	.	
*DRB5*0101*	H	Y	W	F	R	
*DRB5*0102*	H	Y	W	F	R	
*DRB5*0103*	H	Y	W	F	T	
*DRB5*0104*	H	Y	W	F	R	
*DRB5*0105*	H	Y	W	F	R	
*DRB5*0201*	H	Y	W	I	A	
*DRB5*0202*	H	Y	W	I	A	
*DRB5*0203*	H	Y	W	I	A	
*DRB5*0204*	H	Y	W	F	A	
*DRB6*0101*	N	F	W	I	N	
*DRB6*0201*	N	F	W	I	K	
*DRB6*0202*	N	F	W	I	K	

Table 3.23. HLA-DRB pocket for relative position P9

	β9	β57	Anchors/Preferred Residues
*DRB1*0101*	W	D	L,A,I,V,N,F,Y
*DRB1*01021*	W	D	I,L,A,M,Y,W
*DRB1*01022*	W	D	
*DRB1*0103*	W	D	
*DRB1*0104*	.	D	
*DRB1*03011*	E	D	Y,L,F
*DRB1*03012*	E	D	
*DRB1*03021*	E	D	
*DRB1*03022*	E	D	
*DRB1*0303*	.	D	
*DRB1*0304*	E	D	
*DRB1*0305*	.	D	
*DRB1*0306*	E	D	
*DRB1*0307*	E	D	
*DRB1*0308*	E	D	
*DRB1*0311*	E	D	
*DRB1*04011*	E	D	polar, aliphatic, K
*DRB1*04012*	E	D	
*DRB1*0402*	E	D	polar, aliphatic, H
*DRB1*0403*	E	D	
*DRB1*0404*	E	D	polar, aliphatic, K
*DRB1*04051*	E	S	D,E,Q
*DRB1*04052*	.	S	
*DRB1*0406*	E	D	
*DRB1*0407*	E	D	Q,N
*DRB1*0408*	.	D	
*DRB1*0409*	.	S	
*DRB1*0410*	E	S	
*DRB1*0411*	E	S	
*DRB1*0412*	E	S	
*DRB1*0413*	.	D	
*DRB1*0414*	.	D	

Table 3.23. (con't)

	β9	β57	Anchors/Preferred Residues
*DRB1*0415*	E	D	
*DRB1*0416*	.	D	
*DRB1*0417*	.	S	
*DRB1*0418*	.	D	
*DRB1*0419*	.	D	
*DRB1*0420*	.	D	
*DRB1*0421*	E	D	
*DRB1*0422*	E	D	
*DRB1*0423*	E	D	
*DRB1*0701*	W	V	
*DRB1*0801*	E	S	
*DRB1*08021*	E	D	
*DRB1*08022*	E	D	
*DRB1*08031*	E	S	
*DRB1*08032*	E	S	
*DRB1*08041*	E	D	
*DRB1*08042*	.	D	
*DRB1*0805*	E	S	
*DRB1*0806*	E	S	
*DRB1*0807*	.	V	
*DRB1*0808*	E	A	
*DRB1*0809*	.	D	
*DRB1*0810*	E	S	
*DRB1*0811*	E	A	
*DRB1*0812*	E	S	
*DRB1*0813*	E	D	
*DRB1*0814*	E	S	
*DRB1*0815*	E	D	
*DRB1*0816*	E	S	
*DRB1*09011*	.	V	
*DRB1*09012*	K	V	
*DRB1*1001*	E	D	
*DRB1*11011*	E	D	A,G,S,P
*DRB1*11012*	E	D	
*DRB1*11013*	.	D	
*DRB1*1102*	E	D	
*DRB1*1103*	E	D	
*DRB1*11041*	E	D	A,G,S,P
*DRB1*11042*	E	D	
*DRB1*1105*	E	D	
*DRB1*1106*	E	D	
*DRB1*1107*	E	D	
*DRB1*11081*	.	D	
*DRB1*11082*	.	D	
*DRB1*1109*	.	D	
*DRB1*1110*	.	D	
*DRB1*1111*	.	D	
*DRB1*1112*	.	D	
*DRB1*1113*	E	D	
*DRB1*1114*	E	D	
*DRB1*1115*	E	D	
*DRB1*1116*	.	D	
*DRB1*1117*	E	D	
*DRB1*1118*	E	D	
*DRB1*1119*	E	D	
*DRB1*1120*	E	D	
*DRB1*1121*	E	D	
*DRB1*1122*	E	D	
*DRB1*1123*	.	D	
*DRB1*1124*	.	D	
*DRB1*1125*	E	D	
*DRB1*1126*	E	D	

Table 3.23. (con't)

	β9	β57	Anchors/Preferred Residues
*DRB1*1127*	E	D	
*DRB1*1129*	E	D	
*DRB1*1130*	E	D	
*DRB1*1201*	E	V	Y,F,M,I,V
*DRB1*12021*	E	V	
*DRB1*12022*	E	V	
*DRB1*12031*	E	V	
*DRB1*12032*	E	V	
*DRB1*1204*	E	D	
*DRB1*1205*	E	V	
*DRB1*1301*	E	D	Y,F,A,S,T
*DRB1*1302*	E	D	Y,F,A,S,T
*DRB1*13031*	E	S	
*DRB1*13032*	E	S	
*DRB1*1304*	E	S	
*DRB1*1305*	E	D	
*DRB1*1306*	.	D	
*DRB1*1307*	E	D	
*DRB1*1308*	E	D	
*DRB1*1309*	E	D	
*DRB1*1310*	E	D	
*DRB1*1311*	E	D	
*DRB1*1312*	E	S	
*DRB1*1313*	E	S	
*DRB1*1314*	.	D	
*DRB1*1315*	.	D	
*DRB1*1316*	E	D	
*DRB1*1317*	E	D	
*DRB1*1318*	E	D	
*DRB1*1319*	E	D	
*DRB1*1320*	E	D	
*DRB1*1321*	E	S	
*DRB1*1322*	E	D	
*DRB1*1323*	E	D	
*DRB1*1324*	E	D	
*DRB1*1326*	E	D	
*DRB1*1327*	.	D	
*DRB1*1328*	E	D	
*DRB1*1329*	E	D	
*DRB1*1330*	E	S	
*DRB1*1401*	E	A	
*DRB1*1402*	E	D	
*DRB1*1403*	E	D	
*DRB1*1404*	E	A	
*DRB1*1405*	E	D	
*DRB1*1406*	E	D	
*DRB1*1407*	E	A	
*DRB1*1408*	E	D	
*DRB1*1409*	E	D	
*DRB1*1410*	E	A	
*DRB1*1411*	E	D	
*DRB1*1412*	.	D	
*DRB1*1413*	E	S	
*DRB1*1414*	E	D	
*DRB1*1415*	.	D	
*DRB1*1416*	E	A	
*DRB1*1417*	E	D	
*DRB1*1418*	.	D	
*DRB1*1419*	E	D	
*DRB1*1420*	E	D	
*DRB1*1421*	E	D	
*DRB1*1422*	E	A	

Table 3.23. (con't)

	β9	β57	Anchors/Preferred Residues
*DRB1*1423*	E	D	
*DRB1*1424*	.	D	
*DRB1*1425*	E	A	
*DRB1*1426*	E	A	
*DRB1*1427*	E	D	
*DRB1*1428*	E	A	
*DRB1*1429*	E	D	
*DRB1*15011*	W	D	
*DRB1*15012*	W	D	
*DRB1*15021*	W	D	
*DRB1*15022*	.	D	
*DRB1*1503*	W	D	
*DRB1*1504*	.	D	
*DRB1*1505*	W	D	
*DRB1*1506*	.	D	
*DRB1*16011*	W	D	
*DRB1*16012*	W	D	
*DRB1*16021*	W	D	
*DRB1*16022*	.	D	
*DRB1*1603*	W	D	
*DRB1*1604*	W	D	
*DRB1*1605*	.	D	
*DRB1*1606*	W	D	
*DRB1*1608*	W	D	
*DRB3*01011*	E	V	
*DRB3*01013*	.	V	
*DRB3*0102*	E	V	
*DRB3*0201*	E	D	
*DRB3*0202*	E	D	L,V,I,S,G
*DRB3*0203*	E	D	
*DRB3*0204*	E	D	
*DRB3*0205*	E	D	
*DRB3*0206*	E	D	
*DRB3*0301*	E	V	I,L,V
*DRB4*0101101*	E	D	
*DRB4*0102*	.	D	
*DRB4*0103101*	E	D	
*DRB4*0104*	E	D	
*DRB4*0201N*	E	.	
*DRB5*0101*	Q	D	R,K
*DRB5*0102*	Q	D	
*DRB5*0103*	Q	D	
*DRB5*0104*	Q	D	
*DRB5*0105*	Q	D	
*DRB5*0201*	Q	D	
*DRB5*0202*	Q	D	
*DRB5*0203*	Q	D	
*DRB5*0204*	Q	D	
*DRB6*0101*	.	V	
*DRB6*0201*	E	V	
*DRB6*0202*	.	V	

Table 3.24. H2-E pocket for relative position P1

	β85	β86	β89	β90	Anchors/Preferred residues
H2-E$_{\beta}^{d}$	I	S	F	L	W,Y,F,I,L,V
H2-E$_{\beta}^{b}$	I	S	F	L	W,F,Y,I,L,V
H2-E$_{\beta}^{s}$	I	L	F	L	I,V,L,F,Y,W
H2-E$_{\beta}^{k}$	I	F	F	L	I,L,V,F,Y,W
*RT1.B**	G	S	R	T	polar,aliphatic

According to Stern et al[30] and Fremont et al[11]
*The predicted pockets for the relative positions 1, 4, 6, 7, and 9 in the rat sequence (Accession number X56596) refer to those residues which are homologous to comparable mouse residues.

Table 3.25. H2-E pocket for relative position P4

	β13	β70	β71	β74	β78	Anchors/Preferred residues
H2-E$_{\beta}^{d}$	S	D	A	S	Y	R,K,I,V
H2-E$_{\beta}^{b}$	S	Q	K	E	V	L,I,F,V,S,A
H2-E$_{\beta}^{s}$	S	Q	R	A	Y	L,I,V,T,S,N,Q
H2-E$_{\beta}^{k}$	S	Q	K	E	V	I,L,V,F,S,A
RT1.B	G	Q	T	E	V	F,H,Q,K,R,N,T,L,I

Table 3.26. H2-E pocket for relative position P6

	β11	β13	Anchors/Preferred Residues
H2-E$_{\beta}^{d}$	V	S	I,L,V,G
H2-E$_{\beta}^{b}$	C	S	Q,N,S,T,A,H,R,E
H2-E$_{\beta}^{s}$	S	S	Q,N,S,T,A,H,R,E
H2-E$_{\beta}^{k}$	C	S	Q,N,S,T,A,H,R,E
RT1.B	F	G	A,S,V,T,P,L

Table 3.27. H2-E pocket for relative position P7

	β28	β47	β61	β67	β71	Anchors/Preferred Residues
H2-E$_{\beta}^{d}$	E	Y	W	I	A	
H2-E$_{\beta}^{b}$	E	F	W	F	K	
H2-E$_{\beta}^{s}$	E	F	W	F	R	
H2-E$_{\beta}^{k}$	V	F	W	F	K	
RT1.B	I	Y	F	Y	T	large amino acids

Table 3.28. H2-E pocket for relative position P9

	β9	β57	Anchors/Preferred Residues
H2-E$_{\beta}^{d}$	E	D	K,R
H2-E$_{\beta}^{b}$	E	D	K,R
H2-E$_{\beta}^{s}$	E	D	K,R
H2-E$_{\beta}^{k}$	E	D	K,R,G
RT1.B	Y	S	E,D,aliphatic

References

1. Bjorkman PJ, Saper MA, Samraoui B et al. Structure of the human class I histocompatibility antigen, HLA-A2. Nature 1987; 329:506-12.
2. Stern LJ, Wiley DC. Antigenic peptide binding by class I and class II histocompatibility proteins. Structure 1994; 2:245-51.
3. Bouvier M, Wiley DC. Importance of peptide amino and carboxyl termini to the stability of MHC class I molecules. Science 1994; 265:398-402.
4. Collins EJ, Garboczi DN, Wiley DC. Three-dimensional structure of a peptide extending from one end of a class I MHC binding site. Nature 1994; 371:626-9.
5. Guo HC, Jardetzky TS, Garrett TP et al. Different length peptides bind to HLA-Aw68 similarly at their ends but bulge out in the middle. Nature 1992; 360:364-6.
6. Guo HC, Madden DR, Silver ML et al. Comparison of the P2 specificity pocket in three human histocompatibility antigens: HLA-A*6801, HLA-A*0201, and HLA-B*2705. Proc Natl Acad Sci USA 1993; 90:8053-7.
7. Garboczi DN, Madden DR, Wiley DC. Five viral peptide-HLA-A2 co-crystals. Simultaneous space group determination and X-ray data collection. J Mol Biol 1994; 239:581-7.
8. Falk K, Rötzschke O, Stevanović S et al. Allele-specific motifs revealed by sequencing of self-peptides eluted from MHC molecules. Nature 1991; 351:290-6.
9. Falk K, Rötzschke O, Takiguchi M et al. Peptide motifs of HLA-A1, -A11, -A31, and -A33 molecules. Immunogenetics 1994; 40:238-41.
10. DiBrino M, Tsuchida T, Turner RV et al. HLA-A1 and HLA-A3 T cell epitopes derived from influenza virus proteins predicted from peptide binding motifs. J Immunol 1993; 151:5930-5.
11. Silver ML, Guo HC, Strominger JL et al. Atomic structure of a human MHC molecule presenting an influenza virus peptide. Nature 1992; 360:300-1.
12. Young AC, Zhang W, Sacchettini JC et al. The three-dimensional structure of H-2Db at 2.4 A resolution: implications for antigen-determinant selection. Cell 1994; 76:39-50.
13. Smith KJ, Reid SW, Harlos K et al. Bound water structure and polymorphic amino acids act together to allow the binding of different peptides to MHC class I HLA-B53. Immunity 1996; 4:215-28.
14. Fremont DH, Matsumura M, Stura EA et al. Crystal structures of two viral peptides in complex with murine MHC class I H-2Kb. Science 1992; 257:919-27.
15. Falk K, Rötzschke O. Consensus motifs and peptide ligands of MHC class I molecules. Semin Immunol 1993; 5:81-94.
16. Matsumura M, Fremont DH, Peterson PA et al. Emerging principles for the recognition of peptide antigens by MHC class I molecules. Science 1992; 257:927-34.
17. Chelvanayagam G. A roadmap for HLA-A, HLA-B and HLA-C allotype peptide binding specificities. Immunogenetics 1996; 45:15-26.
18. Madden DR, Garboczi DN, Wiley DC. The antigenic identity of peptide-MHC complexes: a comparison of the conformations of five viral peptides presented by HLA-A2 [published erratum appears in Cell 1994; 76:410]. Cell 1993; 75:693-708.
19. Jackson MR, Peterson PA. Assembly and intracellular transport of MHC class I molecules. Annu Rev Cell Biol 1993; 9:207-35.
20. Wang CR, Castano AR, Peterson PA et al. Nonclassical binding of formylated peptide in crystal structure of the MHC class Ib molecule H2-M3. Cell 1995; 82:655-64.
21. Smith KJ, Reid SW, Stuart DI et al. An altered position of the alpha 2 helix of MHC class I is revealed by the crystal structure of HLA-B*3501. Immunity 1996; 4:203-13.
22. Nandi D, Jiang H, Monaco JJ. Identification of MECL-1 (LMP-10) as the third IFN-gamma-inducible proteasome subunit. J Immunol 1996; 156:2361-4.
23. Rammensee HG, Robinson PJ, Crisanti A et al. Restricted recognition of beta 2-microglobulin by cytotoxic T lymphocytes. Nature 1986; 319:502-4.

24. Sun J, Leahy DJ, Kavathas PB. Interaction between CD8 and major histocompatibility complex (MHC) class I mediated by multiple contact surfaces that include the alpha 2 and alpha 3 domains of MHC class I. J Exp Med 1995; 182:1275-80.
25. Saper MA, Bjorkman PJ, Wiley DC. Refined structure of the human histocompatibility antigen HLA-A2 at 2.6 A resolution. J Mol Biol 1991; 219:277-319.
26. Garboczi DN, Gosh P, Utz U et al. Structure of the complex between human T cell receptor, viral peptide and HLA-A2. Nature 1996; 384:134-41.
27. Garcia KC, Degano M, Stanfield RL et al. An alpha-beta T cell receptor structure at 2.5 A and its orientation in the TCR-MHC complex. Science 1996; 274:209-19.
28. Jardetzky TS, Brown JH, Gorga JC et al. Crystallographic analysis of endogenous peptides associated with HLA-DR1 suggests a common, polyproline II-like conformation for bound peptides. Proc Natl Acad Sci USA 1996; 93:734-8.
29. Ghosh P, Amaya M, Mellins E et al. The structure of an intermediate in class II MHC maturation: CLIP bound to HLA-DR3. Nature 1995; 378:457-62.
30. Stern LJ, Brown JH, Jardetzky TS et al. Crystal structure of the human class II MHC protein HLA-DR1 complexed with an influenza virus peptide. Nature 1994; 368:215-21.
31. Brown JH, Jardetzky TS, Gorga JC et al. Three-dimensional structure of the human class II histocompatibility antigen HLA-DR1. Nature 1993; 364:33-9.
32. Rammensee HG. Chemistry of peptides associated with MHC class I and class II molecules. Curr Opin Immunol 1995; 7:85-96.

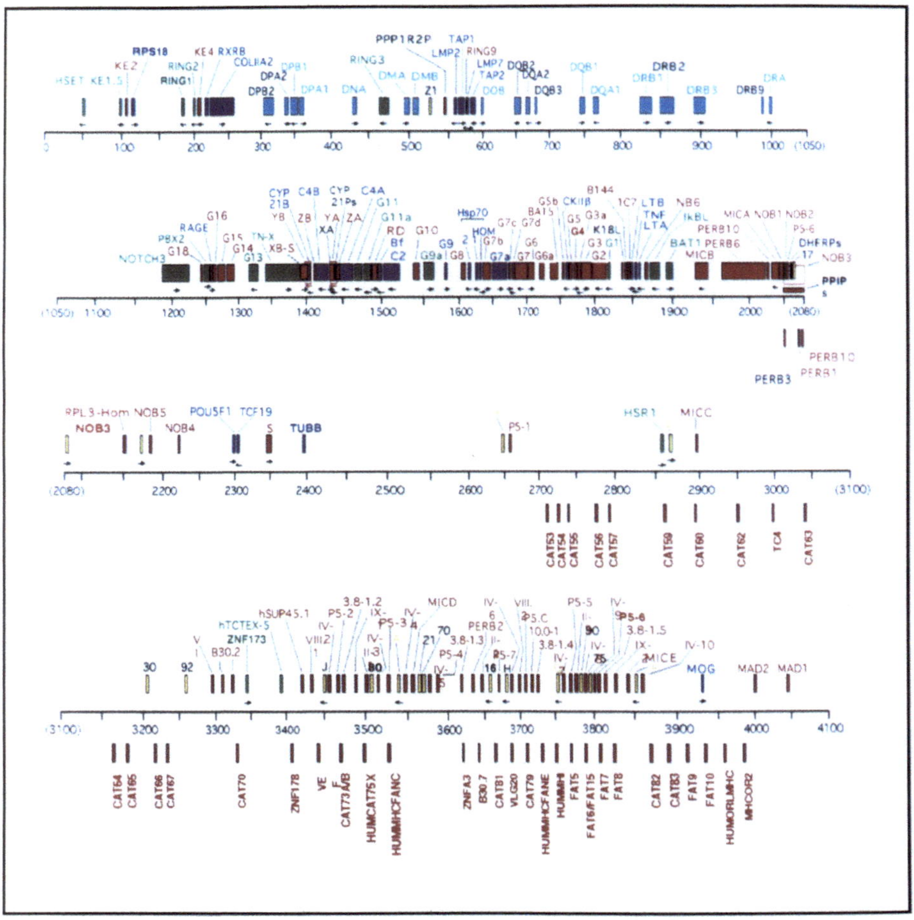

Fig. 2.1. Map of the human chromosome 6. Reprinted with permission from: Campbell RD, Trowsdale J. Immunol Today 1997; 18:Centerfold ©1997 Elsevier Trends Journals.

Fig. [illegible] Reprinted with permission from Campbell [illegible] Copyright [illegible] Elsevier [illegible] journals.

CHAPTER 4

The Function

PART I

PEPTIDE MOTIFS

Amino Acids in Peptide-MHC Interactions

Table 4.1 lists all 20 proteinogenic amino acids present in peptides which interact with MHC molecules. There are different criteria for grouping amino acids, such as the size of side chains, polarity, charge or hydrophobicity. Regarding the specific characteristics that are required in one distinct contact site, usually one of the different sets of amino acids is best at meeting the needs. Although grouped into separate sets in Table 4.1, some of the amino acids are able to fulfill completely different requirements and therefore act as jokers. As an example, T belongs to the set of hydrophilic amino acids. Because of the methyl group at the end of its side chain, it may interact *via* hydrophobic interactions with an MHC pocket which is shaped in such a way that methyl groups fit optimally into it. In this case, T interacts similarly to aliphatic amino acids, which also have a methyl group at the end of their side chains. Another joker is Y, which belongs to the set of large aromatic/hydrophobic amino acids. Its hydroxyl group at the end of the side chain enables Y to interact by hydrogen bonding and therefore act like hydrophilic residues.

Figure 4.1 shows the molecular structure of the 20 amino acids, side chains are pointing upwards. Please note that under physiological conditions around pH 7 all amino groups are protonated ($-NH_3^+$ instead of $-NH_2$), carboxy groups are dissociated ($-COO^-$ instead of $-COOH$) and the nitrogen atom of the imidazole ring in the histidine side chain is protonated ($-NH^+=$ instead of $-N=$).

Peptide Motifs

MHC molecules spend the major part of their lifetime presenting peptides. Usually, MHC proteins are burdened with peptides in an intracellular compartment, which is either the endoplasmic reticulum (ER) in the class I loading pathway or a compartment in the class II pathway referred to as MIIC, which is an intermediate stage between trans-Golgi, endosomes, and lysosomes.

Both MHC class I and class II peptide presentation follows distinct rules known as peptide motifs. The details of peptide binding and presentation by MHC I and MHC II, however, make it advisable for the subject to be treated in two separate chapters. Generally, peptide motifs describe the length of MHC-presented peptides as well as the preference for

MHC Ligands and Peptide Motifs, by Hans-Georg Rammensee, Jutta Bachmann, Stefan Stevanović.

certain amino acids in distinct positions of the bound ligand. If one of these positions is exclusively occupied by a small set of closely related amino acids, the terms anchor amino acids or anchor position are used.

Many scientists have participated in the work of determining peptide motifs of class I and class II molecules, and several different strategies have been employed. Although the peptide motifs of the most common human and mouse MHC molecules have been revealed, the knowledge acquired so far is far from being comprehensive.

MHC I PEPTIDE MOTIFS, PART ONE: LENGTH

Usually, MHC class I motifs stipulate a length of 8-11 amino acids. Length restriction may differ significantly between alleles: while 84% of the HLA-B*2702 ligands and epitopes listed below (Table 4.2) have a length of nine amino acids, only 57% of the HLA-A*1101 ligands and epitopes share this length, and HLA-B8 or H2-K^k may present octamer peptides nearly as often as nonamers. The overall length of all ligands and epitopes comprised in the present listing is from 7-13 amino acids, with only two exceptions.

The length of MHC I ligands can be determined by two technical methods: mass spectrometry[1] and Edman degradation.[2] The latter technique, for years synonymous with sequence analysis, can be employed for the analysis of individual ligands[3] or peptide pools.[4] In each application, the length of peptides is judged in a different way: single peptides divulge their C-terminal amino acid by a sudden breakdown of the amount detected in this very position and by the absence of signals beyond this point. Peptide pools, however, show the same breakdown of most amino acids but a final increase in the amount of few (anchor) amino acids and again no signals in further degradation cycles. Using mass spectrometry, the molecular mass of an analyzed peptide may help to estimate the number of amino acids present, and tandem MS techniques complete the identification of the sequence. Molecular mass analysis may also prove helpful in combination with Edman degradation, because sometimes the C-terminal part of a peptide is hard to characterize among high background and fading signals.

MHC I PEPTIDE MOTIFS, PART TWO: ANCHORS

Peptides are bound by MHC molecules *via* interactions between amino acid side chains and peptide backbones of both counterparts.[5] While every amino acid of a ligand may contribute to tight binding, anchor residues are characterized by their ability to summarize the correspondence of all ligands.[6] As an example, position 1 (P1, which is the N-terminal amino acid) of the listed natural HLA-A*0101 ligands is occupied by 13 different amino acids with completely different properties, such as small, aliphatic, aromatic, acidic, basic or neutral polar side chains. In contrast, their C-terminal amino acid is generally tyrosine, representing a most uniform anchor position among HLA molecules.

Anchor positions are defined by the strict occurrence of amino acids which possess very similar side chains or belong to the same set (Table 4.1). Sometimes there is just one amino acid allowed in an anchor position, like N^5 of H2-D^b ligands, and sometimes a small set of amino acids are capable of anchoring their ligands to the MHC molecule, like the acidic amino acids D and E in position 3 (P3) of HLA-A*0101-bound peptides. The most common HLA class I allele in the Caucasian population, HLA-A*0201, uses aliphatic side chains of ligands as a common element. Of 109 9mer sequences listed, 60 carry L in P2, while M, I, V, A, and T are less frequently used.

Most MHC class I molecules use two anchors. It is interesting that the C-terminal amino acid always serves as an anchor but the N-terminal position never does (at least among the > 70 class I molecules listed). Thus one anchor is fixed at the Ω position, while the majority of motifs use P2 as a second anchor position. There are only a few exceptions among human and mouse motifs: HLA-A*0101 makes use of P3 and HLA-B8 exhibits two additional anchors in P3 and P5, as does HLA-B14 in P2 and P5. The mouse H2-K^b and H2-D^b motifs require anchor amino acids in P5. Although few data are available from other species, it seems that anchor usage is similar in rat, cattle and even chicken.

Chickens are the only exception to a general rule which allows either hydrophobic or basic amino acids in the C-terminal anchor position: the B-F2 motif is characterized by a C-terminal glutamic acid. All other motifs described so far adhere to this rule, with mouse motifs being even more strict by using hydrophobic residues only. Which group of amino acids is admitted to C-terminal positions is most likely determined by the specificity of TAP proteins,[7] which differs between mice and men. The situation is quite different for internal anchor positions in MHC I motifs. Apart from cysteine, any amino acid can be found among residues occupying such anchor positions. Usually, the anchor limitations allow small groups of closely related amino acids, characteristically small, aliphatic, aromatic, hydrophobic, acidic, basic or hydrophilic. Even the grouping of amino acids can differ between the peptide motifs: sometimes the basic amino acids R and K are allowed to be present together (PΩ of HLA-A*6801) and sometimes only R is present (P2 of B*2705).

Several experimental methods are available to identify anchor residues of MHC I molecules:

Sequence analysis of natural ligands (by Edman degradation or tandem MS) and alignment of the sequences obtained reveals anchor positions if the number of ligands characterized is sufficiently high.[3]

Pool sequencing of the whole mixture of ligands eluted from one MHC allele allows for a very rapid and impressive analysis of anchor residues. Multiple sequence analysis of peptide pools represents a breakthrough in MHC peptide motif analysis.[4] It is always fascinating to see how a peptide pool may behave like a single sequence: in anchor positions, ideally one amino acid rises to an overwhelming signal height, while all other amino acid signals drop to an absolute minimum in this cycle of Edman degradation.[8]

Binding studies with synthetic peptides and isolated MHC molecules,[9] or stabilization assays with synthetic peptides and cell lines defective in antigen presentation,[10] are able to define anchor residues. Such experiments may also be carried out employing peptide libraries,[11] which came into fashion simultaneously with peptide motifs in the early 90s.

An elegant method is the use of phage display libraries in binding studies with isolated MHC molecules.[12] This approach was first applied to MHC class II molecules, but it is not restricted to these.

Although all four methods result in the identification of allele-specific contact sites between peptides and MHC class I molecules, analysis of natural ligands has a major advantage over experiments using synthetic peptides or isolated MHC molecules. Only natural ligands have been properly processed, transported, and presented and have thus suffered every selection procedure utilized within the cell for MHC I-restricted peptide presentation. Loading peptides onto MHC molecules from the outside only helps to determine binding motifs, which may differ significantly from peptide motifs[13] (originally referred to as natural ligand motifs), which reflect features of processing and transport events. This is obvious by the fact that C-terminal anchor positions of binding motifs are often much more degenerate compared to peptide motifs; that is, they allow a much broader set of amino acids in this position.

It is worth noting that a small percentage of reported ligands or epitopes does not cling to the rules of peptide motifs. Either length restrictions or anchor rules are violated by these peptides.

MHC I PEPTIDE MOTIFS, PART THREE: AUXILIARY ANCHORS AND PREFERRED RESIDUES

It is hard to draw a line between anchors and auxiliary anchors. Because there is no rule without an exception, almost every ligand table belonging to a peptide motif contains peptides with unusual or wrong amino acids in anchor positions. Unusual amino acids are still related in some way to the correct anchor residues such as A (small, aliphatic) instead of L (aliphatic); wrong amino acids belong to a chemically different group, such as I (aliphatic/hydrophobic) instead of D/E (acidic/hydrophilic). While R is present in P2 of all HLA-B*2702 ligands and epitopes, only 84% of HLA-A*0101 ligands and epitopes carry D or E in P3. On the other hand, 65% of these ligands have S or T in P2, which is regarded as an auxiliary anchor position. The definition of auxiliary anchors states that there is correspondence with amino acids in a major part of ligands, but other residues are tolerated in such positions. If correspondence is still lower, then the respective amino acids are classified as preferred residues.

MHC I PEPTIDE MOTIFS, PART FOUR: UNFAVORABLE RESIDUES

The peptide motif tables only contain amino acids which favor peptide presentation by MHC class I molecules. Residues not mentioned in a certain position may neither improve nor worsen a peptide's probability to be loaded onto MHC molecules, but they may also contribute to much lower binding affinity. Such disadvantageous amino acids can be identified by three methods:

Pool sequencing of natural ligands. Usually, in anchor positions, values of non-anchor residues show an absolute minimum compared to all other degradation cycles. Unfavorable residues can then be identified if this is the case in other positions, too. This kind of analysis is extremely difficult for technical resons. High background values, often present in samples extracted from biological tissue, may prevent the recognition of minimum values. In addition, in the HPLC chromatogram used for the quantitation of amino acids after Edman degradation, very high peaks of single amino acids may conceal small neighboring peaks from analysis.

Alignment of known ligands, whether naturally presented self peptides or T cell epitopes, whose processing and presentation has been proven.

Binding studies with synthetic peptides lead to the determination of deleterious residues[9] detrimental for peptide binding. The model antigen HLA-A*0201 was investigated by several groups in this regard. Usually, large sets of random peptides were used either in competition assays together with radioactively labelled MHC binders and purified MHC molecules,[9] or in MHC stabilization assays using T2 cells defective in TAP transporting,[10] or in β2-microglobulin dissociation assays.[14]

The matter of unfavorable or preferred residues as well as the question of tolerance of unusual amino acids in anchor positions will be discussed in detail below (section on epitope prediction).

MHC II PEPTIDE MOTIFS, PART ONE: LENGTH

Peptide length is far less restricted in MHC classs II ligands compared to class I ligands. Although the majority of ligands and epitopes listed in the motif tables vary in length between 13 and 18 amino acids, self peptides are still presented by MHC II molecules if they are 11 amino acids long, and there are functional T cell epitopes with only nine amino acids. There is no clearcut upper limit to peptide length regarding binding to MHC II; peptides of more than 24 amino acids can often be found. Since the binding cleft harbors only a nine amino acid stretch and since flanking sequences of about three to five more residues on both sides enhance the affinity, the optimal length is in the range of 15-18 amino acids. Between the different HLA-DR, -DQ or -DP molecules and mouse or rat alleles there is no difference in the length of ligands. Most probably, the final length of natural ligands is not dictated by binding affinity, but rather by processing in the intracellular vesicles.[15] This is indicated by the phenomenon of ragged ends: peptides shortened by one or two amino acids at either terminus bind with similar affinities to the MHC class II molecule.

Determining the length of class II ligands is possible by a combination of Edman degradation, database searching, and mass spectrometry. Sequence analysis by Edman degradation alone is very often not sufficient to reach the C-terminal end of the peptide because of increasing background and sample loss over the many cycles. Tandem-MS analysis alone often does not identify the sequence of MHC II ligands, because the interpretation of data obtained from peptides longer than 15 amino acids is rather difficult. After having sequenced the N-terminal part of the ligand this sequence is used to screen a database for the source protein. With the sequence known, determination of the molecular mass of the ligand leads to the identification of the C-terminal residue.

MHC II PEPTIDE MOTIFS, PART TWO: ANCHORS

Unlike MHC I peptide motifs, the preferences for certain amino acids in distinct positions of MHC II ligands cannot be described by the categories anchors, auxiliary anchors, and (other) preferred residues. The strictness of anchor occupancy is much lower compared to class I: the anchor positions of MHC class II molecules are often able to tolerate amino acids belonging to different sets. With such degenerate anchors, there is no need to define secondary anchors or preferred residues. The current anchor definition in MHC class II ligands is based primarily on structural data.[16] Regarding the specificities for certain amino acids, the five pockets determined by X-ray crystal structure analysis differ greatly in their stringency. The range in the number of residues allowed in anchor positions ranges from one (the unique D anchor in P4 of HLA-DRB1*0301 ligands) to more than ten amino acids (the sets polar, charged and aliphatic are allowed in P7 of HLA-DRB1*0401 ligands). A special feature of MHC II-peptide interaction is that often only two to three of four to five possible anchor positions have to be occupied by the appropriate amino acids.[17]

Both the ragged ends of ligands and the degenerate anchor positions impede the determination of MHC II peptide motifs. The different distance between N-terminal amino acid and first anchor residue makes it hard to identify anchor residues by Edman degradation. Alignment of individual ligands is difficult too,[18] because anchor positions are not occupied in a uniform way. Nevertheless, by pool sequence analysis many of the motifs listed below have been determined. Fortunately, there is no complete disorder in the N-terminal part of MHC II ligands, but most of the peptides eluted from MHC II molecules extend out of the binding groove by three to four amino acids, having their first anchor residue in absolute position 4 or 5 of the sequence. As a consequence, in pool sequence analysis anchors are readily recognized by a cluster of a set of amino acids over two sequencing cycles.[17]

As mentioned in the MHC class I paragraph above, binding studies with phage display libraries were helpful in identifying anchor residues.[12] Recently, a similar approach was introduced by the use of synthetic peptide libraries.[19] For the determination of MHC class II peptide motifs, it is much more advisable to employ binding studies than for class I motifs because of the degeneracy of anchors. Nevertheless, processing events play a role in the class II presentation pathway in addition to binding preferences; "a processing motif"[17] is visible within a large number of ligands, and trimming takes place after ligands have bound to class II molecules.[15] Although little is yet known about the influence of cleavage specificities of endosomal proteases, this effect must not be underestimated. After all, ligands or epitopes must not be cut within by proteases. Therefore, similarly to class I motifs, the MHC II peptide motifs appear not to be merely binding motifs.

Motif Tables

Tables 4.2 to 4.4 summarize all MHC I peptide motifs, ligands, T cell epitopes and other binding peptides published until the end of 1996 (and some of 1997). In the first part of each table, a shortcut of the motif based primarily on results of pool sequencing or characterization of individual natural ligands is shown, comprising anchor residues, secondary/auxiliary anchors and preferred and other observed residues.

The second part of the motif tables lists sequences and source proteins of natural ligands, most of which are self peptides; however, some T cell epitopes, too, have been shown to be naturally processed and presented. The third part contains T cell epitopes which are able to bind to the respective MHC molecule and to stimulate T cells, but for these epitopes it is not clear whether they are naturally processed. For some tables, a fourth part is added containing peptides which bind to MHC molecules but whose ability to tease T cells has not yet been proven.

Tables 4.5 to 4.7 compile the peptide motifs of MHC II molecules together with ligands and T cell epitopes. Only peptide motifs which are in accordance to pocket structure have been mentioned. Peptide sequences are aligned in a way that explains the orientation of the ligands within the binding cleft.

Epitope Prediction

Very soon after the knowledge of allele-specific motifs had spread, scientists began to utilize the predictive power of the motifs. Less than nine weeks after the publication of the H2-K^d peptide motif,[4] a paper describing the first motif-based epitope prediction reached Nature's editorial office. Members of Michael Bevan's group had screened the sequence of listeriolysin for the occurrence of H2-K^d anchor residues in nonamer peptides. According to their prediction of potential ligands, they only had to synthesize eleven peptides and to test them with *Listeria monocytogenes*-specific CTL until they knew the listeriolysin epitope.[206]

Between 1991 and 1993, the number of CTL epitopes identified by motif-based prediction doubled every year,[440] and most of the epitopes listed in the motif tables have been characterized with the knowledge of the respective motifs. The situation is quite different for MHC II epitopes. Only very few of the class II-restricted epitopes characterized so far have been identified solely by motif-based prediction.

Experimental epitope mapping procedures are now also feasible on the genetic level,[57] but the classical approach of epitope mapping was to use overlapping peptides covering the whole sequence of a protein.[180] In order to avoid tedious testing of many peptides, for more than twelve years now attempts have been made to predict antigenic sequences presented by MHC molecules. In the beginning of the prediction era, no discrimination was even made between MHC class I and class II restricted antigens. Similar to prediction programs that look for sequences suitable for antibody induction, such methods were based on secondary structure analysis combined with physicochemical properties of amino acids: Over a period of about five years, T cell epitopes were believed to form amphipathic helices.[441]

The use of sequence patterns now looks back on almost ten years of history. First approaches tried to make alternating hydrophilic/hydrophobic residues[442] or just rarely occurring sequence stretches[443] responsible for immunogenicity. Over time, predictions were carried out in order to directly identify epitopes. The question regarding what makes up an epitope can only be answered by T cell receptors (TCR). In spite of a published X-ray crystal structure of a TCR-peptide complex,[444] nowadays it still seems impossible to use such structural properties to directly predict peptides able to bind to a TCR. Therefore, modern prediction methods make a detour by predicting potential MHC ligands. If peptides bind to an MHC molecule (whether class I or class II), it should be possible to raise T cells against this MHC-peptide complex, at least, if it does not belong to a "self" sequence. The procedure of in vitro stimulating T cells with peptides exogenously loaded onto MHC molecules has proved successful in many cases. The only discrepancy between such immunogenic peptides and real T cell epitopes are those intracellular events of processing and transport which are responsible for the decision whether any peptide sequence which might be immunogenic per se meets its MHC counterpart. For this reason we believe that peptide motifs are of higher predictive value if obtained from the analysis of natural ligands; these reflect rules of transport and processing in addition to mere binding characteristics.[6]

Prediction of MHC I-Restricted Epitopes

The main objective of performing theoretical predictions is merely to save time. Instead of synthesizing and testing dozens or even hundreds of peptides a preselection of a small set of peptides is made. However, there are some prerequisites. The sequence of the immunogenic protein (or its gene), the restriction element, and the motif belonging to it, have to be available. With these tools, within less than one hour the selection of the most promising candidate peptides can easily be accomplished.

It is worth noting that theoretical approaches cannot always guarantee success. Motif-based prediction results in a list of peptides that have a high probability of being presented by MHC class I molecules. Although it is the intention of many groups of scientists to improve the motifs as far as possible, the latter will hardly be able to rank every T cell epitope as always taking first place in the scoring. We expect the correct (which is the naturally presented) T cell epitope from any source protein to appear among the top 2% of peptides in the high score list in more than 90% of our predictions. For example, listeriolysin contains 529 amino acids, with 521 possible nonamers cut out of this sequence. The optimal T cell epitope is then expected within the ten high-scoring peptides. Indeed, using the pattern described in the following section, the natural epitope takes third place in the ranking.

Still about 10% of the predictions are not able to identify the respective epitope. This is because of the fact that MHC molecules sometimes refuse to obey their motifs. The occurrence of unusual anchor amino acids can be compensated for by refinement of the motif (see below), but a small percentage of epitopes is not in accordance with any rules of the respective motif. In these cases, the theoretical approach will fail; to identify such epitopes lacking motifs, practical epitope mapping is unavoidable.

Basic and Refined Motifs

From the very beginning of the motif era it was clear that peptide motifs, although quite useful for the identification or the alignment of T cell epitopes are not valid universally: the attempt to align the very few epitopes known in 1991 according to their anchor residues revealed that there was no perfect correspondence in length and anchor amino acids.[4] These findings were confirmed and extended by binding assays using large collections of synthetic peptides and isolated MHC molecules.[9] The human class I molecule HLA-A*0201 emerged as the most intensively analyzed peptide receptor. The basic motif required L/M in P2 and V/L in P9. Several studies verified the existence of amino acids present in both anchor positions but differing from the basic anchor residues, like I/V/A, or T. Still more interesting was the finding that only about 12% of nonamers carrying the proper anchor residues really bound to HLA-A*0201. Therefore, from that time on interest focused on nonanchor positions which were thought to influence tight binding of peptides to MHC molecules. By three different methods (competition assay,[9] T2 binding assay[10] or β2m dissociation assay[14]) amino acids were classified as preferred, neutral or deleterious residues in nonanchor positions.

PREDICTION PROCEDURES

Only for very simple basic motifs and short protein sequences is it advisable to perform predictions without the aid of a computer program. As soon as more complex motif patterns are used (see "Building-Up Patterns" below), or if screened sequences are long protein chains, it becomes essential to employ automated procedures. The most basic program for screening protein sequences with motifs is called MOTIFS, supplied from the Genetics Computer Group[445] and performed on UNIX systems. It is able to list all possible peptides carrying given anchor residues, but it cannot calculate scores. A different MOTIFS program,[446] as well as a no-name program,[14] perform calculation procedures in order to rank all possible peptides from a protein sequence according to their potential to be bound by MHC molecules. The PAP program[447] (originally established for MHC II ligand analysis and epitope prediction) even ranks peptides according to their probability of being processed and presented. It directly translates pool sequencing data of natural ligands into patterns used for screening and includes features of binding, processing and intracellular transport.

The GCG MOTIFS program running on UNIX computers is available from the Genetics Computer Group, Wisconsin. The MOTIFS program running on IBM-compatible PCs is available from Joe D'Amaro, Leiden. The PAP program (also for IBM-PCs) is available from Miles Davenport, Oxford.

BUILDING-UP PATTERNS

The most favorable prediction procedure calculates the scores of every possible peptide from a protein sequence by adding coefficients from a table according to the positions of the amino acids in the peptide. Such coefficients may result directly from binding studies or from pool sequence analysis, or they may be placed arbitrarily in the pattern used for predictions. Although it seems scientifically more correct to directly translate experimental data into a scoring matrix, the disadvantage of this procedure is that only one kind of experiment influences the quality of the prediction. As discussed earlier (MHC I peptide motifs section) each of the experimental methods used for determining peptide motifs has its limitations. Therefore, we recommend that all possible information is collected to build up patterns which result in high probabilities of identifying T cell epitopes.

As a first example, we follow the route of the first motif-based prediction and describe how to compose a pattern suitable for the prediction of H2-K^d-presented nonamer peptides. Experimental data are available from pool sequencing experiments and from alignment of natural ligands. If only a few naturally presented peptides are known, we try to include T cell epitopes in the alignment, although they have been identified mainly by in vitro binding studies. In the case of H2-K^d, we deduce our pattern from the data of the motif Table 4.3. Building a pattern is achieved in four steps according to the four parts of MHC I peptide motifs explained above:

1) Anchor residues. Pool sequencing only shows anchor signals of Y/F in P2 and I/L in P9. All other positions reveal multiple signals and therefore are not anchor positions. Alignment of eight ligands and 25 epitopes confirms Y as the P2 anchor residue, present in 91% of peptides, with F present in another 6%. Both amino acids belong to the same set of aromatic/hydrophobic residues. The only exception in the motif table is a peptide carrying K in P2. According to our (arbitrarily chosen) assessment, anchor valuation is 10 for frequently occurring residues, 8 for amino acids present in a significant portion of ligands, and 6 for rarely occurring amino acids belonging to the same set. The Y coefficient therefore is 10; the coefficient for the rarely occurring F is 6. In the P9 position, alignment of eight ligands and 13 nonamer epitopes reveals that the C-terminal position is occupied by I/L in 76% of the peptides, with 19% of the C-terminal positions occupied by V, and 5% by A. All amino acids belong to the same set of aliphatic/hydrophobic residues. Considering that in epitopes longer than nine amino acids, V and A are also present in PΩ, the P9 anchor coefficients are assessed as follows: The most frequent I/L are valued 10, V is valued 8, and the coefficient for A is 6.

2) Auxiliary or secondary anchors. Neither in pool sequence data, nor by the alignment of individual sequences can auxiliary anchors be identified. Although there seems to be a preference for aliphatic/hydrophobic amino acids in P3 in pools as well as in ligands and epitopes, polar residues such as N, K or Q play such an important role that the requirements of auxiliary anchors are not fulfilled. In our assessment, amino acids frequently occurring in auxiliary anchor positions are valued 6; less frequent residues of the same set have a coefficient of 4.
3) Preferred residues. Such amino acids cause strong signals in pool sequence analysis, and they are present in a significant number of ligands or epitopes. According to the strength of signals or the occurrence in individual sequences, preferred residues have coefficients of 1-4. Most striking is the preference of T in P7, (valued 4); other highly preferred residues are L in P3, S in P1, and P in P4 (all valued 3). Other more or less preferred amino acids are valued 2 or 1, as can be seen in the H2-K^d pattern table (Table 4.8).
4) Unfavorable residues. Pool sequence analysis reveals minimum values of large hydrophobic amino acids in P4 and of aromatic residues F and Y in P5, and S in P6. The level of minimum values of other amino acids is still too high to be judged as unfavorable. Because of the rather small number of individual sequences, unfavorable residues cannot be recognized by alignment alone. The results of pool sequencing, however, are confirmed by the absence of the amino acids mentioned above in the respective positions. Unfavorable residues have a coefficient of -1.

We use the PAP program[447] with our own motif patterns to calculate the probabilities of peptides from a given protein to be presented by MHC I molecules. Table 4.9 shows the predictive power of such analyses. Of eight natural ligands of H2-K^d molecules, one is from an unknown source and can therefore not be calculated. The other seven ligands always occupy one of the top three positions of the prediction (highlighted sequences). It is interesting to observe how the single mutation in position 147 of the sequence of the transplantation antigen P198 gives rise to a high-scoring peptide just by introducing the T in P7. The listeriolysin epitope is the worst one yet, ranking only on the third position in its table and with a relatively low score compared to most other natural ligands.

As the next step, of course, the prediction pattern has to be verified by calculating all epitopes listed in the motif table. This is easily done for the nonamers; almost every epitope listed is among the top scoring peptides and most of them are even in the first rank (data not shown), with only one exception: the ras p21 peptide, with K in P2, reaches a score of only 1.667 and would most probably be missed by such a prediction. To calculate the decamers, a new pattern has to be composed stretching over 10 positions; and 11mers or 8mers (one example each in the listed epitopes) once again are not covered by this approach.

The mouse represents an ideal model system in immunology and problems often arise if data from the mouse have to be transferred to the human system. In spite of the much higher number of known MHC alleles in humans versus mice, the principles of motif-based epitope prediction work equally well in both systems. As a second example, we will build up a prediction pattern suitable for HLA-A*0201. Compared to H2-K^d much more data are available for HLA-A*0201 from pool sequencing, the alignment of huge numbers of natural ligands or T cell epitopes, and from binding studies of several groups. There is, however, little agreement between the different studies (Table 4.10); only four preferred and three deleterious residues in nonanchor positions are common to all studies. Similarly, alignment of 31 natural ligands listed in the motif table shows preferences other than the alignment of 121 T-cell epitopes. Nevertheless, we try to combine all our knowledge in order to compose an optimal pattern for HLA-A*0201-restricted epitope prediction:

1) Anchor residues. From pool sequencing, L/M in P2 and V/L in P9 are the only signals. A minority of ligands and epitopes, as well as binding assays, suggest that other aliphatic residues have to be included. According to the rules outlined above, in P2 only the L coefficient is 10, the less frequent residues I and M are valued 8, while A, V, and T represent exceptional anchor residues with coefficients of 6, respectively. The situation is quite similar in P9, where V and L represent the most common anchor amino acids (coefficient 10), but I is used sometimes by ligands (valued 8), and the other aliphatic/hydrophobic residues A, M and T (each valued 6) are also included.
2) Auxiliary anchors. Unlike the H2-K^d motif, there is a secondary anchor in the HLA-A*0201 motif. Pool sequence data show a strong preference for the aliphatic/hydrophobic residues V, I, and L in P6. This secondary anchor position is confirmed by the alignment of natural ligands (more than 50% of the sequences carry one of these residues in P6) or T cell epitopes, but only partially confirmed by results of binding assays. In P6, V/I/L each have a coefficient of 6.
3) Preferred residues. This category of amino acids is most complicated to compile for the HLA-A*0201 pattern. Each of the four methods which supply data (pool sequencing, ligand alignment, epitope alignment, binding studies) result in rather different options for preferred residues. In our combined approach, data obtained from natural ligand analysis are always of greater importance than data relying merely on MHC binding. Therefore, results from binding assays or T cell epitope analysis always have to be confirmed by natural ligand analysis. Corresponding preferences in P1 are found for A, L, I, Y and S (each coefficient 2), and less frequently for F, G, K and V (each coefficient 1). In P3-P8, several residues are considered as slightly preferred with coefficients 2 or 1 (Table 4.11).
4) Unfavorable residues. Pool sequencing results suggest minimum values of the hydrophilic amino acids E, K, and T in P3 and K in P7, and of hydrophobic residues in P4 and P8. Alignments and binding assays confirm the findings only as far as hydrophilic residues are concerned. The only hydrophobic amino acids hardly present in ligands and epitopes are F and Y in P4 (valued -1), while in P8 hydrophobic residues seem to be tolerated.

The newly built pattern is shown in Table 4.11 and tested for its ability to predict self peptides or T cell epitopes from the sequences of the respective proteins. Table 4.12 shows the 10 best scoring peptides of six predictions: the first three natural ligands (left column in Table 4.12) and the first three T cell epitopes in the HLA-A*0201 motif table (right column in Table 4.12). It is probably just good fortune that in four of the lists the correct ligand/epitope sequence is ranked first. Usually, we do not expect the final epitope on top of such high score lists, but it should be among the 10 high-scoring peptides in most cases.

Table 4.13 contains the prediction patterns of several human and mouse MHC I molecules built up according to the procedure reviewed twice above. All patterns are composed for nonamers. This has been done for two resons: first, pool sequencing and ligand alignment have made it obvious that the majority of ligands and epitopes have a length of nine amino acids. Second, it is easier to expand a pattern than to shorten it. For the prediction of decamers, all values in P1-P3 are kept, and the values in P7-P9 shift by just one position to P8-P10. For the original P4-P6 positions, it seems that for the HLA-A*0201 motif at least, they also shift by one position towards the C-terminal site and become P5-P7. It is not yet clear whether this shift is comparable to decamers of other peptide motifs. In order to avoid mistakes, to build up decamer patterns one should keep P1-P3 and the three C-terminal positions of the nonamer pattern, and leave the central positions without any values (at zero). Thus, the scores of decamers or longer peptides will be lower compared to nonamers, but a ranking is still possible.

PREDICTION OF MHC II RESTRICTED EPITOPES

Peptide motifs proved extremely helpful in the identification of MHC class I-restricted T cell epitopes. For the description of new class II-restricted epitopes, however, conventional epitope-mapping still represents the state of the art. This is mainly because of the highly degenerate anchor positions in MHC class II-presented peptides: if all possible anchor residues of an MHC class II peptide motif were included within a search pattern, a very high number of possible MHC II ligands would be predicted out of any protein sequence. Only few of the class II peptide motifs listed encompass anchor residues specific enough to make motif-based predictions worthwhile, such as HLA-DRB1*0301 with its D anchor in P4, or H2-E^k with R/K in P9. In order to enable predictions of MHC II-restricted epitopes, several authors have proposed methods that not only differentiate between the many possible anchor residues in MHC class II peptide motifs, but also value the role of every amino acid of a peptide sequence in the interaction with the MHC II binding cleft. Three different strategies have been employed:

1) "Side chain scanning."[448] Synthetic designer peptides binding to HLA-DRB*0401 were substituted in each position except P1 with every possible amino acid. The inhibitory effect of such peptides on binding to HLA-DRB1*0401 of the high-affinity ligand Influenza hemagglutinin 307-319 was analyzed, and data from the competition assay were translated into a prediction pattern. The prediction program is available from J. Hammer, Milano.
2) "An empirical method."[447] Data obtained from pool sequence analysis of natural HLA-DR13 ligands were directly transferred into a prediction pattern by averaging the values of sequencing results. The prediction pattern scores the probability of being processed and presented" of every possible peptide within a protein sequence using the PAP program, which is available from M. Davenport, Oxford.
3) "Activity patterns."[19] Similar to the side chain scanning procedure, competition assays against a high-affinity binder to HLA-DRB1*0101 were performed using combinatorial peptide libraries. The inhibitory effects of undecapeptide libraries with one amino acid position fixed in every sublibrary were determined and used to compose a prediction pattern for HLA-DRB1*0101 ligands. The program is available from B. Fleckenstein, Tübingen.

Although such programs proved to be successful in the prediction of peptides binding to the MHC class II molecule examined and in the retrospective description of known T cell epitopes, no new T cell epitopes were determined this way. To our knowledge, the only motif-based prediction of MHC class II epitopes used a rather crude H2-A^b motif[409] to identify epitopes from the sequence of the Sendai virus M protein.[418] Because there were only two degenerate anchor positions required by the motif and because it was not proven that the suggested anchor residues really were responsible for allele-specific binding, this motif has not been included in the listing.

PART II

Antigen Processing

The term antigen processing describes the events between entry of the complete protein (or incompletely translated gene product) into the degradation pathway and the completely assembled MHC protein/peptide complex that has reached its destination, the plasma membrane. Thus, antigen processing includes endo- and exoprotease activity, transport, and chaperoning of MHC ligands or intermediates, chaperoning and assembly of MHC molecules, and transport of the MHC-peptide composites to the cell surface. Since antigen processing pathways for class I[449] and class II[450-452] loading are rather different, both are treated separately. On the other hand, there are considerable intersections between the two pathways, as pointed out below.

THE 'CLASSICAL' MHC I LOADING PATHWAY

The first step is the degradation of proteins situated in the cytosol. This includes not only cytosolic proteins per se, but also misfolded ER proteins re-exported into the cytosol, and, most likely, incomplete translation products not properly targeted into their compartment of destiny. The major proteolytic activity in the cytosol is the proteasome. Proteins bound for degradation within the regular protein-turnover of the cell are coupled with ubiquitin that targets the protein to the 26S proteasome, comprised of the 20S particle and the 19S complex, whereby the latter functions as an adapter between ubiquitin and the proteasome (see Fig. 4.2).[453]

The 20S proteasome is the proteolytically active core of the 26S complex, but it is also active on its own. Based on structural analysis of the proteasome from the archebacterium *Thermoplasma acidophilum*, and on electron microscopic studies, the structure of the mouse or human proteasome has been predicted as follows:[454] Four rings, each consisting of 7 subunits, are stacked in a barrel-like structure (see Fig. 4.2). The two outer rings consist of 7 different α subunits, each ranging between 25 and 30 kD (Table 4.14). Each of the two inner rings consists of seven different β units (22 to 30 kD), three of which carry active threonine proteinase groups, δ, ε, and α_1, also called Z.[455] The latter subunits can be replaced by interferon γ inducible homologs: α by MECL1,[456] δ by LMP2 and ε by LMP7.[452] Thus, the proteasome relevant during immune response accompanied by INFγ production, such as viral infection, contains MECL, LMP2 and LMP7. Therefore, these particles have been called 'immunoproteasomes'.[457] Cells from mice lacking LMP2 or LMP7 show impaired antigen presentation; the exact influence of the INFγ inducible proteasome subunits on proteolytic specificity is not known, however.[458-466] The three active subunits represent chymotrypsin-like, trypsin-like and peptidyl-glutamyl-peptide hydrolase activities.[467]

For protease activity to occur, a protein has to be inserted into the lumen of the proteasome. For the 26S proteasomes, this is achieved by funneling ubiquinated protein through the 19S complex into the 20S proteasome. For the naked 20S proteasome, the intermediate natural substrates are not known; in vitro, however, longer peptides work. Once in the proteasome, the substrates are cleaved into peptides of various length. The cleavage specificity of the proteasome is not obvious, if one looks at the products derived from a fine substrate. Studies using a short fluorogenic substrate of a size representative of three or four amino acids are easy to undertake,[452] but are not very useful for following the role of proteasomes in MHC-I loading, which requires peptides of eight or more amino acids. In cleavage studies using large synthetic peptides the detection of the products requires mass spectrometric analysis. This has limited the number of substrates tested so far; what emerges, though, is a preference for cleavages after hydrophobic residues. However, flanking amino acids must also contribute, since not every hydrophobic residue within a particle stretch is used for cleavage. It has been suggested that the *Thermoplasma* proteasome cuts at two sites of the substrate simultaneously, since the distribution of peptide products observed was centered on hepta- or octapeptides.[454,468] A hepta- or octapeptide in extended formation may span the shortest distance, 28 Å, between two of the active sites, so that both sites may work simultaneously on the substrate and together constitute a molecular rule to produce the peptide of the observed length.

However, kinetic studies have indicated that the mouse or human 20S proteasome preferentially produces single cleavages so that for an internal fragment of a protein to be produced, two subsequent cleavages are necessary.[469] This possibly requires exit of the intermediate product for the proteasome and re-entry, which would make the process of producing internal fragments a rather inefficient one in vivo, with hundreds of different substrates around. Surprisingly, the 20S proteasome can be induced to produce double cleavages by attachment of the PA28 regulator, also called 11S complex.[469] This molecule consists of two homologous subunits forming a hexa- or heptameric ring structure.[470-474] Like the three proteasome subunits LMP2, LMP7 and MECL1, the PA28 regulator is induced by IFNγ; it appears, therefore, that the real 'immunoproteasome', the enzymatic complex centrally involved in producing immunologically relevant MHC class I ligands, is the induced 20S proteasome with PA28 attached. The effect of PA28 on proteasome performance is illustrated with the following examples.[469] A 21mer-peptide from the protein tyrosine kinase JAK1, containing the prominent H2-K^d ligand SYFPEITHI (the first MHC ligand ever to be sequenced directly)[4] is cut by the naked 20S proteasome at several sites, the most dominant products being the peptides 1-7 and 8-21 (see Fig. 4.3). The class I ligand SYFPEITHI (8-14) is also produced, albeit only as a minor product, and with kinetics indicative of two subsequent cleavages. If the PA28 regulator is added to the 20S proteasome, however, the dominant products are SYFPEITHI and the flanking peptides. Thus, 20S/PA28 produces this particular class I ligand very efficiently and in one step, as indicated by its kinetics. However, one step production of this very dominant class I ligand (estimated to occupy 10% of the H2-K^d molecule of the tumor cell P815) does not mean that all class I ligands are produced as efficiently. This is illustrated by another example. A 25-mer peptide from the MCMV pp89 protein containing the H2-L^d ligand and T cell epitope YPHFMPTNL,[236] is cleaved by the naked 20S proteasome such that the dominant products are 1-5 and 16-25 (Fig. 4.3). Upon influence of PA28, the dominant products are internal peptides, the most abundant being PHFMPTNL, short of the Tyr as compared to the H2-L^d ligand YPHFMPTNL. Thus, the dominant product cannot be related to antigen processing. The second dominant one, however, is DMYPHFMPTNL, two amino acids longer than the ligand. The ligand itself is actually also produced, however, as a very minor product only. Thus, it is likely that for this epitope, the relevant peptide produced by the proteasome is an intermediate of processing, DMYPHFMPTNL, which has to be trimmed further by removing the N-terminal D and M residues.

The above mentioned data on 20S/PA28 interaction have been obtained entirely in vitro. However, fibroblasts overexpressing PA28 are much more efficient in presenting the MCMV epitope and other viral antigens to cytotoxic T cells as compared to its normal, nontransfected counterparts.[475] Thus, it is very likely that the processing steps discussed before are the ones used by the relevant target cells. A similar conclusion can be drawn for the results on the JAK1 digests by 20S/PA28. The second dominant product of the in vitro digest is the heptamer FPEITHI. This peptide is also found in a total peptide extract of P815 tumor cells, in addition to the H2-K^d ligand SYFPEITHI.[469] An open question, however, is the nature of the physiological substrate of the 20S/PA28 complex. Native proteins are unlikely to be digested by the proteasome. Possibly, the 26S proteasome digests ubiquinated proteins into large peptides using single cleavage. These peptides could then be used as substrates by 20S/PA28. Alternatively, denatured proteins might be the relevant substrate.

The peptides finally leaving the proteasome make their way to the transporter associated with processing, TAP.[476,477] Since it is unlikely that peptides float around freely in the cytosol, one has to assume that they are either delivered directly from the proteasome to TAP (this would require physical association between proteasome and TAP) or, alternatively, are chaperoned in between. A candidate for such a peptide shuffle is Hsc70, a cytosolic chaperone found to be associated with cellular antigens upon immunization of mice.[478] TAP is a heterodimer of TAP1 and TAP2 chains. Their genes are located within the MHC region. TAP sequences are homologous to the ATP-binding cassette (ABC) family of transport protein. TAP molecules have a certain selectivity for peptide transport.[476,479-482] Most favored are the peptides between 9 and 13 amino acids, and thus roughly of the size produced by 20S/PA28 by double cleavage. However, peptides much longer are also transported, although with lesser efficiency.[483] Other criteria for peptide selection by TAP are the C-terminal amino acid, and amino acids at additional positions within the peptide sequence.[481] None of these criteria, however, is as stringent as an MHC class I anchor. The mouse transporter shows a preference for peptides with a hydrophobic C-terminus, whereas the human TAP does not care about it.[481] The rat possesses two allelic forms of TAP, one having a specificity much like the mouse TAP; the other is as nondiscriminatory as the human TAP, both times with regard to the C-terminus of peptides.[484] For amino acid residues other than the C-terminus, the selectivity is not very pronounced. Depending on the assay used (binding of peptides to TAP, or measurement of actual peptide transport) certain preferred or unfavored residues have been found for certain positions, e.g., Pro at position 2 is unfavorable for transport.[476] By and large, however, transport specificity by TAP is not very pronounced but still a certain influence on the pool of peptides finally presented by MHC I molecules has to be assumed. This is illustrated by the rat, with its two functionally different allelic TAP forms.[484] Identical rat MHC molecules are associated with different sets of peptides, dependent on the TAP allele expressed. On the other hand, the limited sequence polymorphism of mouse and human TAP genes does not seem to have influence on TAP specificity.[485]

Once the peptide has reached the luminal exit of TAP, it has the chance to bind to a newly synthesized MHC I molecule.[449,486] The class I heavy chain is synthesized with a leader sequence so that it starts its appearance as a membrane-bound luminal protein. The nascent heavy chain is first chaperoned by calnexin.[487-490] When the light chain, β2-microglobulin, binds to the heavy chain (HC), calnexin is released, and another chaperone, calreticulin, binds to the HC/ β2m complex and serves as a device for retaining in the ER.[488] The HC/β2m complex then may bind to TAP via an adapter molecule, tapasin, to be loaded by peptides having arrived through the TAP channel.[491] However, not all MHC allelic products have been found to be able to associate with TAP, and the majority of peptides coming in by TAP are not able to bind to the MHC molecule on hand. The latter statement is based on the assumption that the selection of peptides brought into the ER by TAP is not influenced by the MHC molecules coexpressed in the cell.[202] Thus, the processing machine—proteasome, TAP, and accessory molecules—is able to provide the ER lumen with all the peptides possibly required by any of the species' MHC molecules. Of these—e.g., 186 HLA-B, 83 HLA-A and 46 HLA-C allelic products, only up to six are expressible in a cell. Even if one takes into consideration overlaps in peptide specificity of the different MHC molecules, it is still evident that most of the imported peptides do not fit to the MHC molecule present.[202] In addition, some peptides might possess the correct motif but might be a few amino acids too long. Taken together with the observation that some HLA molecules do not associate with TAP, one has to think about the fate of peptides either not fitting to the MHC molecule present, or not yet fitting, or fitting, but not immediately reaching the MHC molecule. Since, again, it seems unlikely that free peptides are floating in the

ER lumen it has been assumed that such peptides are accepted by a chaperone.[478] A primary candidate for such a chaperone is gp96, which has been found, at least functionally, to be associated with many cellular antigens, most likely in the form of peptides.[478,492,493] Indeed, gp96 is an acceptor for the TAP-transported peptides and it has been found to be associated at least with one peptide, independent of the MHC molecules coexpressed.[494] In addition, another peptide acceptor, protein disulfide isomerase (PDI), has been detected that is even more efficient in absorbing peptides brought into the ER lumen by TAP.[494] It is not clear, however, what happens to peptide acceptor-bound peptides in the ER. Possibilities are that motif-containing peptides are shuffled to MHC molecules, possibly after trimming of the peptides has occurred,[495] and that those peptides not containing a suitable MHC motif are either completely degraded by some unknown enzymes or are re-exported into the cytosol, possibly by the protein transporter SEC61.[496] Re-exported peptides may then be completely degraded or imported again into the ER, possibly after cytosolic trimming.[497]

After a nascent MHC I molecule has managed to acquire a peptide, calreticulin releases the fully associated HC/β2m/peptide trimer onto the default pathway of membrane proteins via the Golgi apparatus to the cell surface. Although TAP-mediated delivery is the major source for peptide loading of MHC I molecules, there are some variants of that process. Some peptides are produced inside the ER; these are mainly signal sequence-derived peptides.[32,498] In addition, TAP-deficient cells like RMA-S are still able to present some minor histocompatibility antigen[499] and some particular viral epitopes,[500] so that even TAP-negative cells are able to present at least a few MHC I-associated peptides.

Many of the essential steps required for MHC I assembly and loading can be blocked by action of viruses.[496,501-503] This, on one hand, indicates that viruses suffer from selective pressure by antigen processing and the subsequent immune response; on the other hand, virus-mediated inhibition of particular steps in processing has taught us a lot of the above-mentioned details. Examples for virus-mediated processing defects are as follows: Herpes virus ICP47 molecules attach to the cytosolic side of TAP and thereby block TAP function.[504] A human cytomegalovirus protein, US11, eludes nascent MHC heavy chains to the exporter SEC61, which is followed by cytosolic degradation of the heavy chain.[496] Both mechanisms lead to a reduction of MHC-I expression on the cell surface. An adenovirus protein binds nascent MHC I heavy chains instead of β2-microglobulin and thereby interferes with proper assembly.[505] Many more examples of this category of virus/host cell interactions have been described.

The MHC loading discussed so far is meant for proteins occurring inside the cytosol upon protein synthesis in the cell. However, at least macrophages and dendritic cells, or certain types of these cells, are able to load peptides from phagocytosed or otherwise acquired exogenous antigens to class I molecules.[506,507] Particulate antigens are especially prone to this pathway.[508-510] One route by which this happens is inserting the acquired antigen into the cytosol, and joining of the regular, TAP-dependent class I loading pathway.[511] Alternatively, the exogenous antigen is digested in a brefeldin-insensitive compartment typical for class II-associated processing and is thus loaded to class I molecules.[512,510] The biological significance of this intersecting class I loading pathway is not known; however, loading of external antigen on class I molecules might be useful for vaccine purposes.

MHC CLASS II LOADING

Only a fraction of cell types express class II molecules. The cells having functional significance for their class II expression fall into three categories: Antigen-acquiring presenting cells, mainly macrophages and dendritic cells, B lymphocytes, and thymic epithelial cells. Macrophages and dendritic cells, the so-called professional antigen-presenting cells, are instrumental for primary activation of T cells. The class II molecules on B cells, presenting fragments of the antigen recognized by the B cell, connect the B cell to a T helper cell with specificity for the same antigen. Thymic epithelial cells are involved in positive T cell selection. In addition, a number of other cells expressing class II molecules, mostly in the activated state, like human T cells, or after induction by INFγ, like most of the epithelial cells. The biological significance of class II-expression on the latter cell types is not clear.

Class II molecules start their appearance in cells in the ER.[513,450] The nascent α and β chains are first chaperoned by BiP and then associate with both invariant chains and calnexin, both acting like a chaperone (Fig. 4.4).[450,451] Upon release of calnexin, nonameric structures are left containing 3 αβ pairs and 3 invariant chains. These $(\alpha\beta)_3$ Ii_3 complexes do not bind peptides, since their grooves are occupied by the middle part of Ii, the CLIP (class II-associated invariant chain peptide, residue 81-104 of Ii) region.[514] Directed by the invariant chain, these complexes are exported to endocytic compartments.[515] MHC class II molecules are loaded with peptides in what is considered a special compartment called MIIC, for MHC class II loading compartment.[516-520] Once the $(\alpha\beta)_3$ Ii_3 complex has arrived there, the invariant chain is degraded with the involvement of cathepsin S,[521] until only CLIPs are left occupying the groove. Thus, at this step, αβ heterodimers associated with CLIP occur. Removal of CLIP and its replacement by the final class II ligand takes place under association of HLA-DM molecules.[522-530] The exact mode of DM/class II interaction is not understood; however, DM catalyzes the removal of CLIP and 'edits' the peptide collection to be mounted on class II molecules by enabling only high affinity peptides to replace CLIP.[531-534] The fully assembled class II molecule, consisting of the αβ heterodimer and the bound peptide, are then brought to the cell surface. Some class II molecules still occupied with CLIP also can make their way to the surface;[535,536,17] in cells deficient in DM, most surface class II molecules are loaded with CLIP.[537] The mode of interaction of CLIP and the class II groove is such that CLIP uses a few of the anchors only and avoids unfavorable residues at other positions, so that it can bind to almost all class II molecules, at least with intermediate affinity.[536,538]

The peptides replacing CLIP in the class II loading compartment are derived from protein endogenous to the cell or from exogenous antigens. Endogeneous sources of peptides are predominantly membrane-bound molecules, although cytosolic proteins also contribute.[539] Depending on the cell type, exogenous antigens are brought inside a cellular vesicle by a number of different uptake mechanisms, such as phagocytosis, receptor-mediated uptake, or macropinocytosis or class II recycling.[540-542,513] It is not entirely clear whether degradation of protein for class II loading takes place in the same compartment as the loading itself, or in a separate endolysosome.[451] In any instance, a number of lysosomal proteases is involved in the production of class II ligands. Most notable are endopeptidases like cathepsin D and other cathepsins with an activity optimum in the lower pH range.[543-545] Depending on the antigen, different enzymes play the major role in processing. In addition to endopeptidases, it is likely that exopeptidases contribute in producing the final ligand. One piece of evidence stems from a frequently found Pro residue at position 2 of class II ligands; this Pro is thought to serve as a stop signal for aminopeptidases.[17,289] An elegant series of experiments using the H2-A^k-restricted hen egg white lysozyme epitope expressed with different flanking regions provide compelling evidence for exopeptidase involvement.[15] Most likely, the class II molecule serves as a template for the peptides in that the binding 9-amino acid core is protected from exopeptidase activity whereas the flanking regions outside the groove are prone to degradation.[546-548] Thus, the MHC class II molecule appears to play an instructive role in ligand production, as was anticipated by the determinant protection hypothesis.[549]

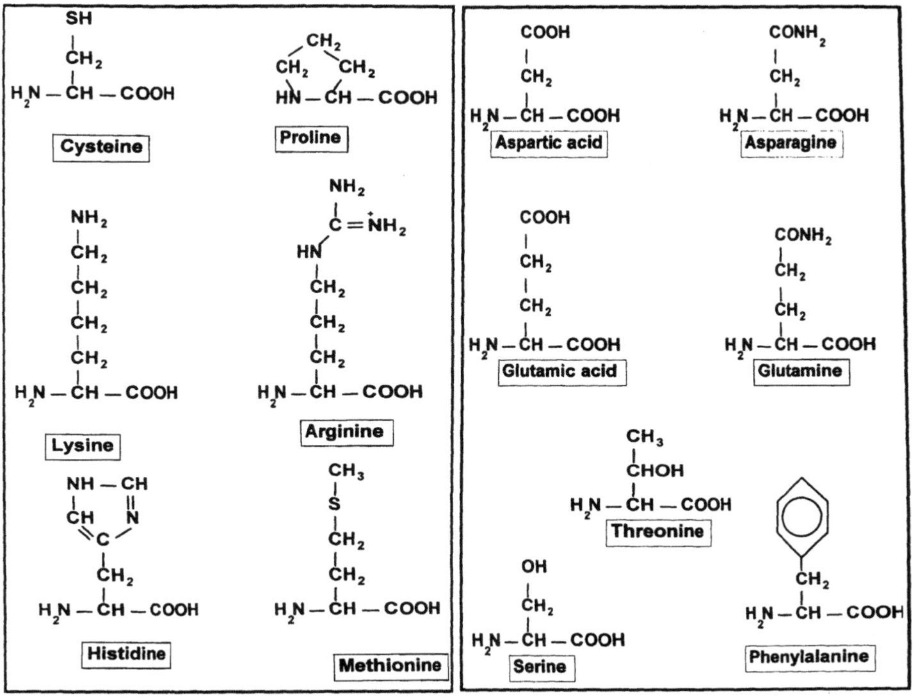

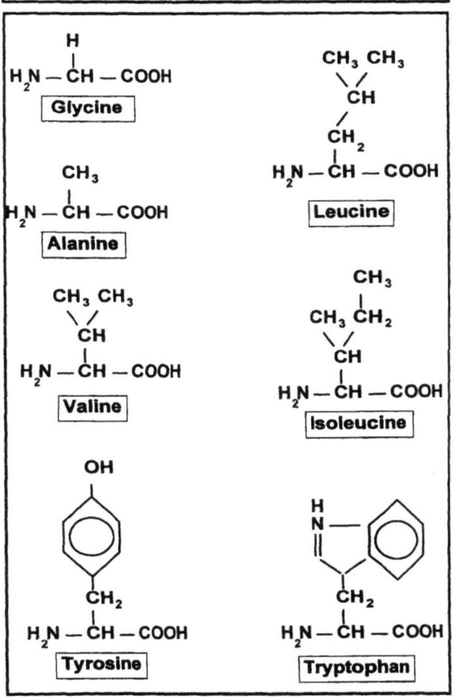

Fig. 4.1. Amino acids.

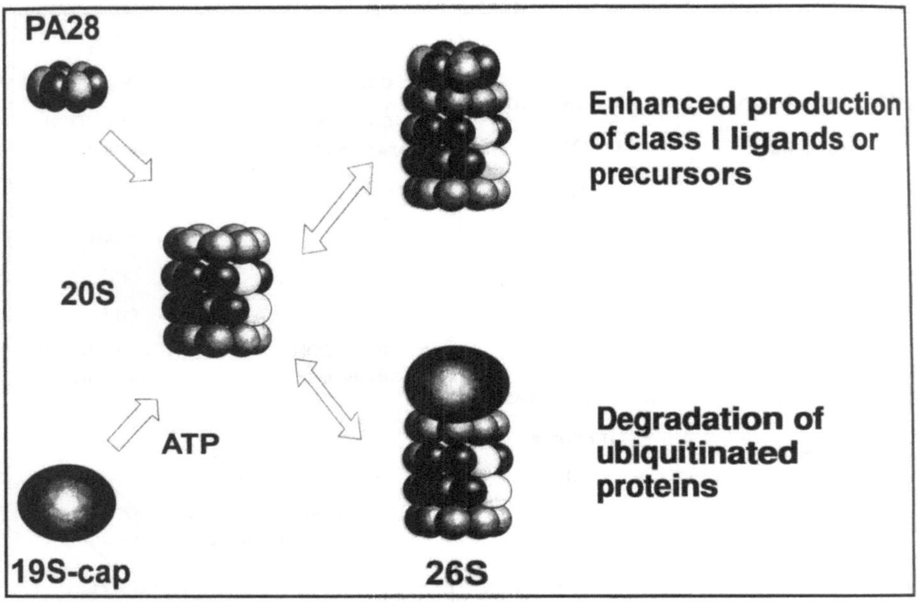

Fig. 4.2. The 20S proteasome and its relation to 19S and PA28 attachments. See text for further details.

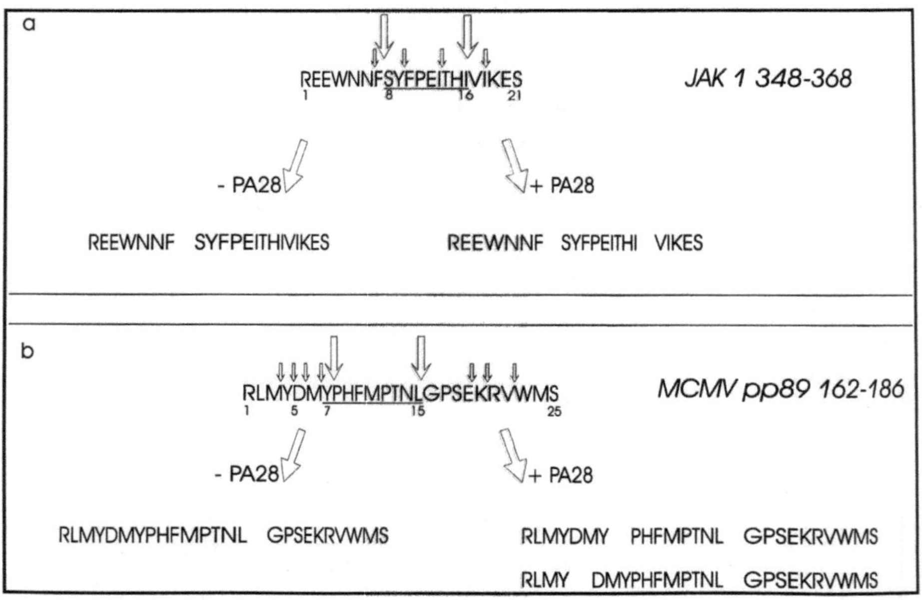

Fig. 4.3. Cleavage of peptides containing the class I ligand SYFPEITHI and YPHFMPTNL; respectively, by the 20S proteasome with and without P28. See text for further details.

Table 4.1. Amino acids

One-letter code	Three-letter code	Full name	Amino acid set
A	Ala	Alanine	small, aliphatic/hydrophobic
C	Cys	Cysteine	
D	Asp	Aspartic acid	charged, acidic/hydrophilic
E	Glu	Glutamic acid	charged, acidic/hydrophilic
F	Phe	Phenylalanine	aromatic/hydrophobic
G	Gly	Glycine	small
H	His	Histidine	charged, basic/hydrophilic
I	Ile	Isoleucine	aliphatic/hydrophobic
K	Lys	Lysine	charged, basic/hydrophilic
L	Leu	Leucine	aliphatic/hydrophobic
M	Met	Methionine	aliphatic/hydrophobic
N	Asn	Asparagine	neutral/hydrophilic
P	Pro	Proline	small
Q	Gln	Glutamine	neutral/hydrophilic
R	Arg	Arginine	charged, basic/hydrophilic
S	Ser	Serine	small, alcoholic/hydrophilic
T	Thr	Threonine	alcoholic/hydrophilic
V	Val	Valine	aliphatic/hydrophobic
W	Trp	Tryptophan	aromatic/hydrophobic
Y	Tyr	Tyrosine	aromatic/hydrophobic

Table 4.2. HLA class I motifs

Amino acids in boldface indicate anchor residues, amino acids in small print indicate that they have not been detected unequivocally, underlined amino acids represent auxillary anchors.

HLA-A1	Position													Source	Ref.
	1	**2**	**3**	4	5	6	7	8	**9**						
Anchor or auxiliary anchor residues		T	**D**				L		**Y**						20, 21, 22
		S	**E**												23,24
Other preferred residues		L		G	G	G									
				I	N	V									
				P	Y	I									
Examples for ligands	A	T	**D**	F	K	F	A	M	**Y**					Cyclin-like protein 135-143	20, 24
	I	A	**D**	M	G	H	L	K	**Y**					Proliferating cell nuclear antigen 241-249	20, 21, 24
	M	I	**E**	P	R	T	L	Q	**Y**					40S ribosomal protein S16 40-48	20, 21
	Y	T	S	D	Y	F	I	S	**Y**					Ets-1 154-162	20, 24
	L	T	**D**	P	G	V	L	D	**Y**					Unknown	20
	V	S	**D**	I	V	G	P	D	G	L	V	**Y**		Fibrillarin 177-188	20, 21
	Y	T	**D**	Y	G	G	L	I	F	N	S	**Y**		Cytochrome C oxidase II 110-121	20, 24
	Q	S	**E**	D	G	S	H	T	I	Q	I	M	**Y**	HLA class I α chain 111-123	20
	Y	L	**D**	D	P	D	L	K	**Y**					Cytosine methyl transferase 238-246	24
	S	T	**D**	H	I	P	I	L	**Y**					Fructose-6-amino transferase 217-225	24
	D	S	**D**	G	S	F	F	L	**Y**					Ig gamma-4 chain C 279-287	24
	G	T	**D**	E	X	R	N	X	**Y**					Unknown	24
	V	S	**D**	P	Y	N	X	K	**Y**					Unknown	25, 24
	V	A	**D**	K	V	H	X	M	**Y**					Unknown	24
	Y	T	A	V	V	P	L	V	**Y**					J-chain 102-110	24
	Y	T	N	P	Q	F	N	V	**Y**					Unknown	24
	E	T	X	X	P	D	W	S	**Y**					Unknown	24
	F	T	**D**	V	N	S	X	X	R	**Y**				Unknown	24
	S	S	**E**	Q	T	F	M	Y	**Y**					Ornithin decarboxylase 309-317	21
	S	T	**E**	P	V	N	I	L	**Y**					Unknown	21
	G	T	**D**	P	G	V	L	I	**Y**					Unknown	21
	S	T	**E**	P	P	M	L	N	**Y**					Unknown	21
	S	L	**E**	P	Q	R	T	Q	**Y**					Unknown	21

	F T **E** V S I R K **Y**	Unknown	21
	K F **D** P V N L V **Y**	Unknown	21
	A V **D** P G G M Y S	Unknown	21
	F G S G A R D X **Y**	Unknown	21
	Y X **E** P Q F L T **Y**	Unknown	21
	A X I P A F I N **Y**	Unknown	21
	I T **E** D M G H L K **Y**	Unknown	23
	E T **D** X X X D R S E **Y**	Unknown	24
	V E **D** F Q Y L Y **Y**	Unknown	26
T cell epitopes	E A **D** P T G H S **Y**	MAGE-1 161-169	27, 28
	V S **D** G G P N L **Y**	Influenza A PB1 591-599	21, 23
	C T **E** L K L S D **Y**	Influenza A NP 44-52	23
	E V **D** P I G H L **Y**	MAGE-3 168-176	29, 30

HLA-A*0201	Position	Source	Ref.
	1 **2** 3 4 5 6 7 8 **9**		
Anchor or auxiliary anchor residues	**L** (2), V (6), **V** (9)		4
	M (2), **L** (9)		
Preferred residues	E (4), K (8)		
	K (4)		
Other residues	I (1), A (3), G (4), I (5), I (6), A (7), E (8)		
	L (1), Y (3), P (4), K (5), L (6), Y (7), S (8)		
	F (1), F (3), D (4), Y (5), T (6), H (7)		
	K (1), P (3), T (4), N (5)		
	M (1), M (3), G (5)		
	Y (1), S (3), F (5)		
	V (1), R (3), V (5)		
	H (5)		
Examples for ligands	S **L** L P A I V E **L**	Protein phosphatase 2A 389-3971	
	Y **L** L P A I V H I	ATP-dependent RNA Helicase 148-156	1
	T **L** W V D P Y E **V**	B cell transloc. gene 1 protein 103-111	1
	S X[2] P S G G X G **V**	Unknown	1
	G X V P F X V S **V**	Unknown	1
	S X X V R A X E **V**	Unknown	1
	K X N E P V X X X	Unknown	1
	A **L** W G F F P V X+	Unknown	1, 31
	L **L** D V P I A A **V**	IP-30 signal sequence 27-35	1
	L L **L** D V P I A A **V**	IP-30 signal sequence 26-35	1, 32

Table 4.2. (con't)

	1	**2**	3	4	5	6	7	8	**9**				Source	Ref.
L	L	**L**	D	V	P	T	A	A	**V**	Q	A		IP-30 signal sequence 26-37	1, 32
L	L	**L**	D	V	P	T	A	A	**V**	Q			IP-30 signal sequence 26-36	32
L	F	R	G	G	P	R	G	L	L	A	V	A	SSRα signal sequence 12-25	33, 32
	M	V	D	G	T	L	L	L	**L**				HLA-E signal sequence 1-9	1
	Y	**M**	N	G	T	M	S	Q	**V**+				Tyrosinase 369-377	34, 35, 36, 37
	M	**L**	L	S	V	P	L	L	**L**	G			Calreticulin signal sequence 1-10	32
	S	**L**	L	G	L	L	V	E	**V***				Unknown	38
	A	**L**	L	P	P	I	N	I	**L***				Unknown	38
	T	**L**	I	K	I	Q	H	T	**L***				Unknown	38
	A	**L**	I	V	G	X	N	D	D*				Unknown	38
	H	**L**	I	D	Y	L	V	T	S*				Carboxypeptidase M 91-99	38
	I	**L**	A	P	P	V	V	K	L	L	**V***		Unknown	38
	A	**L**	F	P	Q	L	V	I	**L***				Unknown	38
	G	I	L	G	F	V	F	T	**L**+				Influenza MP 58-66	4,39,40,41,42
	S	T	B[1]	X	Q	S	G	X	Q				HBV pre-S protein 141-149	43
	X	S	K	K	F	D	Q	S	Q				Unknown	43
	X	Q	Y	T	S	R	M	I					Aldehyde dehydrogenase 5572-5595 (bp)	43
	G	**L**	D	V	L	T	A	K	**V***				Human vinculin 358-366	44
	R	I	L	G	A	V	A	K	**V***				Human vinculin 823-831	44
	Q	V	C	E	R	I	P	T	I*				Human vinculin 983-991	44
	Y	**M**	D	G	T	M	S	Q	**V***				Tyrosinase 369-377	45
	I	**L**	F	G	H	E	N	R	**V**				β-5 GTP binding protein 320-329	46
	I	**L**	M	E	H	I	H	K	**L**				60S ribosomal protein L19 137-145	46
	I	**L**	D	Q	K	I	N	E	**V**				Ornithin decarboxylase 23-31	46
	S	**L**	A	G	G	I	I	G	**V**				hnRNP K 159-167	46
	L	**L**	I	E	N	V	A	S	**L**				Glutathion peroxidase 38-46	46
	V	**L**	I	D	F								Unknown	46
	F	**L**	L										GPIX 8-10	46
	W	A	T	A	E	A							GPIX 11-16	46
	F	**L**	L	W	A	T	A	E					GPIX 8-15	46
	F	**L**	L	W	A	T	A	E	A				GPIX 8-16	46
	X	**L**	P	D	F	G	I	S	Y	**V**			Unknown	46
	X	**L**	I	D	F	A	L	Y	**L**				Unknown	46
	K	K	R	E	E	A	P	S	**L**				Fibrinogen β-chain 51-59	46
	L	E	R	P	E	G	N	E	I				Fibrinogen α-chain 261-269	46
	A	**L**	S	N	L	E	V	K	**L**				Unknown	46

	A **L** N E L L Q H **V**	Talin 777-785	46
	L **L** P P P P	Tyrosin protein kinase 557-562	46
T cell epitopes	I **L** K E P V H G **V**	HIV-1 RT 476-484	4, 31, 47
	I **L** G F V F T L T **V**	Influenza MP 59-68	4, 39
	L **L** F G Y P V Y **V**	HTLV-1 tax 11-19	40
	G **L** S P T V W L S **V**	HBV sAg 348-357	48
	W **L** S L L V P F **V**	HBV sAg 335-343	48
	F **L** P S D F F P S **V**	HBV cAg 18-27	49, 50, 51
	C **L** G G L L T M **V**	EBV LMP-2 426-434	52
	F **I** A G N S A Y E Y **V**	HCMV gp B 618-628	48
	K **L** G E F Y N Q M M	Influenza B NP 85-94	53
	K **L** V A L G I N A **V**	HCV-1 NS3 400-409	54
	D **L** M G Y I P L **V**	HCV MP 17-25	55
	R **L** V T L K D I **V**	HPV11 E7 4-12	56
	M **L** L A V L Y C **L**	Tyrosinase 1-9	34, 35
	A A G I G I L T **V**	Melan A/Mart-1 27-35	57, 58, 59, 68
	Y **L** E P G P V T A	pmel 17/gp100 480-488	60
	I **L** D G T A T L R **L**	pmel 17/gp100 457-466	61
	L **L** D G T A T L R **L**	pmel gp100 457-466	62
	I T D Q V P F S **V**	pmel gp100 209-217	62
	K T W G Q Y W Q **V**	pmel gp100 154-162	62
	T I T D Q V P F S **V**	pmel gp100 208-217	62
	A F H H V A R E **L**	HIV-1 nef 190-198	63
	Y **L** N K I Q N S **L**	*P. falciparum* CSP 334-342	64
	M **M** R K L A I L S **V**	*P. falciparum* CSP 1-10	64
	K A G E F Y N Q M M	Influenza BNP 85-94	65
	N I A E G L R A **L**	EBNA-1 480-488	66
	N **L** R R G T A L A	EBNA-1 519-527	66
	A **L** A I P Q C R **L**	EBNA-1 525-533	66
	V **L** K D A I K D **L**	EBNA-1 575-582	66
	F **M** V F L Q T H I	EBNA-1 562-570	66
	H **L** I V D T D S **L**	EBNA-2 15-23	66
	S **L** G N P S L S **V**	EBNA-2 22-30	66
	P **L** A S A M R M **L**	EBNA-2 126-134	66
	R **M** L W M A N Y I	EBNA-2 132-140	66
	M **L** W M A N Y I **V**	EBNA-2 133-141	66
	I **L** P Q G P Q T A	EBNA-2 151-159	66
	P **L** R P T A P T I	EBNA-2 171-179	66
	P **L** P P A T L T **V**	EBNA-2 205-213	66

Table 4.2. (con't)

	Position													Source	Ref.
	1	**2**	3	4	5	6	7	8	**9**						
	R	**M**	H	L	P	V	L	H	**V**					EBNA-2 246-254	66
	P	**M**	P	L	P	P	S	Q	**L**					EBNA-2 287-295	66
	Q	**L**	P	P	P	A	A	P	A					EBNA-2 294-302	66
	S	**M**	P	E	L	S	P	V	**L**					EBNA-2 381-389	66
	D	**L**	D	E	S	W	D	Y	I					EBNA-2 453-461	66
	P	**L**	P	C	V	L	W	P	**V**					BZLF1 43-51	66
	S	**L**	E	E	C	D	S	E	**L**					BZLF1 167-175	66
	E	**I**	K	R	Y	K	N	R	**V**					BZLF1 176-184	66
	Q	**L**	L	Q	H	Y	R	E	**V**					BZLF1 195-203	66
	L	**L**	Q	H	Y	R	E	V	A					BZLF1 196-204	66
	L	**L**	K	Q	M	C	P	S	**L**					BZLF1 217-225	66
	S	I	I	P	R	T	P	D	**V**					BZLF1 229-237	66
	A	I	M	D	K	N	I	I	**L**					Influenza A NS 1 122-130	67
		I	M	D	K	N	I	I	**L**	K	A			Influenza A NS 1 123-132	67
	L	**L**	A	L	L	S	C	L	T	**V**				HCV MP 63-72	69
	I	**L**	H	T	P	G	C	**V**						HCV MP 105-112	69
	Q	**L**	R	R	H	I	D	L	L	**V**				HCV env E 66-75	69
	D	**L**	C	G	S	V	F	L	**V**					HCV env E 88-96	69
	S	**M**	V	G	N	W	A	K	**V**					HCV env E 172-180	69
	H	**L**	H	Q	N	I	V	D	**V**					HCV NS1 308-316	69
	F	**L**	L	L	A	D	A	R	**V**					HCV NS1 340-348	69
	G	**L**	R	D	L	A	V	A	**V**	E	P	V	**V**	HCV NS2 234-246	69
	S	**L**	L	A	P	G	A	K	Q	N	**V**			HCV NS1 18-28	69
		L	L	A	P	G	A	K	Q	N	**V**			HCV NS1 19-28	69
	F	**L**	L	S	L	G	I	H	**L**					HBV pol 575-583	70
	S	**L**	Y	A	D	S	P	S	**V**					HBV pol 816-824	70
	G	**L**	S	R	Y	V	A	R	**L**					HBV pol 455-463	70
	K	I	F	G	S	L	A	F	**L**					HER-2 369-377	71
	E	**L**	V	S	E	F	S	R	M					HER-2 971-979	71
	K	**L**	T	P	L	C	V	T	**L**					HIV-1 gp160 120-128	72
S	L	**L**	N	A	T	D	I	A	**V**					HIV-1 gp160 814-823	72
	V	**L**	Y	R	Y	G	S	F	S	**V**				pmel gp100 476-485	62
	Y	I	G	E	V	L	V	S	**V**					Non-filament forming class I myosin family (HA-2)**	73
	L	**L**	F	N	I	L	G	G	W	**V**				HCV NS4 192-201	74
	L	**L**	V	P	F	V	Q	W	F	**V**				HBV env 338-347	74
	A	**L**	M	P	I	Y	A	C	I					HBV pol 642-650	74

Y	**L**	V	A	Y	Q	A	T	**V**		HCV NS3 579-587	74
T	**L**	G	I	V	C	P	I	C		HPV16 E7 86-94	74
Y	**L**	L	P	R	R	G	P	R	**L**	HCV core protein 34-43	74
L	**L**	P	I	F	F	C	L	W	**V**	HBV env 378-387	74
Y	**M**	D	D	V	V	L	G	A		HBV Pol 538-546	74
G	T	L	G	I	V	C	P	I		HPV16 E7 85-93	74
L	**L**	A	L	L	S	C	L	T	I	HCV MP 63-72	74
M	**L**	D	L	Q	P	E	T	T		HPV16 E7 12-20	74
S	**L**	M	A	F	T	A	A	**V**		HCV NS4 174-182	75
C	I	N	G	V	C	W	T	**V**		HCV NS3 67-75	75
V	**M**	N	I	L	L	Q	Y	V	**V**	Glutamic acid decarboxylase 114-123	76
I	**L**	T	V	I	L	G	V	**L**		Melan A/Mart-1 32-40	77
F	**L**	W	G	P	R	A	L	**V**		MAGE-3 271-279	78
L	**L**	C	P	A	G	H	A	**V**		HCV NS3 163-171	54
I	**L**	D	S	F	D	P	L	**V**		HCV NS5 239-247	54
L	**L**	L	C	L	I	F	L	**L**		HBV env 250-258	79
L	**L**	D	Y	Q	G	M	L	P	**V**	HBV env 260-269	79
S	I	V	S	P	F	I	P	L	**L**	HBV env 370-379	79
F	**L**	L	T	R	I	L	T	I		HBV env 183-191	80
H	**L**	G	N	V	K	Y	L	**V**		*P. falciparum* TRAP 3-11	81
G	I	A	G	G	L	A	L	**L**		*P. falciparum* TRAP 500-508	81
I	**L**	A	G	Y	G	A	G	**V**		HCV NS4A 236-244	82
G	**L**	Q	D	C	T	M	L	**V**		HCV NS5 714-722	82
T	G	A	P	V	T	Y	S	T	Y	HCV NS3 281-290	83
V	I	Y	Q	Y	M	D	D	**L**		HIV-1RT 179-187	84
V	**L**	P	D	V	F	I	R	C	**V**	N-acetylglucosaminyltransferase V Gnt-V intron	85
V	**L**	P	D	V	F	I	R	C		N-acetylglucosaminyltransferase V Gnt-V intron	85
A	V	G	I	G	I	A	V	**V**		Human CD9	86
L	V	V	L	G	L	L	A	**V**		Human glutamyltransferase	86
A	**L**	G	L	G	L	L	P	**V**		Human G protein coupled receptor 164-172	86
G	**I**	G	I	G	V	L	A	A		HSV-1 gp C 480-488	86
G	A	G	I	G	V	A	V	**L**		HSV-2 gp C 446-454	86
I	A	G	I	G	I	L	A	I		Pseudorabies gpGIII 455-463	86
L	I	V	I	G	I	L	I	**L**		Adenovirus 3 E3 9kD 30-38	86
L	A	G	I	G	L	I	A	A		*S. lincolnensis* lmrA	86
V	D	G	I	G	I	L	T	I		Yeast ysa-1 77-85	86
G	A	G	I	G	V	L	T	A		*B. polymyxa*, β-endoxylanase 149-157	86
A	A	G	I	G	I	I	Q	I		*E. coli* methionine synthase 590-598	86
Q	A	G	I	G	I	L	L	A		*E. coli* hypothetical protein 4-12	86

Table 4.2. (con't)

	Position											Source	Ref.
		1	**2**	3	4	5	6	7	8	**9**			
	K	A	R	D	P	H	S	G	H	F	**V**	CDK4[wt] 22-32	87
	K	A	C	D	P	H	S	G	H	F	**V**	CDK4-R24C 22-32	87
		A	C	D	P	H	S	G	H	F	**V**	CDK4-R24C 23-32	87
		S	**L**	Y	N	T	V	A	T	**L**		HIV-1 gag p17 77-85	88
		E	**L**	V	S	E	F	S	R	**V**		HER-2, M>V substituted 971-979	89
		R	G	P	G	R	A	F	V	T	I	HIV-1 gp160 315-329	90
		H	**M**	W	N	F	I	S	G	I		HCV NS4A 149-157	91
		N	**L**	V	P	M	V	A	T	V	Q	HCMV pp65 495-504	92
		G	**L**	H	C	Y	E	Q	L	**V**		HPV 6b E7 21-30	93
		P	**L**	K	Q	H	F	Q	I	**V**		HPV 6b E7 47-55	93
		L	**L**	D	F	V	R	F	M	G	**V**	EBNA-6 284-293	95
Examples for other binding peptides		A	I	M	E	K	N	I	M	**L**		Influenza Alaska NS 1 122-130	67
		Y	**L**	K	T	I	Q	N	S	**L**		*P. falciparum* cp36 CSP	96
		Y	**L**	N	K	I	Q	N	S	**L**		*P. falciparum* cp39 CSP	96
		Y	**M**	L	D	L	Q	P	E	T	T	HPV16 E7 11-20***	97
		L	**L**	M	G	T	L	G	I	**V**		HPV16 E7 82-90***	97
		T	**L**	G	I	V	C	P	I			HPV16 E7 86-93***	97
		T	**L**	T	S	C	N	T	S	**V**		HIV-1 gp120 197-205	98
		K	**L**	P	Q	L	C	T	E	**L**		HPV16 E6 18-26	97
		T	I	H	D	I	I	L	E	C		HPV16 E6 29-37	97
		L	G	I	V	C	P	I	C	S		HPV16 E7 87-95	97
		V	I	L	G	V	L	L	L	I		Melan A/Mart-1 35-43	68
		A	**L**	M	D	K	S	L	H	**V**		Melan A/Mart-1 56-64	68
		G	I	L	T	V	I	L	G	**V**		Melan A/Mart-1 31-39	68

* Class I ligands allocated to A2 by motif.
** minor H antigen
*** potential T cell antigens
[1] B indicates D or N
[2] X indicates I or L
[+]also a T cell epitope

HLA-A*0202	Position										Source	Ref.
	1	**2**	3	4	5	6	7	8	**9**			
Anchor residues		**L**							**L** **V**			99
Other preferred residues	A F G V I	A	F A	E D	I	I L V T	H Q					
T cell epitopes	M	I	N	A	Y	L	D	K	**L**		*P. falciparum* STARP 523-531	81
	A	A	G	I	G	I	L	T	**V**		Melan A/Mart-1 27-35	100
	F	**L**	P	S	D	F	F	P	S	**V**	HBV cAg 18-27	51

HLA-A*0203	Sequence	Source	Ref.
Motif unknown T cell epitope	S V R D R L A R L	EBNA-3 464-472	101

HLA-A*0204	Position									Source	Ref.
	1	**2**	3	4	5	6	7	8	**9**		
Anchor or auxiliary anchor residues		**L**							**L**		102
Preferred residues				E P		L I					
T cell epitope	A	A	G	I	G	I	L	T	V	Melan A/Mart-1 27-35	100

Table 4.2. (con't)

HLA-A*0205	**Position**										**Source**	**Ref.**
	1	**2**	3	4	5	6	7	8	**9**			
Anchor or auxiliary anchor residues		**V**				I			**L**			103, 99
		L				V						
		I				L						
		M				A						
		Q										
Other preferred residues	F		Y	G	Y	T	Q	K				
	V		P	E	V	H	Y					
	Y		F	D	L	V						
	A		I	K	I							
			M	N								
				P								
Examples for ligands	A	**V**	P	D	E	I	P	P	**L**		HSP90 703-711	99
	F	A	Y	D	G	K	D	Y	I		Human MHC I-α 140-148	99
T cell epitopes	A	A	G	I	G	I	L	T	V		Melan A/Mart-1 27-35	100
	F	**L**	P	S	D	F	F	P	S	V	HBV cAg 18-27	51
HLA-A*0206	**Position**										**Source**	**Ref.**
	1	**2**	3	4	5	6	7	8	**9**			
Anchor or auxiliary anchor residues		**V**							**V**			102
Preferred residues		Q	I	E		L			L			
			L	P								
T cell epitopes	A	A	G	I	G	I	L	T	**V**		Melan A/Mart-1 27-35	100
	F	L	P	S	D	F	F	P	S	**V**	HBV cAg 18-27	51
HLA-A*0207	**Position**										**Source**	**Ref.**
	1	**2**	**3**	4	5	6	7	8	**9**			
Anchor or auxiliary anchor residues		**L**	**D**						**L**			102
Preferred residues			P	E		I						

HLA-A*0209	Sequence	Source	Ref.
Motif unknown T cell epitope	A A G I G I L T V	Melan A/Mart-1 27-35	100

HLA-A*0214	Position										Source	Ref.
	1	**2**	3	4	5	6	7	8	**9**			
Anchor or auxiliary anchor residues		**V,Q** **L**				I,L V,F			**L** **V**			99
Other preferred residues	F,Y V,A	A	I,L M,D Y,P	D,E P,G K		K,N		R,Y	M			
Examples for ligands	F	**V**	L	P	E	L	P	S	**V**		Expressed sequence tag	99
	Y	**V**	I	S	V	V	F	R	**L**		Connexin 32 135-143	99
	F	**Q**	L	E	I	N	V	R	**L**		Unknown	99
	K	**Q**	L	D	D	L	K	V	E	**L**	60S ribosomal protein L35 18-27	99
	H	**L**	P	S	D	F	T	P	A	**V**	Bovine hemoglobin 112-121	99
	I	**L**	M	E	H	I	H	K	**L**		60S ribosomal protein L19 137-145	99
	F	A	Y	D	G	K	D	Y	I		MHC I α chain 140-148	99
	F	A	Y	D	G	K	D	Y	**L**		HLA-E-precursor 137-145	99
	S	T	L	H	L	V	R	**L**			Ubiquitin 65-73	99

HLA-A3	Position									Source	Ref.
	1	**2**	3	4	5	6	7	8	**9**		
Anchor or auxiliary anchor residues		**L** **V** **M**	F Y			I M F V L	I L M F		**K** **Y** **F**		104, 105, 24
Other preferred residues	I				I P V K	T		Q S T K			
Examples for ligands	K	X	F	K	M	I	L	R	**K**	Unknown	104
	K	**L**	F	K	N	I	L	Y	**K**	Unknown	104

Table 4.2. (con't)

	Position											Source	Ref.
	1	**2**	3	4	5	6	7	8	**9**				
	Y	**L**	X	V	R	X	A	X	i	V		Unknown	104
	K	**L**	H	K	Q	R	A	K	S			Unknown	104
	S	**L**	F	K	Q	V	V	T	**K**			Unknown	104
	K	X	F	V	K	X	L	X	**Y**			Unknown	104
	S	**L**	F	N	T	H	L	X	**K**			Unknown	104
	T	**L**	A	N	D	X	V	V	P			Unknown	104
	G	I	F	A	X	X	X	V	K	A		Unknown	104
	T	X	F	V	K	X	L	X	**Y**			Unknown	104
	S	**L**	F	D	H	I	L	X	K	H		Unknown	104
	K	**L**	F	K	V	V	X	N	**Y**			Unknown	104
	K	**L**	Y	E	K	V	Y	T	Y	**K**		Unknown	104
	K	**L**	F	N	I	M	V	T	**Y**			Unknown	104
	K	**L**	F	E	K	V	Y	N	**Y**			Unknown	104
	K	**L**	F	K	V	T	F	S	**Y**			Unknown	104
	G	**L**	F	P	X	Q	F	A	**Y**			Unknown	104
	S	**L**	F	E	L	V	F	X	**Y**			Unknown	104
	S	**L**	X	E	K	T	F	D	**Y**			Unknown	104
	S	**L**	H	K	Y	X	f	e	**Y**			Unknown	104
	K	**M**	F	N	I	T	v	T	**Y**			Unknown	104
	K	**L**	F	V	K	V	y	N	**Y**			Unknown	104
	K	I	V	R	K	P	G	M	A			Unknown	104
	G	P	P	G	V	T	I	V	**K**			Unknown kidney peptide	106
	K	I	K	S	F	E	V	V	**F**			Unknown	26
	A	**L**	L	A	V	G	A	T	**K**			pmel17 gp100 17-25	107
	N	**V**	I	R	D	A	V	T	**Y**			Histon H4 65-73	26
	R	**V**	Y	I	G	R	L	S	**Y**			Splicing factor 3-11	26
	S	**L**	Y	A	S	S	P	G	G	V	**Y**	Vimentin 51-61	26
T cell epitopes	R	**L**	R	D	L	L	L	I	V	T	R	HIV-1 gp41 768-778	108
	Q	**V**	P	L	R	P	M	T	Y	**K**		HIV-1 nef 73-82	109
	T	**V**	Y	Y	G	V	P	V	W	**K**		HIV-1 gp120 36-45	110
	R	**L**	R	P	G	G	K	K	**K**			HIV-1 gag p17 20-29	110
	I	**L**	R	G	S	V	A	H	**K**			Influenza NP 265-273	21
	R	**L**	R	A	E	A	G	V	**K**			EBNA-3 603-611	111
	R	**L**	R	D	L	L	L	I	V	T	R	HIV-1 gp41 770-780	112
	V	Y	Y	G	V	P	V	W	**K**			HIV-1 gp120 38-46	113
	R	**V**	C	E	K	M	A	L	**Y**			HCV NS5 575-583	114

HLA-A*0301	Sequence	Source	Ref.
Motif unknown T cell epitope	K I F S E V T L K	Unknown; mutated (P182L) melanoma peptide 175-183	Wölfel et al., pers. comm.

HLA-A*1101	Position	Source	Ref.
	1 2 3 4 5 6 7 8 **9**		
Anchor or auxiliary anchor residues	2: V, I, F, Y 3: M, L, F, Y, I, A 7: L, I, Y, V, F 9: **K**		115, 20, 24
Other preferred residues	1: A 2: T 3: N, D, E, Q 4: P, G, D, E, K 5: P, I, F, V, M 6: I, V, M 8: R, K, N, E, Q 9: R		
Examples for ligands	A V M K P E A E K R **K**	Unknown	20
	A V I L P P L S P Y F **K**	HSB 66 EST 18-29	20
	A S F D K A K L K **K**	Thymosin β-10 11-20	20
	G Q Y G N P L N **K**	Bovine metalloproteinase 19-27	20
	G V M P S H F S R	40S ribosomal protein S19 93-101	20
	Y F D P A N G K F S **K**	Elongation factor 2 265-275	20
	A T A G D G L I E L R **K**	Prohibitin (rat) 229-240	20, 24
	S T Y Y G S F V T R	Unknown (also presented by A33)	115, 20
	S V L N L V I V **K**	40S ribosomal protein S6 107-115	24
	K V V N P L F E **K**	60S ribosomal protein L7A 25-33	24
	R T Q N V L G E **K**	40S ribosomal protein S3 54-62	24
	G T M T T S X Y **K**	Unknown	24
	A S F D K A K L **K**	Thymosin β-10 11-19	24
	A A M X D T V V F **K**	Unknown	24
	R V E Q A V E S M V **K**	Unknown	24

Table 4.2. (con't)

	Position	Source	Ref.
	1 2 3 4 5 6 7 8 **9**		
	Y V N V N M G L **K***	HBV cAg 88-96	116
T cell epitopes	I V T D F S V I **K**	EBNA-4 416-424	115, 117
	E L N E A L E L **K**	p53 343-351	115
	V P L R P M T Y **K**	HIV-1 nef 74-82	115
	A I F Q S S M T **K**	HIV-1 gag p24 325-333	115
	Q V P L R P M T **Y** **K**	HIV-1 nef 73-82	118
	S T A P P A H G V	Epithelial cell mucin, MUC-1 9-17	119
	T I N Y T I F **K**	HCV NS1 238-246	114
	A A V D L S H F L K E **K**	HIV-1 nef 83-94	120
	G S P A T W T T R	Type IV collagen 51-59	121
	ACQ G V G G P G G H **K**	HIV-1 IIIB p24 349-359	122
* also a T cell epitope			

HLA-A23	Sequence	Source	Ref.
Motif unknown			
T cell epitope	Y I S W C L W W	HCV NS2 109-117	114

HLA-A24	Position									Source	Ref.
	1	**2**	3	4	5	6	7	8	**9**		
Anchor or auxiliary anchor residues		**Y**			I, V	F			**I**, **L**, **F**		105
Other preferred residues		F	N, E, L, M, P, G	D, P, E, K			Q, N	E, K			
Examples for ligands	K	**Y**	P	E	N	F	F	L	**L**	Protein phosphatase 1 113-121	24
	Y	**Y**	E	E	Q	H	P	E	**L**	NK/T cell activation protein 107-115	24
	A	**Y**	V	H	M	V	T	H	**F**	Unknown	24
	V	**Y**	X	K	H	P	V	S	**X**	Unknown	24

T cell epitopes	S **Y** L D S G I H **F***	β-catenin, mutated (proto-oncogen) 29-37	123
	R **Y** L K D Q Q L **L**	HIV gp 41 583-591	124
	A **Y** G L D F Y I **L**	p15 melanoma Ag 10-18	125
	A F L P W H R L F **L**	Tyrosinase 206-215	126
	A F L P W H R L **F**	Tyrosinase 206-214	126
	R **Y** S I F F D Y	EBNA-3 246-253	101

* also a T cell epitope

HLA-A25	**Sequence**	**Source**	**Ref.**
Motif unknown			
T cell epitope	E T I N E E A A E W	HIV-1 gag p24 203-212	127

HLA-A*2902	**Position**	**Source**	**Ref.**
	1 **2** 3 4 5 6 7 8 **9**		
Anchor or auxilliary anchor residues	**E** (2), **Y** (9)		128
Other preferred residues	2: M; 3: F, V,I, A,K, L; 4: P; 5: V; 7: Y; 9: L		
Examples for ligands	X[1] **E** V D V E Y - **Y**	Unknown	128
	X **E** F D T - E S **Y**	Unknown	128
	K **E** I E L I L E **Y**	Unknown	128
	X **E** - P M A E A **-**	Unknown	128
	X **E** D D Q Q Q A L V	Unknown	128
	X **E** K Y I D Q E E L	Human HSP90 α-chain 481-490	128
	X **E** F F P E Y Y **Y** **Y**	Unknown	128
	K **E** F Q E H Y E **Y**	Unknown	128
	X **E** F Q V Y L - Q	Unknown	128
	X **E** I Q I N V Q	Unknown	128
	X **E** V N N V A L L	Unknown	128
	P **E** M S V - - L L	Unknown	128
	X **E** I G A G A T G A	Unknown	128
	K **E** S T L H L V L	Human ubiquitin 64-72	128
	X **E** F P L V V - L	Unknown	128
	X **E** F T L - L A **Y**	Unknown	128

Table 4.2. (con't)

HLA-A*3101	Position											Comments	Ref.
	1	2	3	4	5	6	7	8	**9**				
Anchor or auxiliary anchor residues		L	F			L			**R**				20
		V	L			F							
		Y	Y			V							
		F	W			I							
Other preferred residues	K	T	K	P	P	T	N	L				P1 deduced from individual ligands	
	R	Q	N	D	I	N	V	R					
				E	V	D	R	N					
				G	F	E	F	Q					
				S	L	R	T						
				V	Y		H						
				T	W		L						
							Y						
												Source	
Examples for ligands	L	Q	F	P	V	G	R	V	H	**R**		Histone H2a 23-32	20
	Q	Q	L	Y	W	S	H	P	**R**			40S ribosomal protein S29 (rat) 3-11	20
	R	G	Y	R	P	R	F	R	**R**			CCAAT-binding transcription factor 240-248	20
	K	V	F	G	P	I	H	E	**R**			[GlcNac]-P-transferase 371-379	20
	K	I	M	K	W	N	Y	E	**R**			Unknown	20
	R	Y	M	D	A	W	N	T	Y	S	**R**	Lamin B2	20
T cell epitopes	S	T	L	P	E	T	T	V	V	R	**R**	HBV cAg 141-151	129
	M	S	L	Q	R	Q	F	L	**R**			ORF 3P-gp75 294-321 (bp)	130
	L	L	P	G	G	R	P	Y	**R**			TRP-2 (tyrosinase rel.) 197-205	131

HLA-A*3302	Position									Comments	Ref.
	1	2	3	4	5	6	7	8	**9**		
Anchor or auxiliary anchor residues		A							**R**		20
		I									
		L									
		F									
		Y									
		V									
Preferred residues	D	T	L	P	P	I				P1 deduced from individual ligands	
	E		K			L					
					F						

	1	2	3	4	5	6	7	8	9				Source	Ref.
Other possible residues	M		Q	R	R	R	H	Q						
			W	D	I	D	Y	N						
			E	E	F	H	V	E						
			N	G	P	Y	T	M						
				S	V		S							
				H	L									
				P	W									
Examples for ligands	D	M	A	A	Q	I	T	Q	**R**				HLA class I α-chain 161-169	20
	E	S	G	P	S	I	V	H	**R**				Actin 364-372	20
	T	Y	Y	G	S	F	V	T	**R**				Unknown	20
	D	Y	I	H	I	R	I	Q	Q	**R**			Human protein translation factor-sui homologue 65-74	20
	E	I	M	K	W	N	R	E	**R**				Unknown	20
	T	I	M	P	K	D	I	Q	L	A	R	**R**	Histone 3.1/3.3 118-129	20
T cell epitope	I	V	G	L	N	K	I	V	**R**				HIV gag p24 267-275	132, 133

HLA-A*6801	**Position**												**Source**	**Ref.**
	1	**2**	3	4	5	6	7	8	**9**					
Anchor residues		**V**							**R**					134
		T							**K**					
	D													99
	E													
Examples for ligands	A	**V**	A	A	V	A	A	R	**R**				Unknown	134
	E	**V**	A	P	P	E	Y	H	**R**				Unknown	134
	E	**V**	A	P	P	E	Y	H	R	**K**			Unknown	134
	D	**V**	F	R	D	P	A	L	**K**				60S ribsomal protein L27 98-106	134
	K	**T**	G	G	P	I	Y	K	**R**+				Influenza NP 91-99	134, 135
	E	**V**	I	L	I	D	P	F	H	**K**			Unknown	134
	T	**V**	F	D	A	K	R	L	I	G	**R**		HSP70B / HSC70 66-76	134

Table 4.2. (continued)

	Position											Comments	Ref.
	X	**V**	L	K	X	I	A	K	**R***			Unknown	38
	P	**V**	K	Q	V	V	Y	H	**R***			Unknown	38
	E	S	G	P	S	I	V	H	R	**K***		β-Actin 364-373	38
	T	**T**	X	T	T	T	N	A	**R***			Unknown	38
	D	**T**	T	P	T	X	X	**R***				Unknown	38
T cell epitopes	S	**T**	L	P	E	T	T	V	V	R	**R**	HBV cAg 141-151	129
	F	L	P	S	D	F	F	P	S	V		HBV cAg 18-27	51
Examples for other binding peptides	K	**T**	G	G	P	I	Y	K	**R**			Influenza NP 91-99	96

*Class I ligands allocated to A68.1 by motif.
+Also a T cell epitope

HLA-A*6901	Position											Source	Ref.
	1	**2**	3	4	5	6	7	8	**9**				
Anchor or auxilliary residues		**V**	I			I			**V**				99
		T	F			F			**L**				
		A	L			L							
			M										
Preferred residues	E		V	D	P	V		Y	M				
			Y	E				R					
				R				Q					
				P									
Examples for ligands	E	**T**	F	N	T	P	A	H	Y	**V**		γ actin 126-135	99
	E	**T**	V	A	V	G	V	I	K	A	**V**	Elongation factor 1-α1 431-441	99
	A	**A**	G	I	G	I	L	T	**V**			Melan A/Mart-1 27-35	100

HLA-B7	Position									Source	Ref.
	1	**2**	3	4	5	6	7	8	**9**		
Anchor or auxiliary anchor residues		**P**	R						**L**		136, 105
									F		
Other preferred residues				D	D	F	L				
				G	P	T					

Also detected	A		D	E	I	R	V						
	H		E	H	V	L							
	S		Q	L		I							
			K	K									
			Y	S									
			F	T									
			M	P									
			N										
			A										
Examples for ligands	A	**P**	R	T	V	A	L	T	A			HLA-DP signal sequence 9-17	136
	A	**P**	R	T	V	A	L	T	A	**L**		HLA-DP signal sequence 9-18	136
	A	**P**	R	A	X	X	X	X	X			Unknown	136
	A	**P**	R	X	P	X	T	G	X			Unknown	136
	A	**P**	R	A	S	R	P	S	X			Unknown	136
	A	**P**	R	T	L	V	L	L	**L**			HLA-A2.1 signal sequence 5-13	136
	M	**P**	R	G	V	V	V	T	X			Unknown	136
	S	**P**	R	Y	I	F	T	M	**L**			Topoisomerase II 801-809	136
	A	**P**	A	P	T	V	A	V	X			Unknown	136
	R	**P**	S	G	P	G	P	E	X			Unknown	136
	L	V	M	A	P	R	T	V	**L**			HLA-B7 signal sequence 2-10	136
	R	V	M	A	P	R	A	X	X			Unknown	136
	A	**P**	R	A	F	X	P	X	P	V		Unknown	136
	A	A	S	K	E	R	S	G	V	S	**L**	Histone H1 49-59	136
	A	**P**	R	S	N	G	M	V	X			Unknown	25
	A	**P**	R	Q	P	G	X	M	A			Unknown	25
	A	**P**	A	P	P	P	K	P	M			40S ribosomal protein S26 107-115	25
	A	**P**	Y	G	G	P	X	A	X			Unknown	25
	R	**P**	K	S	N	I	V	L	**L**			CD20 222-230	136
	S	**P**	S	V	D	K	A	R	A	E	**L**	Human SMCY	137

Table 4.2. (con't)

		Position													Source	Ref.
		1	**2**	3	4	5	6	7	8	**9**						
T cell epitopes		T	**P**	G	P	G	V	R	Y	P	**L**				HIV-1 nef 128-137	120
		Q	**P**	R	A	P	I	R	P	I					EBNA-6 881-889	138
		R	**P**	P	I	F	I	R	R	**L**					EBNA-3 379-387	138
		E	**P**	D	V	P	P	G	A	I					EBNA-1 426-434	66
		I	**P**	Q	C	R	L	T	P	**L**					EBNA-1 228-236	66
		G	**P**	G	P	Q	P	G	P	**L**					EBNA-1 546-554	66
		Q	**P**	G	P	L	R	E	S	I					EBNA-1 550-558	66
		R	**P**	Q	K	R	P	S	C	I					EBNA-1 72-80	66
		P	**P**	T	P	L	L	T	V	**L**					EBNA-2 224-232	66
		T	**P**	S	P	P	R	M	H	**L**					EBNA-2 241-249	66
		P	**P**	R	M	H	L	P	V	**L**					EBNA-2 244-252	66
		V	**P**	D	Q	S	M	H	P	**L**					EBNA-2 254-262	66
		P	**P**	S	I	D	P	A	D	**L**					EBNA-2 446-454	66
		L	**P**	C	V	L	W	P	V	**L**					BZLF1 44-52	66
		C	**P**	S	L	D	V	D	S	I	I				BZLF1 222-231	66
		T	**P**	D	V	L	H	E	D	**L**					BZLF1 234-242	66
		G	**P**	R	L	G	V	R	A	T					HCV core protein 40-48	114
		M	**P**	N	D	P	N	R	N	V					P. falciparum CSP 300-308	81
		S	**P**	S	S	N	R	I	R	N	T				Human RAGE-1 from ORF2 11-20	139
		K	**P**	L	D	G	E	Y	F	T	**L**				p53 321-330	140
Examples for other binding peptides		A	**P**	R	M	P	E	A	A	P	R	V			p53 63-73	140
		A	**P**	P	Q	H	L	I	R	V					p53 189-197	140
		L	**P**	E	N	N	V	L	S	P	**L**				p53 26-35	140
		A	**P**	P	Q	H	R	I	R	V					p53 189-197	140
		R	**P**	I	L	T	I	I	T	**L**					p53 249-257	140
		A	**P**	R	M	P	E	A	A	P	P	V			p53 63-73	140
		R	**P**	R	K	L	P	Q	**L**						HPV E6 15-22	141
	RK	T	**P**	R	V	T	G	G	G	A	M	A	G	A	HCMV pp65 415-429	92

HLA-B*0702	Position											Source	Ref.
	1	**2**	3	4	5	6	7	8	**9**				
Anchor or auxiliary anchor residues		**P**							**L**				142, 143
Other preferred residues	A,R	V	R,K	E			Y	F					
Also detected			N,H	L	V	R,T	L						
			F	G,T									
			M,Q										
			L,Y										
Examples for ligands	A	**P**	R	A	S	R	P	S	**L**			Unknown	143
	A	A	S	K	E	R	S	G	V	S	**L**	Histone H1 40-50	143
	R	**P**	R	H	Q	G	V	M	V			β-actin 37-45	143
	A	**P**	R	T	V	A	L	T	A			HLA-DP signal sequence 9-17	143
	R	V	M	A	P	R	A	L	**L**			Unknown	143
	R	**P**	K	S	N	I	V	L	**L**			CD20 222-230	143

HLA-B*0703	Position									Source	Ref.
	1	**2**	3	4	5	6	7	8	**9**		
Anchor or auxiliary anchor residues		**P**	R					E	**L**		142
Other preferred residues	A	N	A	Q	M	R		F			
	R	D	T	E		D					
			Q	I							
			M,F								
			H								

HLA-B*0705	Position									Source	Ref.
	1	**2**	3	4	5	6	7	8	**9**		
Anchor or auxiliary anchor residues		**P**							**L**		142
Other preferred residues	A,R		A,L	G,E					F		
			M,Q	R							
			Y,S								
			I,F								
			K,N								
			E,T								
			W								

Table 4.2. (con't)

HLA-B8	Position									Source	Ref.
	1	2	**3**	4	**5**	6	7	8	**9**		
Anchor residues			**K**		**K**				**L**		144, 145, 146
					R						
Other preferred residues	G		R	E		N	E	E	F		
	L			Q		Q	H	Q	M		
	I			D		H	M	H			
				H		I	N	S			
				L		L	D	L			
				S		Y	Q	V			
				T		V	S	D			
				R		E	T	T			
				G		M	Y				
				K		S					
						T					
						F					
Examples for ligands	H	P	**K**	Y	**K**	T	E	**L**		Tristetraproline 148-155	146
	I	L	**K**	Q	**K**	I	A	d	**I**	IL-6 precursor 161-169	146
	E	L	**K**	V	**K**	N	I	e	**I**	Restin 1273-1281	146
	E	P	**K**	Y	**K**	T	Q	**L**		Yeast PRAI-SCS 95-102	146
	V	P	**K**	L	**K**	V	X	A	**L**	60S ribosomal protein L18 (rat) 94-102	146
	F	A	**K**	P	**R**	V	G	G		Unknown	146
	S	P	**K**	L	**K**	Y	M	Q		Unknown	146
	E	L	**K**	K	**K**	T	N	**I**		Unknown	146
	S	P	**K**	E	**K**	I	X	Y		Unknown	146
	X	A	**K**	E	**K**	L	A	D		Unknown	146
	S	P	**K**	E	**K**	Y	E	X		Unknown	146
	E	L	**K**	E	**K**	T	Q	**L**		Unknown	146
	L	P	**K**	V	**K**	L	A	**L**		Unknown	146
	H	p	**K**	Y	**K**	T	E	**L**		Unknown	146
	V	L	D	L	**K**	I	V	A	**F**	Unknown	146
	G	P	**K**	E	**K**	X	A	**M**		Unknown	146
	G	L	**K**	V	**K**	G	N	E	**F**	Unknown	146
	F	L	**K**	P	**K**	F	V	A	**L**	Unknown	146
	E	L	**K**	I	**K**	V	Y	X	**I**	Unknown	146
	S	L	**K**	E	**K**	V	X	**L**		Unknown	146

	Position	Source	Ref.
	1 2 **3** 4 **5** 6 7 8 **9**		
	E L **K** E **K** X y e **I**	Unknown	146
	I P **K** L **K** N V K r	Unknown	146
	S L **K** I **K** X L	Unknown	146
	D L **K** Q **K** N E **L**	Unknown	146
T cell epitopes	E L **R** S **R** Y W A **I**	Influenza NP 380-388	145
	F L **R** G **R** A Y G **L**	EBNA-3 339-347	147
	E I Y K **R** W I I **L**	HIV gag p24, 262-270	146, 148
	G E I Y **K** R W I **I**	HIV gag p24, 261-269	146, 148
	E I **K** D T K E A **L**	HIV gag p17, 93-101	146, 149
	Y L **K** D Q Q L **L**	HIV gag gp41 586-593	150
	A S **K** N **K** E K A **L**	*P. falciparum* ssp 2 107-115	151
	H S **K** K **K** C D E **L**	HCV NS3 389-397	114
	L R **K** P **K** H K K **L**	*P. falciparum* CSP 105-113	81
	Q A **K** W **R** L Q T **L**	EBNA-3 NP 26-34	101
	G G **K** K **K** Y K **L**	HIV-1 gag p17 24-31	152
Examples for other binding peptides	K N **K** E **K** A L I I	*P. falciparum* TRAP	96
	A Y P L H E Q H G	EBNA-3 325-333	94
	Y I **K** S F V S D A	EBNA-3 158-166	94

HLA-B13	**Sequence**	**Source**	**Ref.**
Motif unknown			
Examples for ligands	A A D D X* F K D	Human oncoprotein c-abl 793-800	43
	A A I G Y M X K	Unknown	43
*: X may be L or I			

HLA-B14	**Position**	**Source**	**Ref.**
	1 **2** <u>3</u> 4 **5** <u>6</u> 7 8 **9** HLA-B14	Position	
Anchor or auxiliary anchor residues	**R** L **R** I **L** **K** Y **H** L F		146

Table 4.2. (con't)

	Position										Source	Ref.
	1	**2**	3	4	**5**	6	7	8	**9**			
Examples for ligands	D	A	Y	R	**r**	I	H	S	**L**		HSrn 234-242	146
	S	G	V	I	T	L	N	T	n		Unknown	146
	A	**R**	Y	D	**R**	S	G	R	Y	I	Unknown	146
	E	**R**	L	K	I	R	G	S	**L**		40S ribosomal protein S25 75-83	146
	D	**R**	H	E	**R**	I	T	K	**L**		Unknown	146
	E	**r**	f	t	x	I	x	g			Unknown	146
	V	X	D	P	X	g	t	g			Unknown	146
	D	**R**	K	L	**R**	I	N	S	**L**		Unknown	146
	E	**R**	Y	P	**R**	Y	N	Q	**L**		Unknown	146
	G	**R**	Y	F	**R**	I	Q	E	Y		Unknown	146
	S	**R**	D	L	**R**	V	i	X	g		Unknown	146
	E	**R**	T	L	**h**	L	v	E	l		Unknown	146
	D	**R**	A								Unknown	146
	S	G	L	G	X	I	T				Unknown	146
	E	**R**	L	K	**R**	L	t	S	**L**		Unknown	146
	S	G	F	I	G	L	T	Q	**L**		Unknown	146
	D	**K**	Y	E	**R**	L	V	Q			Unknown	146
	I	F	F	A	**R**	I	Q	G			Unknown	146
	S	**R**	L	N	X	L					Unknown	146
	D	**R**	Y	I	**H**	A	V	L	**L**		Unknown	146
	D	**R**	L	E	**R**	I	T	Q	**L**		Unknown	146
	T	**R**	Y	E	**H**	P					Unknown	146
	L	F	L	A	**R**	I					Unknown	146
	D	E	L	I	G	I	T	S	**L**		Unknown	146
T cell epitopes	E	**R**	Y	L	K	D	Q	Q	**L**		HIV env gp41 584-592	150
	D	**R**	F	Y	K	T	L	R	A		HIV-1 gag p24 298-306	88

HLA-B*1501 (B62)	Sequence											Source	Ref.
	1	**2**	3	4	5	6	7	8	**9**				
Anchor or auxiliary anchor residues		**Q**			I				**F**				153, 154
		L			V				**Y**				
Other preferred residues	I	M	K	P	G	V	V	Y					
		V	A	E	L	T	T	V					
			N	G	F	G	L	T					
			F	D	T	I	I						
			P				M						
			Y										
			H										
			R										
Examples for ligands	V	**L**	K	P	G	M	V	V	T	**F**		Elongation factor α 1 271-280	153
	Y	**L**	G	E	F	S	I	T	**Y**			40S ribosomal protein S15 114-122	153
	G	**Q**	R	K	G	A	G	S	V			60S ribosomal protein L8 (rat) 7-15	153
	K	I	K	S	F	V	K	V	**Y**			60S ribosomal protein L27 66-74	153
	I	**Q**	P	G	R	G	F	V	L	**Y**		Unknown	153
	S	**Q**	F	G	G	G	S	Q	**Y**			Unknown	153, 154
	G	**Q**	R	K	P	A	T	S	**Y**			60S ribosomal protein L28 (rat) 68-76	153
	V	**Q**	G	P	V	G	L					Collagen α1 1106-1112	153
	G	**Q**	R	K	G	A	G	S	V	**Y**		60S ribosomal protein L8 (human) 7-16	154
T cell epitopes	I	**L**	G	L	N	K	I	V	R	M	**Y**	HIV gag p24 267-277	132
	Q	N	G	A	L	A	I	N	T	**F**		EBNA-6B 213-222 (B62 epitope)	95

HLA-B17	Sequence	Source	Ref
Motif unknown			
T cell epitopes	YHTQGYFPQWQ	HIV-I nef 115-125	120
	TQGYFPQWQNYT	HIV-I nef 117-128	120
	KSLYDEHI	*P.falciparum* LSA-1 1854-1861	81
	GIWGCSGKLICTTAV	HIV-SF2 gp41 593-607	156

HLA-B18	Sequence	Source	Ref.
Motif unknown			
T cell epitopes	GVRYPLTFGWCYKLVP	HIV-I nef 132-147	120
	SDEEEAIVAYTL	CMV immediate early protein E1 978-989	157

Table 4.2. (con't)

HLA-B22	Sequence	Source	Ref.
T cell epitope	ALIWEDLRSLCLFSY	HIV-SF2 gp41 753-767	156

HLA-B27	1	**2**	3	4	5	6	7	8	**9**			Comment / Source	Ref.
Anchor residues		**R**										Different P9 specificities are found in different subtypes	158
												Source	
T cell epitopes	S	**R**	R	Y	P	D	A	V	Y	L	H	MV F protein 437-447	159
	I	**R**	R	G	V	M	L	A	V			Human HSP60 140-148	160
	K	**R**	I	Q	E	I	I	E	Q			Human HSP60 369-377	160
	K	**R**	T	L	K	I	P	A	M			Human HSP60 469-477	160
	G	**R**	N	V	V	L	D	K	S			Yersinia HSP60 35-43	160
	K	**R**	G	I	D	K	A	V	I			Yersinia HSP60 117-125	160
	I	**R**	A	A	S	A	I	T	A			Yersinia HSP60 420-428	160

HLA-B*2702	1	**2**	3	4	5	6	7	8	**9**		Source	Ref.
Anchor residues		**R**							**F** **Y** **I** **L** **W**			158
Other preferred residues	K		F L X	G P K D E Q T S	I K E V M T	I V Y R D H E Q	Y L V T F	K V D E R				
Examples for ligands	S	**R**	D	K	T	I	I	M	**W**		HGNBPβ-subunit 35-43	158
	G	**R**	L	T	K	H	T	K	**F**		60S ribosomal protein L36 (rat) 36-44	158
	R	**R**	F	V	N	V	V	P	T	**F**	Human fau protein 114-123	158
	K	**R**	Y	K	S	I	V	K	**Y**		HFPS 191-199	158
	K	**R**	K	K	A	Y	A	D	**F**		Cytochrome C oxidase 42-50	158
	K	**R**	G	I	L	T	L	K	**Y**		Actin 63-71	158

HLA-B*2702	1	**2**	3	4	5	6	7	8	**9**	Source	Ref.
A	G	**R**	F	G	V	G	N	R	**Y**	Unknown	158
	G	**R**	F	K	L	I	V	L	**Y**	Unknown	158
T cell epitopes	K	**R**	W	I	I	L	G	L	N	HIV gag p24 263-271	161
	L	**R**	S	R	Y	W	A	I		Influenza NP 381-388	162

HLA-B*2704	Sequence	Source	Ref.
Motif unknown T cell epitope	RRRWRRLTV	EBV LMP-2 236-244	168

HLA-B*2705	1	**2**	3	4	5	6	7	8	**9**				Source	Ref.
Anchor or auxiliary anchor residues		**R**							**L**					3, 158
									F					
Other preferred residues	A		L	K	I	I	I	K	Y					
	G		I	Q	V	A	T	N	M					
	K		F	E	L	N	Y	R	I					
	R			G	P	Q	M	E	R					
					G	D	L	Q	H					
						V	W		K					
						K	N							
							V							
							P							
Examples for ligands	G	**R**	L	T	K	H	T	K	**F**				60S ribosomal protein L36 36-44	158
	A	**R**	L	F	G	I	R	A	**K**				HBBCP 190-198	3,158
	R	**R**	L	G	X	Q	Y	R	**R**				Unknown	158
	R	**R**	F	G	D	K	L	N	**F**				Immediate early response gene 87-95	158
	G	**R**	v	F	I	I	K	E					Homologous to Il-1 receptor antagonist	158
	G	**R**	X	X	i	f	X	r	f	G	Y	**H**	Unknown	158
	T	**R**	Y	P	I	L	A	G	**H**				Cytochrome P450 20-28	158
	K	**R**	F	S	F	K	K	S	**F**				Cattle MARCKS homologue 155-163	158
	A	**R**	L	Q	T	A	L	L					Rat core histone 188-196	158
	R	**R**	L	P	I	F	S	R	**L**				TIS 11B protein 325-333	158
	R	**R**	F	M	q	Y	Y	V	**Y**				Homologous to proteasome subunit C5 127-135	158
	R	**R**	I	K	E	I	V	K	K	**H**			HSP86 200-209	158
	R	**R**	M	G	P	P	V	G	G	H	**R**		Ribonucleoprotein L 312-322	158
	R	**R**	I	K	E	I	V	K	**K**				HSP89 α 200-208	3

Table 4.2. (con't)

	Position	Source	Ref.
	1 **2** 3 4 5 6 7 8 **9**		
	G **R** I D K P I L **K**	60S ribosomal protein L8 173-181	3
	R **R** S K E I T V **R**	ATP-dependent RNA helicase 77-85	3
	K **R** F E G L T Q **R**	Unknown	3
	R **R** V K E V V K **k**	HSP 89B 195-203	3
	F **R** Y N G L I H **R**	60S ribosomal protein L28 37-45	3
	R **R** Y Q K S T E **L**	Histone H3.3 52-60	3
	R **R** W L P A G d a	Elongation factor 2 341-349	3
	R **R** I S G V D R **Y**	Unknown	3
	R **R** F T R P E H	Unknown	3
	K K Y Q K S T E **L**	Unknown	163
	R **R** Y D R K Q S G **Y**	60S ribosomal protein L44 39-48	164
	H **R** A Q V I Y T **R**	40S ribosomal protein S25 103-111	164
	K **R** W Q A I Y K Q **F**	Ca^{2+}-dependent protease 172-181	164
	G **R** W P G S S L Y Y	Lamin B receptor 14-23	164
	R **R** F V N V V P T F G **K**	40S ribosomal protein S30 114-125	164
	G **R** I L S G V V T **K**	40S ribosomal protein S11 70-79	164
	G **R** F G S G M N **M**	hnRNA-binding protein M4 360-368	164
	G **R** T F I Q P N **M**	Amidophosphoribosyl transferase precursor 354-362	164
	L **R** F Q S S A V **M**	Histone 83-91	164
	R **R** V L V Q V S **Y**	Met Adenosyltransferase 312-320	164
	R K G G N N K L I **K**	Phosphatidylinositol-3-kinase 373-382	164
	G **R** K T G Q A P G Y	Cytochrome c 38-47	164
	G **R** F E G T S T **K**	Neuronal acetylcholine receptor 141-149	164
	XXLNSQDQQCDSSLVE	Draft-1 protooncogene 1-16	165
T cell epitopes	S **R** Y W A I R T R	Influenza A NP 383-391	3, 166
	G **R** A F V T I G **K**	HIV gp120 314-322	3
	R **R** Y P D A V Y **L**	Measles F protein 438-446	167
	R **R** I Y D L I E **L**	EBNA-6 258-266	168
	K **R** W I I L G L N **K**	HIV-1 gag p24 265-274	166, 132
	R **R** K A M F E D **I**	HSP 60 284-292	169

HLA-B*2709	**Sequence**	**Source**	**Ref.**
Motif unknown			
Examples for ligands	L R Y P M A V G L	60S ribosomal protein L 36 (rat) 3-11	164
	R R L P I F S R L	TIS 11B protein 325-333	164
	R R F G D K L N F	Immediate early response gene 87-95	164

										Source	Ref.
K	R	T	T	V	V	A	Q	L		Int-6 24-32	164
A	R	X[1]	Q	T	A	X	X	V		Unknown	164
G	R	T	L	S	D	Y	N	I		Ubiquitin 53-61	164
G	R	N	S	F	E	V	R	V		p53 266-274	164
G	R	T	F	I	Q	P	N	M		Amidophosphoribosyltransferase precursor 354-362	164
G	R	D	Y	D	V	Y	Q	X		Unknown	164
R	R	Y	N	X	X	P	V	X		Unknown	164
R	R	F	S	P	P	X	R	X	F	Unknown	164

1 X indicates Leu or Ile

HLA-B*35		Position										Source	Ref.
		1	**2**	3	4	5	6	7	8	**9**			
Anchor or auxiliary anchor residues			**P**							**Y**			170, 171
										F			
										M			
										L			
										I			
Other preferred residues		M	A	I	K	D	I	V	E				
			V	L	D	I	Q	N	Q				
			Y	F	E	V	K	E	V				
			R	V	G	T	V	Q	T				
			D	M	P	E	L	T					
				E		G	M	K					
				T		L							
				Y		M							
				N									
T cell epitope s	DDVWT	S	G	S	D	S	D	E	E	L	V	HCMV pp65 397-411	92
		V	**P**	L	D	E	D	F	R	K	**Y**	HIV-1 IIIB RT 273-282	122
		N	**P**	D	I	V	I	Y	Q	**Y**		HIV-1 IIIB RT 25-33	122

HLA-B*3501	Position									Source	Ref.
	1	**2**	3	4	5	6	7	8	**9**		
Anchor or auxiliary anchor residues		**P**							**Y**		170, 171
									F		
									M		
									L		
									I		

Table 4.2. (con't)

	Position											Source	Ref.
	1	**2**	3	4	5	6	7	8	**9**				
Other preferred residues	M	A	I	K	D	I	V	E					
		V	L	D	I	Q	N	Q					
		Y	F	E	V	K	E	V					
		R	V	G	T	V	Q	T					
		D	M	P	E	L	T						
			E		G	M	K						
			T		L								
			Y		M								
			N										
Examples for ligands	A	**P**	R	T	V	A	L	T	A			MHC II DP signal sequence 9-17	26
	R	**P**	R	H	Q	G	V	M	V			Alpha actin 39-47	26
	X	**P**	P	E	R	I	I	K	**Y**			End. Retrovirus?	26
T cell epitopes	K	**P**	K	D	E	L	D	**Y**				*P. falciparum* CSP 368-375	170
	K	S	K	D	E	L	D	**Y**				*P. falciparum* CSP 368-375	170
	K	**P**	N	D	K	S	L	**Y**				*P. falciparum* LSA-1 1850-1857	170
	A	S	R	C	W	V	A	**M**				HCV env E 44-51	172
	Y	**P**	L	H	E	Q	H	G	**M**			EBNA-3 458-466	173
	Q	V	P	L	R	P	M	T	Y	K		HIV nef 72-82	120
	T	**P**	E	G	I	I	P	T	**L**			Dengue virus 4NS3 500-508	174,175
	I	**P**	S	I	N	V	H	H	**Y**			HCMV pp65 123-131	157
	N	**P**	D	I	V	I	Y	Q	**Y**			HIV-1$_{SF2}$ pol 25-33	176
	E	**P**	I	V	G	A	E	T	F	**Y**		HIV-1$_{SF2}$ pol 432-441	176
	E	**P**	I	V	G	A	E	T	**F**			HIV-1$_{SF2}$ pol 432-440	176
	S	**P**	A	I	F	Q	S	S	**M**			HIV-1$_{SF2}$ pol 6-14	176
	V	**P**	L	D	K	D	F	R	K	**Y**		HIV-1$_{SF2}$ pol 59-68	176
	I	**P**	L	T	E	E	A	E	**L**			HIV-1$_{SF2}$ pol 6-14	176
	R	**P**	Q	V	P	L	R	P	M	T	**Y**	HIV-1$_{SF2}$ nef 69-79	176
	F	**P**	V	R	P	Q	V	P	**L**			HIV-1$_{SF2}$ nef 66-74	176
	D	**P**	N	P	Q	E	V	V	**L**			HIV-1$_{SF2}$ env 10-18	176
	R	**P**	I	V	S	T	Q	L	**L**			HIV-1$_{SF2}$ env 7-15	176
Examples for other binding peptides	V	**P**	V	M	P	R	V	P	**L**			HIV gag 100-108	177
	F	**P**	V	T	P	R	V	P	**L**			HIV nef 100-108	177
	L	**P**	L	D	L	S	V	I	**L**			EBV EAD 286-294	177
	L	**P**	I	T	C	E	Y	L	**L**			EBV KR2 102-110	177
	H	**P**	L	T	N	N	L	P	**L**			EBV TEGU 1974-1982	177
	L	**P**	L	Q	I	P	I	P	**L**			EBV TEGU 498-506	177
	V	**P**	V	S	E	T	V	E	**L**			EBV VIMP	177
	T	**P**	V	Q	V	Q	M	C	**L**			EBV VTER 94-102	177
	T	A	V	P	W	N	A	S	W			HIV-1 env gp41 606-614	178
	I	**P**	I	P	K	Q	F	Q	P	**Y**		HTLV-1 pol 122-131	177

													Source	Ref.
	V	**P**	S	S	S	S	T	P	L	L	**Y**		HTLV-1 env 247-257	177
	F	**P**	F	S	L	L	V	D	A	P	G	**Y**	HTLV-1 env 159-170	177
	E	**P**	I	L	R	S	L	A	**Y**				HTLV-2 gag 302-310	177
	T	**P**	L	K	N	T	S	V	**L**				HTLV-1 vprt 81-89	177
	T	**P**	K	D	K	T	K	V	**L**				HTLV-1 gag 333-341	177

HLA-B*3503	Position									Source	**Ref.**
	1	**2**	3	4	5	6	7	8	**9**		
Anchor or auxiliary anchor residues		**P**							**M**		179
									L		
Preferred residues	A	M	E	V	D	Y			F		
		I	G	M	N	T					
		L	N	T	G	N					
		F	D	I							
		V	K	G							
			H								
T cell epitopes	Y	**P**	L	H	E	Q	**H**	**G**	**M**		EBNA-3 458-466
	101										

HLA-B*3701	Position									Source	**Ref.**
	1	**2**	3	4	<u>5</u>	6	7	**8**	**9**		
Anchor or auxiliary anchor residues		**D**			V			**F**	**I**		171
		E			I			**M**	**L**		
								L			
Other preferred residues	K	H			T		Q	T			
	Q	P			R		K	E			
		G			A		Y	N			
		S			D		L	D			
		L			G			Q			
					H			G			
					M			H			
T cell epitopes	E	**D**	L	R	<u>V</u>	L	S	**F**	**I**	Influenza NP 339-347	180
	T	Q	G	Y	F	P	Q	W	Q	HIV nef 117-125	120

Table 4.2. (con't)

HLA-B*3801	**Position**									**Source**	**Ref.**
	1	2	3	4	5	6	7	8	**9**		
Anchor or auxiliary anchor residues		H	D						**F**		181
			E						**L**		
Other preferred residues	I	F	I	G	M	V	Y	K	I		
		P	A	E	T	I	V	Y			
		W	S	P	V	T	N	N			
		Y	N	L	A	K		R			
			M	V	E	R		T			
			V		G	N					
					L	H					
					K						
					S						
Examples for ligands	E	H	A	G	V	I	S	V	**L**	Unknown	181
	T	H	D	E	L	E	D	K	**L**	Unknown	181
	Q	Y	D	E	A	V	A	Q	**F**	Histone binding protein 627-635	181
	Y	F	D	P	A	N	G	K	**F**	Elongation factor 2 265-273	181
	S	H	I	G	D	A	V	V		Cyclin 152-159	181
	Y	H	E	D	I	H	T	Y	**L**	Cyclin A 178-186	181
	T	F	D	V	A	P	S	R	**L**	Pm5 protein 270-278	181
HLA-B*39011	**Position**									**Source**	**Ref.**
	1	**2**	3	4	5	6	7	8	**9**		
Anchor or auxiliary anchor residues		**R**				I			**L**		181
		H				V					
						L					
Other preferred residues			A	D	V	N	N	S	V		
			D	E	Y		Y	K	I		
			I	G	I		F	R	M		
			L	P	L			E			
			F	K	F			T			
			V		T						
			M		G						
			S		K						
			T		N						

	1	2	3	4	5	6	7	8	9	10	11	Source	Ref.
Examples for ligands			Y		P								
	S	**H**	I	G	D	A	V	**V**				Cyclin 152-159	181
	I	**H**	E	P	E	P	H	**I**				CKShs1 protein 59-66	181
	S	**R**	D	K	T	I	I	**M**				GBLP 35-42	181

HLA-B*3902	1	**2**	3	4	5	6	7	8	**9**	Source	Ref.
Anchor or auxiliary anchor residues		**K**			I				**L**		181
		Q			L						
					F						
					V						
Other preferred residues	K		A	G	N	V	V	T	F		
	A		I	P	E	Y	L	S	M		
			F		G	T	T	R			
			V		P	H	Y				
			N		Q	F	N				
			L		S	I	D				
			T		T	M	H				
			Y			P					
			E			R					
			H								
			S								

HLA-B40*	1	**2**	3	4	5	6	7	8	**9**			Source	Ref.
Anchor or auxiliary anchor residues		**E**	F						**L**				38
			I						W				
			V						M				
									A				
									T				
									R				
Examples for ligands	T	**E**	F	P	K	E	R	H	L	R	**L**	Unknown	38
	G	**E**	F	P	N	K	N	X	**L**			Unknown	38
	G	**E**	F	P	N	K	N	X	L	Y	**A**	Unknown	38
	G	**E**	F	P	G	K	I	F	L	Y	**A**	Unknown	38
	W	**E**	F	L	Q	P	I	L	**L**			Unknown	38
	G	**E**	F	I	P	G	N	D	L	H	**R**	Unknown	38
	G	**E**	F	P	P	X	D	N	**W**			Unknown	38

Table 4.2. (con't)

	1	**2**	3	4	5	6	7	8	**9**				Source	Ref.
	E	**E**	F	Y	V	D	L	E	**R**				HLA-DQ α 33-41	38
	N	**E**	F	P	D	I	D	I	**R**				Unknown	38
	A	**E**	F	P	K	X	E	A	**R**				Unknown	38
	A	**E**	I	G	E	V	I	V	L	W	X	**W**	Unknown	38
	A	**E**	I	P	G	E	I	A	**L**				Unknown	38
	G	**E**	I	L	D	V	F	D	**A**				IRE-BP 695-703	38
	F	**E**	I	P	X	L	D	V	**A**				Unknown	38
	D	**E**	V	T	P	Q	P	Q	L	V			Unknown	38
	K	**E**	V	G	V	D	V	A	L	Y	**A**		Unknown	38
	K	**E**	S	T	L	H	L	V	**L**				Ubiquitin 63-71	38
	G	**E**	V	D	V	E	Q	H	**T**				Cyclin B 313-321	38
	H	**E**	E	T	P	P	T	T	S				c-myc 241-249	38

*Motif and ligands deduced by exclusion: Class I ligands from a c-myc transfected B cell line expressing A2, A68, and B40 were sequenced. Those not containing an A2 or A68 motif were thought to contain B40 ligands.

HLA-B*40012 (B60)	1	**2**	3	4	5	6	7	8	**9**			Source	Ref.
Anchor or auxiliary anchor residues		**E**					I		**L**				153
							V						
Other preferred residues			A	P	L	K	L	K					
			V	K	I	N	Y	R					
			I	D	V	P	M	Q					
			L	G	D	V							
			M	N	T	I							
			F	Q	N	D							
			S	T	P	R							
			D		G	Q							
			N		K								
					Q								
Examples for ligands	K	**E**	S	T	L	H	L	V	**L**			Ubiquitin 63-71	153
	H	**E**	A	T	L	R	c	w	A	**L**		MHC class I 221-230	153
	Y	**E**	I	H	D	G	M	N	**L**			HSHM02C05	153
	S	**E**	S	P	I	V	V	V	**L**			Signal peptidase 45-54	153
	I	**E**	V	D	P	D	T	K	E	m	**L**	40S ribosomal protein S17 95-105	153
	G	Q	I	V	G	G	V	Y	**L**			HCV core potein 27-35	182

HLA-B*4006 (B61)	Position									Comments	Ref.
	1	**2**	3	4	5	6	7	8	**9**		
Anchor or auxiliary anchor residues		**E**	F			I			**V**	C-terminal anchor deduced from individual ligands	153
			I								
			L								
			V								
			Y								
			W								
Other preferred residues	G	P	M	E	V	N	Y	K	A	P1 deduced from individual ligands	
	R		T	G	I		V	S	P		
				P	L		L				
				S	M		W				
				N	D		I				
				D	G		T				
				K	V		R				
				A	F		D				
				R	N		Q				
				N	S		G				
				Q	K						
										Source	
Examples for ligands	G	**E**	F	G	G	F	G	S	**V**	IEF (mRNA) 9306 127-135	153
	E	**E**	F	Q	F	I	K	K	A	Associated-microfibril. protein 72-80	153
	G	**E**	F	V	D	L	Y	**V**		40S ribosomal protein S21 6-13	153
	R	**E**	R	R	D	N	Y	**V**		40S ribosomal protein S17 77-84	153
	R	**E**	I	I	I	N	A	**V**		Ribonucl. reductase 290-297	153
	G	**E**	F	S	I	T	Y	K		40S ribosomal protein S15 116-123	153
	G	**E**	H	G	L	i	I	R	**V**	Unknown	153
	R	**E**	M	I	P	F	A	D	i	Unknown	153

HLA-B44	Position									Source	Ref.
	1	**2**	3	4	5	6	7	8	**9**		
Anchor or auxiliary anchor residues		**E**	I	P		V			**Y**		183
Examples for ligands	S	**E**	I	D	L	I	L	G	**Y**	Unknown	183
	S	**E**	I	D	T	V	A	K	**Y**	Unknown	183
	D	**E**	V	G	I	V	T	K	**Y**	Unknown	183
	A	**E**	I	P	T	R	V	N	**Y**	Unknown	183
	A	**E**	I	P	R	T	F	K	**Y**	Unknown	183

Table 4.2. (con't)

	Position										Source	Ref.
	1	**2**	3	4	5	6	7	8	**9**			
	A	**E**	M	G	K	F	K	F	S	**Y**	Unknown	183
	A	**E**	V	D	K	V	T	G	**y**		Unknown	183
	F	**E**	P	T	V	V	K	K	**Y**		Unknown	183
	D	**E**	F	I	G	V	A	L	**Y**		Unknown	183
	D	**E**	I	G	V	I	D	L	**Y**		Unknown	183
	D	**E**	N	P	L	V	K	Q	**Y**		Unknown	183
	A	**E**	V	D	K	V	T	G	R	F	40S ribosomal protein S21 37-46	183
	D	**E**	A	P	A	V	I	s	**Y**		Unknown	183
	S	**E**	A	I	H	T	F	Q	**Y**		Unknown	183
	A	**E**	G	I	V	T	G	Q	**Y**		Unknown	183
	D	**E**	V	P	D	L	E	R	K	**Y**	Unknown	183
	K	**E**	H	V	I	Q	N	A	F*		EBNA-6 335-343	184
	A	A	I	G	Y	M	X	K			Unknown	43
	A	A	D	D	X	F	K	D			Human oncoprotein c-abl 793-800	43
T cell epitopes	G	**E**	I	S	P	L	P	S	L		Influenza NS1 158-166	183
	F	**E**	D	L	R	V	L	S	F		Influenza NP 338-346	183
* also a T cell epitope	E	**E**	N	L	L	D	F	V	R	F	EBNA-6 130-139	189

HLA-B*4402	Position										Source	Ref.
	1	**2**	3	4	5	6	7	8	**9**			
Anchor or		**E**							**F**			185
auxiliary anchor residues									**Y**			
Preferred residues	A	M	I	V	Y							
	S	I										
		L										
		D										
Others	D	N	P									
			R									
			K									
T cell epitopes	G	**E**	I	S	P	L	P	S	L		Influenza NS1 158-166	183
	F	**E**	D	L	R	V	L	S	**F**		Influenza NP 338-346	183
	S	**E**	I	W	R	D	I	D	**F**		Tyrosinase 192-200	186
	M	**E**	V	D	P	I	G	H	L	**Y**	MAGE-3 167-176	187
	E	**E**	K	L	I	V	V	A	**F**		MUM-1	187, 188
	E	**E**	K	L	I	V	V	L	**F**		MUM-1	187, 188
Other binding peptides	L	**E**	L	R	S	R	Y	W	A		Influenza NP 379-387	183
	L	**E**	L	R	S	R	Y	W	A	I	Influenza NP 379-388	183

HLA-B*4403	Position										Source	Ref.
	1	**2**	3	4	5	6	7	8	**9**			
Anchor or		**E**							**Y**			185
auxiliary anchor residues									**F**			
Preferred residues	A	M										
	S	I										
		L										
		V										
		D										
Others		N	I	Y								
			V	F								
			K									
Examples for ligands	A	**E**	D	K	E	N	Y	K	K	**F**	HSP 90 427-436	185
	A	**E**	M	G	K	G	S	F	K	**Y**	Elongation factor 2 48-57	185
T cell epitopes	S	**E**	I	W	R	D	I	D	**F**		Tyrosinase 192-200	186
	M	**E**	V	D	P	I	G	H	L	**Y**	MAGE-3 167-176	187
	E	**E**	K	L	I	V	V	A	**F**		MUM-1	187, 188
	E	**E**	K	L	I	V	V	L	**F**		MUM-1	187, 188

HLA-B*4501	Sequence											Source	Ref.
Motif unknown													
T cell epitope	A	E	E	A	A	G	I	G	I	L	T	Melan-A/Mart-1 24-34	J. Schneider et al, pers. communication
	A	E	E	A	A	G	I	G	I	L		Melan-A/Mart-1 24-33	J. Schneider et al, pers. communication

HLA-B*4601	Position										Source	Ref.
	1	**2**	3	4	5	6	7	8	**9**			
Anchor or		**M**	K	D	P	S	E	V	**Y**			154
auxiliary anchor residues			R,N	E,V	I			A	**F**			
Preferred residues		I	I,P		G	A	G					
			F									
Examples for ligands	F	I	K	D	G	S	S	T	**Y**		Unknown	154
	S	I	R	D	G	V	R	A	**Y**		Unknown	154
	K	**M**	K	E	I	A	E	A	**Y**		Human HSC70/HSP70 126-134	154
	Y	**M**	I	D	P	S	G	V	S	**Y**	Human proteasome S C8 150-159	154
	Y	V	I	P	H	V	H	A	**F**		Unknown	154
	F	A	F	V	T	D	N	T	**Y**		Human cyclin B 269-277	154

Table 4.2. (con't)

HLA-B51	**Sequence**										**Source**	**Ref.**
Motif unknown												
Examples for ligands	D	T	P	L	I	P	L	T	I	F*	EBNA-2 42-51	184
T cell epitopes	R	A	I	E	A	Q	Q	H	L		HIV-1 III gp41 557-565	122
	T	A	F	T	I	P	S	I			HIV-1 IIIB RT 231-238	122
	I	P	L	T	E	E	A	E	L		HIV-1$_{SF2}$ pol 6-14	176
	D	P	N	P	Q	E	V	V	L		HIV-1$_{SF2}$ env 10-18	176

* also a T cell epitope

HLA-B*5101	**Position**									**Source**	**Ref.**
	1	**2**	3	4	5	6	7	8	**9**		
Anchor or auxiliary anchor residues		**A**							**F**		190
		P							**I**		
		G									
Other preferred residues	I	W	I	G	V	N	K	T	W		
	L	F	L	V	T	I	Q		M		
	V		M	I	G	L	R		V		
	Y		F	K	A	K	E		L		
	D		W	E	I	Q					
			Y	D	S						
			V								
			E								
			H								
			D								
			R								
			N								
Examples for ligands	Y	**P**	F	K	P	P	K	**V**		UBC5, yeast 61-68	190
	D	**A**	H	I	Y	L	N	H	**I**	Thymidylate synthase 253-261	190
	T	**G**	Y	L	N	T	V	T	V	GBLP 192-200	190
	d	**A**	Y	A	L	N	H	T	**L**	Unknown	190
	I	**P**	P	E	V	N	R	Q	**L**	Unknown	190

HLA-B*5102	1	**2**	<u>3</u>	4	5	6	7	8	**9**		Source	Ref.
Anchor or auxiliary anchor residues		**P**	Y						**I**			190
		A							**V**			
		G										
Other preferred residues			F	G	V	I	R	T				
			V	E	Q	N	E	R				
			L	K	N	Q	Q	Y				
			I	L	G	T	K					
				T	T							
				Q								
				R								
				N								
				H								
Examples for ligands	Y	**A**	<u>Y</u>	D	G	K	D	Y	**I**		MHC Iα chain 140-148	190
	Y	**P**	<u>E</u>	K	P	P	K	**V**			UBC5, yeast 61-68	190
	L	**P**	P	G	R	I	I	K	X		Unknown	190
	L	**P**	<u>F</u>	T	V	I	L	**v**			CDC25 homol. 560-567	190
	T	**G**	<u>Y</u>	L	N	T	V	T	**V**		GBLP 192-200	190
	F	**A**	<u>Y</u>	D	G	K	D	Y	**I**		MHC Iα chain 140-148	190
	F	**P**	S	E	I	V	G	K	R	**I**	40S ribosomal protein S7/S8A 135-144	190
	M	**P**	W	F	K	G	w	K	**V**		Elongation factor 1α 208-216	190

HLA-B*5103	1	**2**	<u>3</u>	4	5	6	7	8	**9**	Comments	Ref.
Anchor or auxiliary anchor residues		**A**	Y						**V**	Anchor at 9 deduced from individual ligands	190
		P							**I**		
		G							**F**		
Other preferred residues	T	F	F	E	G	I	V				
	V	W	D	L	A	K	M				
	D		L	N	V	T					
				R	N						
				G	Q						
				Q	M						
				T	R						
				V							

Table 4.2. (con't)

											Source	
Examples for ligands	T	**G**	Y	L	N	T	V	T	**V**		GBLP 192-200	190
	D	**A**	H	I	Y	L	N	H	**I**		Thymidilate synthase 253-261	190
	Y	**F**	D	d	t	L	E	D	**F**		Unknown	190
HLA-B*5201					**Position**						**Comments**	**Ref.**
	1	2	3	4	5	6	7	**8**	**9**			
Anchor or		Q	F		L			**I**	**I**		C-terminal anchor at 8 or 9	190
auxiliary anchor residues			Y		I			**V**	**V**			
			W		V							
Other	V	M	I	L	M	K	K	M	M			
preferred residues	L	F	L	I	F	N	E	F	F			
	I	P	P	V	A	L	Q					
			D	P	T	T	Y					
			K	K	G	S						
				E								
				A								
											Source	
Examples for ligands	T	G	Y	L	N	T	V	T	**V**		GBLP 192-200	190
	G	Q	F	K	I	Y	A	**I**			40S ribosomal protein S21 60-67	190
	H	S	T	I	M	P	R	**L**			P1-CDC21 259-266	190
	G	F	Y	P	G	S	I	E	**V**		MHC II β chain 150-158	190
	V	Q	I	F	G	N	K	**M**			RBAP-2 266-273	190
	Y	F	D	P	A	N	G	K	**F**		Elongation factor 2 265-273	190
	L	Q	F	P	V	G	R	**I**			Histone 2a Z 25-32	190
	H	M	Y	I	F	L	H	T	**V**		Unknown	190
T cell epitopes	A	F	H	H	V	A	R	E	L		HIV-1 nef 190-198	63
HLA-B*5301					**Position**						**Source**	**Ref.**
	1	**2**	3	4	5	6	7	8	**9**			
Anchor residues		**P**							**L,I**			170
Other preferred residues	S,Y		F,K	E,I	I,L	Y			**V,M,Y**			
	F,M		N,Q	L,Q								
T cell epitopes	K	**P**	I	V	Q	Y	D	N	**F**		*P. falciparum* LSA-1 1786-1794	170
	T	**P**	Y	D	I	N	Q	M	**L**		HIV-II gag p24 182-190	191
	R	**P**	L	T	D	F	D	Q	G	W	HCV NS1 77-85	114
Examples for ligands	Y	**P**	A	E	I	T	L	T	W		HLA-Aα3 domain	13
	D	**P**	S	G	A	Y	F	A	W		Proteasome C3	13
	E	**P**	E	P	H	I	L	L	**F**		CKShs1 protein	13
	F	**P**	E	H	X	F	P	A	X		Unknown	13

HLA-B*5401	Position									Source	Ref.
	1	**2**	3	4	5	6	7	8	9		
Anchor or auxiliary anchor residues		**P**									143
Other preferred residues	M,F		F,M R,Y N,K L,Q	G	V				A		

HLA-B*5501	Position										Source	Ref.
		1	**2**	3	4	5	6	7	8	9		
Anchor or auxiliary anchor residues			**P**									143
Other preferred residues		A		R,M Y,K N,F L	T H,D	V	F,G	V	M,H	A		
Examples for ligands		A	**P**	R	Q	P	G	L	M	A	Unknown	143
		A	**P**	R	T	V	A	L	T	A	HLA-DP signal sequence 9-17	143
T cell epitopes	V	H	**P**	V	H	A	G	P	I	A	HIV-1 IIIB gag p24 215-223	122

HLA-B*5502	Position									Source	Ref
	1	**2**	3	4	5	6	7	8	9		
Anchor or auxiliary anchor residues		**P**									143
Other preferred residues	A		R,M Y,F H,K L;Q	H	I		V	M,S	A		
Examples for ligands	A	**P**	R	Q	P	G	L	M	A	Unknown	143
	A	**P**	R	T	V	A	L	T	A	HLA-DP signal sequence 9-17	143
	R	**P**	R	H	Q	G	V	M	V	β-actin	143
	I	**P**	Y	H	I	V	N	I	V	serine tRNA ligase 357-365	143, P49591*
	A	**P**	T	G	D	L	P	R	A	LMP-2	143

*swissprot entry

Table 4.2. (con't)

HLA-B*5601	1	**2**	3	4	5	6	7	8	**9**	Source	**Ref.**
Anchor or		**P**									143
auxiliary anchor residues	A		Y						**A**		
Other preferred residues			N	G,T	V,I		V	A,S	L		
			R,F	E				M			
			Q,K								
			H,L								
			M								
Examples for ligands	A	**P**	R	T	V	A	L	T	**A**	HLA-DP signal sequence 9-17	143
	A	**P**	T	G	D	L	P	R	**A**	LMP-2	143
	A	**P**	R	Q	P	G	L	M	**A**	Unknown	143

HLA-B*5801	1	**2**	3	4	5	6	7	8	**9**		Source	**Ref.**
Anchor or		**A**		P	V				**F**			153
auxiliary anchor residues		**S**		E	I				**W**			
		T		K	L							
					M							
					F							
Other	K	G	G	D	A	I	L	N	Y			
preferred residues	R		T	Q	D	V	Y	R				
	I		I	R	N	L	M	K				
			L		T	F	N	T				
			V		Y							
			F		W							
			Y		Q							
			N									
			Q									
Examples for ligands	K	**A**	G	Q	V	V	T	I	**W**		Lamin C 490-498	153
	A	**G**	D	R	T	F	Q	K	**W**		MHC class I 260-268	153
	I	**t**	T	K	A	I	S	R	**F**		Unknown	153
	R	**T**	D	G	K	V	F	Q	**F**		60S ribosomal protein L30 23-31	153
	I	**T**	S	Q	D	V	L	H	S	**W**	Cytochrome C oxidase 154-163	153
	I	**S**	D	S	N	P	F	L	T	Q	Unknown	153
	K	**t**	D	e	V	V	T	L	**F**		Unknown	153
	V	**T**	S	P	L	T	V	E	**W**		MHC class II β 209-217	153
	g	**A**	V	N	V	V	M	T	**f**		Glucose transporter 5 322-330	153

HLA-B*6701	Position 1	2	3	4	5	6	7	8	9	Source	Ref.
Anchor or auxiliary anchor residues		**P**							**L**		143
Other preferred residues	A		F,M Y,I A,L E,N T,Q D,G	G K,E	V	M					

HLA-B*7301	Position 1	2	3	4	5	6	7	8	9	Source	Ref.
Anchor or auxiliary anchor residues		**R**							**P**		192
	N		N,L F,V A,I M,Y H,T D,W K	R P K	V	D	T Y	S			
Other preferred residues			S	G,E	I,Y T		E				
Examples for ligands	N	**R**	A	V	V	G	V	V	A	60S ribosomal protein L8 162-170	192
	N	**R**	R	F	V	N	V	V	**P**	40S ribosomal protein S30 113-121	192

HLA-B*7801	Position 1	2	3	4	5	6	7	8	Comments	Ref.
Anchor or auxiliary anchor residues		**P A G**				I L F V		A	This motif is only partial; the C-terminal anchor has not been determined	190
Other preferred residues			Y D W	F D G L V	D G V N R		A V N K Q	K S		

Table 4.2. (con't)

	1	2	3	4	5	6	7	8	Comments	Ref.
				S Q R N	Q S T		E			

HLA-Cw*0102	1	**2**	3	4	5	6	7	8	**9**	10	Source	Ref.
Anchor or auxiliary anchor residues		**A** **L**							**L**			154
Other preferred residues			P,Q	E,V Y,T S,W A,L N,R F	R,H G	V,I K,H	F					
Examples for ligands	I	**A**	P	T	G	H	S	**L**			Unknown	154
	I	T	P	T	G	T	H	P	**L**		Human granulin 162-170	154
	A	**A**	P	A	Y	S	R	A	**L**		Human HSP27 69-77	154
	F	**A**	P	Y	N	K	P	S	**L**		Unknown	154
	H	L	P	E	T	K	F	S	E	**L**	Unknown	154
	N	**A**	P	W	A	V	T	S	**L**		Human butyryl cholinesterase 256-264	154
	V	**A**	P	W	N	S	L	S	**L**		Human tissue inhibitor of metalloproteinase 125-133	154
	N	X	P	E	R	I	I	T	**L**		Human nucleic acid binding protein 53-61*	154

* if X stands for C

HLA-Cw*0301		1	2	<u>3</u>	<u>4</u>	5	<u>6</u>	7	8	**9**	10	11	12	Source	Ref.
Anchor or auxiliary anchor residues				V I Y L M	P		F Y			**L** **F** **M** **I**					193, 171
Other preferred residues			H R	E N	E R	N	M	Q K S M	T						
T cell epitopes		H	Q	A	I	S	P	R	T	**L**				HIV gag p24 144-152	194
	or	Q	M	V	H	Q	A	I	S	P	R	T	**L**	HIV gag p24 144-152	194

HLA-Cw*0304	Position											Source	Ref.
	1	**2**	3	4	5	6	7	8	**9**				
Anchor or		**A**	V	P			M		**L**				195
auxiliary anchor residues			I	E			E		**M**				
			P										
			Y										
			M										
Other			F,N	G,D	R	G,Y	R						
preferred residues				R									
Examples for ligands	A	**A**	V	D	A	G	M	A	M			Pyrimidine binding protein 168-176	195
	L	**A**	V	H	P	S	G	V	A	L		IFN-induced 15 kD protein 45-54	195
	F	**A**	Y	D	G	K	D	Y	L	T	L	HLA-E 116-126	195

HLA-Cw*0401	Position									Source	Ref.
	1	**2**	3	4	5	<u>6</u>	7	8	**9**		
Anchor or		**Y**				V			**L**		193, 171
auxiliary anchor residues		**P**				I			**F**		
		F				L			M		
Other			D	D	A		A	K			
preferred residues			H	E	H			S			
				P	M			H			
					T						
					R						
T cell epitope	S	**F**	N	C	G	G	E	F	**F**	HIV-1 gp120 380-388	196
	Q	A	S	Q	E	<u>V</u>	K	N	W	HIV-1 p24 gag 308-316	550

HLA-Cw*0601	Position									Source	Ref.
	1	2	3	4	<u>5</u>	<u>6</u>	7	8	**9**		
Anchor or					I	V			**L**		193
auxiliary anchor residues					L	I			**I**		
					F	L			**V**		
					M				**Y**		
Other	I	P	P	P	K	A	R	Y			

Table 4.2. (con't)

	1	2	3	4	5	6	7	8	**9**			Source	Ref.
preferred residues	F	R	I	E		T	K	E					
	K		G	D		S	Q	Q					
	Y		F	Q			N	N					
			Y	L				R					
			K					G					
			N					T					
			A					S					
								K					
T cell epitopes	Y	R	P	R	P	R	R	**Y**				GAGE-1 and GAGE-2 9-16	197

HLA-Cw*0602	1	2	3	4	5	6	7	8	**9**			Source	Ref.
Anchor or auxiliary anchor residues					I	V			**L**				193
					L	I			**I**				
					F	L			**V**				
					M				**Y**				
Other preferred residues	I	P	P	P	K	A	R	Y					
	F	R	I	E		T	K	E					
	K		G	D		S	Q	Q					
	Y		F	Q			N	N					
			Y	L				R					
			K					G					
			N					T					
			A					S					
								K					
Examples for ligands	Y	Q	F	T	G	I	K	K	**Y**			Unknown	193
	V	R	H	D	G	G	N	V	**L**			Unknown	193
	F	A	F	p	I	I	q	R	**V**			Unknown	193
	X	Q	r	T	P	k	A	g	I	Y	**Y**	Unknown	193

HLA-Cw*0702	1	2	3	4	5	6	7	8	9				Source	Ref.
Anchor or auxiliary anchor residues		Y			V	V			**Y**					193
		P			Y	I			**F**					
					I	L			**L**					
					L	M								
					F									
					M									
Other preferred residues		R	P	D	T	A	Y		E					
		D	G	E		R	M		A					
			A	V			N		F					
				Q			R	D						
				P			V		K					
				S			F							
				G			E							
Examples for ligands	K	Y	F	D	E	H	Y	E	**Y**				CKS-2 11-19	193
	R	Y	R	P	G	T	V	A	**L**				Histone H3.3 40-48	193
	N	K	A	D	V	I	L	K	**Y**				Protein synthesis factor eIF-4C 87-95	193
	I	Y	P	q	n	v	i	L	**Y**				Unknown	193
	I	R	K	P	Y	I	w	E	**Y**				Glutamyl-tRNA synthetase 343-351	193
	N	Y	G	G	G	N	Y	G	S	G	S	**Y**	Homologous hnRNP A2 or B1 (S11=N) 277-288	193
	F	Y	P	P	y	I	**Y**						Unknown	193
	X	M	P	P	f	L	d	G					Unknown	193

HLA-Cw8	Sequence	Source	
Motif unknown			
T cell epitopes	N C S F N I S T S I	HIV-1 IIIB gp120 156-165	122
	C T N V S T V Q C	HIV-1 IIIB gp120 241-249	122

HLA-Cw*1601 M	Sequence	Source	Ref.
Motif unknown			
T cell epitopes	S A Y G E P R K L	Mage-1 230-238	25
	A A R A V F L A L	BAGE 2-10	198

Table 4.2. (con't)

HLA-G	1	**2**	3	4	5	6	7	8	**9**			Source	Ref.
Anchor residues		I, L	**P**						**L**				199, 200
Preferred residues	V,M R,K S,G H	V Y,S Q,R H,G	A,I			I,V L,F	Q,M		I				
Examples for ligands	R	**I**	I	P	R	H	L	Q	**L**			Histone H2A 77-85	199, 200
	R	**L**	P	K	D	F	R	I	**L**			Unknown	199
	K	**L**	P	A	Q	F	Y	I	**L**			Unknown	199
	R	H	P	K	Y	K	T	E	**L**			Nuclear protein (TTP) 130-138	200
	H	V	P	E	H	A	V	V	**L**			Rat fatty acid synthase 751-759	200
	M	Q	P	T	H	P	I	R	**L**			HS1 protein 160-168	200
	K	**I**	A	G	Y	V	T	H	**L**			40S ribosomal protein S17 49-57	200
	G	V	P	K	T	H	L	E	**L**			HLA class III gene	200
	K	G	P	P	A	A	L	T	**L**			Cytokine receptor	200
	S	Y	P	T	R	I	A	S	**L**			Unknown	200
	R	**L**	P	D	G	R	V	V	**L**			Interferon binding protein 339-347	200
	K	S	P	A	S	D	T	Y	I	V	F	Nascent polypeptide complex α chain	200
	M	R	P	R	K	A	F	L	**L**			ERP 72 1-9	200
	R	**L**	P	K	D	F	V	D	**L**			Unknown	200
	V	**L**	P	K	L	Y	V	K	**L**			40S ribosomal protein S26 63-71	200

Table 4.3. Mouse class I motifs

H2-K^d	1	**2**	3	4	5	6	7	8	**9**		Source	Ref.
Anchor residues		**Y**							**I**			4
		F							**L**			
									V			
Preferred residues			N	P	M	K	T					
			I			F	N					
			L									
Others	K		A	A	V	H	P	H				
	A		H	E	N	I	H	E				
	R		V	S	D	M	D	K				
	S		R	D	I	Y	E	V				
	V		S	H	L	V	Q	F				
	T		F	N	S	R	S	R				
			E		T	L						
			Q		G							
			K									
			M									
			T									
Examples for ligands	T	**Y**	Q	R	T	R	A	L	**V***		Influenza A NP 147-155	201, 202
	S	**Y**	F	P	E	I	T	H	**I**		Tyrosine kinase JAK1 355-363	4, 203
	K	**Y**	Q	A	V	T	T	T	**L***		Tum-P198 14-22	4, 204, 205
	G	**Y**	K	D	G	N	E	Y	**I***		Listeriolysin O 91-99	206
	K	**Y**	G	V	S	V	Q	D	**I***		*L. monocytogenes* p60 217-225	207
	G	**Y**	L	G	Q	V	T	X	**I**		Unknown	208
	S	**F**	V	D	T	R	T	L	**L**		Collagen 1 α2 4-12	208
	I	**Y**	V	G	N	G	Q	M	**I***		*L. monocytogenes* p60 449-457	209
T cell epitopes	L	**Y**	Q	N	V	G	T	Y	**V**		Influenza JAP HA 204-212	210
	T	**Y**	V	S	V	G	T	S	T	**L**	Influenza JAP HA 210-219	211
	V	**Y**	Q	I	L	A	I	Y	A		Influenza JAP HA 523-531	210
	I	**Y**	A	T	V	A	G	S	**L**		Influenza JAP HA 529-537	210
	T	**Y**	V	S	V	S	T	S	T	**L**	Influenza A HA 210-219	212, 211
	I	**Y**	S	T	V	A	S	S	**L**		Influenza A HA 518-526	212
	R	**Y**	L	E	N	G	K	E	T	**L**	HLA-A24 170-179	4, 213

Table 4.3. (con't)

	Position 1	2	3	4	5	6	7	8	9			Source	Ref.
	1	**2**	3	4	5	6	7	8	**9**				
	R	**Y**	L	K	N	G	K	E	T	**L**		HLA-Cw3 170-179	4, 213
	S	**Y**	I	P	S	A	E	K	**I**			*P. berghei* CSP 252-260	214
	S	**Y**	V	P	S	A	E	Q	**I**			*P. yoelii* CSP 281-289	215
	S	**Y**	I	G	S	I	N	N	**I**			RSV M2 82-90	216
	D	**Y**	A	T	L	G	V	G	**V**			HSV-1 ICP27 448-456	217
	L	**Y**	R	T	F	A	G	N	P	R	A	HSV-1 ICP27 322-332	217
	T	**Y**	K	D	T	V	Q	**L**				Polio VP1 111-118	218
	F	**Y**	D	G	F	S	K	V	P	**L**		Polio VP1 208-217	218
	A	**Y**	I	S	S	G	S	S	T	**L**		Human Ig VH 49-58	211
	N	**Y**	D	N	A	G	T	N	**L**			*P. falciparum* CSP 39-47	219
	K	**Y**	L	K	K	I	K	N	S	**L**		*P. falciparum* CSP 333-342	219
	K	**Y**	L	K	I	K	H	L	**L**			APC frameshift	220
	M	**Y**	A	P	P	I	G	G	Q	**I**		HIV gp120 431-440	221
	T	**Y**	V	S	V	G	T	S	T	**I**		Influenza JAP HA (L219I) 210-219	222
	S	**F**	A	V	A	T	T	A	**L**			MMTV env gp36 474-482	223
	S	**Y**	E	T	F	I	S	R	**L**			MMTV gag p27 425-433	223
	F	**Y**	Q	L	A	K	T	C	P	**V**		p53 mutant 126-135	224
	Y	K	L	V	V	V	G	A	**V**			Mutant ras p21 oncogene (G12V) 4-12	225
	A	M	Q	M	L	K	E	T	**I**			HIV-1SF2 gag p24 199-207	226
	G	**Y**	K	L	I	F	R	T	**I**			*P. aeruginosa* Leu-Val-Ile-binding protein 123-131	227
	Q	**Y**	G	E	G	I	A	T	E	**V**		*P. aeruginosa* Leu-Val-Ile-binding protein 162-171	227
	T	**Y**	S	P	P	L	N	E	**L**			p53 mutant (K129E) 122-130	228
* Also a T cell epitope													

H2-D[d]	Position 1	2	3	4	5	6	7	8	9	Source	Ref.
	1	**2**	**3**	4	5	6	7	8	**9**		
Anchor or auxiliary anchor residues		**G**	**P**		R K				**I** **L** **F**		a,229
Other preferred residues				D E Q		N I L	D E				
Examples for ligands	K	**G**	**P**	I	T	V	Q	**I**		Unknown	229
	V	**G**	**P**	Q	K	N	E	N	**L**	Unknown	229
	S	**G**	**P**	R	K	X	I	X	**L**	Homol. mRNA CD40 mouse	229

	Sequence	Source	Ref.
	A **G** **P** D R T E K X **L**	Unknown	229
	K **G** **P** D K G N E **F**	Homol. metalloproteinase 2 inhibitor	229
	I **G** **P** E R G H N **L**	Homol. hypoxanthine phosphoribosyltransferase	229
	D **G** **P** V R E H N **L**	Homol. urease canavalia ensiformis	229
	K **G** **P** E R X N G **L**	Unknown	229
	S **G** **P** E R G E K **L**	Homol. proliferating cell nucleolar antigen P40	229
	D **G** **P** V R G I S **I**	40S ribosomal protein S17 (rat)	229
	N **G** **P** Q R I Y N **L**	Unknown	229
	S **G** **P** V A L V N F **I**	Unknown	229
	I **G** **P** N R A F N **F**	Unknown	229
	S **G** **P** E R L L S X Y	Homol. heterog. nucl. RNP complex K	229
	V **G** **P** S G K Y F I **L**	Unknown	229
	F **G** **P** Y K L N R **L**	Homol. feline leukemia virus envelope polyprotein	229
	F **G** **P** L K F N V L T	Unknown	229
	A **G** **P** D R F I X X M	Unknown	229
	F **G** **P** Y R F Y V L T	Unknown	229
	S E Q D L N F	Unknown	229
	S X H K E Q P A T	Homol. transforming protein spi-1 human	229
	S X **P** K T D X Q T **L**	Homol. insulin receptor precursor	229
T cell epitopes	**G** **P** P H S N N F G Y	Tum-P35B 4-13	230
	R **G** **P** G R A F V T **I**	HIV gp160 318-327	231, 232
	L M G Y I P L V G A	HCV core protein 18-27	55
	A D L M G Y I P L V	HCV core protein 16-25	233
	M S Y S W T G A L V T P C A E E	HCV NS5 409-424	234
	I **G** **P** G R A F H T	HIV-1$_{SF2}$ gp120 312-320	226

a. Falk and co-workers, unpublished

H2-L^d	**Position**									**Source**	**Ref.**
	1	**2**	3	4	5	6	7	8	**9**		
Anchor residues		**P** **S**							**F** **L** **M**		4,a,235
Other preferred residues			G Q M L	T	T	I K F	F	Q N			
Examples for ligands	Y	**P**	H	F	M	P	T	N	**L***	MCMV pp89 168-176	236
	L	**S**	P	F	P	F	D	**L***		OGDH 105-112	237,238

Table 4.3. (con't)

	Position	Source	Ref.
	1 **2** 3 4 5 6 7 8 **9**		
	VAITRIEQ L **S** P F P F D **L***	OGDH 97-112	237, 238
	X **P** L E A N Y Q X **F**	Unknown	235
	A **P** Q P G M E N **F**	Unknown	235
	Q **P** Q R G R E N **F**	Unknown	235
	X **P** Q P G R E Q	Unknown	235
	X **P** Q P N L Y Q **L**	Unknown	235
	X **P** A X A Y P Y	Unknown	235
	Y **P** N V N I H N **F**	Unknown	235
	X **P** Q K A G G F L **M**	Phosphoglycerate kinase 180-189	235
	Q N H R A L D **L**	P91A tum⁻ (mutant of PA700 S3) 15-22	239
T cell epitopes	R **P** Q A S G V Y **M**	LCMV NP 118-126	240, 241
	I **S** T Q N H R A **L**	Tumor antigen P91A 12-20	242
	L **P** Y L G W L V **F**	Tumor antigen P815 35-43	243
	A **P** T A G A F F **F**	JHMV Nucleocapsid 318-326	244
	Y **P** A L G L H E **F**	Measles NP 281-289	245
	T **P** H P A R I G **L**	*E. coli* β-gal. 876-884	157
	D **P** V I D R L Y **L**	Measles HA 343-351	246
	S **P** G R S F S Y **F**	Measles HA 544-552	246
	L **S** P Y P F D **L**	OGDH 105-112	247
	L **P** Y L G W L V **F**	Mouse mastocytoma P1A 35-43	248
	I **P** Q S L D S W W T S **L**	HBV sAg 28-39	249
	M **P** G R A F V T I	HIV gp120 p18-8 17-25	250, 251
	S **P** S Y V Y H Q **F**	MuLV env gp70 423-431	252
	Q L **S** P Y P F D **L**	OGDH (F108Y) 104-112	253

* Also a T cell epitope
a: Falk and co-workers, unpublished

H2-K^b		1	**2**	3	4	**5**	6	7	**8**	**9**	Source	Ref.
Anchor or auxiliary anchor residues				Y		**F**			**L**			4
						Y			**M**			
									I			
									V			
Other preferred residues		R	N	P	R		T	N				
		I			D		I	Q				
		L			E		E	K				
		S			K		S					
		A			T							
Examples for ligands		R	G	Y	V	**Y**	Q	G	**L***		VSV NP 52-59	254
		S	I	I	N	**F**	E	K	**L***		Ovalbumin 257-264	4, 255, 256
		H	I	Y	E	**F**	P	Q	**L**		Unknown	257
		G	A	Y	E	**F**	T	T	**L***		40 kD-peptide 89-96	258
		E	Q	Y	K	**F**	Y	S	**V***		Murine lipopolysaccharide binding protein	259
		S	L	V	E	L	T	S	**L***		Murine adenosine phospho ribosyl transferase	260
		A	N	Y	D	**F**	**I**	C	**V***		MMTV env gp73 544-551	261
		S	N	Y	L	**F**	T	K	**L**		Tissue specifc Ag (lung)	551
T cell epitopes		I	I	Y	R	**F**	L	L	**I**		Rotavirus VP7 33-40	262
		S	S	I	E	**F**	A	R	**L**		HSV glycoprotein B 498-505	263
	F	A	P	G	N	**Y**	P	A	**L**		SV NP 324-332	264, 265
		K	S	P	W	**F**	T	T	**L**		MuLV env p15E 574-581	266, 267
		V	G	P	V	**F**	P	P	G	**M**	Rotavirus VP6 376-384	268
	Y	S	G	Y	I	**F**	R	D	**L**		Rotavirus VP3 585-593	268
		F	E	Q	N	T	A	Q	A$^+$		MUT 2 tumor antigen	269
		F	E	Q	N	T	A	Q	P$^+$		MUT 1 tumor antigen	269
		V	V	Y	D	**F**	L	K	C		SV40 T 404-411	270
		C	G	S	H	L	V	E	A	**L**	Insulin B chain 7-15	271
		F	A	P	G	N	Y	P	A	**L**	SV9 324-332	272
		D	I	K	V	G	I	E	F		Synthetic peptide	273
		L	S	P	F	P	F	D	**L**		OGDH 105-112	247
		S	S	W	D	**F**	I	T	**V**		MuLV env gp70 189-196	274, Sijts et al. subm.
		Q	T	F	D	**F**	G	R	**L**		HSV-1 UL39 822-829	275
		G	A	Y	R	**F**	T	T	**L**		40 kD peptide, E92R 89-96	258
		S	I	Y	R	**Y**	Y	G	**L**		Synthetic peptide	276
		Y	A	M	I	**Y**	R	N	**L**		Murine mdm2 100-107	277, 282
		T	T	I	H	**Y**	K	Y	**M**		Murine p53 227-234	277

Table 4.3. (con't)

	Position								Source	Ref.
	1	**2**	3	4	5	6	7	8		
	A	H	Y	L	**F**	R	N	**L**	Epitope mimic of a natural tumor Ag	278
	T	H	Y	L	**F**	R	N	**L**	Epitope mimic of a natural tumor Ag	278
	L	I	V	I	**Y**	N	T	**L**	Epitope mimic of natural H-3 miHAg	279
	L	I	Y	E	**F**	N	T	**L**	Epitope mimic of natural H-3 miHAg	279
	I	P	Y	I	**Y**	N	T	**L**	Epitope mimic of natural H-3 miHAg	279
	I	I	Y	I	**Y**	H	R	**L**	Epitope mimic of natural H-3 miHAg	279
	L	I	Y	I	**F**	N	T	**L**	Epitope mimic of natural H-3 miHAg	279
	M	G	L	K	**F**	R	Q	**L**	HBV cAg 93-100	280
	I	M	I	K	**F**	N	R	**L**	Human autoantigen LA (SS-B) 51-58	281
	S	V	V	E	**F**	S	S	**L**	Vector artefact	260
	S	N	F	V	**F**	A	G	**I**	DEAD box protein p68 RNA helicase 547-554	283
	V	Y	D	F	**F**	V	W	**L**	TRP-2 181-188	284

* Also a T cell epitope
+ One of these peptides was found in a total cell extract of K^b-expressing tumor cells

H2-D^b	Position									Source	Ref.
	1	2	3	4	**5**	6	7	8	**9**		
Anchor residues					**N**				**M**		4
									I		
									L		
Preferred residues		M	I	K		L					
			L	E		F					
			P	Q							
			V	V							
Others	A	A	G	D		A	D	F			
	N	Q		T		Y	E	H			
	I	D				T	Q	K			
	F					V	V	S			
	P					M	T	Y			
	S					E	Y				
	T					Q					
	V					H					
						I					
						K					
						P					
						S					
Examples for ligands	A	S	N	E	**N**	M	E	T	**M***	Influenza A34 NP 366-374	4, 201, 180
	I	Q	V	G	**N**	T	R	T	**I***	Yersinia YOP 51 249-257	285

	Sequence	Source	Ref.
	C L S W **N** G P H **L***	Mouse hepatitis virus spike protein 510-518	286
	A A P D **N** R E T F*	miHAg B6 (dom)	287
	A M G V **N** L T S **M**	Cyclin (mouse) 67-75	Dumrese et al. (unpub.)
T cell epitopes	A S N E **N** M D A **M**	Influenza A68 NP 366-374	288
	S A I N **N** Y A Q K **L**	SV 40 T 206-215	289, 290
	C K G V **N** K E Y **L**	SV 40 T 223-231	289, 290
	Q G I N **N** L D N **L**	SV 40 T 489-497	289, 290
	S G P S **N** T P P E **I**	Adenovirus 5 E1A 234-243	291
	F Q P Q **N** G Q F **I**	LCMV NP 396-404	292
	S G V E **N** P G G Y C **L**	LCMV GP 276-286	293
	K A V Y **N** F A T C G	LCMV GP 33-42	294, 295
	R A H Y **N** I V T F	HPV16 E7 49-57	296
	N N L D **N** L R D Y **(L)**	SV 40 T 492-500 (501)	297
	S A L Q **N** A A S **I** A	Myobacterial HSP60 499-508	298
	K D I G **N** I I S D A	Murine HSP60 162-170	298
	F A P G **N** Y P A **L**	SV NP 324-332	299
	V N I R **N** C C Y **I**	Adenovirus 5 E1B 192-200	300
	S G P S **N** I P P E **I**	Adenovirus 5 E1A (T239I) 234-243	300
	T N L L **N** D R V **L**	Murine cyclin D1 20-28	277
	G R P K **N** G C I V	Murine mdm2 441-449	277
	A Q H P **N** A E L **L**	Epitope mimic of a natural tumor antigen	278
	C C L C L T V F **L**	MuLV gag75K 75-83	301
	K Y M C **N** S S C **M**	Mouse p53^{wt} 232-240	302
	W M H H **N** M D L **I**	Mouse UTY protein	303

* Also a T cell epitope

Table 4.3. (con't)

H2-K^k	Position								Comments	Ref.
	1	**2**	3	4	5	6	7	**8**		
Anchor residues		**E**						**I**	C terminus at P8 or P9	304, 305, 306, 307
								V		
Preferred residues	V	D	K	L	A	N	T			
	F	P	N		G	K				
			Y		P	H				
			M		T					
			Q		V					
			I		F					
			L		S					
			F							
			P							
			H							
			T							
			V							
Also detected	E,A			E,H	E		I			
	R,M			Y						
Examples for natural ligands									**Source**	
	H	**E**	T	T	F	N	S	**I**	β Actin 275-282	308
	D	D	H	R	A	G	K	**I**	40S ribosomal protein S24 53-60	308
	Y	**E**	D	T	G	K	T	**I**	Unknown	308
	K	**E**	M	K	A	K	V	**I**	Homol. T cell transcript. Factor 1	308
	E	**E**	E	P	V	K	K	**I**	hnRNP C protein 84-91	308
	S	**E**	I	V	G	K	R	**I**	40S ribosomal protein S7/S8137-144	308
	S	**E**	G	G	S	H	T	**I**	H2-D^{k}112-119	308
	D	**E**	R	T	V	R	K	**I**	Unknown	308
	E	**E**	D	P	V	K	K	**V**	CArG bind. factor A 209-216	308
	E	A	Y	L	G	K	K	**V**	BiP 158-165	308
	T	**E**	L	Q	G	L	N	**V**	Transcription factor NF-E2 35-42	307
	I	P	V	M	G	L	M	**V**	ATPase 653-660	307
	K	P	K	T	S	L	N	**V**	IL-7 receptor α-chain 289-296	307
	Q	**E**	K	I	N	L	N	**V**	Complement C3b 776-783	307
	G	**E**	L	S	Y	L	N	**V**	Cathepsin D 255-262	307
	Q	**E**	L	G	V	G	C	**V**	Phosphoribosyltransferase 15-22	307
	M	**E**	V	F	L	I	C	**V**	NADH-Dehydrogenase 98-105	307

T cell epitopes	F **E** A N G N L **I**	Influenza A HA 259-266	306, 309, 310
	I **E** G G W T G M **I**	Influenza A HA 10-18	306, 309, 310
	S D Y E G R L **I**	Influenza A NP 50-57	311, 312
	F **E** S T G N L **I**	Influenza JAP HA 255-262	313
	S **E** F L L E K R **I**	SV 40 T 560-568	314
	Y **E** N D I E K K **I**	*P. falciparum* CSP 375-383	315
	D **E** L D Y E N D **I**	*P. falciparum* CSP 371-379	315
	T **E** M E K E G K **I**	HIV-1 RT 206-214	316
	V **E** A E I A H Q **I**	Rabies NS 197-205	309, 310
	E **E** G A I V G E **I**	Influenza A NS1 152-160	304
	T **E** N S G K D **I**	Murine SMCY (miHAg H-Y)	317

H2-K[km1]	Position								Source	Ref.
	1	**2**	3	4	5	6	7	**8**		
Anchor or auxiliary anchor residues		**E**						**I**		305
Other preferred residues		Q	K	P	A		R			
		G	N		R		Y			
		P	Q		K					
			G							
			M							
			P							
			Y							

Qa-1[a]	Sequence	Source	Ref.
Motif unknown			
T cell epitope	A M A P R T L L L	MHC class I leader segment 3-11	318

Table 4.3. (con't)

Qa-2	1	2	3	4	5	6	7	8	9		Source	Ref.
Anchor or auxiliary anchor residues		M	N		V	K	**H**		**L**			319, 320
		L	I		I	M			**I**			
		Q	L			I			**F**			
Other preferred residues	K		T	P	L	L	R	E				
	A			E	T	F		Q				
	E			A	E	N		N				
	Q			G	H	Y		D				
				K	M			K				
				S	F			S				
				D	Y			T				
								R				
Examples for ligands	K	Q	N	P	I	A	**H**	Q	**L**		Unknown	320
	A	L	A	E	L	P	**H**	E	**L**		Unknown	320
	K	Q	N	P	T	V	**H**	H	**L**		Unknown	320
	A	G	L	L	G	M	R	S	G	**L**	Unknown	320
	K	L	I	K	V	Y	**H**	S	**L**		Unknown	320
	V	Q	N	X	T	M	**H**	P	**I**		Unknown	320
	R	S	N	G	Q	V	**H**	M	**L**		Unknown	320
	K	L	T	G	I	K	**H**	E	**L**		Cofilin 127-135	320
	A	M	L	A	T	Y	**H**	K	**L**		Unknown	320
	G	Q	L	X	V	X	**H**	K	**L**		Unknown	320
	I	L	M	E	H	I	**H**	K	**L**		60S ribosomal protein L19 137-145	320
	A	Q	N	P	V	L	Y	Q	**I**		Unknown	320
	S	L	I	K	T	V	R	E	M		Unknown	320
	K	M	L	P	V	E	**H**	N	**L**		Unknown	320
	K	Q	L	I	V	T	Y	H	**L**		Unknown	320
	S	V	L	D	D	L	A	L	**L**		Unknown	320
	Y	E	S	P	L	M	X	F	**L**		Unknown	320
	D	L	L	G	T	L	**H**	N	**L**		Unknown	320

H2-M3	Sequence	Comments	Ref.
Examples for ligands	fM Y F I N I L T L	NADH-Dehydrogenase 1-9	321
	fM I V I L*	*L. monocytogenes* Fr 38	322
T cell epitopes	fM F F I N I L T L L V P	ND1α 1-12	323
	fM F F I N A L T L L V P	ND1β 1-12	323
	fM F F I N I L T L L V P ILIAM	ND1α 1-17	324
	fM F F I N A L T L L V P ILIAM	ND1β 1-17	324
	fM F I N R W	COI mitochondrial gene product 1-6	325
	fM I G W I I	*L. monocytogenes* membrane protein LemA 1-6	326
	fM I G W I I A	*L. monocytogenes* membrane protein Lem A 1-7	326

* also a T cell epitope

Table 4.4 Class I motifs of other species

RT1.A[a]	Position										Source	Ref.
	1	**2**	3	4	5	6	7	8	**9**			
Anchor and auxilliary anchor residues		**L,M**							**R**			
Preferred residues		V,I							K			327

RT1.A[l]	Position										Source	Ref.
	1	2	**3**	4	5	6	7	8	**9**			
Anchor or auxiliary anchor residues		A,S V	**F,Y**						**Y,F L,M**			328
Preferred residues	A,S K		L	E,L K,P G,Q	E,D F	R,K	E,D	E,D T				
Also detected	G,Y F,V			D,V	A,S	I,L V	A,S T,V	A,S				
Examples for ligands	G	G	**Y**	G	G	G	Y	D	N	**Y**	Human hnRNP A2 281-290	328
	A	G	**Y**	G	G	Y	E	E	**Y**		Human hnRNP F 238-246	328
	G	S	**Y**	N	D	F	G	N	**Y**		hnRNP A1 257-265	328
	S	A	V	R	N	V	T	S	**F**		Unknown	328
	N	A	**F**	K	E	I	T	T	**M**		TFIIB 116-124	328
	A	A	**F**	F	N	K	T	E	**F**		Unknown	328
	M	S	L	I	I	N	T	F	**Y**		HSP90β 24-32	328
	N	I	**F**	K	F	I	I	P			LDH M chain 115-122	328

Bota-A11	Position									Source	Ref.
	1	**2**	3	4	5	6	7	8	**9**		
Anchor residues		**P**	A		P				**I V**		330

	1	2	3	4	5	6	7	8	9		
Other preferred residues				I,P M,L E,G T	G,A Y	V,I K,Q L,G	L,I V,Y P,G	Q,V F,I E,Y			
Examples for binding epitopes	X	**P**	A	I	P	V	L	Q	**I**	Unknown	330
		q	F	P	G	I	I	V	**V**	Unknown	330
			V	M	A	K	V	F	L	Unknown	330
Bota-A20	**Position**										**Ref.**
	1	**2**	3	4	5	6	7	8	**9**		
Anchor residues		**K**							**R**		331
Other preferred residues	A I		K	D P	D P	K I P V D	I V L	R Q			
Chicken B-F4	**Position**										**Ref.**
	1	**2**	3	4	**5**	6	7	**8**	9		
Anchor residues		**D** **E**			**D** **E**			**E**			332
Chicken B-F12	**Position**										**Ref.**
	1	2	3	4	**5**	6	7	**8**	9		
Anchor residues					**V** **I**			**V**			332
Chicken B-F15	**Position**										**Ref.**
	1	**2**	3	4	5	6	7	**8**	9		
Anchor residues		**R**						**Y**			332

Table 4.4. (con't)

Chicken B-F19	**Position**										**Ref.**
	1	**2**	3	4	5	6	7	**8**	9		
Anchor residues		**R**						Y P L F			332
Patr-A*04	**Sequence**									**Source**	**Ref.**
Motif unknown											
T cell epitopes	K	H	P	D	A	T	Y	S	R	HCV-1 NS1 205-213	333
	G	D	F	D	S	V	I	D	C	HCV-1 NS3 440-448	333
Patr-A*11	**Sequence**									**Source**	**Ref.**
Motif unknown											
T cell epitope	S	W	A	I	K	W	E	Y		HCV-1 NS1 328-335	155
Patr-B*01	**Sequence**									**Source**	**Ref.**
Motif unknown											
T cell epitope	Y	T	G	D	F	D	S	V	I	HCV-1 NS3 438-446	155
Patr-B*13	**Sequence**									**Source**	**Ref.**
T cell epitopes	T	R	P	P	L	G	N	W	F	HCV-1 NS1 159-167	155
	V	P	H	P	N	I	E	E	V	HCV-1 NS3 351-359	155
Patr-B*16	**Sequence**									**Source**	**Ref.**
Motif unknown											
T cell epitopes	G	D	F	D	S	V	I	D	C	HCV-1 NS3 440-448	155
	G	N	A	S	R	C	W	V	A	HCV-1 env E 118-126	155

Papa-A*06	Position	Source	Ref.
Motif unknown			
T cell epitopes	K H P D A T Y S R	HCV-1 NS1 205-213	333

Mamu-A*01	Sequence	Source	Ref.
Motif unknown			
T cell epitopes	E G C T P Y D I N Q M L	SIV gag p11C 179-190	334

SLA (haplotype d/d)	Sequence	Source	Ref.
T cell epitopes	ENALLVALF	Classical swine fever virus CSFV 2276-2284	335

HCMV class I homolog UL18	Position	Source	Ref.
	1 **2** 3 4 5 6 7 8 **9**		
Anchor or preferred residues	**M** P **L**		336
	L I		
	F		
Examples for ligands	L **M** T T V H A I T A T Q K T V	Hamster 3-PGAL-dehydrogenase 172-186	336
	I **L** P D G T X K **F**	Rat β-galactosidase	336
	I **M** G P N Y T P G K K E D L Y LKPIQ	Hamster elongation factor 429-444	336
	I **M** E E T G K X **F**	Human expressed sequence tag clone	336
	L **M** P N G P M R **L**	Human expressed sequence tag clone	336
	V **M** G G H A I R **I**	Rat cathepsin B	336
	I **L** P E Q G L M L T	Mouse phospholipase A 2-activating protein 102-111	336
	A **L** P H A I L R L D	Human β actin 170-179	336
	N **L** P P H I I R **L**	Human ubiquitin carrier protein E2	336
	M **M** N T D L S R I L K S P E I QR	Rat 60S ribosomal protein L4	336
	A **L** P H A I L R **L**	Human β actin 170-178	336
	T F A P S T I **F**	Human ribophorin II	336

Table 4.5 HLA class II motifs

HLA-DRB1*0101		Relative position										Source	Ref.
		1	2	3	**4**	5	**6**	7	8	**9**			
Anchor residues		**Y,V L,F I,A M,W**			**L,A I,V M,N Q**		**A,G S,T P**			**L,A I,V N,F Y**			337, 17, 16, 338
Examples for ligands	VGSD	**W**	R	F	**L**	R	**G**	Y	H	Q	YA	HLA-A2 103-117	339
	VGSD	**W**	R	F	**L**	R	**G**	Y	H	Q	YAYDG	HLA-A2 103-120	339
	VGSD	**W**	R	F	**L**	R	**G**	Y	H	Q	Y	HLA-A2 103-116	339
	GSD	**W**	R	F	**L**	R	**G**	Y	H	Q	YA	HLA-A2 104-117	339
	LPKPPKPVSK	**M**	R	M	**A**	T	**P**	L	L	M	QALPM	Invariant chain 97-120	339
	IPAD	**L**	R	I	**I**	S	**A**	N	G	C	K	Na+-K+-ATPase 199-216	339
	RVE	**Y**	H	F	**L**	S	**P**	Y	V	S	PKESP	Transferrin receptor 680-696	339
	YKHT	**L**	N	Q	**I**	D	**S**	V	K	**V**	WPRRPT	Cattle fetuin 56-74	339
	AILE	**F**	R	A	**M**	A	Q	F	S	R	KTD	Unknown	340
	PK	**Y**	V	K	**Q**	N	**T**	L	K	**L**	AT*	Influenza HA 306-318	16
	STPE	**F**	T	I	**L**	N	**T**	F	H	**I**	PSFTI	Apolipoprotein B 2646-2663	338
	HPNQPF	**Y**	I	L	K	P	Q	M	P	W	ELW	Sialyltransferase 288-305	338,341
	XXPAF	**Y**	M	L	K	G	K	L	Q	**Y**	XL	Unknown	338
	LDHK	**F**	D	L	**M**	Y	**A**	K	R	**A**	FVHWY	Tubulin α1 chain 391-408	338,341
	LAT	**W**	T	I	**Q**	G	**A**	A	N	**A**	LSGDVW	Transferrin receptor 737-754	338,341
	LPKPPKPVSK	**M**	R	M	**A**	T	**P**	L	L	M	QAL	Invariant chain 97-118	341
T cell epitopes	ER	**V**	R	L	**L**	E	R	C	I	**Y**	NQE	DRB1*0101-chain 22-35	342,341
	TGKENT	**I**	K	I	**Q**	E	**G**	S	G	**L**	SKEEI	*M. leprae* HSP 70 468-487	343
	HQSL	**V**	I	K	**L**	M	**P**	N	I	T	LL	Measles virus fusion protein 51-65	344

* Alignment determined by structural analysis

HLA-DRB1*0102		Relative position										Source	Ref.
		1	**2**	**3**	**4**	**5**	**6**	**7**	**8**	**9**			
Anchor or auxiliary anchor residues		**I, L V,M**			**A, L, M**		**A, G S, T P**			**I, L A, M, Y, W**			338
Examples for ligands	YIPHV	**M**	A	Y	**A**	A	C	I	G	**A**	NRDH	Alkaline phosphatase 479-496	338,341
	LPKPPKPVSK	**M**	R	M	**A**	T	**P**	L	L	**M**	QAL	Invariant chain 97-118	338,341
	DLNP	**L**	I	K	**L**	S	**G**	A	Y	**L**	VDDSD	Mannose-6-phosphate receptor 185-202	338,341
	SPN	**I**	V	I	**A**	L	**S**	G	N	K	ADLANK	Ras-related protein Rab-5A 123-140	338,341
	LPNIPVQT	**I**	S	R	**A**	A	**A**	E	K	**L**	F	Transferrin receptor 335-352	338,341
	IF	**V**	K	T	**L**	T	**G**	K	T	**I**	TLEVEPS	Ubiquitin 3-20	338,341

HLA-DRB1*0301 (DR17)		Relative position										Source	Ref.
		1	**2**	**3**	**4**	**5**	**6**	**7**	**8**	**9**			
Anchor or auxiliary anchor residues		**L,I F,M V**			**D**		**K, R E,Q N**			**Y,L F**			144, 345, 346
Examples for ligands	ISNQ	**L**	T	L	**D**	S	**N**	T	K	**Y**	FHKLN	Apolipoprotein B 2877-2894	144
	ISNQ	**L**	T	L	**D**	S	**N**	T	K	**Y**	FHKL	Apolipoprotein B 2877-2893	144
	ISNQ	**L**	T	L	**D**	S	**N**	T	K	**Y**	FHK	Apolipoprotein B 2877-2892	144
	VDT	**F**	L	E	**D**	V	**K**	N	L	**Y**	HSEA	α1-Antitrypsin 149-164	144
	KPRA	**I**	V	V	**D**	P	V	H	G	**F**	MY	LDL-Receptor 518-532	144
	KQT	**I**	S	P	**D**	Y	**R**	N	M	I		IgG2a, Membrane domain 384-395	144
	YPD	**F**	I	M	**D**	P	**K**	E	K	D	KV	Unknown	144
	NIQ	**L**	I	N	**D**	Q	**E**	V	A	R	FD	Unknown	144
	LLS	**F**	V	R	**D**	L	**N**	Q	Y	R	ADI	Transferrin receptor 618-632	144
	LPKPPKPVSK	**M**	R	M	A	T	P	L				Invariant chain 97-113	347, 18, 348
	LPKPPKPVSK	**M**	R	M	A	T	P	L	L	M	QALP	Invariant chain 97-119	347, 18, 348
	LPKPPKPVSK	**M**	R	M	A	T	P	L	L	M	QALPM	Invariant chain 97-120	347, 18, 348
	PKPPKPVSK	**M**	R	M	A	T	P	L				Invariant chain 98-113	347, 18, 348
	PKPPKPVSK	**M**	R	M	A	T	P	L	L	M	QA	Invariant chain 98-117	347, 18, 348
	KPPKPVSK	**M**	R	M	A	T	P	L	L	M	Q	Invariant chain 99-116	347, 18, 348
	KPPKPVSK	**M**	R	M	A	T	P	L	L	M	QALPM	Invariant chain 99-119	347, 18, 348
	VDDTQF	**V**	R	F	**D**	S	D	A	A	S	Q	HLA-A30 52-67	18
	ATKYGN	**M**	T	E	**D**	H	V	M	H	**L**	LQNA	Invariant chain 131-149	18
	VFLL	**L**	L	A	**D**	K	V	P	E	T	SLS	ACh receptor 289-304	18

Table 4.5. (con't)

		Position										Source	Ref.
		1	**2**	**3**	**4**	**5**	**6**	**7**	**8**	**9**			
	LNK	**I**	L	L	**D**	E	**Q**	A	Q	W	K	ICAM-2 64-76	18
	GPPKLD	**I**	R	K	E	E	**K**	Q	I	M	IDIFH	IFNγ receptor 128-147	18
	GPPKLD	**I**	R	K	E	E	**K**	Q	I	M	IDIFHP	IFNγ receptor 128-148	18
	GFKA	**I**	R	P	**D**	K	**K**	S	N	P	IIRTV	Cyt-b5 155-172	18
	YAN	**I**	L	L	**D**	R	**R**	V	P	Q	TDMTF	Apolipoprotein B 1207-1224	18
	NLF	**L**	K	S	**D**	G	**R**	I	K	**Y**	TLNKNSLK	Apolipoprotein B 1276-1295	18
	IPDNLF	**L**	K	S	**D**	G	**R**	I	K	**Y**	TLNKN	Apolipoprotein B 1273-1292	18
	IPDNLF	**L**	K	S	**D**	G	**R**	I	K	**Y**	TLNK	Apolipoprotein B 1273-1291	18
	IPDNLF	**L**	K	S	**D**	G	**R**	I	K	**Y**	TLN	Apolipoprotein B 1273-1290	144, 18
	IPDNLF	**L**	K	S	**D**	G	**R**	I	K	**Y**	TL	Apolipoprotein B 1273-1289	18
	NLF	**L**	K	S	**D**	G	**R**	I	K	**Y**	TLNK	Apolipoprotein B 1276-1291	18
	NLF	**L**	K	S	**D**	G	**R**	I	K	**Y**	TLN	Apolipoprotein B 1276-1290	18
	VTT	**L**	N	S	**D**	L	**K**	Y	N	A	LDLTN	Apolipoprotein B 1294-1310	18
	V	G	S	**D**	W	**R**	F	L	R	G	YHQYA	HLA-A2 103-117	18
T cell epitopes	GDVV	A	V	V	**D**	I	**K**	E	K	G	KDKWIELK	Lo1 pol. 171-190	345
	KT	**I**	A	Y	**D**	E	**E**	A	R	R		*M. bovis* HSP65 3-13	349

HLA-DRB1*0401 (DR4Dw4)		Relative position										Source	Ref.
		1	2	3	**4**	5	**6**	**7**	8	**9**			
Anchor or preferred residues		**F,Y W,I, L,V M**			**F,W I,L V,A D,E no R,K**		**N,S T,Q H,R**	**pol.* chg.* ali.***		**pol.* ali.* K**			350, 351, 352, 353, 354
Examples for ligands		**F**	V	R	**F**	D	**S**	**D**	A	**A**	SQRMEP	HLA-A2 33-47	350
	VDDTQ	**F**	V	R	**F**	D	**S**	**D**	A	**A**	SQRM	HLA-A2 52-69	350
		F	V	R	**F**	D	**S**	**D**	A	**A**	SQRM	HLA-A2 33-45	350
	VDDTQ	**F**	V	R	**F**	D	**S**	**D**	A	**A**	SPRGEP...	HLA-C 52-?	350
	DGKD	**Y**	I	A	**L**	N	E	**D**	L	S	S	HLA-B44 143-156	350
	LSS	**W**	T	A	**A**	D	**T**	**A**	A	Q	ITQ	HLA-B44 154-168	350
	LSS	**W**	T	A	**A**	D	**T**	**A**	A	Q	IT	HLA-B44 154-167	350
	IY	**F**	R	N	Q	K	G	**S**	H	S	GLQPTGFL	HLA-DR4b 252-270	350

	DVA	**F**	V	K	**D**	Q	**T**	**V**	I	Q	NTD	Cattle transferrin 68-82	350
	YDHN	**F**	V	K	**A**	I	**N**	**A**	I	Q	KSW	Cathepsin C 170-185	350
	KHKV	**Y**	A	C	**E**	V	**T**	**H**	Q	G	...	Igκ chain C region 80-?	350
	HKV	**Y**	A	C	**E**	V	**T**	**H**	Q	G	L...	Igκ chain C region 81-?	350
	DGP	**F**	R	I	**I**	T	V	P	A	**A**	LDY	Unknown	350
	TGN	**Y**	R	I	**E**	S	V	**L**	S	S		Sphingolipid activator protein 3 165-176	350
	GERA	**M**	T	K	**D**	N	**N**	**L**	L	G	...	HSC 70 445-?	350
	XXX	**Y**	E	X	**A**	L	**S**	**L**	P	S	K...	Unknown	350
	GSLF	**V**	Y	N	**I**	T	**T**	**N**	K	**Y**	KAFLKQ	VLA-4 229-247	18
	SPEDF	**V**	Y	Q	**F**	K	G	**M**	C	**Y**	F	HLA-DQβ 3.2 chain 24-38	18
	AAPYEKEVP	**L**	S	A	**L**	T	**N**	**I**	L	S	AQL	PAI-1 261-281	18
	GVYF	**Y**	L	Q	**W**	G	**R**	**S**	T	**L**	VSVS	Ig heavy chain 121-?	18
	AEALERM	**F**	L	S	**F**	P	**T**	**T**	K	T		Cattle hemoglobin 26-41	18
	LRS	**W**	T	A	**A**	D	**T**	**A**	A	Q	ITQRKWEAA	HLA-Cw9 130-150	18
	DLSS	**W**	T	A	**A**	D	**T**	**A**	A	Q	ITQRKWEAA	HLA-Bw62 129-150	18
	APSP	**L**	P	E	T	T	E	**N**	V	V	CALG	HLA-DRα chain 182-198	18
		V	Y	P	**E**	V	**T**	**V**	Y	P	AKT	HLA-DR4β*0401 124-135	355
		V	Y	P	**E**	V	**T**	**V**	Y	P	AK	HLA-DR4β*0401 124-134	355
	PGQPPRL	**L**	I	Y	**D**	A	**S**	**N**	R	**A**	TGIPA	Igκ chain V-region 60-80	355
	KPGQPPRL	**L**	I	Y	**D**	A	**S**	**N**	R	**A**	TGIPA	Igκ chain V-region 59-80	355
	**pEPPRL	**L**	I	Y	**D**	A	**S**	**N**	R	**A**	TGIPA	Igκ chain V-region 61-80	355
	pEPPRL	**L**	I	Y	**D**	A	**S**	**N**	R	**A**	TG	Igk chain V-region 71-77	355
	LSS	**W**	T	A	**A**	D	**T**	**A**	A	Q	ITQ	HLA-B62 130-144	356
T cell epitopes	E	**F**	V	V	**E**	F	D	**L**	P	G	IKA	*M. leprae* HSP18 38-50	357
	AK	**F**	Y	R	**D**	P	**T**	**A**	F	G	SG	Link 61-73	354
	LL	E	S	I	Q	Q	**N**	**L**	L	K	AEKGN	Chlamydial histone-like protein hc-1 13-28	358
	QN	**L**	L	K	**A**	E	K	G	N	K	AAAQR	Chlamydial histone-like protein hc-1 19-34	358
	AG	**F**	K	G	**E**	Q	G	P	K	G	EP	Bovine type II collagen 276-288	359
	Q	N	I	L	**L**	S	**N**	**A**	P	**L**	GPQFP	Tyrosinase 56-70	360
	D	**Y**	S	Y	**L**	Q	D	**S**	D	P	DSFQD	Tyrosinase 448-462	360
		M	N	I	**L**	L	**Q**	Y	V	V	KSFD	Human GAD65 115-127	361
	IA	**F**	T	S	**E**	H	**S**	**H**	F	S	LK	Human GAD65 274-286	361
		A	T	G	**F**	K	**Q**	**S**	S	K	ALQRPVAS	bcr-abl p210, b3a2	362

* pol.: polar; chg.: charged; ali.: aliphatic
**p: pyroglutamic acid

Table 4.5. (con't)

HLA-DRB1*0402 (DR4Dw10)		Relative position										Source	Ref.
		1	2	3	**4**	5	**6**	**7**	8	**9**			
Anchor or preferred residues		V,I L,M			Y,F, W I,L, M R,N no D,E		N,Q S,T K	R,K H,N Q,P		pol.* ali.* H			350, 354
Examples for ligands	GPDGR	**L**	L	R	G	H	**N**	**Q**	F	**A**	YDGKDY...	HLA-B38 128-?	350
	GPDGR	**L**	L	R	G	H	**N**	**Q**	F	**A**	YDGKD	HLA-B38 128-146	350
	GPDGR	**L**	L	R	G	H	**N**	**Q**	F	**A**	YDGK	HLA-B38128-145	350
	GPDGR	**L**	L	R	G	H	**N**	**Q**	F	**A**	YDG	HLA-B38 128-144	350
	GR	**L**	L	R	G	H	**N**	**Q**	F	**A**	YDGK	HLA-B38 131-145	350
	I	**I**	K	G	V	R	**K**	**S**	N	**A**	AERRG	HLA-DRα 238-252	350
		I	Y	F	**R**	N	**Q**	**K**	G	**H**	SGLQPTGFLS	HLA-DR4β 248-266	350
		I	Y	F	**R**	N	**Q**	**K**	G	**H**	SGLQP	HLA-DR4β 248-261	350
				F	**R**	N	**Q**	**K**	G	**H**	SGLQP	HLA-DR4β 250-261	350
	F	**I**	Y	F	**R**	N	**Q**	**K**	G	**H**	SGLQPTGFLS	HLA-DR4β 249-266	350
	LPKPPKPVSK	**M**	R	M	A	T	P	L	L	**Q**		Invariant chain 97-?	350
	FDQK	**I**	V	E	**W**	D	**S**	**R**	K	**S**	KYFE	BLAST-1 62-78	350
	DQK	**I**	V	E	**W**	D	**S**	**R**	K	**S**	KYF	BLAST-1 63-77	350
	IKI	**I**	S	K	**I**	E	**N**	**H**	E	G	VRR	Pyruvate kinase 264-278	350
	IKI	**I**	S	K	**I**	E	**N**	**H**	E	G	VR	Pyruvate-kinase 264-277	350
	FGR	**I**	G	R	**L**	V	**T**	**R**	A	**A**	FNSG	GAPDH 9-24	350
	FGR	**I**	G	R	**L**	V	**T**	**R**	A	**A**	FN	GAPDH 9-22	350
	GFGR	**I**	G	R	**L**	V	**T**	**R**	A	**A**	FNSG	GAPDH 9-24	350
	CNE	**I**	I	N	**W**	L	D	**K**	N	**Q**		HSC70 574-585	350
	QPD	**L**	R	Y	**L**	F	L	**N**	G	**N**		Leucine-rich α2-glycoprotein 200-211	350
	MHHWL	**L**	F	E	**M**	S	R	**H**	S	**L**	E	Invariant chain 185-199	355
	HHWL	**L**	F	E	**M**	S	R	**H**	S	**L**	E	Invariant chain 186-199	355
	WL	**L**	F	E	**M**	S	R	**H**	S	**L**	EQKP	Invariant chain 188-202	355
	SPEEQDF	**L**	T	K	H	A	**S**	**H**	T	G	SWIG	IgE Fc receptor 203-222	355
	EQDF	**L**	T	K	H	A	**S**	**H**	T	G	SWIG	IgE Fc receptor 206-222	355
	QDF	**L**	T	K	H	A	**S**	**H**	T	G	SWIG	IgE Fc receptor 207-222	355
	FDQK	**I**	V	E	**W**	D	**S**	**R**	K	**S**	KYF	CD48 62-77	355

	FDQK	**I**	V	E	**W**	D	**S**	**R**	K	**S**	KYFE	CD48 62-78	355
	FDQK	**I**	V	E	**W**	D	**S**	**R**	K	**S**	KYFES	CD48 62-79	355
	FDQK	**I**	V	E	**W**	D	**S**	**R**	K	**S**	K	CD48 62-75	355
	GPDG	R	L	L	**R**	G	H	**N**	Q	F	AYDGK	HLA-B39 128-145	363
	GPDG	R	L	L	**R**	G	H	**N**	Q	F	AYD	HLA-B39 128-143	363
	GPDG	R	L	L	**R**	G	H	**N**	Q	F	AYDGKDY	HLA-B39 128-147	363
	VGPDG	R	L	L	**R**	G	H	**N**	Q	F	AYD	HLA-B39 127-143	363
	FGRI	G	R	L	V	T	R	A	A	F	NS	GAPDH 9-23	363
	GFGRI	G	R	L	V	T	R	A	A	F	N	GAPDH 8-22	363
T cell epitope	LNSK	**I**	A	F	K	I	V	S	Q	E	PA	Desmoglein 3 190-204	364

* pol: polar; ali: aliphatic

HLA-DRB1*0403 (DR4Dw13)	**Sequence**	**Source**	**Ref.**
Motif unknown T cell epitope	EVWVTPVIGSQA	Rubella virus peptid E1 273-284	365

HLA-DRB1*0404 (DR4Dw14)		**Relative position**										**Source**	**Ref.**
		1	2	3	**4**	5	**6**	**7**	8	**9**			350,354
Anchor or preferred residues		**V,I L,M**			**F,Y, W,I L,V M,A D,E no R,K**		**N,T S,Q R**	**pol.* chg.* ali.***		**pol.* ali.* K**			
Examples for ligands	GSHS	**M**	R	Y	**F**	H	**T**	**A**	M	**S**	RPGRGE	HLA-B60 1-13	350
	SHS	**M**	R	Y	**F**	H	**T**	**A**	M	**S**	RPGRGE	HLA-B60 2-13	350
	YDNS	**L**	K	I	**I**	S	**N**	**A**	S	C	TTN	GAPDH 139-154	350
	AN	**I**	A	V	**D**	K	A	**N**	L	E	IMTKR	HLA-DRα 86-101	355
	LAN	**I**	A	V	**D**	K	A	**N**	L	E	IMTKR	HLA-DRα 85-101	355
	QGALAN	**I**	A	V	**D**	K	A	**N**	L	E		HLA-DRα 82-96	355
	QGALAN	**I**	A	V	**D**	K	A	**N**	L	E	IM	HLA-DRα 82-98	355
	AQGALAN	**I**	A	V	**D**	K	A	**N**	L	E	IMT	HLA-DRα 81-99	355
	KDY	**I**	A	L	N	E	D	**L**	R	**S**		HLA-A α 145-156	355
	KDY	**I**	A	L	N	E	D	**L**	R	**S**	WT	HLA-A α 145-158	355

Table 4.5. (con't)

	Relative position										Source	Ref.
	1	2	3	**4**	5	**6**	**7**	8	**9**			
KDY	**I**	A	L	N	E	D	**L**	R	**S**	WTA	HLA-A α 145-159	355
DY	**I**	A	L	N	E	D	**L**	R	**S**	WTAAD	HLA-A α 146-161	355
DY	**I**	A	L	N	E	D	**L**	R	**S**	WTAA	HLA-A α 146-160	355
DY	**I**	A	L	N	E	D	**L**	R	**S**	WT	HLA-A α 146-158	355
TPDF	**I**	V	P	**L**	T	D	**L**	R	**I**	PS	Apolipoprotein B 2614-2628	355
TPDF	**I**	V	P	**L**	T	D	**L**	R	**I**	P	Apolipoprotein B 2614-2627	355
PDF	**I**	V	P	**L**	T	D	**L**	R	**I**	P	Apolipoprotein B 2615-2627	355
PDF	**I**	V	P	**L**	T	D	**L**	R	**I**	PSVQ	Apolipoprotein B 2615-2630	355
F	**I**	V	P	**L**	T	D	**L**	R	**I**	PS	Apolipoprotein B 2617-2628	355
FQTPDF	**I**	V	P	**L**	T	D	**L**	R	**I**	PSVQI	Apolipoprotein B 2612-2631	355
EIKILN	**I**	F	G	**V**	I	K	G	F	**V**	EP	Transferrin receptor 383-399	355
EIKILN	**I**	F	G	**V**	I	K	G	F	**V**	E	Transferrin receptor 383-398	355
IKILN	**I**	F	G	**V**	I	K	G	F	**V**	EPD	Transferrin receptor 384-400	355
IKILN	**I**	F	G	**V**	I	K	G	F	**V**	EP	Transferrin receptor 384-399	355
IKILN	**I**	F	G	**V**	I	K	G	F	**V**	E	Transferrin receptor 384-398	355
MGQKDSY	**V**	G	D	**E**	A	**Q**	**S**	K	R		Cytoplasmic actin 47-62	355
TLKYP	**I**	E	H	G	I	V	**T**	N	W	DD	Cytoplasmic actin 66-81	355
YP	**I**	E	H	G	I	V	**T**	N	W	DDM	Cytoplasmic actin 69-82	355
VAPEEHPVL	**L**	T	E	**A**	P	L	**N**	P	**K**	A	Cytoplasmic actin 96-114	355
AVFPSI	**V**	G	R	P	R	H	**Q**	G	**V**	MV	Cytoplasmic actin 28-48	355
KPGKAPK	**L**	L	I	**Y**	A	A	**S**	S	**L**	...	Igκ chain 39-?	355
APK	**L**	L	I	**Y**	A	A	**S**	S	**L**	...	Igκ chain 43-?	355
	S	H	S	**M**	R	Y	F	H	**T**	AMSRP	HLA-B*4001 27-40	363
G	S	H	S	**M**	R	Y	F	H	**T**	AMSRPG	HLA-B*4001 26-41	363
	S	H	S	**M**	R	Y	F	H	**T**	AMSRPG	HLA-B*4001 27-41	363
G	S	H	S	**M**	R	Y	F	H	**T**	AMSRPGRG	HLA-B*4001 26-43	363
	S	H	S	**M**	R	Y	F	Y	**T**	AVSRP	HLA-Cw*03 27-40	363
	S	H	S	**M**	R	Y	F	Y	**T**	AVSRPG	HLA-Cw*03 27-41	363
G	S	H	S	**M**	R	Y	F	Y	**T**	AVSRPG	HLA-Cw*03 26-41	363
G	S	H	S	**M**	R	Y	F	Y	**T**	AVSRPGR	HLA-Cw*03 26-42	363
	S	H	S	**M**	R	Y	F	Y	**T**	AVSRPGRG	HLA-Cw*03 27-43	363
	P	G	K	**A**	P	K	R	L	**I**	YAA	Igκ chain V region A30 63-74	363

* pol: polar; ali: aliphatic; chg: charged

HLA-DRB1*0405 (DR4Dw15)		Relative position										Source	Ref.
		1	2	3	**4**	5	**6**	7	8	**9**			
Anchor or preferred residues		**F,Y** W,V I,L **M**			**V,I** L,M D,E		**N,S** T,Q K,D	**pol.*** chg.* ali.*		**D,E**			**350**
Examples for ligands	YPTQRAR	**Y**	Q	W	**V**	R	C	**N**	P	**D**	SNS	PGSG 1-19	350
	QRAR	**Y**	Q	W	**V**	R	C	**N**	P	**D**	SNS	PGSG 4-19	350
	RAR	**Y**	Q	W	**V**	R	C	**N**	P	**D**	SNS	PGSG 5-19	350
	KPPQ	**Y**	I	A	**V**	H	V	**V**	P	**D**	Q	MIF 32-45	350
	FRE	**F**	K	L	S	K	V	W	R	**D**	QH	Transferrin receptor 173-186	350
	FRE	**F**	K	L	S	K	V	W	R	**D**	Q	Transferrin receptor 173-185	350
	RE	**F**	K	L	S	K	V	W	R	**D**	QH	Transferrin receptor 174-186	350
	RE	**F**	K	L	S	K	V	W	R	**D**	Q	Transferrin receptor 174-185	350
	VEPDH	**Y**	V	V	**V**	G	A	**Q**	R	**D**	A	Transferrin receptor 397-411	350
	EPDH	**Y**	V	V	**V**	G	A	**Q**	R	**D**	A	Transferrin receptor 398-411	350
	THY	**Y**	A	V	A	V	V	**K**	K	**D**	TDFK	Transferrin 92-107	350
	KELK	**I**	D	I	**I**	P	**N**	P	Q	**E**	R	HSP90β 68-81	350
	YLL	**Y**	Y	T	**E**	F	**T**	P	T	**E**	KD	β_2-microglobulin 83-96	350
	LL	**Y**	Y	T	**E**	F	**T**	P	T	**E**	KDEY	β_2-microglobulin 84-98	350
	CAIHAKR	**V**	T	I	**M**	P	**K**	**D**	I	**Q**	LA...	Histone H3 110-?	350
	APNT	**F**	K	T	**L**	D	**S**	W	R	**D**		ras-related protein RAB-7 (rat) 86-98	350
	VADK	**I**	Q	L	**I**	N	**N**	**M**	L	**D**		Phosphoglycerate kinase 216-228	350
	GSTV	**F**	D	N	**L**	P	**N**	P	E	I	**D**GDYYGW	Unknown	366
	XXXQ	**Y**	I	A	**V**	H	V	**V**	P	**D**	QT	Homol. MIF 32-46	366
	SDPIL	**Y**	R	P	**V**	A	V	**A**	L	**D**		PKM2 99-112	366
		V	P	I	Q	R	A	**V**	Y	**Q**	NVVVNNPXD	Unknown	366
	SPGTGA	**Y**	Y	V	**L**	L	**N**	**...**				Unknown	366
	KPPQ	**Y**	I	A	**V**	H	V	**V**	P	**D**	QLM	MIF 32-47	367
	KPPQ	**Y**	I	A	**V**	H	V	**V**	P	**D**	QL	MIF 32-46	367
	KPPQ	**Y**	I	A	**V**	H	V	**V**	P	**D**	Q	MIF 32-45	367
	DPIL	**Y**	R	P	**V**	A	V	**A**	L	**D**	TKGPE	PKM2 101-118	367
	DPIL	**Y**	R	P	**V**	A	V	**A**	L	**D**	TKGP	PKM2 101-117	367
	DNPQTHY	**Y**	A	V	A	V	V	**K**	K	**D**	TDFKL	Transferrin 88-108	367
	DNPQTHY	**Y**	A	V	A	V	V	**K**	K	**D**	TDFK	Transferrin 88-107	367
	NPQTHY	**Y**	A	V	A	V	V	**K**	K	**D**	TDFKL	Transferrin 89-108	367

Table 4.5. (con't)

		Relative position										Source	Ref.
	1	2	3	**4**	5	**6**	**7**	8	**9**				
	NPQTHY	**Y**	A	V	A	V	V	**K**	K	**D**	TDFK	Transferrin 89-107	367
	DNPQTHY	**Y**	A	V	A	V	V	**K**	K	**D**		Transferrin 88-103	367
	THY	**Y**	A	V	A	V	V	**K**	K	**D**	TDF	Transferrin 92-106	367
	LL	**Y**	Y	T	**E**	F	**T**	P	T	**E**	KDEY	β_2-microglobulin 84-98	367
	L	**Y**	Y	T	**E**	F	**T**	P	T	**E**	KD	β_2-microglobulin 85-96	367
	XXXXKK	**V**	V	V	Y	L	**Q**	**K**	L	**D**	T	Cathepsin C 58-73	367
	KK	**V**	V	V	Y	L	**Q**	**K**	L	**D**	TAYD	Cathepsin C 62-76	367
	K	**V**	V	V	Y	L	**Q**	**K**	L	**D**	TAYD	Cathepsin C 63-76	367
	KP	**Y**	N	E	A	K	**T**	X	F	**D**	KY	Apolipoprotein B-100 3218-3230	367
T cell epitope	IDG	**L**	E	V	**D**	V	P	G	I	**D**	PNA	Dermatophagoides pteronyssinus Der p II 58-73	368

* pol.: polar; chg.: charged; ali.: aliphatic

HLA-DRB1*0407 (DR4Dw13)		Relative position										Source	Ref.
		1	2	3	**4**	5	**6**	7	8	**9**			
Anchor or preferred residues		**F,Y W**			**A V,K**		**N,T D,S**			**Q N**			369
Examples for ligands	DLRS	**W**	T	A	**A**	D	**T**	A	A	**Q**	I	HLA class I 153-166	369
	DLRS	**W**	T	A	**A**	D	**T**	A	A	**Q**	ITQ	HLA class I 153-168	369
	LRS	**W**	T	A	**A**	D	**T**	A	A	**Q**	IT	HLA class I 154-167	369
	MRY	**F**	Y	T	**A**	V	**S**	R	P	G		HLA class I 29-40	369
	VDDTQ	**F**	V	R	F	D	**S**	D	A	A		HLA class I 28-41	369
	YDHN	**F**	V	K	**A**	I	**N**	A	I	**Q**	KS	Cathepsin C (rat) homol. 170-184	369
	YPTQRAR	**Y**	Q	W	**V**	R	C	N	P	D	SNS	PGSG 28-46	369
	SGTD	**F**	T	L	T	I	**S**	R	L	E	PE	Igκ chain precursor 88-102	369
	GPTT	**Y**	K	V	T	S	**S**	L	Q	I	KE	IgM μ chain homol. 173-187	369
	LPS	**Y**	E	E	**A**	L	**S**	L	P	S	KT	Unknown	369

HLA-DRB1*0701	Sequence	Source	Ref.
Motif unknown			
Ligands	RPAGDGTFQKWASVVVPSGQ	HLA-A29 234-253	18
	RPAGDGTFQKWASVVV	HLA-A29 234-249	18
	GDGTFQKWASVVVPSGQEQRYT	HLA-A29 237-258	18
	GDGTFQKWASVVVPSGQE	HLA-A29 237-254	18
	GTFQKWASVVVPSG	HLA-A29 239-252	18
	GTFQKWASVVVPSGQ	HLA-A29 239-253	18
	GTFQKWASVVVPSGQEQRYTCHV	HLA-A29 239-261	18
	RETQISKTNTQTYRENL	HLA-B44 83-99	18
	RETQISKTNTQTYREN	HLA-B44 83-98	18
	RETQISKTNTQTYRE	HLA-B44 83-97	18
	RSNYTPITNPPEVTVLTNSPVELREP	HLA-DRα 101-126	18
	GALANIAVDKANLEIMTKRSN	HLA-DRα 58-78	18
	SLQSPITVEWRAQSESAQSKMLSGIGGFVL	HLA-DQa 179-?	18
	VTQYLNATGNRWCSWSLSQAR	4F2 318-338	18
	VTQYLNATGNRWCSWSL	4F2 318-334	18
	TSILCYRKREWIK	LIF receptor 854-866	18
	PAFRFTREAAQDCEV	Thromboxane-A synthase 406-420	18
	GDMYPKTWSGMLVGALCALAGVLTI	K+ channel protein 492-516	18
	TPSYVAFTDTERLIGDA	HSP70 38-54	18
	TPSYVAFTDTERLIG	HSP70 38-52	18
	VPGLYSPCRAFFNKEELL	EBV MCP 1264-1282	18
	VPGLYSPCRAFFNK	EBV MCP 1264-1277	18
	KVDLTFSKQHALLCSDYQADYES	Apolipoprotein B-100 1586-1608	18
	KVDLTFSKQHALLCS	Apolipoprotein B-100 1586-1600	18
	FSHDYRGSTSHRL	Apolipoprotein B-100 1942-1954	18
	LPKYFEKKRNTII	Apolipoprotein B-100 2077-2089	18
	APVLISQKLSPIYNLVPVK	Complement C9 465-483	18
	VGSDWRFLRGYHQYAYDG	HLA-A2 103-120	18
	PKPPKPVSKMRMATPLLMQALP	Invariant chain 98-119	18
	APSPLPETTENVVCALGLTV	HLA-DRα 182-200	18
	KHKVYACEVTHQGL	Igκ chain 188-201	18

Table 4.5. (con't)

HLA-DRB1*0801	Sequence	Source	Ref.
Motif unknown			
Examples for ligands	APSPLPETTENVVCALG	HLA-DRα 182-198	18
	SETVFLPREDHLFRKFHYLPFLP	HLA-DRα 158-180	18
	RHNYELDEAVTLQ	HLA-DPβ 80-92	18
	DPQSGALYISKVQKEDNSTYI	LAM Blast-1 88-108	18
	GALYISKVQKEDNSTYI	LAM Blast-1 92-108	18
	DPVPKPVIKIEKIEDMDD	LAM Blast-1 129-146	18
	DPVPKPVIKIEKIED	LAM Blast-1 129-143	18
	FTFTISRLEPEDFAVYYC	Igκ chain 63-80	18
	FTFTISRLEPEDFAV	Igκ chain 63-77	18
	DPVEMRRLNYQTPG	LAR 1302-1316	18
	YQLLRSMIGYIEELAPIV	LIF receptor 709-726	18
	GNHLYKWKQIPDCENVK	IFN-α receptor 271-287	18
	LPFFLFRQAYHPNNSSPVCY	IL-8 receptor 169-188	18
	RPSMLQHLLR	Ca^{2+} release channel 2614-1623	18
	DDFMGQLLNGRVLFPVNLQLGA	CD35 359-380	18
	IPRLQKIWKNYLSMNKY	CD75 106-122	18
	EPFLYILGKSRVLEAQ	Calcitonin receptor 38-53	18
	NRSEEFLIAGKLQDGLLH	TIMP-1 101-118	18
	RSEEFLIAGKLQDGLL	TIMP-1 102-117	18
	SEEFLIAGKLQDGLL	TIMP-1 103-117	18
	NRSEEFLIAGKL	TIMP-1 101-112	18
	QAKFFACIKRSDGSCAWYRGAAPPKQEF	TIMP-2 187-214	18
	QAKFFACIKRSDGSCAWYR	TIMP-2 187-205	18
	DRPFLFVVRHNPTGTVLFM	PAI-1 378-396	18
	MPHFFRLFRSTVKQVD	PAI-1 133-148	18
	QNFTVIFDTGSSNLWVPSVYCTSP	Cathepsin E 89-112	18
	QNFTVIFDTGSSNLWV	Cathepsin E 89-104	18
	TAFQYIIDNKGIDSDAS	Cathepsin S 189-205	18
	DEYYRRLLRVLRAREQIV	Cystatin SN 41-58	18
	EAIYDICRRNLDIERPT	Tubulin α-1 chain 207-223	18
	EAIYDICRRNLDI	Tubulin α-1 chain 207-219	18
	HELEKIKKQVEQEKCEIQAAL	Myosin β heavy chain 1027-1047	18
	AEVYHDVAASEFF...	α-enolase 23-?	18

	KRSFFALRDQIPDL	c-myc 371-385	18
	RQYRLKKISKEEKTPGC	K-ras 164-180	18
	KNIFHFKVNQEGLKLSNDMM	Apolipoprotein B-100 1724-1743	18
	KNIFHFKVNQEGLKLS	Apolipoprotein B-100 1724-1739	18
	YKQTVSLDIQPYSLVTTLNS	Apolipoprotein B-100 1780-1799	18
	STPEFTILNTLHIPSFT	Apolipoprotein B-100 2646-1662	18
	TPEFTILNTLHIPSFTID	Apolipoprotein B-100 2647-2664	18
	TPEFTILNTLHIPSFT	Apolipoprotein B-100 2647-2662	18
	SNTKYFHKLNIPQLDF	Apolipoprotein B-100 2885-2900	18
	LPFFKFLPKYFEKKRNT	Apolipoprotein B-100 2072-2088	18
	LPFFKFLPKYFEKKR	Apolipoprotein B-100 2072-2086	18
	WNFYYSPQSSPDKKL	Apolipoprotein B-100 4022-4036	18
	DVIWELLNHAQEHFGKDKSKE	Cattle transferrin 261-281	18
	DVIWELLNHAQEHFG	Cattle transferrin 261-275	18
	DVIWELLNHAQEH	Cattle transferrin 261-273	18
	IALLLMASQEPQRMSRNFVR	von Willebrand factor 617-636	18
	IALLLMASQEPQRM	von Willebrand factor 617-630	18
T cell epitope	DKREMWMACIKELH	HCMV-IE1 162-175	370

HLA-DRB1*08032	**Sequence**	**Source**	**Ref.**
Motif unknown			
T cell epitopes	DPRRRSRNLGKVIDTFTCGL	HCV NP 111-130	182
	SVNYATGNLPGCSFSIFLLA	HCV NP 161-180	182

HLA-DRB1*0901		**Relative position**										**Source**	**Ref.**
		1	2	3	**4**	5	6	7	8	9			
Anchor residues (preliminary)		**W,Y**			**A, V**								371, 372
		F, L			**S**								
Examples for ligands	KRK	**W**	E	A	**A**	H	A	A	E	Q	QR	HLA-A11 143-156	372
	GAK	**F**	K	T	**S**	A	Q	H	A	L		Neuropeptide Y-like receptor 306-317	372
	NPGGYVA	**Y**	S	K	**A**	A	T	V	T	G		Transferrin receptor 215-230	372
	NNAK	**Y**	A	I	**S**	M	A	R	K	I	GA	L plastin 581-595	372
	NKVD	**L**	T	F	**S**	K	Q	H	A	L	L	Apolipoprotein B-100 1585-1598	372
	VEKY	**Y**	A	Y	**A**	E	N	D	V	E	K	Unknown	372

Table 4.5. (con't)

		Relative position										Source	Ref.
		1	2	3	**4**	5	6	7	8	9			
	FPKY	**Y**	I	G	**S**	Q	E	K	I	L	Q	Unknown	372
	FPKD	**Y**	A	G	**A**	A	L	E	R	L		Unknown	372
	FSYD	**Y**	R	G	**S**	R	S	A	E	L	M	Unknown	372
	SPKY	**Y**	V	L	**A**	K	A	F	V	Y	P	Unknown	372
	KPKA	**Y**	Q	L	**S**	A	I	N	M	I	QYR	Unknown	372
	KPQ	**Y**	V	F	**A**	L	P	G	Q	L		Unknown	372
	EPKD	**F**	V	Y	**A**	L	N	L	T	Q	TQTLNP	Unknown	372

HLA-DR11 or Dw52	**Sequence**	**Source**	**Ref.**
Motif unknown			
Ligands	SXVITLNTNVGLYXQS	Homol. Apolipoprotein 3345-3360	373
	DPXQDELQKLNAXDP	Unknown	373
	XPELNKVARAAAEVAG	Homol. Transferrin receptor	373

HLA-DRw52	**Sequence**	**Source**	**Ref.**
Motif unknown			
T cell epitopes	KDAGISVESEIDHVVLVGGST	*M. leprae* HSP70 298–317	343

HLA-DRw52 or HLA-DQ2	**Sequence**	**Source**	**Ref.**
Motif unknown			
T cell epitope	ERNTTIPTKRSETFTTADDN	*M. leprae* HSP 70 388-407	343

HLA-DR17 or DRw52	**Sequence**	**Source**	**Ref.**
Motif unknown			
Ligands	TFDEIASGFRQGGASQ	Glucose transporter 459-474	18
	YGYTSYDTFSWAFL	Na+ channel protein 384-397	18
	GQVKKNNHQEDKIE	CD45 1071-1084	18
	TGHGARTSTEPTTDY	EBV gp220 592-606	18
	KELKRQYEKKLRQ	EBV tegument p140 1395-1407	18
	SPLQALDFFGNGPPVNYKTGNL	IP30 38-59	18

HLA-DRB1*1101		Relative position										Source	Ref.
		1	2	3	**4**	5	**6**	7	8	**9**			
Anchor residues		**W,Y F**			**L, V, M,A, F, V**		**R,K, H**			**A,G, S,P**			352,373, 338
Examples for ligands	IDF	**Y**	T	S	**I**	T	**R**	A	R	F	EE	HSC 70 291-305	373
	CPAG	**Y**	T	C	N	V	**K**	A	R	**S**	CEK	Granulin D 41-56	373
	VNH	**F**	I	A	E	F	**K**	R	K	H	KKD	Homol. HSC70 238-252	373
	VNH	**F**	I	A	E	F	**K**	R	K	H	K	Homol. HSC70 238-250	373
	MR	**Y**	F	H	T	S	V	S	R	**P**	GRGEP	HLA-Bw61 5-20	373
	KHKV	**Y**	A	C	E	V	T	H	Q	**G**	LS	Homol. Ig κ–chain 190-204	373
	TPT	**L**	V	E	**V**	S	**R**	S	L	**G**	KVGTRC	Cattle serum albumin 419-436	338
	IGRY	**Y**	T	V	**F**	D	**R**	D	N	N	RVGFA	Cathepsin D 221-238	338
	TT	**Y**	K	K	**V**	V	F	R	K	Y	LDSTFTK	Coagulation factor V 39-56	338
	CPAG	**Y**	T	C	N	V	**K**	A	R	**S**	CEKEV	Granulin D 41-58	338
	VGSDWR	**F**	L	R	G	Y	**H**	Q	Y	**A**	YDG	HLA-A2 103-120	338
	VP	**Y**	R	Y	**L**	Q	**R**	R	K	K	KGKADGG	Membrane cofactor prot. 315-332	338
	DLHS	**Y**	V	V	**M**	N	**H**	G	R	**S**	YTAIS	Nidogen 429-446	338
	SGR	**F**	F	T	**V**	K	L	P	V	**A**	LDPGAK	Ribophorin I 86-103	338
	LP	**F**	F	I	**V**	A	L	V	L	**P**	FCESSCH	Serotonin receptor 359-376	338
	ERPT	**Y**	T	N	**L**	N	**R**	L	**I**	**G**	QIVSS	Tubulin α-chain 220-237	338
T cell epitope		I	I	H	R	G	**K**	P	F	Q	LEAV	Der pII 28-40	374

HLA-DRB1*1104		Relative position										Source	Ref.
		1	2	3	**4**	5	**6**	7	8	**9**			
Anchor residues		**I L V**			**L,V M, A,F** Y		**R K,H**			**A,G S,P**			338
Examples for ligands	SPLAL	**I**	K	G	**M**	T	**R**	P	L	**S**	TLIS	Apolipoprotein 196-213	338

Table 4.5. (con't)

		Relative position										Source	Ref.
		1	2	3	**4**	5	**6**	7	8	**9**			
	TPK	**I**	Q	V	**Y**	S	**R**	H	P	**A**	ENGKSN	β_2-microglobulin 4-21	338
	TPT	**L**	V	E	**V**	S	**R**	S	L	**G**	KVGTRC	Cattle serum albumin 419-436	338
	GPVDE	**V**	R	E	**L**	Q	**K**	A	I	**G**	AVPL	Cathepsin D 134-151	338
	NPTNT	**V**	F	D	**A**	K	**R**	L	I	**G**	RRFD	HSC70 62-79	338
	DPGS	**L**	L	S	**L**	F	**R**	R	L	**S**	DQRSK	Lymphocyte activ. antigen 414-431	338
	KPG	**V**	I	F	**L**	T	**K**	R	S	R	QVCADP	Macrophage inflam. prot. 47-64	338
	IPE	**L**	N	K	**V**	A	**R**	A	A	**A**	EVAGQF	Transferrin receptor 580-597	338
	EPE	**I**	T	I	**L**	N	V	K	L	Q	PA	Unknown	338

HLA-DRB1*1201		Relative position										Source	Ref.
		1	2	**3**	4	5	**6**	7	8	**9**			
Anchor residues		**I,L F,Y V**		**L,M N,V A**			**V,Y F,I N,A**			**Y,F M,I V**			17
Examples for ligands	GPDGRL	**L**	R	G	Y	D	Q	F	A	**Y**	DGK	HLA-B38 104-121	17
	GPDGRL	**L**	R	G	H	N	Q	Y	A	**Y**	D	HLA class I 104-119	17
	TGT	**I**	K	**L**	L	N	E	N	S	**Y**	VP	Transferrin receptor 142-155	17
	T	**I**	K	**L**	L	N	E	N	S	**Y**	VPR	Transferrin receptor 144-156	17
	FTGT	**I**	K	**L**	L	N	E	N	S	**Y**	VPR	Transferrin receptor 141-156	17
	DFTGT	**I**	K	**L**	L	N	E	N	S	**Y**	VPR	Transferrin receptor 140-156	17
	SDEK	**I**	R	**M**	N	R	**V**	V	R	N	NLR	Valosin-cont. protein p97 78-93	17
	SSV	**I**	T	**L**	N	T	**N**	V	G	L	YXQT	Homol. to apolipoprotein	17
	EAL	**I**	H	Q	L	K	**I**	N	P	**Y**	VLS	Unknown	17
	AHL	**F**	K	Q	N	K	**V**	V	H	**V**	NG	Dihydrolipoamide dehydrogenase 138-152	a

a: Falk et al. unpublished

HLA-DRB1*1301		Relative position										Source	Ref.
		1	2	3	**4**	5	**6**	7	8	**9**			
Anchor residues		**I,L,** **V**			**L** **V** **M** **A** **W** **Y**		**R** **K**			**Y** **F** **A** **S** **T**			338, 375
Examples for ligands	TPK	**I**	Q	V	**Y**	S	**R**	H	P	**A**	ENGKSN	β_2-microglobulin 21-38	338
	TPK	**I**	Q	V	**Y**	S	**R**	H	P	**A**	ENGKS	β_2-microglobulin 21-37	375
	TPK	**I**	Q	V	**Y**	S	**R**	H	P	**A**	ENGK	β_2-microglobulin 21-36	375
	TPK	**I**	Q	V	**Y**	S	**R**	H	P	**A**	ENG	β_2-microglobulin 21-35	375
	TPK	**I**	Q	V	**Y**	S	**R**	H	P	**A**	EN	β_2-microglobulin 21-34	375
	IDS	**V**	K	V	**W**	P	**R**	R	P	**T**	GEVYDI	Cattle fetuin 45-62	338
	TER	**V**	R	L	**V**	T	**R**	H	I	**Y**	NREEYV	HLA-DQB1*06 53-70	338
	TER	**V**	R	L	**V**	T	**R**	H	I	**Y**	NREE	HLA-DQB1*06 53-68	375
	TER	**V**	R	L	**V**	T	**R**	H	I	**Y**	NRE	HLA-DQB1*06 53-67	375
	TER	**V**	R	L	**V**	T	**R**	H	I	**Y**	NR	HLA-DQB1*06 53-66	375
	FYPGQIK	**V**	R	W	**F**	R	N	D	Q	E	ET	HLA-DQB1*0604 123-140	338
	CPEKW	**I**	N	F	Q	R	**K**	C	Y	**Y**	FGKG	CD23 163-180	338
	DA	**V**	L	R	**F**	N	G	A	P	**T**	ANFQQDV	Sialyltransferase 206-223	338
	GPDGRL	**L**	R	G	H	D	Q	Y	A	**Y**	DGKDY	HLA-B7 104-123	375
	GPDGRL	**L**	R	G	H	D	Q	Y	A	**Y**	DGKD	HLA-B7 104-122	375
	LPKPPKP	**V**	S	K	**M**	R	M	A	T	P	LLMQALPM	Invariant chain 97-120	375
	LPKPPKP	**V**	S	K	**M**	R	M	A	T	P	LLMQALP	Invariant chain 97-119	375

HLA-DRB1*1302	Relative position									Source	Ref.
	1	2	3	**4**	5	**6**	7	8	**9**		
Anchor residues	**Y,F** **V** **A** **I**			**L,V** **M** **A** **W** **Y**		**R** **K**			**Y,F** **A,S** **T**		338, 375

Table 4.5. (con't)

		Relative position										Source	Ref.
		1	2	3	**4**	5	**6**	7	8	**9**			
Examples for ligands	TPK	**I**	Q	V	**Y**	S	**R**	H	P	**A**	ENGKSN	β_2-microglobulin 21-38	338
	AGA	**V**	V	A	**A**	V	**R**	W	R	R	KSSDRK	HLA-A33 323-340	338
	RYF	**Y**	T	A	**M**	S	**R**	P	G	R	GEPRFI	HLA-B44 6-23	338
	DVGEFRA	**V**	T	E	**L**	G	**R**	P	D	E	EY	HLA-DR13 β chain 43-60	338
	DVGEYRA	**V**	T	E	**L**	G	**R**	P	D	E	EY	HLA-DR52 β chain 43-60	338
	TER	**V**	R	L	**V**	T	**R**	H	I	**Y**	NREEYV	HLA-DQB1*06 53-70	338
	TTAYFL	**Y**	Q	Q	Q	G	**R**	L	D	K	LTV	Invariant chain 66-83	338
	TTAYFL	**Y**	Q	Q	Q	G	**R**	L	D	K		Invariant chain 66-80	375
	LPKPPKP	**V**	S	K	**M**	R	M	A	T	P	LLMQALPM	Invariant chain 97-120	375
	ES	**F**	L	X	**Y**	K	**K**	G	I	**Y**		Cathepsin L-like 237-247	338
	XPAF	**Y**	M	L	K	G	**K**	L	Q	**Y**	ELQY	Unknown	338
	GPE	**Y**	W	D	R	E	T	Q	K	**Y**	KRQAQ	HLA-C 56-72	375
	GPE	**Y**	W	D	R	E	T	Q	K	**Y**	KRQA	HLA-C 56-71	375
	GPE	**Y**	W	D	R	E	T	Q	K	**Y**	KRQ	HLA-C 56-70	375
	APR	**F**	K	H	**L**	R	**K**	Y	T	**Y**	NYEA	Apolipoprotein B-100 43-58	375
	SSVIT	L	N	V	G	L	Y	D	Q	**S**	DIAK	Apolipoprotein B-100 3342-3361	375
	SSVIT	L	N	V	G	L	Y	D	Q	**S**	D	Apolipoprotein B-100 3342-3358	375
	DPTLDHH	W	H	L	**W**	K	**K**	T	Y	G	KQYKE	Cathepsin S 21-42	375
	DPTLDHH	W	H	L	**W**	K	**K**	T	Y	G	KQYK	Cathepsin S 21-41	375
	NPGG	**Y**	V	A	**Y**	S	**K**	A	A	**T**	VTGKL	Transferrin receptor 215-232	375
	NPGG	**Y**	V	A	**Y**	S	**K**	A	A	**T**	VTG	Transferrin receptor 215-230	375
T cell epitopes	QY	**I**	K	A	N	S	**K**	F	I	G	ITE	Tetanus toxin 830-843	376
	ET	T	V	V	R	R	**R**	G	R	**S**		HBV core 145-155	377
	H	T	A	L	R	Q	A	I	**L**	C	W	HBV core 52-62	377
		V	G	L	K	I	**R**	Q	**L**	L	W	HBV core 93-103	377

HLA-DRB1*1405	Sequence	Source	Ref.
Motif unknown			
T cell epitope	EEYLILSARDVLAVVSK	Bacillus Calmette-Guérin protein BCGap 84-100	378

HLA-DRB1*1501 (DR2b)		Relative position										Source	Ref.
		1	2	3	**4**	5	6	**7**	8	9			
Anchor residues		**L**			**F**			**I**					
		V			**Y**			**L**					
		I			**I**			**V**					
								M					
								F					379, 380
Examples for ligands	EAEQ	**L**	R	A	**Y**	L	D	G	T	G	VE	HLA-A3 152-166	379
		L	E	E	**F**	G	R	**F**	A	S	FEAQG	HLA-DRα 45-58	379
	D	**V**	G	V	**Y**	R	A	**V**	T	P	QGRPDA	HLA-DQw6 43-58	379
T cell epitopes	PV	**V**	H	F	**F**	K	N	**I**	V	T		MBP 85-95	380
	V	**I**	G	L	**Y**	G	N	G	V			Flavivirus NS3 prot. 146-154	381
	WTTCQS	**I**	A	F	P	S	K	T	S	A	SIGSL	Proteolipid protein 30-49	382
	LFCGCG	H	E	A	L	T	G	T	E	K	LIETY	Proteolipid protein 180-199	382

HLA-DRB1*1502	Sequence	Source	Ref.
Motif unknown T cell epitope	KPFQLEAVFEANQNT	Dermatophagoides pteronyssinus Der pII 33-47	368

HLA-DR2	Sequence	Source	Ref.
Motif unknown T cell epitope	AGLTLSLLVICSYLFISRG	EBV lytic Ag BHRF1 171-189	383

HLA-DR3	Sequence	Source	Ref.
Motif unknown T cell epitopes	RHMGSDWSIEIDGKKYTAQE	*M. leprae* HSP70 71-90	343
	DSDKNPLFLDEQLIRAEFQR	*M. leprae* HSP70 261-280	343
	QPSVQIQVYQGEREIASHNK	*M. leprae* HSP70 408-427	343

Table 4.5. (con't)

HLA-DRB3*0202(DR52Dw25)		**Relative position**										**Source**	**Ref.**
		1	2	3	**4**	5	**6**	7	8	**9**			
Anchor residues		**Y,F I,L**			**N**		**A,S P,D E**			**L,V I,S G**			338
Examples for ligands	KSSV	**I**	T	L	**N**	T	N	A	E	**L**	FNQSD	Apolipoprotein 3344-3361	338
	KDY	**I**	A	L	**N**	E	**D**	L	R	**S**	WTAADT	HLA-A1 119-136	338
	IQAE	**F**	Y	L	**N**	P	**D**	Q	S	**G**	EFMFD	HLA-DRα 33-50	338
	LER	**Y**	I	Y	**N**	R	**E**	E	F	**V**	RFDSDVGE	HLA-DPw4β 25-44	338
	VIDW	**L**	V	S	**N**	Q	**S**	V	R	N	RQEGL	Pleckstrin 161-178	338
	SLDK	**F**	L	A	**N**	V	**S**	T	V	**L**	TGKYR	Hemoglobin-like 124-141	338

HLA-DRB3*0301 (DR52Dw26)		**Relative position**										**Source**	**Ref.**
		1	2	3	**4**	5	**6**	7	8	**9**			
Anchor residues		**I,L** V			**N**		**A,S** P,D E			**I,L V**			338
Examples for ligands	AQV	**I**	I	L	**N**	H	**P**	G	Q	**I**	SAGYAP	Elongation factor Tu 342-359	338
	VPPEVT	**V**	L	T	**N**	S	**P**	V	E	**L**	REP	HLA-DRα chain 110-127	338
	FPPSSEE	**L**	Q	A	**N**	K	**A**	T	L	**V**	CL	Igλ chain 11-28	338
T cell epitope	TPQ	**L**	T	K	**N**	A	G	V	L	T		Japanese cedar pollen Ag, Cry J I 356-367	384

HLA-DRB4	**Sequence**	**Source**	**Ref.**
Motif unknown			
T cell epitopes	AKYDAFVTALTE	*Lolium perenne* lol p9 105-116	385
	ETYKFIPSLEAA	*Lolium perenne* lol p9 193-207	385

HLA-DRB4*0101	Sequence	Source	Ref.
Motif unknown T cell epitope	NNAKYAISMARKIGA	L-plastin 581-595	386

HLA-DRB5*0101(DR2a)		Relative position										Source	Ref.
		1	2	3	**4**	5	6	7	8	**9**			
Anchor or preferred residues		**F,Y L,M**			**Q,V I,M**					**R,K**			379, 380
Examples for ligands	DVGV	**Y**	R	A	**V**	T	P	Q	G	**R**	P	HLA-DQw6 43-56	379
	DVGV	**Y**	R	A	**V**	T	P	Q	G	**R**	PDA	HLA-DQw6 43-58	379
	DSDVGV	**Y**	R	A	**V**	T	P	Q	G	**R**	PD	HLA-DQw6 41-57	379
	DSDVGV	**Y**	R	A	**V**	T	P	Q	G	**R**	PDA	HLA-DQw6 41-58	379
	DSDVGV	**Y**	R	A	**V**	T	P	Q	G	**R**	PDAEY	HLA-DQw6 41-60	379
	AAD	**M**	A	A	**Q**	I	T	K	R	**K**	WEAAH	HLA-A3 135-151	379
	TAAD	**M**	A	A	**Q**	I	T	K	R	**K**	WEA	HLA-A3 134-149	379
	DVGE	**F**	A	A	**V**	T	E	K	R	**R**	PDAEYW	HLA-DR2b 43-61	379
T cell epitopes	PK	**Y**	V	K	**Q**	N	T	L	**K**	L	AT	Influenza HA 306-318	387
		L	Q	A	A	P	A	L	D	**K**	L	HSP65 418-427	379, 388
	VHF	**F**	K	N	**I**	V	T	P	**R**	T	P	MBP 87-99	389
	ASD	**Y**	K	S	A	H	K	G	F	**K**	GVD	MBP 131-145	379
	KG	**F**	K	G	**V**	D	A	Q	G	T	LSKI	MBP 139-153	379
	WTTCQS	**I**	A	F	P	S	K	T	S	A	SIGSL	Proteolipid protein 30-49	382
	LFCGCG	H	E	A	L	T	G	T	E	**K**	LIETY	Proteolipid protein 180-199	382

HLA-DR2 (DRB5*0101 or DRB1*1501)	Sequence	Source	Ref.
cannot be specified/Motif unknown Examples for ligands			
	NIVIKRSNSTAATNEVPEVTVFS	HLA-DQα 97-119	18
	NIVIKRSNSTAATNEV	HLA-DQα 97-112	18
	SDVGVYRAVTPQGRPDAE	HLA-DQβ 42-59	18

Table 4.5 (con't)

HLA-DR2 (DRB5*0101 or DRB1*1501)	Sequence	Source	Ref.
	DVGVYRAVTPQGRPDAE	HLA-DQβ 43-59	18
	DVGVYRAVTPQGRPD	HLA-DQβ 43-57	18
	RVQPKVTVYPSKTQPLQH	HLA-DRB1*1501 94-111	18
	RVQPKVTVYPSKTQP	HLA-DRB1*1501 94-108	18
	LSPIHIALNFSLDPQAPVDSHGLRPALHYQ	Fibronectin receptor α 586-616	18
	DGILYYYQSGGRLRRPVN	K+ channel protein 173-190	18
	IQNLIKEEAFLGITDEKTEG	Mannose binding protein 174-193	18
	EHHIFLGATNYIYVLNEEDLQKV	MET protooncogene 59-81	18
	QELKNKYYQVPRKGIQA	Guanylate binding protein 2 434-450	18
	FPKSLHTYANILLDRRVPQTD	Apolipoprotein B100 1200-1220	18
	FPKSLHTYANILLDRRVPQ	Apolipoprotein B100 1200-1218	18
	LWDYGMSSSPHVLRNR	Factor VIII 1775-1790	18

HLA-DR7	Sequence	Source	Ref.
Motif unknown T cell epitope	AKIELSSSQSTSVNLPYITV	*M. leprae* HSP70 241-260	343

HLA-DQA1*0501/DQB1*0301 (DQ7)		Relative position										Source	Ref.
		1	2	3	4	**5**	6	**7**	8	9			
Anchor residues		**F,Y I,M L,V**				**V,L I,M Y**		**Y,F M,L V,I**					17
Preferred residues		A	A	A	A								
Examples for ligands	TPL	**L**	M	Q	A	**L**	P	**M**	G	A	LPQG	Invariant chain 111-126	17
	TPL	**L**	M	Q	A	**L**	P	**M**	G	A	LPQ	Invariant chain 111-125	17
	KPPKPVSKMR	**M**	A	T	P	**L**	L	**M**	Q	A		Invariant chain 99-117	17
	LPKPPKPVSKMR	**M**	A	T	P	**L**	L	**M**				Invariant chain 97-115	17
	IPE	**L**	N	K	V	A	R	A	A	A		Transferrin receptor 579-597	17
	DVEV	**Y**	R	A	V	T	P	**L**	G	P	EVAGQF	HLA-DQβ chain 43-55	17

HLA-DQA1*0301/DQB1*0301 (DQ3.1)		Relative position										Source	Ref.
		1	2	3	**4**	5	**6**	7	8	9			
Anchor residues		**D,E W**			**A,G S,T**		**ali.***						390,391 a
Examples for ligands	HKLQ	**D**	A	S	**A**	E	**V**	E	R	L	RR	BST-2 128-142	a
	TAA	**D**	T	A	**A**	Q	**I**	T	Q	R		HLA-B44 158-169	a
	STF	**D**	A	G	**A**	G	**I**	A	L	N	DH	GAPDH 292-305	a
	LNF	**D**	F	Q	**A**	K	Q	L	S	D	P	Apolipoprotein B-100 2804-2816	a

a Friede et al., unpublished results
ali: aliphatic

HLA-DQA1*0501/DQB1*0201 (DQ2)		Relative position										Source	Ref.
		1	2	3	**4**	5	**6**	**7**	8	**9**			
Anchor residues		**F,W Y,I L,V**			**D,E L,V I,**		**P,D E (H) (H)**	**D,E**		**F,W Y,I L,V M**			392
Examples for ligands	EPRAPW	**I**	E	Q	**E**	G	**P**	**E**	Y	**W**		HLA class Ia 46-60	392
	PRAPW	**I**	E	Q	**E**	G	**P**	**E**	Y			HLA class Iα 47-59	392
	EPRAPW	**I**	E	Q	**E**	G	**P**	**E**	Y			HLA class Iα 46-59	392
	EPRAPW	**I**	E	Q	**E**	G	**P**	**E**				HLA class Iα 46-58	392
	ED	**I**	V	A	**D**	H	V	A	S	**Y**	GVNL	HLA-DQα *0501 1-15	392
	ED	**I**	V	A	**D**	H	V	A	S	**Y**		HLA-DQα *0501 1-11	392
		I	E	Q	**E**	G	**P**	**E**	Y	**W**		HLA class Iα 52-60	392
		Y	Q	S	Y	G	**P**	S	G	Q	YTHEFD	HLA-DQα *0501 16-30	392
	EDIEI	**I**	P	I	G	E	**E**					CD20 260-270	392
	DIEI	**I**	P	I	G	E	**E**					CD20 261-270	392
	AAPSVF	**I**	F	P	P	S	**D**	**E**	Q	**L**	K	Igk chain 111-126	392
	KPPKP	**V**	S	K	M	R	M	A	T	P		Invariant chain 99-112	392
	RMATP	**L**	L	M	Q	A	L	P	M	G	AL	Invariant chain 108-123	392
	RMATP	**L**	L	M	Q	A	L					Invariant chain 108-118	392

Table 4.5 (con't)

		Relative position										Source	Ref.
		1	2	3	**4**	5	**6**	**7**	8	**9**			
T cell epitopes	MATP	**L**	L	M	Q	A	L	P	M	G	AL	Invariant chain 109-123	392
	WT	S	S	N	**V**	M	**E**	**E**	R	**Y**		OVA 267-276	392
	KPLLI	**I**	A	E	**D**	V	**E**	G	E	**Y**		*M. bovis* 65 kDa 243-255	392
	NNQ	**V**	V	S	**L**	K	**P**	**E**	I	**I**	VDQY	Rabies virus NP 11-25	392
	D	A	W	R	**E**	G	**E**	**E**	F	**V**	VEF	*M. leprae* 18 kDa 31-43	392
	YLT	**F**	L	P	S	A	**D**	**E**	I	**Y**	DCKV	HLA-DQα*0301 153-168	392
	I	A	S	N	**E**	N	M	**D**	A	**M**	ESSTLY	Influenza NP 265-279	392
	IDV	**W**	L	G	G	L	A	**E**	N	**F**	LPY	Thyroid peroxidase 632-645	392
		Y	Q	S	Y	G	**P**	S	G	Q	YTHEFD	HLA-DQα*0501 16-30	392

HLA-DPA1*0201/DPB1*0401 (DPw4)		Relative position											Source	Ref.
		1	2	3	4	5	6	**7**	8	9	**10**			
Anchor residues		**F,L** **Y,M** **I,V** **A**						**F,L** **Y,M** **V,I** **A**			**V,Y** **I,A** **L**			17
Examples for ligands	EKK	**Y**	F	A	A	T	Q	**F**	E	P	**L**	AARL	Unknown	17
	KK	**Y**	F	A	A	T	Q	**F**	E	P	**L**	AARL	Unknown	17
	EKK	**Y**	F	A	A	T	Q	**F**	E	P	**L**		Unknown	17
	GPG	**A**	P	A	D	V	Q	**Y**	D	L	**Y**	LNVANRR	IL-3 Receptor α-chain 127-146	17

HLA-DPA1*0102/DPB1*0201		Relative position										Source	Ref.
		1	2	3	4	**5**	6	7	**8**	9			
Anchor residues		**F,L** **M,V** **W,Y**				**F,L** **M,Y**			**I,A** **M,V**				393
Examples for ligands	ADEKKF	**W**	G	K	Y	**L**	Y	E	**I**	A	RRHP	Bovine serum albumin 152-170	393
	GEP	**L**	S	Y	T	R	F	S	**L**	A	RQVDG	Transferrin receptor 15-31	393
	LPSQA	**F**	E	Y	I	**L**	Y	N	K	G		Cathepsin H 185-198	393

Table 4.6 Mouse class II motifs

H2-E^d		1	2	3	4	5	6	7	8	9		Source	Ref.
Anchor or preferred residues		**I,L V,F Y,W**			**I,L V,F S,A**		**Q,N A,S T,H R,E**			**K,R G**			394, 395, 396, 397
Examples for ligands	HPPHIE	**I**	Q	M	**L**	K	**N**	G	K	**K**		β2-microglobulin 42-56	396
	DNRM	**V**	H	F	**I**	A	**E**	F	K	**R**	K	HSC70 234-248	396
	TPTL	**V**	E	A	**A**	R	**N**	L	G	**R**	VG	Serum albumin 347-361	396
	VNKE	**I**	Q	N	**A**	V	**Q**	G	V	**K**	HI	Clusterin 41-55	396
	GFPT	**I**	Y	F	**S**	P	**A**	N	K	**K**	L	ER60 448-461	394
	IP	**L**	I	M	**L**	I	**N**	K	A	**R**	NKAE	Unknown	394
	YDRN	T	K	S	P	L	F	V	G	**K**	V	α1-antitryp. 397-410	394
		F	A	E	**F**	G	**T**	L	K	**K**	AAVHYDRSG	Unknown	394
	LH	**L**	G	Y	**L**	P	**N**	Q	L	F	**R**	(human) DEAD box protein	394
	IPGGP	**V**	R	L	C	P	G	R	I	**R**		Bovine fetuin 342-355	394
T cell epitopes	RADL	**I**	A	Y	**L**	K	**Q**	A	T	**K**		MCC 91-103	395
	RADL	**I**	A	Y	**L**	K	**Q**	A	T	A	**K**	PCC 91-104	395
	LEDARR	**L**	K	A	**I**	Y	**E**	K	K	**K**		λrep 12-26	398
	QD	**I**	L	I	R	L	F	K	S	H	PETL	SWMb 26-40	398
	VTV	**L**	T	A	**L**	G	**A**	I	L	**K**	K	SWMb 66-78	399
		L	T	A	**L**	G	G	I	L	**K**		EqMb 69-77	395
		L	T	A	**L**	G	**T**	I	L	**K**		MoMb 69-77	395
		I	T	A	**F**	N	**E**	G	L	**K**		MoHb 68-76	395
	KVFGR	C	E	L	**A**	A	**A**	M	K	**R**	HGLD	HEL 1-18	398, 400
	SALLSSD	**I**	T	A	**S**	V	**N**	C	A	**K**		HEL 81-96	399
		W	V	A	W	R	**N**	R	C	**K**	GTD	HEL 108-119	399
	VEK	**Y**	G	P	E	A	**S**	A	F	T	**K**KMVENAK	SNase 51-70	398
	RTDKYGRG	**L**	A	Y	**I**	Y	**A**	D	G	**K**	MVN	SNase 81-100	398
	HEHQ	**L**	R	K	**S**	E	**A**	Q	A	**K**	KEKLNIW	SNase 121-140	401
		I	A	K	**F**	G	**T**	A	F	**K**		LLO 218-226	395

Table 4.6 (con't)

H2-E^d		Relative position										Source	Ref.
		1	2	3	**4**	5	**6**	7	8	**9**			
Anchor or preferred residues		**W,Y** **F,I** **L,V**			**K,R** **I,V**		**I,L** **V,G**			**K,R**			394
Examples for ligands	SQLELR	**W**	K	S	**R**	H	**I**	K	E	**R**		IL-2R. γ chain 168-182	394
	LELR	**W**	K	S	**R**	H	**I**	K	E	**R**		IL-2R. γ chain 170-182	394
	ERAEA	**W**	R	Q	**K**	L	H	G	**R**	L		Apolipoprotein E prec. 222-236	394
	RAEA	**W**	R	Q	**K**	L	H	G	**R**	L		Apolipoprotein E prec. 223-236	394
	AQ	**F**	M	W	**I**	I	R	K	**R**	I	QLP	Unknown	394
	SLDEH	**Y**	H	I	**R**	V	H	L	V	**K**		Apolipoprotein B homolog 2211-2224	394
	GQFY	**F**	L	I	**R**	K	R	I	H	L	**R**	*C. elegans* cDNA homolog 74-87	394
	LV	**V**	D	N	G	S	**G**	M	C	**K**	AGF	Actin B 8-21	394
T cell epitopes	ALWFRNH	**F**	V	F	G	G	**G**	T	**K**	V	TV	Ig λ chain 91-108	402
	KYLEFISEA	**I**	I	H	**V**	L	H	S	**R**			SWMb 102-118	399
	NKALE	**L**	F	R	**K**	D	**I**	A	A	**K**	Y	SWMb 132-146	387
	W	**V**	A	W	**R**	N	R	C	**K**	G	TD	HEL 108-119	399, 403
	A	**Y**	V	Y	**K**	P	N	N	T	H	EQHLRKSE	SNase 112-129	339
	SS	**F**	E	R	F	E	**I**	F	P	**K**		Influenza PR8 HA 109-119	399
	LEDARR	**L**	K	A	**I**	Y	E	K	K	**K**		λrep 12-26	399
	EK	**I**	R	L	**R**	P	**G**	G	K	**K**	K	HIV-1 gag p17 17-28	401
		Y	V	T	Q	F	H	P	P	H	I	β_2-microglobulin 46-55	404
	K	**Y**	V	K	Q	N	T	L	**K**	L		Influenza HA 307-316	405
	RLS	**F**	Q	L	**V**	R	P	P	N	M	TP	Rotavirus major capsid protein VP6 289-302	406

H2-E^s	Relative position									Comments	Ref.
	1	2	3	**4**	5	**6**	7	8	**9**		
Anchor or preferred residues	**I,V** **L,F** **Y,W**			**L,I** **V,T** **S,N** **Q**		**Q,N** **S,T** **A,H** **R,E**			**K,R**	This motif has been predicted based on prediction of pocket structure and comparison with H2-E^k and H2-E^b Motifs	394

												Source	
Examples for ligands		L	Y	V	L	K	I	G	K	K	DG	Carboxypeptidase A 44-54	396
	HPPHIE	I	Q	M	L	K	N	G	K	K		β^2-microglobulin 42-56	396
	EGEC	V	E	W	L	H	R	Y	L	K	NG	H2-L^d 160-174	396
	MQKEITA	L	A	P	S	T	M	K	I	K	II	β-actin 286-303	396
	CT	F	A	I	C	W	L	P	F	H	VFFL	Substance P receptor 255-269	396
	EGSLI	V	E	K	I	M	Q	S	S	S	E	HSP60 478-492	396
T cell epitopes	DL	I	A	Y	L	K	Q	A	T	K		MCC 93-103	398, 395

H2-E^b		Relative position										Comments	Ref.
		1	2	3	**4**	5	**6**	7	8	**9**			
Anchor or preferred residues		W,F Y,I L,V			L,I F,S A		Q,N A,S T,H R,E			K,R		This motif has been predicted based on prediction of pocket structure and comparison with H2-E^k and H2-E^b Motifs	394
												Source	
Examples for ligands	SPSYV	Y	H	Q	F	E	R	R	A	K	YK	MuLV env protein 454-469	407
	SPSYV	Y	H	Q	F	E	R	R	A	K	YKREPVSL	MuLV env protein 454-475	407
	SPSYV	Y	H	Q	F	E	R	R	A	K		MuLV env protein 454-467	407
	GK	Y	L	Y	E	I	A	R	R	H	PYFY	BSA 141-155	407
	XPQS	Y	L	I	H	E	X	X	X	I	S	Unknown	407
T cell epitopes	RTDKYGRG	L	A	Y	I	Y	A	D	G	K	MVN	Snase 81-100	398, 395
	DL	I	A	Y	L	K	Q	A	T	K		MCC 93-103	398, 395

H2-A^u	Sequence	Sources	Ref.
Motif unknown			
T cell epitopes	ASQKRPSQRHG	MBP 1-11	408

Table 4.6. (con't)

H2-A^s	Sequence	Sources	Ref.
Motif unknown			
Ligands	IRLKITDSGPRVPIGPN	MuLV env 255-269	409
	IRLKITDSGPRVPIG	MuLV env 255-267	409
	WQSQSITCNVAHPASST	IgG2a 194-210	409
	NVEVHTAQTQTHREDY	IgG2a 281-296	409
	KPTEVSGKLVHANFGT	Transferrin receptor 203-218	409
	XPYMFADKVVHLPGSQ	Unknown	409
T cell epitope	ARSALILRGSVAHKSCLPACVYGP	Influenza PR8 NP 260-283	410

H2-A^b	Sequence	Sources	Ref.
Motif unknown			
Ligands	HNEGFYVCPGPHRP	MuLV env 145-158	407
	ASFEAQGALANIAVDKA	H2-Eα 52-68	407
	KPVSQMRMATPLLMR	Invariant chain 86-100	407
	NYNAYNATPATLAVD	Unknown	407,409
	RPDAEYWNSQPE	H2-Aβ 55-66	407
	XNADFKTPATLTVDKP	IgG Vμ 59-74	407
T cell epitopes	VTGSPICTAPDLNLGGTCPS	*M. leprae* 28 kD protein 121-140	411
	VTGSVVCTTAAGNVNIAIGG	*M. tuberculosis* 19 kD protein 61-80	411
	MEVGWYRSPFSRVVHLYRNGK	Myelin oligodendrocyte gp 35-55	412
	ISNYCQIYPPNANKI	Der pI 113-127	413
	DLRQMRTVTPIRMQG	Der pI 15-29	413
	NNKTPHAIAAIS	Cholera toxin B subunit 89-100	414
	ELESPFILLADK	*Yersinia enterocolitica* HSP60 214-225	415
	VKEVAAKANDAAG	*Yersinia enterocolitica* HSP60 74-86	415
	FQDAYNAAGGHNAVF	*M. tuberculosis* MPT59 248-254	416
	HNGNQLDKYRSITVRV	Staphylococcal enterotoxin B 121-136	417
	IFNANKVALAPQCLPV	SV M protein 146-161	418
	FRYYPNVVAKNIGRIR	SV M protein 331-346	418
	SVQRNLPFDRTTVMAAFTGNTEG	Influenza PR8 NP 413-435	410
	ARSALILRGSVAHKSCLPACVYGP	Influenza PR8 NP 260-283	410

H2-A^d	Sequence	Source	Ref.
Motif unknown			
Ligands	WANLMEKIQASVATNPI	Apolipoprotein E 268-284	419
	WANLMEKIQASVATNP	Apolipoprotein E 268-283	419
	DAYHSRAIQVVRARKQ	Cys-C 40-55	419
	ASFEAQGALANIAVDKA	H2-Eα^d 52-68	419
	ASFEAQGALANIAVDK	H2-Eα^d 52-67	419
	EEQTQQIRLQAEIFQAR	Apolipoprotein E 236-252	419
	EQTQQIRLQAEIFQAR	Apolipoprotein E 237-252	419
	KPVSQMRMATPLLMRPM	Invariant chain 85-101	419
	VPQLNQMVRTAAEVAGQX	Tf receptor 442-459	419
	ISQAVHAAHAEINE	Ovalbumin 323-336	419
	LEDARRLKAIYEKKK	λ repressor 12-26	419
T cell epitopes	FWRGENGRKTRIAYERMCNILKGK	Influenza PR8 NP 206-229	410
	TELKLSDYEGRLIQNS	Influenza PR8 NP 45-60	410

H2-A^k		Relative position											Source	Ref.
		1	2	3	**4**	5	**6**	7	8	9	10			
Anchor or preferred residues		**D**			**I,V**		**E**							420
		N			**L,N**		**Q**							
Examples for ligands	EDE	**N**	L	Y	E	G	L	N	L	D	D	CSMY	MB1 177-193	420
	SFL	**D**	A	W	**V**	C	**E**	Q	L	A	T		Fcε Receptor II 298–310	420
	YILY	**N**	K	G	**I**	M	G	E	D	S	Y	PY	Cathepsin H 77-92	420
	VRF	**D**	S	D	**V**	G	**E**	F	R	A	V	TEL	H2-Aβ^k 37-53	420
	DPFKG	**D**	D	Y	**N**	E	**E**	N	P	T	E	PS	DNA-B 92-108	420
	AILL	**D**	K	G	**N**	K	**E**	F	L	S	A	G	IL-1 Receptor 185-199	420
	DGST	**D**	Y	G	**I**	L	**Q**	I	N	S	R		HEL 48-61	421
	DGST	**D**	Y	G	**I**	L	**Q**	I	N	S			HEL 48-60	421
	DGST	**D**	Y	G	**I**	L	**Q**	I	N	S	R	W	HEL 48-62	421
		D	Y	G	**I**	L	**Q**	I	N	S	R	WW(C)	HEL 52-63 (64)	421
	IIAN	**D**	Q	G	**N**	R	T	T	P	S	Y		HSP70 28-41	421
	TPRR	G	E	V	Y	T	C	H	V	E	H	P	H2-Aβ^k 165-179	421
	KVHGS	L	A	R	A	G	K	V	R	G	Q	TPKVAKQ	40S ribosomal protein S30 1-22	421
	AGKVR	G	Q	T	P	K	V	A	K	Q	E	KKKKKT	40S ribosomal protein S30 9-28	421

Table 4.6. (con't)

		Relative position											Source	Ref.
		1	2	3	**4**	5	**6**	7	8	9	10			
	EPLVPL	**D**	N	H	**I**	P	**E**	N	A	Q	P	G	Ryudocan 84-100	421
		X	Q	L	G	A	**Q**	N	E	M	L	XPL	Unknown	396
	XXKKGT	**D**	F	Q	**L**	N	**Q**	L	E				Transferrin 100-113	396
	KGT	**D**	F	Q	**L**	N	**Q**	L	E	G	K	KG	Transferrin 103-117	396
	FVRF	**D**	S	D	**V**	G	**E**	F	R	A	V	TEL	H2-Aβ^k 37-53	396
	YILY	**N**	K	G	**I**	M	G	E	D	S	Y	PY	Cathepsin H 72-92	396
	XPL	A	L	Q	F	A	**E**	L	P	V	N	KG	Unknown	396
	XNL	R	F	D	S	D	V	G	E	F	R	AV	H2-Eβ^k 33-47	396
	EDE	**N**	L	Y	E	G	L	N	L	D	D	CSMYY	MBI 177-194	396
	XX	X	F	V	H	Q	F	Q	P	F	c	yF	H2-Aβ^k 3-17	396
		Q	F	Q	P	F	X	Y	F	T	N	T	H2-Aβ^k 10-20	396
T-cell epitope		A	R	S	A	L	I	L	R	G	S	VAHKSCLPACVYGP	Influenza PR8 NP 260-283	410

H2-A^{g7}	Relative position									Source	Ref.
Motif according to Reizis et al	1	2	3	**4**	5	**6**	**7**	8	**9**		
Anchor residues											
Preferred residues				**L**		**A**	**R**		**E**		422
						T	**A**				
				Y							
				A							
				T							
Motif according to Harrison et al											
Anchor and preferred residues				**K**		**I**			**Y**		423
						M			**R,F**		
						L			**D,L**		
									K		

	Sequence	Source	Ref.
Examples for ligands	KPKATAEQLKTVMDD	Serum albumin 560-574	208
	GHNYVTAIRNQQEG	Transferrin 55-68	208
	ETTEESLRNYYEQ	hnRNP B1 & A2 31-43	208
	VVMRDPASKRSRGFGF	hnRNP A2 & B1 51-66	208
	VVMRDPQTKRSRGFGF	hnRNP A1 44-59	208
	PKEPEQLRKLFIGGL	hnRNP A1 7-21	208
	VVYPWTQRYFDSF	β globin major 33-45	208
T cell epitopes	AAAMKRHGLDNYRGYSLGNW	HEL 9-29	424
	SVNCAKKIVSDGNGM	HEL 90-104	425
	SRLSKVAPVIKARMMEYGTT	GAD65 524-543	426
	IPPSLRYLLDNEERMSRLSK	GAD65 509-528	427
	NMYAMMIARFKMFPEVKEKG	GAD65 247-266	427
	ISQAVHAAHAEINEAGR	OVA 323-339	428
	LEDARRLKAIYEKKK	λ repressor 12-26	428
	PGYPIRALVGDEQED	MOG 8-22	429
	DYEYLINVIHAFQYV	PLP 56-70	429
	YLATASTMDHARHGFLPRHRDTGI	MBP12-35	429
	VLGGGCALLRCIPALDSLTPANED	HSP65 (p277) 437-460	430
	KNSLINYLEQIHRGVKGFVR	Carboxypeptidase H 362-382	430
	FSPAVGVDFELESFSERKEEEKEEL	Carboxypeptidase H 440-464	430
	SHLVEALYLVCGERG	Insulin B chain 9-23	431
	DTGHGLRLIHYSYGAGSTEKGDI	TCR Vβ8.2 38-60	432
	DSGKGLRLIYYSITENDLQKGDL	TCR Vβ6 38-60	432
	IIIEVLKKRHSG	Myoglobin 110-121	432
	LTALGTILKK	Myoglobulin 69-78	432
	KVHGSLARAGKVRGQTPKVAKQ	40S ribosomal protein S30 1-22	432
	MEVGWYRSPFSRVVHLVRNGK	MOG 35-55	433

Table 4.7 Rat class II motifs

RT1.B^{l}		1	2	3	4	5	6	7	8	9		Source	Ref.
Anchor and auxiliary anchor residues				**T,S, V**	**F,H, Q**		**A,S, V,T**			**E, D**			329, 434
Also detected		pol.* ali.*		A,M, W,Y, F,I,L	Q,K R,N T,L, I		P,L	lar.*	M, W, Y,F, I,L, V,G A,P, C,S, T	ali.*			
Examples for ligands													
	TIPTKQ	T	Q	**T**	**F**	T	**T**	Y	S	**D**	NQP	HSP70 420-437	329
	LDPQN	Q	H	**T**	**F**	E	**A**	R	D	L		Nucleobindin 140-153	329
	DIPAYS	Q	D	**T**	**F**	K	**V**	H	Y	**E**	N	Ribophorin I 203-218	329
	ERGY	S	F	**T**	T	T	**A**	E	R	**E**	IVR	Actin 195-210	329

T cell epitopes

	Q	K	**S**	**Q**	R	**S**	Q	D	**E**	NPV	GBP 73-84	435
FV	S	M	**V**	T	T	**A**	C	H	**E**	FFEHE	S100β (rat) 76-91	436
			T	**F**	G	L	Q	L	**E**	LT	*M. tuberculosis* HSP65 180-188	437
DAV	R	N	A	K	A	**A**	V	E	**E**	GIV	*M. tuberculosis* HSP65 396-410	437
ALPK	Q	I	A	**F**	N	**S**	G	L	**E**	PG	*M. tuberculosis* HSP65 446-460	437
K	L	E	L	**Q**	S	**A**	L	E	**E**	AEASLEH	Cardiac myosin α (rat)1539-1555	438
T	L	T	**V**	N	N	**A**	R	P	**E**		TCR β 77-86	439
	Q	K	**S**	**Q**	R	**S**	Q	D	**E**	NPV	MBP (guinea pig) 72-85	434
	Q	K	**S**	**Q**	R	**T**	Q	D	**E**	NPV	MBP (rat) 72-85	434
KVCGSN	L	L	**S**	I	C	K	T	A	**E**	FQMTFHLFI	PLP (rat) 217-240	434
TESPFKNTEI	S	F	K	L	G	Q	E	F	**E**	ETTADNR	Myelin P2 (bovine) 53-78	434
FVSMV	T	T	A	C	H	E	F	F	**E**	HE	S100β (rat) 76-91	434
S	W	E	G	V	G	**V**	V	P	**D**		IRBP (bovine) 1181-1191	434
KLE	L	Q	**S**	A	L	E	E	A	**E**	ASLEH	Myosin (rat) 1539-1555	434
DGDFAI	V	H	M	T	K	L	L	L	**D**	Y	Acetyl-Choline receptor (torpedo fish) 97-11	434
	T	F	G	L	Q	L	E	L	T		HSP65 180-188	434
QK	S	Q	R	S	Q	D	E	N	P	V	MBP 72-85	434
IS	Q	A	**V**	**H**	A	**A**	H	A	**E**	INEAGR	OVA 323-339	434
PL	G	F	F	P	D	H	Q	L	**D**	PAFG	HBV pre-S1 protein 10-24	434
EQ	N	V	R	S	A	G	E	L	**E**	L	Lol. P1 121-132	434
			N	T	D	G	S	T	**D**	YGILQINSR	HEL 46-61	434
VHFF	K	N	I	V	T	P	R	T	P		MBP 87-99	434
QHG	Y	W	R	R	Q	**A**	R	F	K	PGKGG	Avian infectious bronchitis virus 67-83	434
HNTN	G	V	**T**	A	A	**S**	S	H	**E**		Influenza HA 130-142	434

*pol: polar, ali: aliphatic, lar: large

Table 4.8. Pattern used for the prediction of H2-K^d nonamers.

AA	P1	**P2**	P3	P4	P5	P6	P7	P8	**P9**
A	0	0	1	0	1	2	0	0	**6**
C	0	0	0	0	0	0	0	0	0
D	0	0	0	1	0	0	0	0	0
E	0	0	0	0	0	0	1	1	0
F	0	**6**	0	-1	-1	0	0	0	0
G	0	0	0	2	0	2	0	0	0
H	0	0	0	0	0	0	0	0	0
I	1	0	1	-1	0	1	0	0	**10**
K	2	0	1	0	0	2	2	0	0
L	0	0	3	-1	1	0	0	1	**10**
M	0	0	0	-1	0	0	0	0	0
N	0	0	0	0	0	0	0	0	0
P	0	0	0	3	0	0	0	0	0
Q	0	0	2	0	0	0	1	0	0
R	1	0	0	0	0	0	0	0	0
S	3	0	0	2	2	-1	1	2	0
T	2	0	0	2	1	0	4	0	0
V	0	0	2	1	2	1	0	0	**8**
W	0	0	0	0	0	0	0	0	0
X	0	0	0	0	0	0	0	0	0
Y	0	**10**	0	0	-1	0	0	1	0

Table 4.9. H2-K^d motif-based prediction from source proteins of reported natural ligands

Protein: jak1, mouse			**Protein: listeriolysin, *L. monocytogenes***		
Pos.	**Score**	**Sequence**	**Pos.**	**Score**	**Sequence**
367	3.444	SYFPEITHI	439	2.889	NYDPEGNEI
702	3.000	SYLEDKDLV	479	2.778	VYAKECTGL
991	3.000	DYLGSRQYV	91	2.667	GYKDGNEYI
40	2.556	FYLLDREPL	413	2.556	AYTDGKINI
141	2.556	KRVPEATPL	192	2.444	KYAQAYPNV
777	2.556	SFGTTLWEI	196	2.333	AYPNVSAKI
95	2.444	ITVDDKTSL	220	2.333	KFGTAFKAV
285	2.444	IFETSMLLI	224	2.333	AFKAVNNSL

Protein: p60, *L. monocytogenes*			**Protein: collagen 1 α2**		
Pos.	**Score**	**Sequence**	**Pos.**	**Score**	**Sequence**
449	3.111	IYVGNGQMI	3	3.111	SFVDTRTLL
217	3.000	KYGVSVQDI	1203	2.444	DFSTGETCI
236	3.000	IYVGQKLAI	1253	2.222	SSKEMATQL
401	2.889	KYVFAKAGI	17	2.111	SCLATCQYL
476	2.667	KYLVGFGRV	312	2.111	TGAKGATGL
403	2.444	VFAKAGISL	23	2.000	QYLQSGSVR
439	2.444	DYGSGISHV	195	2.000	KGQPGAQGV
94	2.222	SGAGVDNSI	1138	2.000	DYEVDATLK

Protein: tum-P198			**Protein: Influenza A nucleoprotein**		
Pos.	**Score**	**Sequence**	**Pos.**	**Score**	**Sequence**
147*	3.333	KYQAVTTTL	39	2.889	FYIQMCTEL
147	2.889	KYQAVTATL	147	2.667	TYQRTRALV
46	2.556	FYRNKLKYL	257	2.333	TFLARSALI
166	2.556	HYRKKKQIL	25	2.222	IRASVGKMI
110	2.222	PYDKKKRMV	218	2.222	AYERMCNIL
19	1.778	AAIVAKQVL	290	2.222	DFEREGYSL
117	1.778	MVVPAALKV	345	2.222	SFIKGTKVV
186	1.778	KKICKFTEV	182	2.111	AVKGVGTMV

*Table 4.10. Evaluating the influence of residues in nonanchor positions of HLA-A*0201 binding peptides*

Study		P1	P2	P3	P4	P5	P6	P7	P8	P9
Binding studies (1) (Ruppert et al., 1993)	associated with good binding	Y F W		Y F W	S T C	Y F W		A	P	
	associated with no binding	D E P		D E R K H			R K H	D E R K H		
Binding studies (2) (Parker et al., 1994)	associated with good binding	K		W F Y L V		Y F W K	F Y E V	F W		
	associated with no binding	D H		K E R	F I		K W	G R	V	
Binding studies (3) (Drijfhout et al., 1995)	associated with good binding	K Y T		Y W M A	D E T	I T V H W Y	V C Q	Q T A	Y P R	
	associated with no binding	D		R		R N D	H D	R D	V F	
Pool sequencing of natural ligands (Falk et al., 1991)	auxiliary anchors or preferred residues	I L F K M Y V		A Y F P M S R	**E** **K** G P D T	I K Y N G F V H	**V** I L **T**	A Y H	**K** E S	
Comparison of individual ligands (unpublished)	preferred in ligands	I Y L M F A S		L D F S V	G E P S	L G T N D A	I P V L	L V P A H	E H K G S T L	
	absent in ligands	E Q P N H V		C H R T Y	K D F R Y	R E Q S	D H N Q R Y	G K M R	D P N V	

Table 4.11. Pattern used for the prediction of *HLA-A*0201* ***nonamers.***

AA	P1	**P2**	P3	P4	P5	P6	P7	P8	**P9**
A	2	**6**	2	0	0	0	2	1	**6**
C	0	0	0	0	0	0	0	0	0
D	-1	0	0	1	0	0	0	0	0
E	-1	0	-1	2	0	0	0	2	0
F	1	0	1	-1	1	0	0	0	0
G	1	0	0	2	2	0	0	1	0
H	0	0	0	0	0	0	1	0	0
I	2	**8**	2	0	0	6	0	0	**8**
K	1	0	-1	0	1	0	-1	2	0
L	2	**10**	2	0	1	6	1	0	**10**
M	0	**8**	1	0	0	0	0	0	**6**
N	0	0	1	0	0	0	1	0	0
P	0	0	0	2	1	0	1	0	0
Q	0	0	0	0	0	0	0	0	0
R	0	0	0	0	0	0	0	0	0
S	2	0	0	0	0	0	0	2	0
T	0	**6**	-1	0	0	2	0	2	**6**
V	1	**6**	0	0	0	6	2	0	**10**
W	0	0	1	0	0	0	0	0	0
X	0	0	0	0	0	0	0	0	0
Y	2	0	1	-1	1	0	1	0	0

*Table 4.12. HLA-A*0201 motif-based prediction of self peptides and T cell epitopes*

self peptides from p68 (helicase)			T cell epitopes from HIV-1 RT		
Pos.	**Score**	**Sequence**	**Pos.**	**Score**	**Sequence**
148	3.556	[YLLPAIVHI]	476	3.556	[ILKEPVHGV]
466	3.444	AINPKLLQL	718	3.111	LVSAGIRKV
127	3.000	VALSGLDMV	794	3.111	HLEGKVILV
178	3.000	ELAQQVQQV	426	3.000	KLVGKLNWA
297	3.000	YIHINIGAL	448	3.000	KLLRGTKAL
145	2.889	TLSYLLPAI	534	3.000	QLTEAVQKI
171	2.778	LVLAPTREL	960	3.000	PLWKGPAKL
455	2.778	DLISVLREA	193	2.889	LTEEKIKAL
299	2.667	HINIGALEL	294	2.889	YTAFTIPSI
308	2.667	SANHNILQI	423	2.889	DIQKLVGKL
self peptides from protein phosphatase 2A			**T cell epitopes from Flu A matrix protein**		
Pos.	**Score**	**Sequence**	**Pos.**	**Score**	**Sequence**
402	4.000	[SLLPAIVEL]	58	3.556	[GILGFVFTL]
87	3.667	CLLPPLESL	23	2.778	EIAQRLEDV
343	3.444	ALASVIMGL	47	2.778	KTRPILSPL
364	3.444	LLPLFLAQL	51	2.778	ILSPLTKGI
11	3.222	PIAVLIDEL	55	2.778	LTKGILGFV
324	3.222	QILPCIKEL	180	2.778	VLASTTAKA
38	3.111	ALALGVERT	142	2.667	VAFGLVCAT
359	3.000	NTIEHLLPL	3	2.556	LLTEVETYV
446	3.000	CMAWLVDHV	2	2.444	SLLTEVETY
449	3.000	WLVDHVYAI	6	2.444	EVETYVLSI
self peptides from B cell transloc. protein			**T cell epitopes from HTLV-1 tax**		
Pos.	**Score**	**Sequence**	**Pos.**	**Score**	**Sequence**
10	3.000	TMIGEIAAA	72	3.222	ALQFLIPRL
96	3.000	RLLPSELTL	128	3.222	TLGQHLPTL
43	2.778	SLQELLAEH	168	3.222	ITWPLLPHV
7	2.667	RAATMIGEI	16	3.111	[LLFGYPVYV]
75	2.667	KMDPLIGQA	238	3.111	GLLPFHSTL
103	2.667	[TLWVDPYEV]	183	3.000	QLGAFLTNV
11	2.556	MIGEIAAAV	195	3.000	RIEELLYKI
14	2.556	EIAAAVSFI	35	2.889	PISGGLCSA
36	2.556	QLQTFSQSL	317	2.889	YTNIPISLL
71	2.222	RINHKMDPL	68	2.778	VIGSALQFL

Table 4.13. Pattern for the prediction of HLA class I ligands.

HLA-A*0101

AA	P1	P2	**P3**	P4	P5	P6	P7	P8	**P9**
A	1	0	0	0	0	0	0	0	0
C	0	0	0	0	0	0	0	0	0
D	0	0	**10**	0	0	0	0	0	0
E	0	0	**10**	0	0	0	0	0	0
F	1	0	0	0	0	3	0	0	0
G	0	0	0	1	2	1	0	0	0
H	0	0	0	0	0	0	0	0	0
I	0	0	0	0	0	0	4	0	0
K	0	0	0	0	0	0	0	2	0
L	0	1	0	0	0	0	6	2	0
M	0	0	0	0	0	0	0	1	0
N	0	0	0	0	0	1	0	0	0
P	0	0	0	4	1	0	0	0	0
Q	0	0	0	0	2	0	0	0	0
R	0	0	0	0	0	1	0	0	0
S	2	4	0	0	0	0	0	0	0
T	0	6	0	0	0	0	0	0	0
V	1	0	0	0	2	1	0	1	0
W	0	0	0	0	0	0	0	0	0
X	0	0	0	0	0	0	0	0	0
Y	2	0	0	0	1	0	0	0	**10**

HLA-A*0301

AA	P1	**P2**	P3	P4	P5	P6	P7	P8	**P9**
A	0	0	0	0	0	0	0	0	0
C	0	0	0	0	0	0	0	0	0
D	0	0	0	0	0	0	0	0	0
E	0	0	0	1	0	0	0	0	0
F	0	0	6	0	0	0	2	0	**6**
G	1	0	0	2	1	0	0	0	0
H	0	0	0	0	0	0	0	0	0
I	1	**8**	0	0	0	1	1	0	0
K	3	0	0	2	2	0	0	2	**8**
L	0	**10**	0	0	0	0	2	0	0
M	0	**6**	0	0	0	1	0	0	0
N	0	0	0	2	0	0	0	0	0
P	0	0	0	1	0	0	0	0	0
Q	0	0	0	0	0	0	0	0	0
R	0	0	0	0	0	0	0	1	0
S	2	0	0	0	0	0	0	1	0
T	0	0	0	0	0	2	0	2	0
V	0	**8**	0	1	1	2	2	1	0
W	0	0	0	0	0	0	0	0	0
X	0	0	0	0	0	0	0	0	0
Y	0	0	4	0	0	0	0	0	**10**

HLA-A24

AA	P1	**P2**	P3	P4	P5	P6	P7	P8	**P9**
A	1	0	0	0	0	0	0	0	0
C	0	0	0	0	0	0	0	0	0
D	0	0	0	1	1	0	0	0	0
E	0	0	1	1	0	0	0	1	0
F	0	**6**	0	0	0	1	0	0	**10**
G	0	0	0	0	0	0	0	0	0

Table 4.13. (con't)

HLA-A*1101

AA	P1	P2	P3	P4	P5	P6	P7	P8	**P9**
A	2	0	0	0	0	0	0	0	0
C	0	0	0	0	0	0	0	0	0
D	0	0	0	0	0	0	0	0	0
E	0	0	0	1	0	0	0	0	0
F	0	0	6	0	0	0	2	0	**6**
G	1	0	0	2	1	0	0	0	0
H	0	0	0	0	0	0	0	1	0
I	1	0	0	0	2	0	0	0	**8**
K	1	0	0	1	0	0	0	1	0
L	0	0	2	0	0	0	0	1	**10**
M	0	0	0	0	0	0	0	0	0
N	0	0	0	0	0	0	0	0	0
P	0	0	1	1	0	0	0	0	0
Q	0	0	0	0	0	0	0	0	0
R	0	0	0	0	0	0	0	0	0
S	0	0	0	0	0	0	0	0	0
T	0	0	0	0	0	0	0	0	0
V	0	0	0	0	2	0	0	0	0
W	0	0	0	0	0	0	0	0	0
X	0	0	0	0	0	0	0	0	0
Y	0	**10**	0	0	0	0	0	0	0

HLA-A*3101

AA	P1	P2	P3	P4	P5	P6	P7	P8	**P9**
A	1	0	0	0	0	0	0	0	0
C	0	0	0	0	0	0	0	0	0
D	0	0	0	1	0	0	0	0	0
E	0	0	0	1	0	0	0	1	0
F	0	6	6	0	0	0	2	0	0
G	0	0	0	1	0	0	0	0	0
H	0	0	0	0	0	0	1	0	0
I	1	4	0	0	1	1	0	0	0
K	2	0	1	0	0	0	0	0	0
L	0	6	4	0	0	0	0	1	0
M	0	0	4	0	0	0	0	0	0
N	0	0	1	0	0	0	0	0	0
P	0	0	0	1	2	0	0	0	0
Q	0	4	0	0	0	0	0	1	0
R	1	0	0	1	0	0	0	0	**10**
S	0	0	0	0	0	0	0	0	0
T	0	4	0	0	0	0	0	0	0
V	1	6	-1	0	0	0	1	0	0
W	0	0	0	0	1	0	0	0	0
X	0	0	0	0	0	0	0	0	0
Y	0	4	4	0	0	0	1	0	0

HLA-A*3302

AA	P1	P2	P3	P4	P5	P6	P7	P8	**P9**
A	0	4	0	0	0	0	0	0	0
C	0	0	0	0	0	0	0	0	0
D	1	0	0	1	0	0	0	0	0
E	4	0	0	1	0	0	0	1	0
F	0	6	0	-1	1	2	0	0	0
G	0	0	0	1	0	0	0	0	0
H	0	0	0	0	0	0	0	0	0
I	0	4	2	-1	2	1	0	0	0
K	0	-1	2	1	2	0	0	0	0
L	0	4	3	0	0	1	0	0	0
M	2	0	2	0	0	0	0	0	0

Table 4.13. (con't)

HLA-A*3302

AA	P1	P2	P3	P4	P5	P6	P7	P8	**P9**
N	0	0	0	0	0	1	0	1	0
P	0	0	0	2	2	0	0	0	0
Q	0	0	1	0	0	0	0	2	0
R	0	0	0	0	0	0	0	0	**10**
S	0	0	-1	1	1	0	0	0	0
T	1	6	-1	0	0	0	2	1	0
V	0	6	0	-1	0	0	3	0	0
W	0	0	1	0	1	0	1	0	0
X	0	0	0	0	0	0	0	0	0
Y	0	6	0	0	0	0	1	0	0

HLA-A*6801

AA	P1	**P2**	P3	P4	P5	P6	P7	P8	**P9**
A	0	0	1	0	0	0	1	0	0
C	0	0	0	0	0	0	0	0	0
D	2	0	0	0	0	0	0	0	0
E	3	0	0	0	0	0	0	0	0
F	0	0	1	0	0	0	0	0	0
G	0	0	1	0	0	0	0	0	0
H	0	0	0	0	0	0	1	1	0
I	0	0	0	0	0	1	0	0	0
K	0	0	0	0	0	0	0	1	**10**
L	0	0	0	0	0	0	0	0	0
M	0	0	0	0	0	0	0	0	0
N	0	0	0	0	0	0	0	0	0
P	0	0	0	0	1	0	0	0	0
Q	0	0	0	0	0	0	0	0	0
R	0	0	0	0	0	0	0	1	**10**
S	0	0	0	0	0	0	0	0	0
T	1	**8**	0	0	0	0	0	0	0
V	0	**10**	0	0	1	0	0	0	0
W	0	0	0	0	0	0	0	0	0
X	0	0	0	0	0	0	0	0	0
Y	0	0	0	0	0	0	1	0	0

HLA-A*6901

AA	P1	**P2**	P3	P4	P5	P6	P7	P8	**P9**
A	2	**10**	0	0	0	0	0	0	0
C	0	0	0	0	0	0	0	0	0
D	0	0	0	1	0	0	0	0	0
E	0	0	0	1	0	0	0	0	0
F	0	0	2	0	0	1	0	0	0
G	0	0	0	0	0	0	0	0	0
H	0	0	0	0	0	0	0	0	0
I	0	0	1	0	0	2	0	0	0
K	0	0	1	0	0	0	0	0	0
L	0	0	0	0	0	1	0	0	**6**
M	0	0	1	0	0	0	0	0	**6**
N	0	0	0	0	0	0	0	0	0
P	0	0	0	0	1	0	0	0	0
Q	0	0	0	0	0	0	0	0	0
R	0	0	0	1	0	0	0	0	0
S	0	0	0	0	0	0	0	0	0
T	0	**10**	0	0	0	0	0	0	0
V	0	**10**	1	0	0	1	0	0	**10**
W	0	0	0	0	0	0	0	0	0
X	0	0	0	0	0	0	0	0	0
Y	0	0	1	0	0	0	0	1	0

Table 4.13. (con't)

HLA-B7

AA	P1	**P2**	P3	P4	P5	P6	P7	P8	**P9**
A	2	0	1	1	0	0	1	1	0
C	0	0	0	0	0	0	0	0	0
D	0	0	1	0	0	0	0	0	0
E	1	0	0	0	0	0	0	1	0
F	0	0	0	0	0	1	0	0	**6**
G	0	0	1	2	0	1	0	0	0
H	0	0	0	0	0	0	0	0	0
I	1	0	0	0	0	0	0	0	**6**
K	1	0	0	1	0	0	0	0	0
L	0	0	0	0	0	0	2	0	**10**
M	0	0	1	0	0	0	0	0	0
N	0	0	0	0	0	0	0	0	0
P	0	**10**	0	1	3	0	1	1	0
Q	0	0	0	0	0	0	0	0	0
R	1	0	2	0	0	1	0	0	0
S	0	0	2	0	0	0	0	0	0
T	0	0	0	0	0	1	1	0	**6**
V	0	0	0	0	0	1	2	1	**6**
W	0	0	0	0	0	0	0	0	0
X	0	0	0	0	0	0	0	0	0
Y	0	0	0	0	0	0	0	0	0

HLA-B8

AA	P1	P2	**P3**	P4	**P5**	P6	P7	P8	**P9**
A	0	4	0	0	0	0	0	1	0
C	0	0	0	0	0	0	0	0	0
D	0	0	0	0	0	0	0	0	0
E	2	0	0	2	0	0	0	1	0
F	1	0	0	0	0	0	0	0	**6**
G	1	0	0	0	0	0	0	0	0
H	1	0	0	0	0	0	0	0	0
I	1	4	0	0	0	1	0	0	**6**
K	0	0	**10**	0	**10**	0	1	0	0
L	0	6	0	1	0	0	0	0	**10**
M	0	0	0	0	0	0	0	0	0
N	0	0	0	0	0	1	0	0	0
P	0	6	0	0	0	0	0	0	0
Q	0	0	0	0	0	0	0	0	0
R	0	0	**6**	0	**8**	0	0	0	0
S	2	0	0	0	0	0	0	0	0
T	0	0	0	0	0	0	0	0	0
V	1	0	0	1	0	1	1	0	0
W	0	0	0	0	0	0	0	0	0
X	0	0	0	0	0	0	0	0	0
Y	0	0	0	1	0	0	0	0	0

Table 4.13. (con't)

HLA-B*1501

AA	P1	**P2**	P3	P4	P5	P6	P7	P8	**P9**
A	0	0	1	0	0	0	0	0	0
C	0	0	0	0	0	0	0	0	0
D	0	0	0	1	0	0	0	0	0
E	0	0	0	1	0	0	0	0	0
F	0	0	2	0	0	0	0	0	**8**
G	1	0	0	1	1	1	0	0	0
H	0	0	0	0	0	0	0	0	0
I	1	**8**	1	0	0	0	0	0	0
K	0	0	2	1	0	0	0	0	0
L	0	**10**	0	0	0	0	0	0	0
M	0	**8**	0	0	0	0	0	0	0
N	0	0	1	0	0	0	0	0	0
P	0	0	0	1	0	0	0	0	0
Q	0	**10**	0	0	0	0	0	0	0
R	0	0	2	0	0	0	0	0	0
S	1	0	0	0	0	0	0	0	0
T	0	0	0	0	0	0	1	1	0
V	1	**8**	0	0	0	0	1	1	0
W	0	0	0	0	0	0	0	0	0
X	0	0	0	0	0	0	0	0	0
Y	0	0	1	0	0	0	0	0	**10**

HLA-B*2702

AA	P1	**P2**	P3	P4	P5	P6	P7	P8	**P9**
A	0	0	1	0	0	1	0	0	0
C	0	0	0	0	0	0	0	0	0
D	0	0	0	1	0	0	0	0	0
E	0	0	-1	1	0	0	0	1	0
F	0	0	3	0	0	0	0	0	**10**
G	2	0	0	1	0	0	0	0	0
H	0	0	0	0	0	0	0	0	0
I	0	0	2	0	1	2	1	0	**6**
K	2	0	0	3	0	0	0	2	**6**
L	0	0	2	0	1	0	1	0	0
M	0	0	1	0	0	0	1	0	0
N	0	0	0	0	0	0	0	1	0
P	0	0	0	1	1	0	0	0	0
Q	0	0	0	1	0	0	0	1	0
R	0	**10**	0	0	0	0	0	0	0
S	0	0	0	0	0	0	0	0	0
T	0	0	0	0	1	0	0	0	0
V	0	0	0	0	1	1	1	0	0
W	0	0	3	0	0	0	0	0	**10**
X	0	0	0	0	0	0	0	0	0
Y	0	0	3	0	0	0	1	0	**10**

Table 4.13. (con't)

H2-D^b AA	P1	**P2**	**P3**	P4	P5	P6	P7	P8	**P9**
A	0	0	0	0	0	0	0	0	0
C	0	0	0	0	0	0	0	0	0
D	1	0	0	1	0	0	0	0	0
E	0	0	0	2	0	0	1	0	0
F	1	0	0	0	0	1	0	0	**8**
G	0	**10**	0	0	0	2	0	0	0
H	0	0	0	0	0	0	1	0	0
I	0	0	0	0	0	0	1	0	**6**
K	1	0	0	1	4	0	0	1	0
L	0	0	0	0	0	1	0	0	**10**
M	0	0	0	0	0	0	0	0	0
N	0	0	0	0	0	0	2	3	0
P	0	0	**10**	0	0	0	0	0	0
Q	0	0	0	1	0	0	0	0	0
R	0	0	0	0	6	0	0	0	0
S	0	0	0	0	0	0	0	1	0
T	0	0	0	0	0	0	0	0	**6**
V	1	0	0	1	0	0	0	1	0
W	0	0	0	0	0	0	0	0	0
X	0	0	0	0	0	0	0	0	0
Y	0	0	0	0	0	0	1	0	0

H2-L^b AA	P1	**P2**	P3	P4	P5	P6	P7	P8	**P9**
A	0	0	1	1	1	0	0	0	0
C	0	0	0	0	0	0	0	0	0
D	0	0	0	0	0	0	0	0	0
E	0	0	0	0	0	0	1	0	0
F	0	0	0	1	0	1	1	0	**10**
G	0	0	1	0	2	0	0	0	0
H	0	0	1	0	0	0	1	0	0
I	0	0	0	0	0	0	0	0	**6**
K	0	0	0	0	0	0	0	0	0
L	1	0	0	1	0	1	1	0	**10**
M	0	0	0	0	0	0	0	0	**6**
N	0	0	0	0	1	0	0	2	0
P	0	**10**	1	2	0	0	0	0	0
Q	0	0	2	0	0	0	0	0	0
R	0	0	0	1	0	1	0	0	0
S	0	**8**	0	0	1	0	0	0	0
T	0	0	1	0	0	0	1	0	0
V	0	0	0	0	0	0	1	1	0
W	0	0	0	0	0	1	0	0	0
X	0	0	0	0	0	0	0	0	0
Y	1	0	1	0	0	0	0	1	0

Table 4.13. (con't)

H2-K^b AA	P1	P2	P3	P4	**P5**	**P6**	P7	**P8**
A	1	1	0	0	0	0	0	0
C	0	0	0	0	0	0	0	0
D	0	0	0	1	0	0	0	0
E	0	0	0	1	0	1	0	0
F	0	0	0	0	**10**	0	0	0
G	0	1	0	0	0	0	0	0
H	0	0	0	0	0	0	0	0
I	1	1	1	0	0	1	0	**6**
K	0	0	0	1	0	0	1	0
L	1	0	0	0	0	0	0	**10**
M	0	0	0	0	0	0	0	**6**
N	0	1	0	0	0	0	1	0
P	0	0	1	0	0	0	0	0
Q	0	0	0	0	0	0	1	0
R	1	0	0	1	0	1	0	0
S	1	1	0	0	0	1	0	0
T	0	0	0	0	0	1	1	0
V	0	0	0	0	0	0	0	**6**
W	0	0	0	0	0	0	0	0
X	0	0	0	0	0	0	0	0
Y	0	0	**6**	0	**10**	0	0	0

H2-D^b AA	P1	P2	P3	P4	**P5**	P6	P7	P8	**P9**
A	2	1	0	0	0	1	0	0	**6**
C	0	0	0	0	0	0	0	0	0
D	0	0	0	1	0	0	1	0	0
E	0	0	0	1	0	0	1	0	0
F	0	0	0	0	0	0	0	0	**6**
G	0	1	1	1	0	1	0	0	0
H	0	0	0	0	0	0	0	0	0
I	0	0	2	0	0	0	0	0	**10**
K	0	0	0	1	0	0	0	0	0
L	0	0	1	0	0	2	0	0	**10**
M	0	1	0	0	0	0	0	0	0
N	0	0	0	0	**10**	0	0	0	0
P	0	0	2	0	0	0	0	0	0
Q	0	1	0	1	0	0	1	0	0
R	0	0	0	0	0	0	0	0	0
S	1	0	0	0	0	0	0	1	0
T	0	0	0	0	0	0	1	1	0
V	0	0	1	1	0	0	0	0	**6**
W	0	0	0	0	0	0	0	0	0
X	0	0	0	0	0	0	0	0	0
Y	0	0	0	0	0	0	0	0	0

Table 4.14. The subunits of the 20S proteasome

Human gene	MW	p1	Chromosomal locus	GDB	Rat symbol[a]	Yeast gene	Essential
α-type subunits							
HC2[a]	29555	6.16		PSMA1	RC2	PRE5	+
Pros30[a]	30239	6.56	11q15.1	PSMA1			
HC3	25898	7.29	6q27	PSMA2	RC3	Y7	-
HC8	28433	5.06	14q23	PSMA3	RC8	PRS1	+
HC9	29483	7.69		PSMA4	RC9	Y13	+
Zeta	26425	4.59		PSMA5	rZeta	PUP2	+
Pros27 (Iota)	27374	5.97	14q13	PSMA6	rIota	PRS2	+
XAPC7-S[a]	27900	8.69		PSMA7	RC6-1-S	PRE6	+
XAPC7-L[a]				PSMA7	RC6-I-L		
β-type subunits							
HC5	26489	8.20	7p12-13	PSMB1	RC5	PRS3	+
HC7-I	22836	6.61		PSMB2	RC7-I	PRE1	+
HC10-II	22931	6.15		PSMB3	RC10-II	PUP3	+
HN3	29192	5.63		PSMB4	RN3	PRE4	+
X (MB1, e)	22897	8.67	14q11.2	PSMB5	rX	PRE2	+
Y (Delta)	25315	4.65	17p13	PSMB6	rDelta	PRE3	+
Z	29965	7.61	9q34.11-34.12	PSMB7		PUP1	+
LMP7-E1[a]	29769	5.46	6p21	PSMB8			-
LMP7-E2[a]	30354	7.18	6p21	PSMB8	RC1		-
LMP2	23245	4.75	6p21	PSMB9	rLMP2		-
MECL1	28936	7.73	16q22.1	PSMB10			

[a]These three pairs of subunits (HC2 and Pros30, XAPC7-S and XAPC7-L, LMP7-E1 and LMP7-E2) are almost identical. Therefore their mRNAs may arise by alternative splicing or use of different transcription initiation sites.
[b]GDB: human genome database. Adapted from ref 452.

References

1. Hunt DF, Henderson RA, Shabanowitz J et al. Characterization of peptides bound to the class I MHC molecule HLA-A2.1 by mass spectrometry. Science 1992; 255:1261-3.
2. Stevanović S, Jung G. Multiple sequence analysis: pool sequencing of synthetic and natural peptide libraries. Anal Biochem 1993; 212:212-20.
3. Jardetzky TS, Lane WS, Robinson RA et al. Identification of self peptides bound to purified HLA-B27. Nature 1991; 353:326-9.
4. Falk K, Rötzschke O, Stevanović S et al. Allele-specific motifs revealed by sequencing of self-peptides eluted from MHC molecules. Nature 1991; 351:290-6.
5. Fremont DH, Matsumura M, Stura EA et al. Crystal structures of two viral peptides in complex with murine MHC class I H-2K^b. Science 1992; 257:919-27.
6. Rammensee HG, Falk K, Rötzschke O. Peptides naturally presented by MHC class I molecules. Annu Rev Immunol 1993; 11:213-44.
7. Androlewicz MJ, Cresswell P. How selective is the transporter associated with antigen processing? Immunity 1996; 5:1-5.
8. Stevanović S. Multiple sequence analysis of MHC ligands. In: Levkovits I, ed. Immunology Methods Manual. San Diego: Academic Press Ltd., 1997: 589-602.
9. Ruppert J, Sidney J, Celis E et al. Prominent role of secondary anchor residues in peptide binding to HLA-A2.1 molecules. Cell 1993; 74:929-37.
10. Drijfhout JW, Brandt RMP, D'Amaro J et al. Detailed motifs for peptide binding to HLA-A*0201 derived from large random sets of peptides using a cellular binding assay. Hum Immunol 1995; 43:1-12.
11. Udaka K, Wiesmüller K-H, Kienle S et al. Tolerance to amino acid variations in peptides binding to the major histocompatibility complex class I protein H-2K^b. J Biol Chem 1995; 270:24130-4.
12. Hammer J, Takacs B, Sinigaglia F. Identification of a motif for HLA-DR1 binding peptides using M13 display libraries. J Exp Med 1992; 176:1007-13.
13. Davenport MP, Smith KJ, Barouch D et al. HLA class I binding motifs derived from random peptide libraries differ at the COOH terminus from those of eluted peptides. J Exp Med 1997; 185:367-71.
14. Parker KC, Bednarek MA, Coligan JE. Scheme for ranking potential HLA-A2 binding peptides based on independent binding of individual peptide side-chains. J Immunol 1994; 152:163-75.
15. Nelson CA, Vidavsky I, Viner NJ et al. Amino terminal trimming of peptides for presentation on major histocompatibility complex class II molecules. Proc Natl Acad Sci U S A 1997; 94:628-33.
16. Stern LJ, Brown JH, Jardetzky TS et al. Crystal structure of the human class II MHC protein HLA-DR1 complexed with an influenza virus peptide. Nature 1994; 368:215-21.
17. Falk K, Rötzschke O, Stevanović S et al. Pool sequencing of natural HLA-DR, DQ, and DP ligands reveals detailed peptide motifs, constraints of processing, and general rules. Immunogenetics 1994; 39:230-42.
18. Chicz RM, Urban RG, Gorga JC et al. Specificity and promiscuity among naturally processed peptides bound to HLA-DR alleles. J Exp Med 1993; 178:27-47.
19. Fleckenstein B, Kalbacher H, Müller C et al. New ligands binding to the human leukocyte antigen class II molecule DRB1*0101 based on the activity pattern of an undecapeptide library. Eur J Biochem 1996; 240:71-7.
20. Falk K, Rötzschke O, Takiguchi M et al. Peptide motifs of HLA-A1, -A11, -A31, and -A33 molecules. Immunogenetics 1994; 40:238-41.
21. DiBrino M, Tsuchida T, Turner RV et al. HLA-A1 and HLA-A3 T cell epitopes derived from influenza virus proteins predicted from peptide binding motifs. J Immunol 1993; 151:5930-5.
22. Sette A, Sidney J, del Guercio MF et al. Peptide binding to the most frequent HLA-A class I alleles measured by quantitative molecular binding assays. Mol Immunol 1994; 31:813-22.
23. DiBrino M, Parker KC, Shiloach J et al. Endogenous peptides with distinct amino acid anchor residue motifs bind to

HLA-A1 and HLA-B8. J Immunol 1994; 152: 620-31.
24. Kubo RT, Sette A, Grey HM et al. Definition of specific peptide motifs for four major HLA-A alleles. J Immunol 1994; 152:3913-24.
25. Engelhard VH. Structure of peptides associated with MHC class I molecules. Curr Opin Immunol 1994; 6:13-23.
26. Stevanović S, Pomer S, Rammensee H-G. Oberflächenantigene im Nierenzellkarzinom-Präsentation von MHC I-gebundenen Selbstpeptiden. Akt Urol 1995; Sonderheft:45-6.
27. Traversari C, van der Bruggen P, Luescher IF et al. A nonapeptide encoded by human gene MAGE-1 is recognized on HLA-A1 by cytolytic T lymphocytes directed against tumor antigen MZ2-E. J Exp Med 1992; 176:1453-7.
28. van der Bruggen P, Traversari C, Chomez P et al. A gene encoding an antigen recognized by cytolytic T lymphocytes on a human melanoma. Science 1991; 254:1643-7.
29. Gaugler B, van den Eynde B, van der Bruggen P et al. Human gene MAGE-3 codes for an antigen recognized on a melanoma by autologous cytolytic T lymphocytes. J Exp Med 1994; 179: 921-30.
30. Celis E, Tsai V, Crimi C et al. Induction of anti-tumor cytotoxic T lymphocytes in normal humans using primary cultures and synthetic peptide epitopes. Proc Natl Acad Sci U S A 1994; 91: 2105-9.
31. Henderson RA, Cox AL, Sakaguchi K et al. Direct identification of an endogenous peptide recognized by multiple HLA-A2.1-specific cytotoxic T cells. Proc Natl Acad Sci U S A 1993; 90:10275-9.
32. Henderson RA, Michel H, Sakaguchi K et al. HLA-A2.1-associated peptides from a mutant cell line: a second pathway of antigen presentation. Science 1992; 255:1264-6.
33. Wei ML, Cresswell P. HLA-A2 molecules in an antigen-processing mutant cell contain signal sequence-derived peptides. Nature 1992; 356:443-6.
34. Wölfel T, Van Pel A, Brichard V et al. Two tyrosinase nonapeptides recognized on HLA-A2 melanomas by autologous cytolytic T lymphocytes. Eur J Immunol 1994; 24:759-64.
35. Robbins PF, el Gamil M, Kawakami Y et al. Recognition of tyrosinase by tumor-infiltrating lymphocytes from a patient responding to immunotherapy [published erratum appears in Cancer Res 1994; 54:3952]. Cancer Res 1994; 54:3124-6.
36. Brichard V, Van Pel A, Wölfel T et al. The tyrosinase gene codes for an antigen recognized by autologous cytolytic T lymphocytes on HLA-A2 melanomas. J Exp Med 1993; 178:489-95.
37. Engelhard VH, Appella E, Benjamin DC et al. Mass spectrometric analysis of peptides associated with the human class I MHC molecules HLA-A2.1 and HLA-B7 and identification of structural features that determine binding. Chem Immunol 1993; 57:39-62.
38. Harris PE, Colovai A, Liu Z et al. Naturally processed HLA class I bound peptides from c-myc-transfected cells reveal allele-specific motifs. J Immunol 1993; 151:5966-74.
39. Gotch F, McMichael A, Rothbard J. Recognition of influenza A matrix protein by HLA-A2-restricted cytotoxic T lymphocytes. Use of analogues to orientate the matrix peptide in the HLA-A2 binding site. J Exp Med 1988; 168:2045-57.
40. Utz U, Koenig S, Coligan JE et al. Presentation of three different viral peptides, HTLV-1 Tax, HCMV gB, and influenza virus M1, is determined by common structural features of the HLA-A2.1 molecule. J Immunol 1992; 149:214-21.
41. Falk K, Rötzschke O, Stevanović S et al. Analysis of a naturally occurring HLA class I-restricted viral epitope. Immunology 1994; 82:337-42.
42. Bednarek MA, Sauma SY, Gammon MC et al. The minimum peptide epitope from the influenza virus matrix protein. Extra and intracellular loading of HLA-A2. J Immunol 1991; 147:4047-53.
43. Kobayashi H, Sato K, Miyokawa N et al. Analysis of naturally processed human histocompatibility leukocyte antigen class I-bound peptides from hepatocellular carcinoma tissues in vivo. Jpn J Cancer Res 1995; 86:962-8.

44. di Marzo Veronese F, Arnott D, Barnaba V et al. Autoreactive cytotoxic T lymphocytes in human immunodeficiency virus type 1-infected subjects. J Exp Med 1996; 183:2509-16.
45. Skipper JC, Hendrickson RC, Gulden PH et al. An HLA-A2-restricted tyrosinase antigen on melanoma cells results from posttranslational modification and suggests a novel pathway for processing of membrane proteins. J Exp Med 1996; 183:527-34.
46. Diehl, M. Untersuchungen zur Peptidpräsentation gewebsspezifischer HLA-Moleküle 1995; Phillips-Universität Marburg.
47. Walker BD, Flexner C, Birch Limberger K et al. Long-term culture and fine specificity of human cytotoxic T-lymphocyte clones reactive with human immunodeficiency virus type. Proc Natl Acad Sci U S A 1989; 86:9514-8.
48. Nayersina R, Fowler P, Guilhot S et al. HLA A2 restricted cytotoxic T lymphocyte responses to multiple hepatitis B surface antigen epitopes during hepatitis B virus infection. J Immunol 1993; 150:4659-71.
49. Bertoletti A, Costanzo A, Chisari FV et al. Cytotoxic T lymphocyte response to a wild type hepatitis B virus epitope in patients chronically infected by variant viruses carrying substitutions within the epitope. J Exp Med 1994; 180:933-43.
50. Bertoletti A, Chisari FV, Penna A et al. Definition of a minimal optimal cytotoxic T-cell epitope within the hepatitis B virus nucleocapsid protein. J Virol 1993; 67:2376-80.
51. del Guercio MF, Sidney J, Hermanson G et al. Binding of a peptide antigen to multiple HLA alleles allows definition of an A2-like supertype. J Immunol 1995; 154:685-93.
52. Lee SP, Thomas WA, Murray RJ et al. HLA A2.1-restricted cytotoxic T cells recognizing a range of Epstein-Barr virus isolates through a defined epitope in latent membrane protein LMP2. J Virol 1993; 67:7428-35.
53. Robbins PA, Lettice LA, Rota P et al. Comparison between two peptide epitopes presented to cytotoxic T lymphocytes by HLA-A2. Evidence for discrete locations within HLA-A2. J Immunol 1989; 143:4098-103.
54. Cerny A, McHutchison JG, Pasquinelli C et al. Cytotoxic T lymphocyte response to hepatitis C virus-derived peptides containing the HLA A2.1 binding motif. J Clin Invest 1995; 95:521-30.
55. Shirai M, Okada H, Nishioka M et al. An epitope in hepatitis C virus core region recognized by cytotoxic T cells in mice and humans. J Virol 1994; 68: 3334-42.
56. Tarpey I, Stacey S, Hickling J et al. Human cytotoxic T lymphocytes stimulated by endogenously processed human papillomavirus type 11 E7 recognize a peptide containing a HLA-A2 (A*0201) motif. Immunology 1994; 81:222-7.
57. Coulie PG, Brichard V, Van Pel A et al. A new gene coding for a differentiation antigen recognized by autologous cytolytic T lymphocytes on HLA-A2 melanomas. J Exp Med 1994; 180:35-42.
58. Kawakami Y, Eliyahu S, Delgado CH et al. Cloning of the gene coding for a shared human melanoma antigen recognized by autologous T cells infiltrating into tumor. Proc Natl Acad Sci U S A 1994; 91:3515-9.
59. Kawakami Y, Eliyahu S, Sakaguchi K et al. Identification of the immunodominant peptides of the MART-1 human melanoma antigen recognized by the majority of HLA-A2-restricted tumor infiltrating lymphocytes. J Exp Med 1994; 180:347-52.
60. Cox AL, Skipper J, Chen Y et al. Identification of a peptide recognized by five melanoma-specific human cytotoxic T cell lines. Science 1994; 264:716-9.
61. Kawakami Y, Eliyahu S, Delgado CH et al. Identification of a human melanoma antigen recognized by tumor-infiltrating lymphocytes associated with in vivo tumor rejection. Proc Natl Acad Sci U S A 1994; 91:6458-62.
62. Kawakami Y, Eliyahu S, Jennings C et al. Recognition of multiple epitopes in the human melanoma antigen gp100 by tumor-infiltrating T lymphocytes associated with in vivo tumor regression. J Immunol 1995; 154:3961-8.
63. Hadida F, Haas G, Zimmermann N et al.

CTLs from lymphoid organs recognize an optimal HLA-A2-restricted and HLA-B52-restricted nonapeptide and several epitopes in the C-terminal region of HIV-1 Nef. J Immunol 1995; 154: 4174-86.
64. Blum-Tirouvanziam U, Servis C, Habluetzel A et al. Localization of HLA-A2.1-restricted T cell epitopes in the circumsporozoite protein of Plasmodium falciparum. J Immunol 1995; 154:3922-31.
65. Robbins PA, Garboczi DN, Strominger JL. HLA-A*0201 complexes with two 10-Mer peptides differing at the P2 anchor residue have distinct refolding kinetics. J Immunol 1995; 154:703-9.
66. Stuber G, Dillner J, Modrow S et al. HLA-A0201 and HLA-B7 binding peptides in the EBV-encoded EBNA-1, EBNA-2 and BZLF-1 proteins detected in the MHC class I stabilization assay. Low proportion of binding motifs for several HLA class I alleles in EBNA-1. Int Immunol 1995; 7:653-63.
67. Man S, Newberg MH, Crotzer VL et al. Definition of a human T cell epitope from influenza A nonstructural protein 1 using HLA-A2.1 transgenic mice. Int Immunol 1995; 7:597-605.
68. Rivoltini L, Kawakami Y, Sakaguchi K et al. Induction of tumor-reactive CTL from peripheral blood and tumor-infiltrating lymphocytes of melanoma patients by in vitro stimulation with an immunodominant peptide of the human melanoma antigen MART-1. J Immunol 1995; 154:2257-65.
69. Shirai M, Arichi T, Nishioka M et al. CTL responses of HLA-A2.1-transgenic mice specific for hepatitis C viral peptides predict epitopes for CTL of humans carrying HLA-A2.1. J Immunol 1995; 154:2733-42.
70. Rehermann B, Fowler P, Sidney J et al. The cytotoxic T lymphocyte response to multiple hepatitis B virus polymerase epitopes during and after acute viral hepatitis. J Exp Med 1995; 181:1047-58.
71. Fisk B, Blevins TL, Wharton JT et al. Identification of an immunodominant peptide of HER-2/neu protooncogene recognized by ovarian tumor-specific cytotoxic T lymphocyte lines. J Exp Med 1995; 181:2109-17.
72. Dupuis M, Kundu SK, Merigan TC. Characterization of HLA-A 0201-restricted cytotoxic T cell epitopes in conserved regions of the HIV type 1 gp160 protein. J Immunol 1995; 155:2232-9.
73. den Haan JM, Sherman NE, Blokland E et al. Identification of a graft versus host disease-associated human minor histocompatibility antigen. Science 1995; 268:1476-80.
74. Wentworth PA, Vitiello A, Sidney J et al. Differences and similarities in the A2.1-restricted cytotoxic T cell repertoire in humans and human leukocyte antigen-transgenic mice. Eur J Immunol 1996; 26:97-101.
75. Cerny A, Fowler P, Brothers MA et al. Induction in vitro of a primary human antiviral cytotoxic T cell response. Eur J Immunol 1995; 25:627-30.
76. Panina-Bordignon P, Lang R, van Endert PM et al. Cytotoxic T cells specific for glutamic acid decarboxylase in autoimmune diabetes. J Exp Med 1995; 181: 1923-7.
77. Castelli C, Storkus WJ, Maeurer MJ et al. Mass spectrometric identification of a naturally processed melanoma peptide recognized by $CD8^+$ cytotoxic T lymphocytes. J Exp Med 1995; 181:363-8.
78. van der Bruggen P, Bastin J, Gajewski T et al. A peptide encoded by human gene MAGE-3 and presented by HLA-A2 induces cytolytic T lymphocytes that recognize tumor cells expressing MAGE-3. Eur J Immunol 1994; 24:3038-43.
79. Rehermann B, Pasquinelli C, Mosier SM et al. Hepatitis B virus (HBV) sequence variation of cytotoxic T lymphocyte epitopes is not common in patients with chronic HBV infection. J Clin Invest 1995; 96:1527-34.
80. Rehermann B, Lau D, Hoofnagle JH et al. Cytotoxic T lymphocyte responsiveness after resolution of chronic hepatitis B virus infection. J Clin Invest 1996; 97:1655-65.
81. Aidoo M, Lalvani A, Allsopp CE et al. Identification of conserved antigenic components for a cytotoxic T lymphocyte-inducing vaccine against malaria. Lancet 1995; 345:1003-7.

82. Battegay M, Fikes J, Di Bisceglie AM et al. Patients with chronic hepatitis C have circulating cytotoxic T cells which recognize hepatitis C virus-encoded peptides binding to HLA-A2.1 molecules. J Virol 1995; 69:2462-70.
83. Kurokohchi K, Akatsuka T, Pendleton CD et al. Use of recombinant protein to identify a motif-negative human cytotoxic T-cell epitope presented by HLA-A2 in the hepatitis C virus NS3 region. J Virol 1996; 70:232-40.
84. Harrer E, Harrer T, Barbosa P et al. Recognition of the highly conserved YMDD region in the human immunodeficiency virus type 1 reverse transcriptase by HLA-A2-restricted cytotoxic T lymphocytes from an asymptomatic long-term nonprogressor. J Infect Dis 1996; 173:476-9.
85. Guilloux Y, Lucas S, Brichard VG et al. A peptide recognized by human cytolytic T lymphocytes on HLA-A2 melanomas is encoded by an intron sequence of the N-acetylglucosaminyltransferase V gene. J Exp Med 1996; 183:1173-83.
86. Loftus DJ, Castelli C, Clay TM et al. Identification of epitope mimics recognized by CTL reactive to the melanoma/melanocyte-derived peptide MART-1. J Exp Med 1996; 184:647-57.
87. Wölfel T, Hauer M, Schneider J et al. A p16INK4a-insensitive CDK4 mutant targeted by cytolytic T lymphocytes in a human melanoma. Science 1995; 269: 1281-4.
88. Yang OO, Kalams SA, Rosenzweig M et al. Efficient lysis of human immunodeficiency virus type 1-infected cells by cytotoxic T lymphocytes. J Virol 1996; 70:5799-806.
89. Fisk B, Savary C, Hudson JM et al. Changes in an HER-2 peptide upregulating HLA-A2 expression affect both conformational epitopes and CTL recognition: implications for optimization of antigen presentation and tumor-specific CTL induction. J Immunother Emphasis Tumor Immunol 1995; 18:197-209.
90. Alexander-Miller MA, Parker KC, Tsukui T et al. Molecular analysis of presentation by HLA-A2.1 of a promiscuously binding V3 loop peptide from the HIV-1 envelope protein to human cytotoxic T lymphocytes. Int Immunol 1996; 8:641-9.
91. Wentworth PA, Sette A, Celis E et al. Identification of A2-restricted hepatitis C virus-specific cytotoxic T lymphocyte epitopes from conserved regions of the viral genome. Int Immunol 1996; 8:651-9.
92. Wills MR, Carmichael AJ, Mynard K et al. The human cytotoxic T-lymphocyte (CTL) response to cytomegalovirus is dominated by structural protein pp65: frequency, specifity, and T-cell receptor usage of pp65-specific CTL. J Virol 1996; 70:7569-79.
93. Tarpey I, Stacey S, Hickling J et al. Human cytotoxic T lymphocytes stimulated by endogenously processed human papillomavirus type 11 E7 recognize a peptide containing a HLA-A2 (A*0201) motif. Immunology 1994; 81:222-7.
94. Steven NM, Leese AM, Annels NE et al. Epitope focusing in the primary cytotoxic T cell response to Epstein-Barr virus and its relationship to T cell memory. J Exp Med 1996; 184:1801-13.
95. Kerr BM, Kienzle N, Burrows JM et al. Identification of Type B-specific and cross-reactive cytotoxic T-lymphocyte responses to Epstein-Barr virus. J Virol 1996; 70:8858-64.
96. Plebanski M, Allsopp CE, Aidoo M et al. Induction of peptide-specific primary cytotoxic T lymphocyte responses from human peripheral blood. Eur J Immunol 1995; 25:1783-7.
97. Ressing ME, Sette A, Brandt RM et al. Human CTL epitopes encoded by human papillomavirus type 16 E6 and E7 identified through in vivo and in vitro immunogenicity studies of HLA-A*0201-binding peptides. J Immunol 1995; 154: 5934-43.
98. Altuvia Y, Schueler O, Margalit H. Ranking potential binding peptides to MHC molecules by a computational threading approach. J Mol Biol 1995; 249:244-50.
99. Barouch D, Friede T, Stevanović S et al. HLA-A2 subtypes are functionally distinct in peptide binding and presentation. J Exp Med 1995; 182:1847-56.
100. Fleischhauer K, Tanzarella S, Wallny H et al. Multiple HLA-A alleles can present

an immunodominant peptide of the human melanoma antigen Melan-A/MART-1 to a peptide-specific HLA-A*0201+ cytotoxic T cell line. Journal of Immunology 1996; 157:787-97.
101. Burrows SR, Gardner J, Khanna R et al. Five new cytotoxic T cell epitopes identified within Epstein-Barr virus nuclear antigen 3. J Gen Virol 1994; 75:2489-93.
102. Sudo T, Kamikawaji N, Kimura A et al. Differences in MHC class I self peptide repertoires among HLA-A2 subtypes. J Immunol 1995; 155:4749-56.
103. Rötzschke O, Falk K, Stevanović S et al. Peptide motifs of closely related HLA class I molecules encompass substantial differences. Eur J Immunol 1992; 22: 2453-6.
104. DiBrino M, Parker KC, Shiloach J et al. Endogenous peptides bound to HLA-A3 possess a specific combination of anchor residues that permit identification of potential antigenic peptides. Proc Natl Acad Sci U S A 1993; 90:1508-12.
105. Maier R, Falk K, Rötzschke O et al. Peptide motifs of HLA-A3, -A24, and -B7 molecules as determined by pool sequencing. Immunogenetics 1994; 40: 306-8.
106. Poindexter NJ, Naziruddin B, McCourt DW et al. Isolation of a kidney-specific peptide recognized by alloreactive HLA-A3-restricted human CTL. J Immunol 1995; 154:3880-7.
107. Skipper JCA, Kittlesen DJ, Hendrickson RC et al. Shared epitopes for HLA-A3-restricted melanoma-reactive human CTL include a naturally processed epitope from Pmel-17/gp100. J Immunol 1996; 157:5027-33.
108. Takahashi K, Dai LC, Fuerst TR et al. Specific lysis of human immunodeficiency virus type 1-infected cells by a HLA-A3.1-restricted $CD8^+$ cytotoxic T-lymphocyte clone that recognizes a conserved peptide sequence within the gp41 subunit of the envelope protein. Proc Natl Acad Sci U S A 1991; 88:10277-81.
109. Koenig S, Fuerst TR, Wood LV et al. Mapping the fine specificity of a cytolytic T cell response to HIV-1 nef protein. J Immunol 1990; 145:127-35.
110. Venet A, Walker BD. Cytotoxic T-cell epitopes in HIV/SIV infection. AIDS 1993; 7 Suppl 1:S117-26.
111. Hill AB, Lee SP, Haurum JS et al. Class I major histocompatibility complex-restricted cytotoxic T lymphocytes specific for Epstein-Barr virus (EBV)-transformed B lymphoblastoid cell lines against which they were raised. J Exp Med 1995; 181:2221-8.
112. Safrit JT, Andrews CA, Zhu T et al. Characterization of human immunodeficiency virus type 1-specific cytotoxic T lymphocyte clones isolated during acute seroconversion: recognition of autologous virus sequences within a conserved immunodominant epitope. J Exp Med 1994; 179:463-72.
113. Johnson RP, Hammond SA, Trocha A et al. Induction of a major histocompatibility complex class I-restricted cytotoxic T-lymphocyte response to a highly conserved region of human immunodeficiency virus type 1 (HIV-1) gp120 in seronegative humans immunized with a candidate HIV-1 vaccine. J Virol 1994; 68:3145-53.
114. Koziel MJ, Dudley D, Afdhal N et al. HLA class I-restricted cytotoxic T lymphocytes specific for hepatitis C virus. Identification of multiple epitopes and characterization of patterns of cytokine release. J Clin Invest 1995; 96:2311-21.
115. Zhang QJ, Gavioli R, Klein G et al. An HLA-A11-specific motif in nonamer peptides derived from viral and cellular proteins. Proc Natl Acad Sci U S A 1993; 90:2217-21.
116. Tsai SL, Chen MH, Yeh CT et al. Purification and characterization of a naturally processed hepatitis B virus peptide recognized by CD8+ cytotoxic T lymphocytes. J Clin Invest 1996; 97:577-84.
117. Gavioli R, Kurilla MG, de Campos Lima PO et al. Multiple HLA A11-restricted cytotoxic T-lymphocyte epitopes of different immunogenicities in the Epstein-Barr virus-encoded nuclear antigen 4. J Virol 1993; 67:1572-8.
118. Couillin I, Connan F, Culmann Penciolelli B et al. HLA-dependent variations in human immunodeficiency virus Nef protein alter peptide/HLA binding. Eur J Immunol 1995; 25:728-32.
119. Domenech N, Henderson RA, Finn OJ.

Identification of an HLA-A11-restricted epitope from the tandem repeat domain of the epithelial tumor antigen mucin. J Immunol 1995; 155:4766-74.
120. Culmann B, Gomard E, Kieny MP et al. Six epitopes reacting with human cytotoxic CD8+ T cells in the central region of the HIV-1 NEF protein. J Immunol 1991; 146:1560-5.
121. Merkel F, Kalluri R, Marx M et al. Autoreactive T-cells in Goodpasture's syndrome recognize the N-terminal NC1 domain on alpha 3 type IV collagen. Kidney Int 1996; 49:1127-33.
122. Sipsas NV, Kalams SA, Trocha A et al. Identification of type-specific cytotoxic T lymphocyte responses to homologous viral proteins in laboratory workers accidentally infected with HIV-1. J Clin Invest 1997; 99:752-62.
123. Robbins PF, el Gamil M, Li YF et al. A mutated beta-catenin gene encodes a melanoma-specific antigen recognized by tumor infiltrating lymphocytes. J Exp Med 1996; 183:1185-92.
124. Dai LC, West K, Littaua R et al. Mutation of human immunodeficiency virus type 1 at amino acid 585 on gp41 results in loss of killing by CD8+ A24-restricted cytotoxic T lymphocytes. J Virol 1992; 66:3151-4.
125. Robbins PF, el Gamil M, Li YF et al. Cloning of a new gene encoding an antigen recognized by melanoma-specific HLA-A24-restricted tumor-infiltrating lymphocytes. J Immunol 1995; 154:5944-50.
126. Kang X, Kawakami Y, el Gamil M et al. Identification of a tyrosinase epitope recognized by HLA-A24-restricted, tumor-infiltrating lymphocytes. J Immunol 1995; 155:1343-8.
127. van Baalen CA, Klein MR, Huisman RC et al. Fine-specificity of cytotoxic T lymphocytes which recognized conserved epitopes of the GAG protein of human immunodeficiency virus type 1. J Gen Virol 1996; 77:1659-65.
128. Boisgerault F, Khalil I, Tieng V et al. Definition of the HLA-A29 peptide ligand motif allows predicition of potential T-cell epitopes from the retinal soluble antigen, a candidate autoantigen in birdshot retinopathy. Proc Natl Acad Sci U S A 1996; 93:3466-70.
129. Missale G, Redeker A, Person J et al. HLA-A31- and HLA-Aw68-restricted cytotoxic T cell responses to a single hepatitis B virus nucleocapsid epitope during acute viral hepatitis. J Exp Med 1993; 177:751-62.
130. Wang RF, Parkhurst MR, Kawakami Y et al. Utilization of an alternative open reading frame of a normal gene in generating a novel human cancer antigen. J Exp Med 1996; 183:1131-40.
131. Wang R, Appella E, Kawakami Y et al. Identification of TRP-2 as a human tumor antigen recognized by cytotoxic T lymphocytes. J Exp Med 1996; 184:2207-16.
132. Buseyne F, McChesney M, Porrot F et al. Gag-specific cytotoxic T lymphocytes from human immunodeficiency virus type 1-infected individuals: Gag epitopes are clustered in three regions of the p24gag protein. J Virol 1993; 67:694-702.
133. Buseyne F, Riviere Y. HIV-specific CD8+ T-cell immune responses and viral replication. AIDS 1993; 7 Suppl 2:S81-5.
134. Guo HC, Jardetzky TS, Garrett TP et al. Different length peptides bind to HLA-Aw68 similarly at their ends but bulge out in the middle. Nature 1992; 360:364-6.
135. Silver ML, Guo HC, Strominger JL et al. Atomic structure of a human MHC molecule presenting an influenza virus peptide. Nature 1992; 360:367-9.
136. Huczko EL, Bodnar WM, Benjamin D et al. Characteristics of endogenous peptides eluted from the class I MHC molecule HLA-B7 determined by mass spectrometry and computer modeling. J Immunol 1993; 151:2572-87.
137. Wang W, Meadows LR, den Haan JM et al. Human H-Y: a male-specific histocompatibility antigen derived from the SMCY protein. Science 1995; 269:1588-90.
138. Hill A, Worth A, Elliott T et al. Characterization of two Epstein-Barr virus epitopes restricted by HLA-B7. Eur J Immunol 1995; 25:18-24.
139. Gaugler B, Brouwenstijn N, Vantomme V et al. A new gene coding for an anti-

gen recognized by autologous cytolytic T lymphocytes on a human renal carcinoma. Immunogenetics 1996; 44:323-30.
140. Gnjatić S, Bressac de Paillerets B, Guillet JG et al. Mapping and ranking of potential cytotoxic T epitopes in the p53 protein: effect of mutations and polymorphism on peptide binding to purified and refolded HLA molecules. Eur J Immunol 1995; 25:1638-42.
141. Ellis JR, Keating PJ, Baird J et al. The association of an HPV16 oncogene variant with HLA-B7 has implications for vaccine design in cervical cancer binding of a peptide antigen to multiple HLA alleles allows definition of an A2-like supertype. Nat Med 1995; 1:464-70.
142. Smith KD, Epperson DF, Lutz CT. Alloreactive cytotoxic T-lymphocyte-defined HLA-B7 subtypes differ in peptide antigen presentation. Immunogenetics 1995; 43:27-37.
143. Barber LD, Gillece-Castro B, Percival L et al. Overlap in the repertoires of peptides bound in vivo by a group of related class I HLA-B allotypes. Curr Biol 1995; 5:179-90.
144. Malcherek G, Falk K, Rötzschke O et al. Natural peptide ligand motifs of two HLA molecules associated with myasthenia gravis. Int Immunol 1993; 5:1229-37.
145. Sutton J, Rowland Jones S, Rosenberg W et al. A sequence pattern for peptides presented to cytotoxic T lymphocytes by HLA B8 revealed by analysis of epitopes and eluted peptides. Eur J Immunol 1993; 23:447-53.
146. DiBrino M, Parker KC, Margulies DH et al. The HLA-B14 peptide binding site can accommodate peptides with different combinations of anchor residues. J Biol Chem 1994; 269:32426-34.
147. Burrows SR, Sculley TB, Misko IS et al. An Epstein-Barr virus-specific cytotoxic T cell epitope in EBV nuclear antigen 3 (EBNA 3). J Exp Med 1990; 171:345-9.
148. Phillips RE, Rowland Jones S, Nixon DF et al. Human immunodeficiency virus genetic variation that can escape cytotoxic T cell recognition. Nature 1991; 354:453-9.
149. Achour A, Picard O, Zagury D et al. HGP-30, a synthetic analogue of human immunodeficiency virus (HIV) p17, is a target for cytotoxic lymphocytes in HIV-infected individuals. Proc Natl Acad Sci U S A 1990; 87:7045-9.
150. Johnson RP, Trocha A, Buchanan TM et al. Identification of overlapping HLA class I-restricted cytotoxic T cell epitopes in a conserved region of the human immunodeficiency virus type 1 envelope glycoprotein: definition of minimum epitopes and analysis of the effects of sequence variation. J Exp Med 1992; 175:961-71.
151. Wizel B, Houghten RA, Parker KC et al. Irradiated sporozoite vaccine induces HLA-B8-restricted cytotoxic T lymphocyte responses against two overlapping epitopes of the Plasmodium falciparum sporozoite surface protein 2. J Exp Med 1995; 182:1435-45.
152. Phillips RE, Rowland-Jones S, Nixon DF et al. Human immunodeficiency virus genetic variation that can escape cytotoxic T cell recognition. Nature (London) 1991; 354:453-559.
153. Falk K, Rötzschke O, Takiguchi M et al. Peptide motifs of HLA-B58, B60, B61, and B62 molecules. Immunogenetics 1995; 41:165-8.
154. Barber LD, Percival L, Valiante NM et al. The inter-locus recombinant HLA-B*4601 has high selectivity in peptide binding and functions characteristic of HLA-C. J Exp Med 1996; 184:735-40.
155. Kowalski H, Erickson AL, Cooper S et al. Patr-A and B, the orthologues of HLA-A and B, present hepatitis C virus epitopes to $CD8^+$ cytotoxic T cells from two chronically infected chimpanzees. J Exp Med 1996; 183:1761-75.
156. Carmichael A, Jin Y, Sissons P. Analysis of the human *env*-specific cytotoxic T-lymphocyte (CTL) response in natural human immunodeficiency virus Type 1 infection: Low prevalence of broadly cross-reactive *env*-specific CTL. J Virol 1996; 70:8468-76.
157. Gavin MA, Gilbert MJ, Riddell SR et al. Alkali hydrolysis of recombinant proteins allows for the rapid identification of class I MHC-restricted CTL epitopes. J Immunol 1993; 151:3971-80.
158. Rötzschke O, Falk K, Stevanović S et al.

Dominant aromatic/aliphatic C-terminal anchor in HLA-B*2702 and B*2705 peptide motifs. Immunogenetics 1994; 39: 74-7.
159. Verjans GM, Janssen R, UytdeHaag FG et al. Intracellular processing and presentation of T cell epitopes, expressed by recombinant Escherichia coli and Salmonella typhimurium, to human T cells. Eur J Immunol 1995; 25:405-10.
160. Huang F, Hermann E, Wang J et al. A patient-derived cytotoxic T-lymphocyte clone and two peptide-dependent monoclonal antibodies recognize HLA-B27-peptide complexes with low stringency for peptide sequences. Infect Immun 1996; 64:120-7.
161. Nietfield W, Bauer M, Fevrier M et al. Sequence constraints and recognition by CTL of an HLA-B27-restricted HIV-1 gag epitope. J Immunol 1995; 154: 2189-97.
162. Tussey LG, Rowland Jones S, Zheng TS et al. Different MHC class I alleles compete for presentation of overlapping viral epitopes. Immunity 1995; 3:65-77.
163. Shepherd JC, Schumacher TN, Ashton Rickardt PG et al. TAP1-dependent peptide translocation in vitro is ATP dependent and peptide selective [published erratum appears in Cell 1993; 75:613]. Cell 1993; 74:577-84.
164. Fiorillo MT, Meadows L, D'Amato M et al. Susceptibility to ankylosing spondylitis correlates with the C-terminal residue of peptides presented by various HLA-B27 subtypes. Eur J Immunol 1997; 27: 368-73.
165. Frumento G, Harris PE, Gawinowicz MA et al. Sequence of a prominent 16-residue self-peptide bound to HLA-B27 in a lymphoblastoid cell line. Cell Immunol 1993; 152:623-6.
166. Huet S, Nixon DF, Rothbard JB et al. Structural homologies between two HLA B27-restricted peptides suggest residues important for interaction with HLA B27. Int Immunol 1990; 2:311-6.
167. van Binnendijk RS, Versteeg van Oosten JP, Poelen MC et al. Human HLA class I- and HLA class II-restricted cloned cytotoxic T lymphocytes identify a cluster of epitopes on the measles virus fusion protein. J Virol 1993; 67:2276-84.
168. Brooks JM, Murray RJ, Thomas WA et al. Different HLA-B27 subtypes present the same immunodominant Epstein-Barr virus peptide. J Exp Med 1993; 178: 879-87.
169. Cerrone MC, Ma JJ, Stephens RS. Cloning and sequence of the gene for heat shock protein 60 from Chlamydia trachomatis and immunological reactivity of the protein. Infect Immun 1991; 59: 79-90.
170. Hill AV, Elvin J, Willis AC et al. Molecular analysis of the association of HLA-B53 and resistance to severe malaria. Nature 1992; 360: 434-9.
171. Falk K, Rötzschke O, Grahovać B et al. Peptide motifs of HLA-B35 and -B37 molecules [published erratum appears in Immunogenetics 1994; 39:379]. Immunogenetics 1993; 38:161-2.
172. Koziel MJ, Dudley D, Wong JT et al. Intrahepatic cytotoxic T lymphocytes specific for hepatitis C virus in persons with chronic hepatitis [published erratum appears in J Immunol 1993; 150:2563]. J Immunol 1992; 149: 3339-44.
173. Lee SP, Morgan S, Skinner J et al. Epstein-Barr virus isolates with the major HLA B35.01-restricted cytotoxic T lymphocyte epitope are prevalent in a highly B35.01-positive African population. Eur J Immunol 1995; 25:102-10.
174. Livingston PG, Kurane I, Dai LC et al. Dengue virus-specific, HLA-B35-restricted, human CD8+ cytotoxic T lymphocyte (CTL) clones. Recognition of NS3 amino acids 500 to 508 by CTL clones of two different serotype specificities. J Immunol 1995; 154:1287-95.
175. Zivny J, Kurane I, Leporati AM et al. A single nine-amino acid peptide induces virus-specific, CD8+ human cytotoxic T lymphocyte clones of heterogeneous serotype specificities. J Exp Med 1995; 182:853-63.
176. Shiga H, Shioda T, Tomiyama H et al. Identification of multiple HIV-1 cytotoxic T-cell epitopes presented by human leukocyte antigen B35 molecules. AIDS 1996; 10:1075-83.
177. Schönbach C, Ibe M, Shiga H et al. Fine tuning of peptide binding to HLAB*3501

molecules by nonanchor residues. J Immunol 1995; 154:5951-8.
178. Ferris RL, Buck C, Hammond SA et al. Class I-restricted presentation of an HIV-1 gp41 epitope containing an N-linked glycosylation site. Implications for the mechanism of processing of viral envelope proteins. J Immunol 1996; 156: 834-40.
179. Steinle A, Falk K, Rötzschke O et al. Motif of HLA-B*3503 peptide ligands. Immunogenetics 1996; 43:105-7.
180. Townsend AR, Rothbard J, Gotch FM et al. The epitopes of influenza nucleoprotein recognized by cytotoxic T lymphocytes can be defined with short synthetic peptides. Cell 1986; 44:959-68.
181. Falk K, Rötzschke O, Takiguchi M et al. Peptide motifs of HLA-B38 and B39 molecules. Immunogenetics 1995; 41: 162-4.
182. Kaneko T, Nakamura I, Kita H et al. Three new cytotoxic T cell epitopes identified within the hepatitis C virus nucleoprotein. J Gen Virol 1996; 77:1305-9.
183. DiBrino M, Parker KC, Margulies DH et al. Identification of the peptide binding motif for HLA-B44, one of the most common HLA-B alleles in the Caucasian population. Biochemistry 1995; 34: 10130-8.
184. Moss DJ, Burrows SR, Khanna R et al. Immune surveillance against Epstein-Barr virus. Semin Immunol 1992; 4:97-104.
185. Fleischhauer K, Avila D, Vilbois F et al. Characterization of natural peptide ligands for HLA-B*4402 and -B*4403: implications for peptide involvement in allorecognition of a single amino acid change in the HLA-B44 heavy chain. Tissue Antigens 1994; 44:311-7.
186. Brichard VG, Herman J, Van Pel A et al. A tyrosinase nonapeptide presented by HLA-B44 is recognized on a human melanoma by autologous cytolytic T lymphocytes. Eur J Immunol 1996; 26:224-30.
187. Herman J, van der Bruggen P, Luescher IF et al. A peptide encoded by the human MAGE3 gene and presented by HLA-B44 induces cytolytic T lymphocytes that recognize tumor cells expressing MAGE3. Immunogenetics 1996; 43:377-83.
188. Coulie PG, Lehmann F, Lethe B et al. A mutated intron sequence codes for an antigenic peptide recognized by cytolytic T lymphocytes on a human melanoma. Proc Natl Acad Sci U S A 1995; 92: 7976-80.
189. Khanna R, Burrows SR, Kurilla MG et al. Localization of Epstein-Barr virus cytotoxic T cell epitopes using recombinant vaccinia: implications for vaccine development. J Exp Med 1992; 176:169-76.
190. Falk K, Rötzschke O, Takiguchi M et al. Peptide motifs of HLA-B51, -B52 and -B78 molecules, and implications for Behcet's disease. Int Immunol 1995; 7:223-8.
191. Gotch F, McAdam SN, Allsopp CE et al. Cytotoxic T cells in HIV2 seropositive Gambians. Identification of a virus-specific MHC-restricted peptide epitope. J Immunol 1993; 151:3361-9.
192. Barber LD, Percival L, Parham P. Characterization of the peptide-binding specificity of HLA-B*7301. Tissue Antigens 1996; 47:472-7.
193. Falk K, Rötzschke O, Grahovać B et al. Allele-specific peptide ligand motifs of HLA-C molecules. Proc Natl Acad Sci U S A 1993; 90:12005-9.
194. Littaua RA, Oldstone MB, Takeda A et al. An HLA-C-restricted CD8+ cytotoxic T-lymphocyte clone recognizes a highly conserved epitope on human immunodeficiency virus type 1 gag. J Virol 1991; 65:4051-6.
195. Tzeng C, Adams EJ, Gumperz JE et al. Peptides bound endogenously by HLA-Cw*0304 expressed in LCL 721.221 cells include a peptide derived from HLA-E. Tissue Antigens 1996; 48:325-8.
196. Johnson RP, Trocha A, Buchanan TM et al. Recognition of a highly conserved region of human immunodeficiency virus type 1 gp120 by an HLA-Cw4-restricted cytotoxic T-lymphocyte clone. J Virol 1993; 67:438-45.
197. van den Eynde B, Peeters O, De Backer O et al. A new family of genes coding for an antigen recognized by autologous cytolytic T lymphocytes on a human melanoma. J Exp Med 1995; 182:689-98.

198. Boel P, Wildmann C, Sensi ML et al. BAGE: a new gene encoding an antigen recognized on human melanomas by cytolytic T lymphocytes. Immunity 1995; 2:167-75.
199. Diehl M, Münz C, Keilholz W et al. Nonclassical HLA-G molecules are classical peptide presenters. Current Biology 1996; 6:305-14.
200. Lee N, Malacko AR, Ishitani A et al. The membrane-bound and soluble forms of HLA-G bind identical sets of endogenous peptides but differ with respect to TAP association. Immunity 1995; 3:591-600.
201. Rötzschke O, Falk K, Deres K et al. Isolation and analysis of naturally processed viral peptides as recognized by cytotoxic T cells. Nature 1990; 348:252-4.
202. Falk K, Rötzschke O, Deres K et al. Identification of naturally processed viral nonapeptides allows their quantification in infected cells and suggests an allele-specific T cell epitope forecast. J Exp Med 1991; 174:425-34.
203. Harpur AG, Zimiecki A, Wilks AF et al. A prominent natural H-2 Kd ligand is derived from protein tyrosine kinase JAK1. Immunol Lett 1993; 35:235-7.
204. Sibille C, Chomez P, Wildmann C et al. Structure of the gene of tum- transplantation antigen P198: a point mutation generates a new antigenic peptide. J Exp Med 1990; 172:35-45.
205. Wallny HJ, Deres K, Faath S et al. Identification and quantification of a naturally presented peptide as recognized by cytotoxic T lymphocytes specific for an immunogenic tumor variant. Int Immunol 1992; 4:1085-90.
206. Pamer EG, Harty JT, Bevan MJ. Precise prediction of a dominant class I MHC-restricted epitope of Listeria monocytogenes. Nature 1991; 353:852-5.
207. Pamer EG. Direct sequence identification and kinetic analysis of an MHC class I-restricted Listeria monocytogenes CTL epitope. J Immunol 1994; 152:686-94.
208. Reich EP, von Grafenstein H, Barlow A et al. Self peptides isolated from MHC glycoproteins of nonobese diabetic mice. J Immunol 1994; 152:2279-88.
209. Sijts AJ, Neisig A, Neefjes J et al. Two Listeria monocytogenes CTL epitopes are processed from the same antigen with different efficiencies. J Immunol 1996; 156:683-92.
210. Braciale TJ, Braciale VL, Winkler M et al. On the role of the transmembrane anchor sequence of influenza hemagglutinin in target cell recognition by class I MHC-restricted, hemagglutinin-specific cytolytic T lymphocytes. J Exp Med 1987; 166:678-92.
211. Cao W, Myers Powell BA, Braciale TJ. Recognition of an immunoglobulin VH epitope by influenza virus-specific class I major histocompatibility complex-restricted cytolytic T lymphocytes. J Exp Med 1994; 179:195-202.
212. Kuwano K, Braciale TJ, Ennis FA. Localization of a cross-reactive CTL epitope to the transmembrane region on the hemaglutinin of influenza H1 and H2 viruses. FASEB J 1988; 2:2221.
213. Maryanski JL, Pala P, Corradin G et al. H-2-restricted cytolytic T cells specific for HLA can recognize a synthetic HLA peptide. Nature 1986; 324:578-9.
214. Romero P, Maryanski JL, Corradin G et al. Cloned cytotoxic T cells recognize an epitope in the circumsporozoite protein and protect against malaria. Nature 1989; 341:323-6.
215. Weiss WR, Mellouk S, Houghten RA et al. Cytotoxic T cells recognize a peptide from the circumsporozoite protein on malaria-infected hepatocytes. J Exp Med 1990; 171:763-73.
216. Kulkarni AB, Morse HC III, Bennink JR et al. Immunization of mice with vaccinia virus-M2 recombinant induces epitope-specific and cross-reactive K^d-restricted $CD8^+$ cytotoxic T cells. J Virol 1993; 67:4086-92.
217. Banks TA, Nair S, Rouse BT. Recognition by and in vitro induction of cytotoxic T lymphocytes against predicted epitopes of the immediate-early protein ICP27 of herpes simplex virus. J Virol 1993; 67:613-6.
218. Kutubuddin M, Simons J, Chow M. Poliovirus-specific major histocompatibility complex class I-restricted cytolytic T-cell epitopes in mice localize to neutralizing antigenic regions. J Virol 1992; 66: 5967-74.

219. Blum-Tirouvanziam U, Beghdadi-Rais C, Roggero MA et al. Elicitation of specific cytotoxic T cells by immunization with malaria soluble synthetic polypeptides. J Immunol 1994; 153:4134-41.
220. Townsend A, Ohlen C, Rogers M et al. Source of unique tumour antigens. Nature 1994; 371:662.
221. Renggli J, Valmori D, Romero JF et al. $CD8^+$ T-cell protective immunity induced by immunization with Plasmodium berghei CS protein-derived synthetic peptides: evidence that localization of peptide-specific CTLs is crucial for protection against malaria. Immunol Lett 1995; 46:199-205.
222. Cao W, Tykodi SS, Esser MT et al. Partial activation of $CD8^+$ T cells by a self-derived peptide. Nature 1995; 378:295-8.
223. Wei WZ, Gill RF, Jones RF et al. Induction of cytotoxic T lymphocytes to murine mammary tumor cells with a Kd-restricted immunogenic peptide. Int J Cancer 1996; 66:659-63.
224. Ciernik F, Berzofsky JA, Carbone DP. Induction of cytotoxic T lymphocytes and antitumor immunity with DNA vaccines expressing single T cell epitopes. J Immunol 1996; 156:2369-75.
225. Abrams SI, Stanziale SF, Lunin SD et al. Identification of overlapping epitopes in mutant ras oncogene peptides that activate $CD4^+$ and $CD8^+$ T cell responses. Eur J Immunol 1996; 26:435-43.
226. Doe B, Selby M, Barnett S et al. Induction of cytotoxic T lymphocytes by intramuscular immunization with plasmid DNA is facilitated by bone marrow-derived cells. Proc Natl Acad Sci U S A 1996; 93:8578-83.
227. Yamazaki H, Tanaka M, Nagoya M et al. Epitope selection in major histocompatibility complex class I-mediated pathway is affected by the intracellular localization of an antigen. Eur J Immunol 1997; 27:347-53.
228. Bertholet S, Iggo R, Corradin G. Cytotoxic T lymphocyte responses to wild-type and mutant mouse p53 peptides. Eur J Immunol 1997; 27:798-801.
229. Corr M, Boyd LF, Padlan EA et al. H-2Dd exploits a four residue peptide binding motif. J Exp Med 1993; 178:1877-92.
230. Szikora JP, Van Pel A, Boon T. Tum-mutation P35B generates the MHC-binding site of a new antigenic peptide. Immunogenetics 1993; 37:135-8.
231. Takahashi H, Cohen J, Hosmalin A et al. An immunodominant epitope of the human immunodeficiency virus envelope glycoprotein gp160 recognized by class I major histocompatibility complex molecule-restricted murine cytotoxic T lymphocytes. Proc Natl Acad Sci U S A 1988; 85:3105-9.
232. Bergmann C, Stohlmann SA, McMillan M. An endogenously synthesized decamer peptide efficiently primes cytotoxic T cells specific for the HIV-1 envelope glycoprotein. Eur J Immunol 1993; 23:2777-81.
233. Rehermann B, Chang K, McHutchison JG et al. Quantitative analysis of the peripheral blood cytotoxic T lymphocyte response in patients with chronic hepatitis C virus infection. J Clin Invest 1996; 98:1432-40.
234. Shirai M, Chen M, Arichi T et al. Use of intrinsic and extrinsic helper epitopes for in vivo induction of anti-hepatitis C virus cytotoxic T lymphocytes (CTL) with CTL epitope peptide vaccines. J Infect Dis 1996; 173:24-31.
235. Corr M, Boyd LF, Frankel SR et al. Endogenous peptides of a soluble major histocompatibility complex class I molecule, $H\text{-}2L^{ds}$: sequence motif, quantitative binding, and molecular modeling of the complex. J Exp Med 1992; 176: 1681-92.
236. Reddehase MJ, Rothbard JB, Koszinowski UH. A pentapeptide as minimal antigenic determinant for MHC class I-restricted T lymphocytes. Nature 1989; 337:651-3.
237. Udaka K, Tsomides TJ, Eisen HN. A naturally occurring peptide recognized by alloreactive CD8+ cytotoxic T lymphocytes in association with a class I MHC protein. Cell 1992; 69:989-98.
238. Udaka K, Tsomides TJ, Walden P et al. A ubiquitous protein is the source of naturally occurring peptides that are recognized by a $CD8^+$ T-cell clone. Proc Natl Acad Sci U S A 1993; 90:11272-6.
239. McCormick D, Stauss HJ, Thorpe C et al. Major histocompatibility complex and

T cell receptor interaction of the P91 tum- peptide. Eur J Immunol 1996; 26:2895-902.
240. Whitton JL, Tishon A, Lewicki H et al. Molecular analyses of a five-amino-acid cytotoxic T-lymphocyte (CTL) epitope: an immunodominant region which induces nonreciprocal CTL cross-reactivity. J Virol 1989; 63:4303-10.
241. Schulz M, Aichele P, Schneider R et al. Major histocompatibility complex binding and T cell recognition of a viral nonapeptide containing a minimal tetrapeptide. Eur J Immunol 1991; 21:1181-5.
242. Lurquin C, Van Pel A, Mariame B et al. Structure of the gene of tum- transplantation antigen P91A: the mutated exon encodes a peptide recognized with Ld by cytolytic T cells. Cell 1989; 58:293-303.
243. Lethé B, van den Eynde B, Van Pel A et al. Mouse tumor rejection antigens P815A and P815B: two epitopes carried by a single peptide. Eur J Immunol 1992; 22:2283-8.
244. Bergmann C, McMillan M, Stohlman S. Characterization of the Ld-restricted cytotoxic T-lymphocyte epitope in the mouse hepatitis virus nucleocapsid protein. J Virol 1993; 67:7041-9.
245. Beauverger P, Buckland R, Wild TF. Measles virus antigens induce both type-specific and canine distemper virus cross-reactive cytotoxic T lymphocytes in mice: localization of a common L^d-restricted nucleoprotein epitope. J Gen Virol 1993; 74:2357-63.
246. Beauverger P, Buckland R, Wild F. Measles virus hemagglutinin induces an L^d-restricted $CD8^+$ cytotoxic T lymphocyte response to two specific epitopes. Virology 1994; 200:281-3.
247. Wu MX, Tsomides TJ, Eisen HN. Tissue distribution of natural peptides derived from a ubiquitous dehydrogenase, including a novel liver-specific peptide that demonstrates the pronounced specificity of low affinity T cell reactions. J Immun 1995; 154:4495-502.
248. van den Eynde B, Mazarguil H, Lethé B et al. Localization of two cytotoxic T lymphocyte epitopes and three anchoring residues on a single nonameric peptide that binds to $H\text{-}2L^d$ and is recognized by cytotoxic T lymphocytes against mouse tumor P815. Eur J Immunol 1994; 24:2740-5.
249. Schirmbeck R, Melber K, Kuhrober A et al. Immunization with soluble hepatitis B virus surface protein elicits murine H-2 class I-restricted $CD8^+$ cytotoxic T lymphocyte responses in vivo. J Immunol 1994; 152:1110-9.
250. Bergmann CC, Stohlman SA. Specificity of the H-2 L(d)-restricted cytotoxic T-lymphocyte response to the mouse hepatitis virus nucleocapsid protein. J Virol 1996; 70:3252-7.
251. Bergmann CC, Tong L, Cua RV et al. Cytotoxic T cell repertoire selection—A single amino acid determines alternative class I restriction. J Immunol 1994; 152:5603-12.
252. Huang AYC, Gulden PH, Woods AS et al. The immunodominant major histocompatibility complex class I-restricted antigen of a murine colon tumor derives from an endogenous retroviral gene product. Proc Natl Acad Sci U S A 1996; 93:9730-5.
253. Sykulev Y, Joo M, Vturina I et al. Evidence that a single peptide-MHC complex on a target cell can elicit a cytolytic T cell response. Immunity 1996; 4:565-71.
254. van Bleek GM, Nathenson SG. Isolation of an endogenously processed immunodominant viral peptide from the class I H-2Kb molecule. Nature 1990; 348: 213-6.
255. Rötzschke O, Falk K, Stevanović S et al. Exact prediction of a natural T cell epitope. Eur J Immunol 1991; 21:2891-4.
256. Carbone FR, Moore MW, Sheil JM et al. Induction of cytotoxic T lymphocytes by primary in vitro stimulation with peptides. J Exp Med 1988; 167:1767-79.
257. Wallny HJ. Untersuchungen zur Rolle der MHC-Klasse-I-Moleküle bei der Prozessierung von Nebenhistokompatibilitätsantigenen 1992; Universität Tübingen.
258. Brossart P, Bevan MJ. Selective activation of Fas/Fas ligand-mediated cytotoxicity by a self peptide. J Exp Med 1996; 183:2449-58.
259. Tallquist MD, Yun TJ, Pease LR. A single T cell receptor recognizes structurally

distinct MHC/peptide complexes with high specificity. J Exp Med 1996; 184: 1017-26.
260. Malarkannan S, Gonzalez F, Nguyen V et al. Alloreactive CD8+ T cell can recognize unusual, rare, and unique processed peptide/MHC complexes. J Immunol 1996; 157:4464-73.
261. Malarkannan S, Serwold T, Nguyen V et al. The mouse mammary tumor virus *env* gene is the source of a CD8+ T-cell-stimulating peptide presented by a major histocompatibility complex class I molecule in a murine thymoma. Proc Natl Acad Sci USA 1996; 93:13991-6.
262. Franco MA, Prieto I, Labbe M et al. An immunodominant cytotoxic T cell epitope on the VP7 rotavirus protein overlaps the H2 signal peptide. J Gen Virol 1993; 74:2579-86.
263. Bonneau RH, Salvucci LA, Johnson DC et al. Epitope specificity of H-2Kb-restricted, HSV-1-, and HSV-2-cross-reactive cytotoxic T lymphocyte clones. Virology 1993; 195:62-70.
264. Kast WM, Roux L, Curren J et al. Protection against lethal Sendai virus infection by in vivo priming of virus-specific cytotoxic T lymphocytes with a free synthetic peptide. Proc Natl Acad Sci U S A 1991; 88:2283-7.
265. Schumacher TN, De Bruijn ML, Vernie LN et al. Peptide selection by MHC class I molecules. Nature 1991; 350:703-6.
266. Sijts AJ, Ossendorp F, Mengede EA et al. Immunodominant mink cell focus-inducing murine leukemia virus (MuLV)-encoded CTL epitope, identified by its MHC class I-binding motif, explains MuLV-type specificity of MCF-directed cytotoxic T lymphocytes. J Immunol 1994; 152:106-16.
267. White HD, Roeder DA, Green WR. An immunodominant Kb-restricted peptide from the p15E transmembrane protein of endogenous ecotropic murine leukemia virus (MuLV) AKR623 that restores susceptibility of a tumor line to anti-AKR/gross MuLV cytotoxic T lymphocytes [published erratum appears in J Virol 1994; 68:3452]. J Virol 1994; 68:897-904.
268. Franco MA, Lefévre P, Willems P et al. Identification of cytotoxic T cell epitopes on the VP3 and VP6 rotavirus proteins. J Gen Virol 1994; 75:589-96.
269. Mandelboim O, Berke G, Fridkin M et al. CTL induction by a tumour-associated antigen octapeptide derived from a murine lung carcinoma. Nature 1994; 369:67-71.
270. Mylin LM, Deckhut AM, Bonneau RH et al. Cytotoxic T lymphocyte escape variants, induced mutations, and synthetic peptides define a dominant H-2K^b-restricted deteriminant in Simian Virus 40 tumor antigen. Virology 1995; 208:159-72.
271. Sheil JM, Shepherd SE, Klimo GF et al. Identification of an autologous insulin B chain peptide as a target antigen for H-2Kb-restricted cytotoxic T lymphocytes. J Exp Med 1992; 175:545-52.
272. Liu T, Zhou X, Orvell C et al. Heat-inactivated Sendai virus can enter multiple MHC class I processing pathways and generate cytotoxic T lymphocyte responses in vivo. J Immunol 1995; 154: 3147-55.
273. Walden P, Wiesmuller KH, Jung G. Elucidation of T-cell epitopes: a synthetic approach with random peptide libraries. Biochem Soc Trans 1995; 23:678-81.
274. Neisig A, Roelse J, Sijts AJ et al. Major differences in transporter associated with antigen presentation (TAP)-dependent translocation of MHC class I-presentable peptides and the effect of flanking sequences. J Immunol 1995; 154:1273-9.
275. Salvucci LA, Bonneau RH, Tevethia SS. Polymorphism within the herpes simplex virus (HSV) ribonucleotide reductase large subunit (ICP6) confers type specificity for recognition by HSV type 1-specific cytotoxic T lymphocytes. J Virol 1995; 69:1122-31.
276. Udaka K, Wiesmüller K, Kienle S et al. Self-MHC restricted peptides recognized by an alloreactive T lymphocyte clone. Journal of Immunology 1996; 157:670-8.
277. Dahl AM, Beverley PC, Stauss HJ. A synthetic peptide derived from the tumor-associated protein mdm2 can stimulate autoreactive, high avidity cytotoxic T lymphocytes that recognize naturally processed protein. J Immunol 1996; 157:239-46.

278. Blake J, Johnston JV, Hellstrom KE et al. Use of combinatorial peptide libraries to construct functional mimics of tumor epitopes recognized by MHC class I-restricted cytolytic T lymphocytes. J Exp Med 1996; 184:121-30.
279. Gundlach BR, Wiesmüller KH, Junt T et al. Specificity and degeneracy of minor histocompatibility antigen-specific MHC-restricted CTL. J Immunol 1996; 156:3645-51.
280. Kuhöber A, Pudollek HP, Reifenberg K et al. DNA immunization induces antibody and cytotoxic T cell responses to hepatitis B core antigen in H-2b mice. J Immunol 1996; 156:3687-95.
281. Chen W, Ede JN, Jackson DC et al. CTL Recognition of an altered peptide associated with asparagine bond rearrangement—implications for immunity and vaccine design. J Immunol 1996; 157: 1000-5.
282. Sadovnikova E, Stauss HJ. Peptide-specific cytotoxic T lymphocytes restricted by nonself major histocompatibility complex class I molecules: Reagents for tumor immunotherapy. Proc Natl Acad Sci U S A 1996; 93:13114-8.
283. Dubey P, Hendrickson RC, Meredith SC et al. The immunodominant antigen of an ultraviolet-induced regressor tumor is generated by a somatic point mutation in the DEAD box helicase p68. J Exp Med 1997; 185:695-706.
284. Bloom M., Perry-Lalley D, Robbins PF et al. Identification of tyrosinase-related Protein 2 as a tumor rejection antigen for the B16 melanoma. J Exp Med 1997; 185:453-9.
285. Starnbach MN, Bevan MJ. Cells infected with Yersinia present an epitope to class I MHC-restricted CTL. J Immunol 1994; 153:1603-12.
286. Bergmann CC, Yao Q, Lin M et al. The JHM strain of mouse hepatitis virus induces a spike protein-specific Db-restricted cytotoxic T cell response. J Gen Virol 1996; 77:315-25.
287. Perreault C, Jutras J, Roy DC et al. Identification of an immunodominant mouse minor histocompatibility antigen (MiHA). T cell response to a single dominant MiHA causes craft-versus-host disease. J Clin Invest 1996; 98:622-8.
288. Cerundolo V, Elliott T, Elvin J et al. The binding affinity and dissociation rates of peptides for class I major histocompatibility complex molecules. Eur J Immunol 1991; 21:2069-75.
289. Max H, Halder T, Kropshofer H et al. Characterization of peptides bound to extracellular and intracellular HLA-DR1 molecules. Hum Immunol 1993; 38: 193-200.
290. Tevethia SS, Lewis M, Tanaka Y et al. Dissection of H-2D^{b}-restricted cytotoxic T-lymphocyte epitopes on simian virus 40 T antigen by the use of synthetic peptides and H-2D^{bm} mutants. J Virol 1990; 64:1192-200.
291. Kast WM, Offringa R, Peters PJ et al. Eradication of adenovirus E1-induced tumors by E1A-specific cytotoxic T lymphocytes. Cell 1989; 59:603-14.
292. Yanagi Y, Tishon A, Lewicki H et al. Diversity of T-cell receptors in virus-specific cytotoxic T lymphocytes recognizing three distinct viral epitopes restricted by a single major histocompatibility complex molecule. J Virol 1992; 66:2527-31.
293. Oldstone MB, Whitton JL, Lewicki H et al. Fine dissection of a nine amino acid glycoprotein epitope, a major determinant recognized by lymphocytic choriomeningitis virus-specific class I-restricted H-2Db cytotoxic T lymphocytes. J Exp Med 1988; 168:559-70.
294. Oldstone MB, Tishon A, Eddleston M et al. Vaccination to prevent persistent viral infection. J Virol 1993; 67:4372-8.
295. Klavinskis LS, Whitton JL, Joly E et al. Vaccination and protection from a lethal viral infection: identification, incorporation, and use of a cytotoxic T lymphocyte glycoprotein epitope. Virology 1990; 178:393-400.
296. Feltkamp MC, Smits HL, Vierboom MP et al. Vaccination with cytotoxic T lymphocyte epitope-containing peptide protects against a tumor induced by human papillomavirus type 16-transformed cells. Eur J Immunol 1993; 23:2242-9.
297. Alsheikhly AR. Interaction of in vitro- and in vivo-generated cytotoxic T cells with SV40 T antigen: analysis with syn-

thetic peptides. Scand J Immunol 1994; 39:467-79.
298. Zügel U, Schoel B, Yamamoto S et al. Crossrecognition by CD8 T cell receptor alpha beta cytotoxic T lymphocytes of peptides in the self and the mycobacterial hsp60 which share intermediate sequence homology. Eur J Immunol 1995; 25:451-8.
299. Haurum JS, Tan L, Arsequell G et al. Peptide anchor residue glycosylation: effect on class I major histocompatibility complex binding and cytotoxic T lymphocyte recognition. Eur J Immunol 1995; 25:3270-6.
300. Toes RE, Offringa R, Blom RJ et al. An adenovirus type 5 early region 1B-encoded CTL epitope-mediating tumor eradication by CTL clones is down-modulated by an activated ras oncogene. J Immunol 1995; 154:3396-405.
301. Chen W, Qin H, Chesebro B et al. Identification of a *gag*-encoded cytotoxic T-lymphocyte epitope from FBL-3 leukemia shared by Friend, Moloney, and Rauscher murine leukemia virus-induced tumors. J Virol 1996; 70:7773-82.
302. Lacabanne V, Viguier M, Guillet J et al. A wild-type p53 cytotoxic T cell epitope is presented by mouse hepatocarcinoma cells. Eur J Immunol 1996; 26:2635-9.
303. Greenfield A, Scott D, Pennisi D et al. An H-YD^b epitope is encoded by a novel mouse Y chromosome gene. Nature Genetics 1996; 14:474-8.
304. Cossins J, Gould KG, Smith M et al. Precise prediction of a Kk-restricted cytotoxic T cell epitope in the NS1 protein of influenza virus using an MHC allele-specific motif. Virology 1993; 193:289-95.
305. Norda M, Falk K, Rötzschke O et al. Comparison of the H-2Kk- and H-2Kkm1-restricted peptide motifs. J Immunother 1993; 14:144-9.
306. Gould KG, Scotney H, Brownlee GG. Characterization of two distinct major histocompatibility complex class I Kk-restricted T-cell epitopes within the influenza A/PR/8/34 virus hemagglutinin. J Virol 1991; 65:5401-9.
307. Burrows GG, Ariail K, Celnik B et al. Variation in H-2K^k peptide motif revealed by sequencing naturally processed peptides from T-cell hybridoma class I molecules. J of Neurosci Res 1996; 45:803-11.
308. Brown EL, Wooters JL, Ferenz CR et al. Characterization of peptide binding to the murine MHC class I H-2K^k molecule. Sequencing of the bound peptides and direct binding of synthetic peptides to isolated class I molecules. J Immunol 1994; 153:3079-92.
309. Larson JK, Wunner WH, Otvos L, Jr. et al. Identification of an immunodominant epitope within the phosphoprotein of rabies virus that is recognized by both class I-and class II-restricted T cells. J Virol 1991; 65:5673-9.
310. Gould KG, Scotney H, Townsend AR et al. Mouse H-2k-restricted cytotoxic T cells recognize antigenic determinants in both the HA1 and HA2 subunits of the influenza A/PR/8/34 hemagglutinin. J Exp Med 1987; 166:693-701.
311. Bastin J, Rothbard J, Davey J et al. Use of synthetic peptides of influenza nucleoprotein to define epitopes recognized by class I-restricted cytotoxic T lymphocytes. J Exp Med 1987; 165:1508-23.
312. Gould K, Cossins J, Bastin J et al. A 15 amino acid fragment of influenza nucleoprotein synthesized in the cytoplasm is presented to class I-restricted cytotoxic T lymphocytes. J Exp Med 1989; 170: 1051-6.
313. Sweetser MT, Morrison LA, Braciale VL et al. Recognition of pre-processed endogenous antigen by class I but not class II MHC-restricted T cells. Nature 1989; 342:180-2.
314. Rawle FC, O'Connell KA, Geib RW et al. Fine mapping of an H-2K^k restricted cytotoxic T lymphocyte epitope in SV40 T antigen by using in-frame deletion mutants and a synthetic peptide. J Immunol 1988; 141:2734-9.
315. Kumar S, Miller LH, Quakyi IA et al. Cytotoxic T cells specific for the circumsporozoite protein of Plasmodium falciparum. Nature 1988; 334:258-60.
316. Hosmalin A, Clerici M, Houghten R et al. An epitope in human immunodeficiency virus 1 reverse transcriptase recognized by both mouse and human cytotoxic T lymphocytes. Proc Natl Acad Sci U S A 1990; 87:2344-8.

317. Scott DM, Ehrmann IE, Ellis PS et al. Identification of a mouse male-specific transplantation antigen, H-Y. Nature 1995; 376:695-8.
318. Aldrich CJ, DeCloux A, Woods AS et al. Identification of a Tap-dependent leader peptide recognized by alloreactive T cells specific for a class Ib antigen. Cell 1994; 79:649-58.
319. Rötzschke O, Falk K, Stevanović S et al. Qa-2 molecules are peptide receptors of higher stringency than ordinary class I molecules. Nature 1993; 361:642-4.
320. Joyce S, Tabaczewski P, Angeletti RH et al. A nonpolymorphic major histocompatibility complex class Ib molecule binds a large array of diverse self-peptides. J Exp Med 1994; 179:579-88.
321. Wang C, Castano AR, Peterson PA et al. Nonclassical binding of formylated peptide in crystal structure of the MHC class Ib molecule H2-M3. Cell 1995; 82: 655-64.
322. Gulden PH, Fischer III P, Sherman NE et al. A Listeria monocytogenes pentapeptide is presented to cytolytic T lymphocytes by the H2-M3 MHC class Ib molecule. Immunity 1996; 5:73-9.
323. Fischer-Lindahl K, Hermel E, Loveland BE et al. Maternally transmitted antigen of mice: a model transplantation antigen. Annu Rev Immunol 1991; 9:351-72.
324. Loveland B, Wang CR, Yonekawa H et al. Maternally transmitted histocompatibility antigen of mice: a hydrophobic peptide of a mitochondrially encoded protein. Cell 1990; 60:971-80.
325. Morse MC, Bleau G, Dabhi VM et al. The COI mitochondrial gene encodes a minor histocompatibility antigen presented by H2-M3. J Immunol 1996; 156:3301-7.
326. Lenz LL, Dere B, Bevan MJ. Identification of an H2-M3-restricted Listeria epitope: Implications for Antigen presentation by M3. Immunity 1996; 5:63-72.
327. Thorpe CJ, Moss DS, Powis SJ et al. An analysis of the antigen binding site of RT1.A[a] suggests an allele-specific motif. Immunogenetics 1995; 41:329-31.
328. Reizis B, Schild H, Stevanović S et al. Peptide binding motifs of the MHC class I molecules (RT1.A[l]) of the Lewis rat. Immunogenetics 1997; 45:278-9.
329. Reizis B, Mor F, Eisenstein M et al. The peptide binding specificity of the MHC class II I-A molecule of the Lewis rat, RT1B[l]. Int Immunol 1996; 8:1825-32.
330. Hedge NR, Ellis SA, Gaddum RA et al. Peptide motif of the cattle MHC class I antigen BoLA-A11. Immunogenetics 1995; 42:302-3.
331. Bamford AI, Douglas A, Friede T et al. Peptide motif of a cattle MHC class I molecule. Immunol Lett 1995; 45:129-36.
332. Kaufman J, Volk H, Wallny HJ. A "minimal essential MHC" and an "unrecognized MHC": two extremes in selection for polymorphism. Immunol Rev 1995; 143: 63-88.
333. Cooper S, Kowalski H, Erickson AL et al. The presentation of a hepatitis C viral peptide by distinct major histocompatibility complex class I allotypes from two chimpanzee species. J Exp Med 1996; 183:663-8.
334. Yasutomi Y, Koenig S, Woods RM et al. A vaccine-elicited, single viral epitope-specific cytotoxic T lymphocyte response does not protect against intravenous, cell-free simian immunodeficiency virus challenge. J Virol 1995; 69:2279-84.
335. Pauly T, Elbers K, König M et al. Classical swine fever virus-specific cytotoxic T lymphocytes and identification of a T cell epitope. J Gen Virol 1995; 76:3039-49.
336. Fahnestock ML, Johnson JL, Feldman RM et al. The MHC class I homolog encoded by human cytomegalovirus binds endogenous peptides. Immunity 1995; 3:583-90.
337. Hammer J, Takacs B, Sinigaglia F. Identification of a motif for HLA-DR1 binding peptides using M13 display libraries. J Exp Med 1992; 176:1007-13.
338. Verreck FA, van de Poel A, Drijfhout JW et al. Natural peptides isolated from Gly86/Val86-containing variants of HLA-DR1, -DR11, -DR13, and -DR52. Immunogenetics 1996; 43:392-7.
339. Chicz RM, Urban RG, Lane WS et al. Predominant naturally processed peptides bound to HLA-DR1 are derived from MHC-related molecules and are heterogeneous in size. Nature 1992; 358:764-8.
340. Kropshofer H, Max H, Muller CA et al. Self-peptide released from class II HLA-

DR1 exhibits a hydrophobic two-residue contact motif. J Exp Med 1992; 175: 1799-803.

341. Verreck FAW, Vermeulen C, v.d.Poel A et al. The generation of SDS-stable HLA DR dimers is independent of efficient peptide binding. Int Immunol 1996; 8:397-404.

342. Colovai AI, Liu Z, Harris PE et al. Allopeptide-specific T cell reactivity altered by peptide analogs. J Immunol 1997; 158:48-54.

343. Adams E, Basten A, Rodda S et al. Human T-cell clones to the 70-Kilodalton heat shock protein of Mycobacterium leprae define mycobacterium-specific epitopes rather than shared epitopes. Infection and Immunity 1997; 65:1061-70.

344. Muller CP, Ammerlaan W, Fleckenstein B et al. Activation of T cells by the ragged tail of MHC class II-presented peptides of the measles virus fusion protein. Int Immunol 1996; 8:445-56.

345. Geluk A, van Meijgaarden KE, Southwood S et al. HLA-DR3 molecules can bind peptides carrying two alternative specific submotifs. J Immunol 1994; 152:5742-8.

346. Geluk A, van Meijgaarden KE, Janson AA et al. Functional analysis of DR17(DR3)-restricted mycobacterial T cell epitopes reveals DR17-binding motif and enables the design of allele-specific competitor peptides. J Immunol 1992; 149:2864-71.

347. Riberdy JM, Newcomb JR, Surman MJ et al. HLA-DR molecules from an antigen-processing mutant cell line are associated with invariant chain peptides. Nature 1992; 360:474-7.

348. Sette A, Ceman S, Kubo RT et al. Invariant chain peptides in most HLA-DR molecules of an antigen-processing mutant. Science 1992; 258:1801-4.

349. Hawes GE, Struyk L, Godthelp BC et al. Limited restriction in the TCR-alpha beta V region usage of antigen-specific clones. Recognition of myelin basic protein (amino acids 84-102) and Mycobacterium bovis 65-kDa heat shock protein (amino acids 3-13) by T cell clones established from peripheral blood mononuclear cells of monozygotic twins and HLA-identical individuals. J Immunol 1995; 154:555-66.

350. Friede T, Gnau V, Jung G et al. Natural ligand motifs of closely related HLA-DR4 molecules predict features of rheumatoid arthritis associated peptides. Biochimica et Biophysica Acta 1996; 1316:85-101.

351. Sette A, Sidney J, Oseroff C et al. HLA DR4w4-binding motifs illustrate the biochemical basis of degeneracy and specificity in peptide-DR interactions. J Immunol 1993; 151:3163-70.

352. Hammer J, Valsasnini P, Tolba K et al. Promiscuous and allele-specific anchors in HLA-DR-binding peptides. Cell 1993; 74:197-203.

353. Hill CM, Liu A, Marshall KW et al. Exploration of requirements for peptide binding to HLA DRB1*0101 and DRB1*0401. J Immunol 1994; 152: 2890-8.

354. Hammer J, Gallazzi F, Bono E et al. Peptide binding specificity of HLA-DR4 molecules: correlation with rheumatoid arthritis association. J Exp Med 1995; 181:1847-55.

355. Kirschmann DA, Duffin KL, Smith CE et al. Naturally processed peptides from rheumatoid arthritis associated and nonassociated HLA-DR alleles. J Immunol 1995; 155:5655-62.

356. Adibzadeh M, Friccius H, Bornhak S et al. Role of three quantitatively dominant endogenous peptides from HLA-DRB1*0401 molecules in class II specific allreactivity. Transplant Immunology 1994; 2:293-9.

357. McNicholl JM, Whitworth WC, Oftung F et al. Structural requirements of peptide and MHC for DR(alpha, beta 1*0401)-restricted T cell antigen recognition. J Immunol 1995; 155:1951-63.

358. Gaston JSH, Deane KHO, Jecock RM et al. Identification of 2 *Chlamydia trachomatis* antigens recognized by synovial fluid T cells from patients with Chlamydia induced reactive arthritis. J Rheumatol 1996; 23:130-6.

359. Fugger L, Rothbard JB, Sonderstrup McDevitt G. Specificity of an HLA-DRB1*0401-restricted T cell response to type II collagen. Eur J Immunol 1996; 26:928-33.

360. Topalian SL, Gonzales MI, Parkhurst M et al. Melanoma-specific CD4+T cells

recognize nonmutated HLA-DR-restricted tyrosinase epitopes. J Exp Med 1996; 183:1965-71.

361. Wicker LS, Chen S, Nepom GT et al. Naturally processed T cell epitopes from human glutamic acid decarboxylase identified using mice transgenic for the Type 1 diabetes-associated human MHC Class II allele, DRB1*0401. J Clin Invest 1996; 98:2597-603.

362. ten Bosch GJA, Joosten AM, Kessler JH et al. Recognition of BCR-ABL Positive leukemic blasts by human CD4+ T cells elicited by primary in vitro immunization with a BCR-ABL breakpoint peptide. Blood 1996; 88:3522-7.

363. Hayden JB, McCormack AL, Yates III JR et al. Analysis of naturally processed peptides eluted from HLA DRB1*0402 and *0404. J Neurosci Res 1996; 45:795-802.

364. Wucherpfennig KW, Yu B, Bhol K et al. Structural basis for major histocompatibility complex (MHC)-linked susceptibility to autoimmunity: charged residues of a single MHC binding pocket confer selective presentation of self-peptides in pemphigus vulgaris. Proc Natl Acad Sci U S A 1995; 92:11935-9.

365. Ou D, Mitchell LA, Domeier ME et al. Characterization of the HLA-restrictive elements of a rubella virus-specific cytotoxic T cell clone: influence of HLA-DR4β chain residue 74 polymorphism on antigenic peptide-T cell interaction. Int Immunol 1996; 8:1577-86.

366. Matsushita S, Takahashi K, Motoki M et al. Allele specificity of structural requirement for peptides bound to HLA-DRB1*0405 and -DRB1*0406 complexes: implication for the HLA-associated susceptibility to methimazole-induced insulin autoimmune syndrome. J Exp Med 1994; 180:873-83.

367. Kinouchi R, Kobayasi H, Sato K et al. Peptide motifs of HLA-DR4/DR53 (DRB1*0405/DRB4*0101) molecules. Immunogenetics 1994; 40:376-8.

368. Okano M, Nagano T, Nakada M et al. Epitope analysis of HLA-DR-restricted helper T-cell responses to DER P II, a major allergen molecule of dermatophagoides pteronyssinus. Allergy 1996; 51:29-35.

369. Davenport MP, Godkin A, Friede T et al. A distinctive peptide binding motif for HLA-DRB1*0407, an HLA-DR4 subtype not associated with rheumatoid arthritis. Immunogenetics 1997; 45:229-32.

370. Gautier N, Chavant E, Prieur E et al. Characterization of an epitope of the human cytomegalovirus protein IE1 recognized by a CD4+ T cell clone. Eur J Immunol 1996; 26:1110-7.

371. Fujisao S, Matsushita S, Nishi T et al. Identification of HLA-DR9 (DRB1*0901) binding peptide motifs using a phage fUSE5 random peptide library. Human Immunology 1996; 45:131-6.

372. Futaki G, Kobayashi H, Sato K et al. Naturally processed HLA-DR9/DR53 (DRB1*0901/DRB4*0101)-bound peptides. Immunogenetics 1995; 42:299-301.

373. Newcomb JR, Cresswell P. Characterization of endogenous peptides bound to purified HLA-DR molecules and their absence from invariant chain-associated alpha beta dimers. J Immunol 1993; 150:499-507.

374. Tsitoura DC, Holter W, Cerwenka A et al. Induction of anergy in human T helper 0 cells by stimulation with altered T cell antigen receptor ligands. J Immunol 1996; 156:2801-8.

375. Davenport MP, Quinn CL, Chicz RM et al. Naturally processed peptides from two disease-resistance-associated HLA-DR13 alleles show related sequence motifs and the effects of the dimorphism at position 86 of the HLA-DR beta chain. Proc Natl Acad Sci U S A 1995; 92:6567-71.

376. Boitel B, Blank U, Mege D et al. Strong similarities in antigen fine specificity among DRB1* 1302-restricted tetanus toxin tt830-843-specific TCRs in spite of highly heterogeneous CDR3. J Immunol 1995; 154:3245-55.

377. Diepolder HM, Jung M, Wierenga E et al. Anergic TH1 clones specific for hepatitis B virus (HBV) core peptides are inhibitory to other HBV core-specific CD4+ T cells in vitro. J Virol 1996; 70:7540-8.

378. Matsushita S, Yokomizo H, Kohsaka H et al. Diversity of a human CD4+ T cell repertoire recognizing one TCR ligand. Immunoly Letters 1996; 51:191-4.

379. Vogt AB, Kropshofer H, Kalbacher H et

al. Ligand motifs of HLA-DRB5*0101 and DRB1*1501 molecules delineated from self-peptides. J Immunol 1994; 153:1665-73.
380. Wucherpfennig KW, Sette A, Southwood S et al. Structural requirements for binding of an immunodominant myelin basic protein peptide to DR2 isotypes and for its recognition by human T cell clones. J Exp Med 1994; 179:279-90.
381. Kurane I, Okamoto Y, Dai LC et al. Flavivirus-cross-reactive, HLA-DR15-restricted epitope on NS3 recognized by human CD4+ CD8- cytotoxic T lymphocyte clones. J Gen Virol 1995; 76:2243-9.
382. Markovic Plese S, Fukaura H, Zhang J et al. T cell recognition of immunodominant and cryptic proteolipid protein epitopes in humans. J Immunol 1995; 155:982-92.
383. White CA, Cross SM, Kurilla MG et al. Recruitment during infectious mononucleosis of CD3+CD4+CD8+ virus-specific cytotoxic T cells which recognise Epstein-Barr virus lytic antigen BHRF1. Virology 1996; 219:489-92.
384. Ikagawa S, Matsushita S, Chen YZ et al. Single amino acid substitutions on a Japanese cedar pollen allergen (Cry j 1)-derived peptide induced alterations in human T cell responses and T cell receptor antagonism. J Allergy Clin Immunol 1996; 97:53-64.
385. Blaher B, Suphioglu C, Knox RB et al. Identification of T-cell epitopes of Lol p 9, a major allergen of ryegrass (*Lolium perenne*) pollen. J Allergy Clin Immunol 1996; 98:124-32.
386. Kobayashi H, Kokubo T, Abe Y et al. Analysis of anchor residues in a naturally processed HLA-DR53 ligand. Immunogenetics 1996; 44:366-71.
387. O'Sullivan D, Arrhenius T, Sidney J et al. On the interaction of promiscuous antigenic peptides with different DR alleles. Identification of common structural motifs. J Immunol 1991; 147:2663-9.
388. Anderson DC, van Schooten WC, Barry ME et al. A Mycobacterium leprae-specific human T cell epitope cross-reactive with an HLA-DR2 peptide. Science 1988; 242:259-61.
389. Martin R, Howell MD, Jaraquemada D et al. A myelin basic protein peptide is recognized by cytotoxic T cells in the context of four HLA-DR types associated with multiple sclerosis. J Exp Med 1991; 173:19-24.
390. Kwok WW, Domeier ME, Raymond FC et al. Allele-specific motifs characterize HLA-DQ interactions with a diabetes-associated peptide derived from glutamic acid decarboxylase. J Immunol 1996; 156:2171-7.
391. Sidney J, Oseroff C, del Guercio MF et al. Definition of a DQ3.1-specific binding motif. J Immunol 1994; 152:4516-25.
392. Vartdal F, Johannsen BH, Friede T et al. The peptide binding motif for the disease associated HLA-DQ (α1*0501, β1*0201) molecule. European Journal of Immunology 1996; 26:2764-72.
393. Rötzschke O, Falk K. Origin, structure and motifs of naturally processed MHC class II ligands. Curr Opin Immunol 1994; 6:45-51.
394. Schild H, Grüneberg U, Pougialis G et al. Natural ligand motifs of H-2E molecules are allele specific and illustrate homology to HLA-DR molecules. Int Immunol 1995; 7:1957-65.
395. Reay PA, Kantor RM, Davis MM. Use of global amino acid replacements to define the requirements for MHC binding and T cell recognition of moth cytochrome c (93-103). J Immunol 1994; 152:3946-57.
396. Marrack P, Ignatowicz L, Kappler JW et al. Comparison of peptides bound to spleen and thymus class II. J Exp Med 1993; 178:2173-83.
397. Leighton J, Sette A, Sidney J et al. Comparison of structural requirements for interaction of the same peptide with I-Ek and I-Ed molecules in the activation of MHC class II-restricted T cells. J Immunol 1991; 147:198-204.
398. Altuvia Y, Berzofsky JA, Rosenfeld R et al. Sequence features that correlate with MHC restriction [published erratum appears in Mol Immunol 1994; 31:703]. Mol Immunol 1994; 31:1-19.
399. Spouge JL, Guy HR, Cornette JL et al. Strong conformational propensities enhance T cell antigenicity. J Immunol 1987; 138:204-12.
400. Adorini L, Appella E, Doria G et al. Mechanisms influencing the immuno-

dominance of T cell determinants. J Exp Med 1988; 168:2091-104.
401. Sette A, Buus S, Appella E et al. Prediction of major histocompatibility complex binding regions of protein antigens by sequence pattern analysis. Proc Natl Acad Sci U S A 1989; 86:3296-300.
402. Bogen B, Snodgrass R, Briand JP et al. Synthetic peptides and beta-chain gene rearrangements reveal a diversified T cell repertoire for a lambda light chain third hypervariable region. Eur J Immunol 1986; 16:1379-84.
403. Adorini L, Sette A, Buus S et al. Interaction of an immunodominant epitope with Ia molecules in T-cell activation. Proc Natl Acad Sci U S A 1988; 85: 5181-5.
404. Guery JC, Sette A, Appella E et al. Constitutive presentation of dominant epitopes from endogenous naturally processed self-beta 2-microglobulin to class II-restricted T cells leads to self-tolerance. J Immunol 1995; 154:545-54.
405. Fahrer AM, Geysen HM, White DO et al. Analysis of the requirements for class II-restricted T cell recognition of a single determinant reveals considerable diversity in the T cell response and degeneracy of peptide binding to I-E^d. J Immunol 1995; 155:2849-57.
406. Baños DM, Lopez S, Arias CF et al. Identification of a T-helper cell epitope on the rotavirus VP6 protein. J Virol 1996; 71:419-26.
407. Rudensky AY, Preston Hurlburt P, Hong SC et al. Sequence analysis of peptides bound to MHC class II molecules. Nature 1991; 353:622-7.
408. Samson MF, Smilek DE. Reversal of acute experimental autoimmune encephalomyelitis and prevention of relapses by treatment with a myelin basic protein peptide analogue modified to form long-lived peptide-MHC complexes. J Immunol 1995; 155:2737-46.
409. Rudensky AY, Preston Hurlburt P, al Ramadi BK et al. Truncation variants of peptides isolated from MHC class II molecules suggest sequence motifs. Nature 1992; 359:429-31.
410. Brett SJ, Tite JP. Both H-2- and non-H-2-linked genes influence influenza nucleoprotein epitope recognition by $CD4^+$ T cells. Immunology 1996; 87:42-8.
411. Harris DP, Vordermeier HM, Singh M et al. Cross-recognition by T cells of an epitope shared by two unrelated mycobacterial antigens. Eur J Immunol 1995; 25:3173-9.
412. Mendel I, Kerlero de Rosbo N, Ben-Nun A. Delineation of the minimal encephalitogenic epitope within the immunodominant region of myelin oligodendrocyte glycoprotein: diverse Vβ gene usage by T cells recognizing the core epitope encephalitogenic for T cell receptor $V\beta^b$ and T cell receptor $V\beta^a$ H-2^b mice. Eur J Immunol 1996; 26:2470-9.
413. Kristensen NM, Hoyne GF, Hayball JD et al. Induction of T cell responses to the invariant chain derived peptide CLIP in mice immunized with the group 1 allergen of house dust mite. Int Immunol 1996; 8:1091-8.
414. Cong Y, Bowdon HR, Elson CO. Identification of an immunodominant T cell epitope on cholera toxin. Eur J Immunol 1996; 26:2587-95.
415. Noll A, Autenrieth IB. Yersinia-hsp60-reactive T cells are efficiently stimulated by peptides of 12 and 13 amino acid residues in a MHC class II (I-A^b)-restricted manner. Clin Exp Immunol 1996; 105: 231-7.
416. Yanagisawa S, Koike M, Kariyone A et al. Mapping of $M\beta 11^+$ helper T cell epitopes on mycobacterial antigen in mouse primed with *Mycobacterium tuberculosis.* Int Immunol 1997; 9:227-37.
417. Wen R, Broussard DR, Surman S et al. Carboxy-terminal residues of major histocompatibility complex class II-associated peptides control the presentation of the bacterial superantigen toxic shock syndrome toxin-1 to t cells. Eur J Immun 1997; 27:772-81.
418. Cole GA, Tao T, Hogg TL et al. Binding motifs predict major histocompatibility class II-restricted epitopes in the Sendai virus M protein. J Virol 1995; 69:8057-60.
419. Hunt DF, Michel H, Dickinson TA et al. Peptides presented to the immune system by the murine class II major histocompatibility complex molecule I-A^d. Science 1992; 256:1817-20.

420. Nelson CA, Viner NJ, Young SP et al. A negatively charged anchor residue promotes high affinity binding to the MHC Class II molecule I-A^k. J Immunol 1996; 157:755-62.
421. Nelson CA, Roof RW, McCourt DW et al. Identification of the naturally processed form of hen egg white lysozyme bound to the murine major histocompatibility complex class II molecule I-Ak. Proc Natl Acad Sci U S A 1992; 89: 7380-3.
422. Reizis B, Eisenstein M, Bockova J et al. Molecular characterization of the diabetes-associated mouse MHC class II protein, I-A^{g7}. Int Immunol 1997; 9:43-51.
423. Harrison LC, Honeyman MC, Trembleau S et al. A peptide binding motif for I-A^{g7}, the class II MHC molecule of NOD and BIOZZI ABH mice. [In Press] J Exp Med 1997.
424. Hurtenbach U, Lier E, Adorini L et al. Prevention of autoimmune diabetes in nonobese diabetic mice by treatment with a class II major histocompatibility complex-blocking peptide. J Exp Med 1993; 177:1499-594.
425. Deng H, Apple M, Clare-Salzler M et al. Determinant capture as a possible mechanism of protection afforded by major histocompatibility complex class II molecules in autoimmune disease. J Exp Med 1993; 178:1675-80.
426. Chen S, Whiteley PJ, Freed DC et al. Responses of NOD congenic mice to a glutamic acid decarboxylase-derived peptide. J Autoimmunity 1994; 7:635-41.
427. Kaufman DL, Clare Salzler M, Tian J et al. Spontaneous loss of T-cell tolerance to glutamic acid decarboxylase in murine insulin-dependent diabetes. Nature 1993; 366:69-72.
428. Smilek DE, Lock CB, McDevitt HO. Antigen recognition and peptide-mediated immunotherapy in autoimmune disease. Immunol Rev 1990; 118:37-71.
429. Amor S, O'Neill JK, Morris MM et al. Encephalitogenic epitopes of myelin basic protein, proteolipid protein, myelin oligodendrocyte glycoprotein for experimental allergic encephalomyelitis induction in Biozzi ABH (H-2Ag7) mice share an amino acid motif. J Immunol 1996; 156:3000-8.
430. Carrasco-Marin E, Shimizu J, Kanagawa O et al. The class II MHC I-A^{g7} molecules from nonobese diabetic mice are poor peptide binders. J Immunol 1996; 156:450-8.
431. Daniel D, Wegmann DR. Protection of nonobese diabetic mice from diabetes by intranasal or subcutaneous administration of insulin peptide B-(9-23). Proc Natl Acad Sci U S A 1996; 93:956-60.
432. Ridgway WM, Fasso M, Lanctot A et al. Breaking self-tolerance in nonobese diabetic mice. J Exp Med 1996; 183:1657-62.
433. Bernard CCA, Johns TG, Slavin A et al. Myelin oligodendrocyte glycoprotein: a novel candidate autoantigen in multiple sclerosis. J Mol Med 1997; 75:77-88.
434. Wauben MHM, van der Kraan M, Grosfeld-Stulemeyer MC et al. Definition of an extended MHC class II-peptide binding motif for the autoimmune disease-associated Lewis rat RT1.B^L molecule. Int Immunol 1997; 9:281-90.
435. Mannie MD, Paterson PY, U'Prichard DC et al. The N- and C-terminal boundaries of myelin basic protein determinants required for encephalitogenic and proliferative responses of Lewis rat T cells. J Neuroimmunol 1990; 26:201-11.
436. Kojima K, Berger T, Lassmann H et al. Experimental autoimmune panencephalitis and uveoretinitis transferred to the Lewis rat by T lymphocytes specific for the S100 beta molecule, a calcium binding protein of astroglia. J Exp Med 1994; 180:817-29.
437. Anderton SM, van der Zee R, Noordzij A et al. Differential mycobacterial 65-kDa heat shock protein T cell epitope recognition after adjuvant arthritis-inducing or protective immunization protocols. J Immunol 1994; 152:3656-64.
438. Wegmann KW, Zhao W, Griffin AC et al. Identification of myocarditogenic peptides derived from cardiac myosin capable of inducing experimental allergic myocarditis in the Lewis rat. The utility of a class II binding motif in selecting self-reactive peptides. J Immunol 1994; 153:892-900.
439. Broeren CP, Lucassen MA, van Stipdonk MJ et al. CDR1 T-cell receptor beta-chain peptide induces major histocom-

patibility complex class II-restricted T-T cell interactions. Proc Natl Acad Sci U S A 1994; 91:5997-6001.
440. Stevanović S, Rammensee HG. Identification of T-cell epitopes using allele-specific ligand motifs. Behring Inst Mitt 1994; 7-13.
441. DeLisi C, Berzofsky JA. T-cell antigenic sites tend to be amphipathic structures. Proc Natl Acad Sci USA 1985; 82:7048-52.
442. Rothbard JB, Taylor WR. A sequence pattern common to T cell epitopes. EMBO J 1988; 7:93-100.
443. Claverie JM, Kourilsky P, Langlade-Demoyen P et al. T-immunogenic peptides are constituted of rare sequence patterns. Use in the identification of T epitopes in the human immunodeficiency virus gag protein. Eur J Immunol 1988; 18:1547-653.
444. Garcia KC, Degano M, Stanfield RL et al. An alphabeta T cell receptor structure at 2.5 A and its orientation in the TCR-MHC complex. Science 1996; 274:209-19.
445. Devereux J, Haeberli P, Smithies O. A comprehensive set of sequence analysis programs for the VAX. Nucleic Acids Res 1984; 12:387-95.
446. D'Amaro J, Houbiers JGA, Drijfhout JW et al. A computer program for predicting possible cytotoxic T lymphocyte epitopes based on HLA class I peptide-binding motifs. Hum Immunol 1995; 43:13-8.
447. Davenport MP, Ho Shon IAP, Hill AVS. An empirical method for the prediction of T-cell epitopes. Immunogenetics 1995; 42:392-7.
448. Hammer J, Bono E, Gallazzi F et al. Precise prediction of major histocompatibility complex class II-peptide interaction based on peptide side chain scanning. J Exp Med 1994; 180:2353-8.
449. Lehner PJ, Cresswell P. Processing and delivery of peptides presented by MHC class I molecules. Curr Opin Immunol 1996; 8:59-67.
450. Busch R, Mellins ED. Developing and shedding inhibitions: how MHC class II molecules reach maturity. Curr Opin Immunol 1996; 8:51-8.
451. Pieters J. MHC class II restricted antigen presentation. Curr Opin Immunol 1997; 9:89-96.
452. Coux O, Tanaka K, Goldberg AL. Structure and functions of the 20S and 26S proteasomes. Annu Rev Biochem 1996; 65:801-47.
453. Goldberg AL. Functions of the proteasome: the lysis at the end of the tunnel. Science 1995; 268:522-3.
454. Lowe J, Stock D, Jap B et al. Crystal structure of the 20S proteasome from the archaeon T. acidophilum at 3.4 Å resolution. Science 1995; 268:533-9.
455. Seemüller E, Lupas A, Stock D et al. Proteasome from Thermoplasma acidophilum: a threonine protease. Science 1995; 268:579-82.
456. Nandi D, Jiang H, Monaco JJ. Identification of MECL-1 (LMP-10) as the third IFN-gamma-inducible proteasome subunit. J Immunol 1996; 156:2361-4.
457. Tanaka K. Role of proteasomes modified by interferon-gamma in antigen processing. J Leukoc Biol 1994; 56:571-5.
458. Kuckelkorn U, Frentzel S, Kraft R et al. Incorporation of major histocompatibility complex—encoded subunits LMP2 and LMP7 changes the quality of the 20S proteasome polypeptide processing products independent of interferon-gamma. Eur J Immunol 1995; 25:2605-11.
459. Sibille C, Gould KG, Willard Gallo K et al. LMP2+ proteasomes are required for the presentation of specific antigens to cytotoxic T lymphocytes. Curr Biol 1995; 5:923-30.
460. Groettrup M, Ruppert T, Kuehn L et al. The interferon-gamma-inducible 11 S regulator (PA28) and the LMP2/LMP7 subunits govern the peptide production by the 20 S proteasome in vitro. J Biol Chem 1995; 270:23808-15.
461. Van Kaer L, Ashton Rickardt PG, Eichelberger M et al. Altered peptidase and viral-specific T cell response in LMP2 mutant mice. Immunity 1994; 1:533-41.
462. Gaczynska M, Rock KL, Spies T et al. Peptidase activities of proteasomes are differentially regulated by the major histocompatibility complex-encoded genes for LMP2 and LMP7. Proc Natl Acad Sci U S A 1994; 91:9213-7.

463. Fehling HJ, Swat W, Laplace C et al. MHC class I expression in mice lacking the proteasome subunit LMP-7. Science 1994; 265:1234-7.
464. Zhou X, Momburg F, Liu T et al. Presentation of viral antigens restricted by H-2Kb, Db or Kd in proteasome subunit LMP2- and LMP7-deficient cells. Eur J Immunol 1994; 24:1863-8.
465. Driscoll J, Brown MG, Finley D et al. MHC-linked LMP gene products specifically alter peptidase activities of the proteasome. Nature 1993; 365:262-4.
466. Arnold D, Driscoll J, Androlewicz M et al. Proteasome subunits encoded in the mhc are not generally required for the processing of peptides bound by MHC class-I molecules. Nature 1992; 360: 171-4.
467. Orlowski M, Wilk S. A multicatalytic protease complex from pituitary that forms enkephalin and enkephalin containing peptides. Biochem Biophys Res Commun 1981; 101:814-22.
468. Wenzel T, Eckerskorn C, Lottspeich F et al. Existence of a molecular ruler in proteasomes suggested by analysis of degradation products. FEBS Lett 1994; 349:205-9.
469. Dick TP, Ruppert T, Groettrup M et al. Coordinated dual cleavages induced by the proteasome regulator PA28 lead to dominant MHC ligands. Cell 1996; 86: 253-62.
470. Gray CW, Slaughter CA, DeMartino GN. PA28 activator protein forms regulatory caps on proteasome stacked rings. J Mol Biol 1994; 236:7-15.
471. Ahn JY, Tanahashi N, Akiyama K et al. Primary structures of two homologous subunits of PA28, a gamma-interferon-inducible protein activator of the 20S proteasome. FEBS Lett 1995; 366:37-42.
472. Realini C, Dubiel W, Pratt G et al. Molecular cloning and expression of a gamma-interferon-inducible activator of the multicatalytic protease. J Biol Chem 1994; 269:20727-32.
473. Hoffman L, Rechsteiner M. Activation of the multicatalytic protease. The 11 S regulator and 20 S ATPase complexes contain distinct 30-kilodalton subunits. J Biol Chem 1994; 269:16890-5.
474. Dubiel W, Pratt G, Ferrell K et al. Purification of an 11 S regulator of the multicatalytic protease. J Biol Chem 1992; 267:22369-77.
475. Groettrup M, Soza A, Eggers M et al. A role for the proteasome regulator PA28 alpha in antigen presentation. Nature 1996; 381:166-8.
476. Momburg F, Neefjes JJ, Hämmerling GJ. Peptide selection by MHC-encoded TAP transporters. Curr Opin Immunol 1994; 6:32-7.
477. Howard JC. Supply and transport of peptides presented by class I MHC molecules. Curr Opin Immunol 1995; 7: 69-76.
478. Srivastava PK, Udono H, Blachere NE et al. Heat shock proteins transfer peptides during antigen processing and CTL priming. Immunogenetics 1994; 39:93-8.
479. van Endert PM, Riganelli D, Greco G et al. The peptide-binding motif for the human transporter associated with antigen processing. J Exp Med 1995; 182: 1883-95.
480. Neefjes J, Gottfried E, Roelse J et al. Analysis of the fine specificity of rat, mouse and human TAP peptide transporters. Eur J Immunol 1995; 25:1133-6.
481. Momburg F, Roelse J, Howard JC et al. Selectivity of MHC-encoded peptide transporters from human, mouse and rat. Nature 1994; 367:648-51.
482. Schumacher TN, Kantesaria DV, Heemels MT et al. Peptide length and sequence specificity of the mouse TAP1/TAP2 translocator. J Exp Med 1994; 179:533-40.
483. Koopmann JO, Post M, Neefjes JJ et al. Translocation of long peptides by transporters associated with antigen processing (TAP). Eur J Immunol 1996; 26: 1720-8.
484. Powis SJ, Young LL, Joly E et al. The rat cim effect: TAP allele-dependent changes in a class I MHC anchor motif and evidence against C-terminal trimming of peptides in the ER. Immunity 1996; 4:159-65.
485. Obst R, Armandola EA, Nijenhuis M et al. TAP polymorphism does not influence transport of peptide variants in mice and humans. Eur J Immunol 1995; 25:2170-6.

486. Cresswell P, Androlewicz MJ, Ortmann B. Assembly and transport of class I MHC-peptide complexes. Ciba Found Symp 1994; 187:150-69.
487. Suh WK, Mitchell EK, Yang Y et al. MHC class I molecules form ternary complexes with calnexin and TAP and undergo peptide-regulated interaction with TAP via their extracellular domains. J Exp Med 1996; 184:337-48.
488. Williams DB, Watts TH. Molecular chaperones in antigen presentation. Curr Opin Immunol 1995; 7:77-84.
489. Rajagopalan S, Brenner MB. Calnexin retains unassembled major histocompatibility complex class I free heavy chains in the endoplasmic reticulum. J Exp Med 1994; 180:407-12.
490. Jackson MR, Cohen Doyle MF, Peterson PA et al. Regulation of MHC class I transport by the molecular chaperone, calnexin (p88, IP90). Science 1994; 263: 384-7.
491. Sadasivan B, Lehner PJ, Ortmann B et al. Roles for calreticulin and a novel glycoprotein, tapasin, in the interaction of MHC class I molecules with TAP. Immunity 1996; 5:103-14.
492. Arnold D, Faath S, Rammensee HG et al. Cross-priming of minor histocompatibility antigen-specific cytotoxic T cells upon immunization with the heat shock protein gp96. J Exp Med 1995; 182:885-9.
493. Nieland TJ, Tan MC, Monne van Muijen M et al. Isolation of an immunodominant viral peptide that is endogenously bound to the stress protein GP96/GRP94. Proc Natl Acad Sci U S A 1996; 93: 6135-9.
494. Lammert E, Stevanović S, Brunner J et al. Protein disulfide isomerase is the dominant acceptor for peptides translocation into the endoplasmic reticulum. [In Press] Eur J Immunol.
495. Falk K, Rötzschke O, Rammensee HG. Cellular peptide composition governed by major histocompatibility complex class I molecules. Nature 1990; 348: 248-51.
496. Wiertz EJ, Jones TR, Sun L et al. The human cytomegalovirus US11 gene product dislocates MHC class I heavy chains from the endoplasmic reticulum to the cytosol. Cell 1996; 84:769-79.
497. Roelse J, Gromme M, Momburg F et al. Trimming of TAP-translocated peptides in the endoplasmic reticulum and in the cytosol during recycling. J Exp Med 1994; 180:1591-7.
498. Wei ML, Cresswell P. HLA-A2 molecules in an antigen-processing mutant cell contain signal sequence-derived peptides. Nature 1992; 356:443-6.
499. Rötzschke O, Falk K, Faath S et al. On the nature of peptides involved in T cell alloreactivity. J Exp Med 1991; 174: 1059-71.
500. Hosken NA, Bevan MJ. An endogenous antigenic peptide bypasses the class I antigen presentation defect in RMA-S. J Exp Med 1992; 175:719-29.
501. Fruh K, Ahn K, Peterson PA. Inhibition of MHC class I antigen presentation by viral proteins. J Mol Med 1997; 75:18-27.
502. Levitskaya J, Coram M, Levitsky V et al. Inhibition of antigen processing by the internal repeat region of the Epstein-Barr virus nuclear antigen-1. Nature 1995; 375:685-8.
503. Rotem Yehudar R, Groettrup M, Soza A et al. LMP-associated proteolytic activities and TAP-dependent peptide transport for class 1 MHC molecules are suppressed in cell lines transformed by the highly oncogenic adenovirus 12. J Exp Med 1996; 183:499-514.
504. Tomazin R, Hill AB, Jugovic P et al. Stable binding of the herpes simplex virus ICP47 protein to the peptide binding site of TAP. EMBO J 1996; 15: 3256-66.
505. Korner H, Burgert HG. Down-regulation of HLA antigens by the adenovirus type 2 E3/19K protein in a T-lymphoma cell line. J Virol 1994; 68:1442-8.
506. Reimann J, Bohm W, Schirmbeck R. Alternative processing pathways for MHC class I-restricted epitope presentation to CD8+ cytotoxic T lymphocytes. Biol Chem Hoppe Seyler 1994; 375:731-6.
507. Harding CV, Song R, Griffin J et al. Processing of bacterial antigens for presentation to class I and II MHC-restricted T lymphocytes. Infect Agents Dis 1995; 4:1-12.
508. Pfeifer JD, Wick MJ, Roberts RL et al. Phagocytic processing of bacterial anti-

gens for class I MHC presentation to T cells. Nature 1993; 361:359-62.
509. Schirmbeck R, Bohm W, Melber K et al. Processing of exogenous heat-aggregated (denatured) and particulate (native) hepatitis B surface antigen for class I-restricted epitope presentation. J Immunol 1995; 155:4676-84.
510. Liu T, Zhou X, Orvell C et al. Heat-inactivated Sendai virus can enter multiple MHC class I processing pathways and generate cytotoxic T lymphocyte responses in vivo. J Immunol 1995; 154: 3147-55.
511. Kovacsovics-Bankowski M, Rock KL. A phagosome-to-cytosol pathway for exogenous antigens presented on MHC class I molecules. Science 1995; 267:243-6.
512. Zhou X, Liu T, Franksson L et al. Characterization of TAP-independent and brefeldin A-resistant presentation of Sendai virus antigen to CD8+ cytotoxic T lymphocytes. Scand J Immunol 1995; 42:66-75.
513. Cresswell P. Assembly, transport, and function of MHC class II molecules. Annu Rev Immunol 1994; 12:259-93.
514. Cresswell P. Invariant chain structure and MHC class II function. Cell 1996; 84:505-7.
515. Pieters J, Bakke O, Dobberstein B. The MHC class II-associated invariant chain contains two endosomal targeting signals within its cytoplasmic tail. J Cell Sci 1993; 106:831-46.
516. Tulp A, Verwoerd D, Dobberstein B et al. Isolation and characterization of the intracellular MHC class II compartment. Nature 1994; 369:120-6.
517. Pieters J, Horstmann H, Bakke O et al. Intracellular transport and localization of major histocompatibility complex class II molecules and associated invariant chain. J Cell Biol 1991; 115:1213-23.
518. Harding CV. Intracellular organelles involved in antigen processing and the binding of peptides to class II MHC molecules. Semin Immunol 1995; 7: 355-60.
519. Copier J, Kleijmeer MJ, Ponnambalam S et al. Targeting signal and subcellular compartments involved in the intracellular trafficking of HLA-DMB. J Immunol 1996; 157:1017-27.
520. Robbins NF, Hammond C, Denzin LK et al. Trafficking of major histocompatibility complex class II molecules through intracellular compartments containing HLA-DM. Hum Immunol 1996; 45: 13-23.
521. Riese RJ, Wolf PR, Bromme D et al. Essential role for cathepsin S in MHC class II-associated invariant chain processing and peptide loading. Immunity 1996; 4:357-66.
522. Weber DA, Evavold BD, Jensen PE. Enhanced dissociation of HLA-DR-bound peptides in the presence of HLA-DM. Science 1996; 274:618-20.
523. Vogt AB, Kropshofer H, Moldenhauer G et al. Kinetic analysis of peptide loading onto HLA-DR molecules mediated by HLA-DM. Proc Natl Acad Sci U S A 1996; 93:9724-9.
524. Pierre P, Denzin LK, Hammond C et al. HLA-DM is localized to conventional and unconventional MHC class II-containing endocytic compartments. Immunity 1996; 4:229-39.
525. Sanderson F, Thomas C, Neefjes J et al. Association between HLA-DM and HLA-DR in vivo. Immunity 1996; 4:87-96.
526. Mellins E, Kempin S, Smith L et al. A gene required for class II-restricted antigen presentation maps to the major histocompatibility complex. J Exp Med 1991; 174:1607-15.
527. Morris P, Shaman J, Attaya M et al. An essential role for HLA-DM in antigen presentation by class II major histocompatibility molecules. Nature 1994; 368: 551-4.
528. Fling SP, Arp B, Pious D. HLA-DMA and -DMB genes are both required for MHC class II/peptide complex formation in antigen-presenting cells. Nature 1994; 368:554-8.
529. Mellins E, Smith L, Arp B et al. Defective processing and presentation of exogenous antigens in mutants with normal HLA class II genes. Nature 1990; 343:71-4.
530. Sloan VS, Cameron P, Porter G et al. Mediation by HLA-DM of dissociation of peptides from HLA-DR. Nature 1995; 375:802-6.
531. Kropshofer H, Vogt AB, Moldenhauer G et al. Editing of the HLA DR peptide rep-

ertoire by HLA DM. EMBO J 1996; 15:6144-6154.
532. Katz JF, Stebbins C, Appella E et al. Invariant chain and DM edit self peptide presentation by major histocompatibility complex (MHC) class II molecules. J Exp Med 1996; 184:1747-1753.
533. Vanham SM, Gruneberg U, Malcherek G et al. Human histocompatibility leukocyte antigen (HLA) DM edits peptides presented by HLA DR according to their ligand binding motifs. J Exp Med 1996; 184:2019-2024.
534. Kropshofer H, Hämmerling GJ, Vogt AB. How HLA-DM edits the MHC class II peptide repertoire: survival of the fittest? Immunology Today 1997; 18:77-82.
535. Chicz RM, Urban RG, Gorga JC et al. Specificity and promiscuity among naturally processed peptides bound to HLA-DR alleles. J Exp Med 1993; 178:27-47.
536. Malcherek G, Gnau V, Jung G et al. Supermotifs enable natural invariant chain-derived peptides to interact with many major histocompatibility complex-class II molecules. J Exp Med 1995; 181:527-36.
537. Riberdy JM, Newcomb JR, Surman MJ et al. HLA-DR molecules from an antigen-processing mutant cell line are associated with invariant chain peptides. Nature 1992; 360:474-7.
538. Ghosh P, Amaya M, Mellins E et al. The structure of an intermediate in class II MHC maturation: CLIP bound to HLA-DR3. Nature 1995; 378:457-62.
539. Pinet V, Malnati MS, Long EO. Two processing pathways for the MHC class II-restricted presentation of exogenous influenza virus antigen. J Immunol 1994; 152:4852-60.
540. Pinet V, Vergelli M, Martin R et al. Antigen presentation mediated by recycling of surface HLA-DR molecules. Nature 1995; 375:603-6.
541. Long EO. Antigen processing for presentation to CD4+ T cells. New Biol 1992; 4:274-82.
542. Malnati MS, Marti M, LaVaute T et al. Processing pathways for presentation of cytosolic antigen to MHC class II-restricted T cells. Nature 1992; 357:702-4.
543. Mizuochi T, Yee ST, Kasai M et al. Both cathepsin B and cathepsin D are necessary for processing of ovalbumin as well as for degradation of class II MHC invariant chain. Immunol Lett 1994; 43: 189-93.
544. Matsunaga Y, Saibara T, Kido H et al. Participation of cathepsin B in processing of antigen presentation to MHC class II. FEBS Lett 1993; 324:325-30.
545. Rodriguez GM, Diment S. Role of cathepsin D in antigen presentation of ovalbumin. J Immunol 1992; 149:2894-8.
546. Hansen AS, Noren O, Sjostrom H et al. A mouse aminopeptidase N is a marker for antigen-presenting cells and appears to be co-expressed with major histocompatibility complex class II molecules. Eur J Immunol 1993; 23:2358-64.
547. Mouritsen S, Meldal M, Werdelin O et al. MHC molecules protect T cell epitopes against proteolytic destruction. J Immunol 1992; 149:1987-93.
548. Rötzschke O, Falk K. Origin, structure and motifs of naturally processed MHC class II ligands. Curr Opin Immunol 1994; 6:45-51.
549. Werdelin O. Determinant protection. A hypothesis for the activity of immune response genes in the processing and presentation of antigens by macrophages. Scand J Immunol 1986; 24:625-36.
550. Buseyne F. Stevanović S, Rammensee HG et al. Characterization of an HIV-1 $p24^{gag}$ epitope recognized by a $CD8^+$ cytotoxic T-cell clone. Immunol Letters 1997; 55:145-149.
551. Falk K, Rötzschke O. Consensus motifs and ligands of MHC class I molecules. Sem Immunol 1993; 5:81-94.

CHAPTER 5

Recognition by Immune Cells

NATURAL KILLER CELLS

Natural killer cells have a different way of looking at MHC molecules as compared to T-cells. The relationship between NK cells and MHC molecules was originally proposed by Klaas Kärre's 'missing self' hypothesis which assumed that NK cells screen other cells for the absence of MHC molecules.[1-5] This hypothesis has been proven correct in essence.[5] NK cells express group-specific receptors for MHC molecules.[6] These receptors can be either inhibitory (killer inhibitory receptors, KIR), or activatory. In addition, NK cells express activatory receptors that recognize structures expressed on many cell types. If an NK cell binds to a normal MHC expressing cell, both inhibitory and activatory receptors are engaged. This leads to a dominant inhibitory effect so that no activation takes place. If a target cell has lost MHC expression, however, the inhibitory receptor does not find its ligand, and as a consequence, the target cell is killed. A number of KIRs both on human and mouse cells have been identified.[7,8] Originally, receptors of different gene families were discovered in mice and humans and only recently evidence that the two families exist in both species has been provided.[6,8-11] Therefore, the best known mouse receptors are of the lectin receptor type, whereas the most intensively studied human ones belong to the immunoglobulin superfamily. Each of the mouse receptors, Ly49 A, B, C, D, E, F, G, and H, is specific for a different selection of H-2 molecules (see Table 5.1). Similarly, each of the human receptors, NKAT1 through NKAT4, recognizes a certain epitope on the HLA class I molecule that defines its recognition pattern (Table 5.1).[8,12-14] Each NK cell expresses several KIRs; their combination, relative density, and functional significance is dependent on inheritance and selection processes during their ontogeny, details of which are not well known, however.[15-19]

Thus, NK cells serve to survey proper expression of MHC molecules on cells. If a cell stops to express MHC, e.g., upon interference of MHC assembly by viral infection, NK cells are activated and kill the altered cell. Since KIRs are group-specific, NK cells can be able to detect cells that have lost only one of the MHC molecules. Possibly, NK cells are also able to detect gross differences in peptide presentation by MHC molecules, although peptide-dependent NK recognition is rarely reported.[20,21] Thus, NK cells can be looked at as a back-up mechanism stepping in when infected or transformed cells escape the surveillance of MHC restricted T cells. Recently, KIR expressing $\gamma\delta$ T cells have been found to serve a similar function in surveillance against MHC-loosing lymphocytes (P. Fisch, personal communication). In addition to their back-up mechanism, NK cells play an important role

---

MHC Ligands and Peptide Motifs, by Hans-Georg Rammensee, Jutta Bachmann, Stefan Stevanović.

in initiation and regulation of specific immune responses via their production of cytokines, most notably INFγ and their activation by IL-12.[22,23]

ANTIGEN-SPECIFIC T CELLS

The immune cells principally dealing with MHC presented peptides are the $\alpha\beta$ T cells.[24] $\gamma\delta$ T cells are specialized on other forms of antigens.[25,26] Thus, this chapter will consider $\alpha\beta$ T cells only.

The majority of peptides presented by MHC class I or class II molecules on antigen-presenting cells or other cells are self peptides that do not lead to an immune response, since T cells are tolerant against most of the self peptides.[27,28] The basis of such tolerance can be central clonal deletion of self reactive T cells, as is the case for peptides presented in sufficient amounts in the thymus.[522] For other peptides derived from peripheral proteins, deletion or anergy may occur in the peripheral lymphoid system. However, T cells reactive against some peptides of the latter category can occur under certain conditions, such that self tolerance is not absolute.[30]

On the other hand, the mere presentation of a foreign antigen on antigen-presenting cells does not necessarily lead to a T cell response. Required are a productive interaction between the $\alpha\beta$ T cell receptor and the MHC-peptide complex, the structure of which has been elucidated recently.[31,32] Productive means that the interaction is able to initiate full T cell activation (T cell receptor-agonist interaction), in contrast to the partial activation that is initiated by TCR-antagonist peptides and that may lead to T cell anergy or deletion. What distinguishes the two possibilities at the structural level is not fully understood, most likely seems a structural change in the TCR upon ligand binding that induces further signal transduction.[31] In addition to TCR ligand binding, several additional interactions between T cell and antigen-presenting cell have to take place before activation can occur. These fall into two categories, engagement of costimulatory receptors of T cells with their ligands on the antigen-presenting cell, and binding of cytokines to their receptors on both T cell and APC. Expression of both cytokine and ligands depends on the activation state of antigen-presenting cells and is usually associated with some kind of 'stress', e.g., a wound or tissue damage.[30] One of the principal co-stimulatory interactions between T cells and APCs is that between the CD28 receptor on the T cell and the B7 ligand on APC (reviewed in refs. 33,34). The CD28/B7 system is complex insofar as a CD28 homologue on the T cell side, CTLA-4, acts in a counteractive way by downregulating the T cell response. On the other hand, there are two costimulatory ligands, B7-1 and B7-2, on the APC side, each of which is specialized. In a primary response, B7-2 plays the dominant role, whereas in an ongoing response, both ligands are involved. The third factor regulating T cell activation, after TCR engagement and costimulation, are cytokines, the combinations of which decide which class of T cell mediated immune response is going to develop. Once the requirement for productive T cell activation is fulfilled, signal transduction in the T cell finally leads to specific gene activation. The signalling process is mediated via cytoplasmic domains of the TCR/CD3 complex located in CD3γ, δ, and ε chains and on the invariant ζ chain.[35] The intracellular tails of these chains contain an ITAM motif (immunoglobulin receptor family tyrosine-based activation motif) with a core of a duplicated YXXL sequence. This motif allows interaction with intracellular tyrosine kinases and thus is crucial for the subsequent signalling events. The cascade now following is intersecting with the cascade initiated by costimulatory receptors and eventually leads to activation of the transcription factors NFκB, AP-1 or NFAT that now activate cytokine or other T cell genes.

According to their functional significance, $\alpha\beta$ T cells can be grouped into three primary categories, $CD8^+$, $CD4^+Th_1$, and $CD4^+$ Th_2 cells.[36] On top of this rough classification, however, there are a number of intermediate types, such as the Th_2-like $CD8^+$ cells.[37]

$CD8^+$ T cells recognize peptide presented by MHC I molecules. This selection is brought about by binding of CD8 to a conserved site on the MHC I molecule, the α3 domain,[38] and selection upon TCR engagement of thymic class I molecules during T cell maturation.[39-42] All cell types expressing MHC I molecules are able to present peptides, and therefore $CD8^+$ T cells can check every cell for expression of aberrant peptide, e.g., after virus infection.[43]

The function of $CD8^+$ T cells is to destroy cells expressing aberrant peptides, either by direct lysis or by activation of other effector cells upon cytokine release. Direct lysis by $CD8^+$ T cells is mediated either by target-directed release of perforin that leads to pores formed in the membrane of the attacked cells, or by induction of apoptosis in the target cell via Fas/Fas ligand interaction.[44,43] The cytokines typically produced by $CD8^+$ T cells are IFNγ, TNFα, and TNFβ.[45] Apart from representing a major branch of cellular immunity, $CD8^+$ T cells play a role in immune regulation by their release of cytokines and by inhibiting T cell responses against self peptides presented by these MHC I molecules. $CD4^+$ Th_1 cells, recognizing peptides presented by class II molecules, are characterized by release of a similar combination of cytokines as are $CD8^+$ cells.[45,36] Leitcytokines are IFNγ and TNFβ. Together with $CD8^+$ cells, $CD4Th_1$ cells represent most of the antigen specific part of cellular immunity, mediating delayed type hypersensitivity reaction (DTH)[46,47] and other forms of tissue damage upon cytokine-induced activation of effector cells such as macrophages and granulocytes.[48] In addition, $CD4^+$ Th_1 cells play a role in B cell activation, the regulation of isotype switch, and in the regulation of Th_2 cells.[34] $CD4^+$ Th_2 cells are the principal T helper cells, activating and regulating B cells via cytokine release and CD80/CD40L interactions.[49,50] Leitcytokines of Th_2 cells are IL4 and CD40L.[45] Isotype expression like IgG1, IgA, and IgE are controlled by Th_2 cytokines. In addition, Th_2 cells regulate the activation of Th_1 cells. Thus, the two $CD4^+$ T cell subsets are able to control each other.[46]

ALLOREACTIVITY AND TRANSPLANTATION

The term alloreactivity in general describes the immune reaction against allogeneic tissue, that is, tissue from a different individual of the same species. Xenoreactivity, in contrast, stands for the reaction against tissue of a different species. In a narrower sense, the term alloreactivity is used for the immune reaction against foreign MHC molecules.[51-53]

Alloreactivity is an extremely strong immune response. It was the phenomenon leading to the discovery of MHC molecules in the first half of the 20th century.[54,55] Why this reaction has to be that strong that the frequency of T cells reacting against a given foreign MHC molecule is in the range of 1 in 1000 is not fully understood.[51] Positive selection in the thymus aims at T cells able to recognize peptides in context with self MHC molecules, and does not explain the high frequency of alloreactive T cells.[56,57] The old hypothesis by Jerne (published in the starting article of the European Journal of Immunology) that germ line T cell receptors are directed against all possible MHC molecules of the species is not correct in its details but contains the grain that the somatic generation of TCR diversity has been selected to be biased towards recognition of MHC molecules. A more naive and mechanistic interpretation for the strong alloreactivity comes from considering the three-dimensional structure of the TCR/peptide/MHC trimeric complex: Half of the contact area of the TCR surface is occupied by MHC surface,[31] and this surface is strongly influenced by MHC polymorphism. The other half of the TCR surface contacts the peptide, and the peptide content of the MHC groove is also heavily influenced by MHC polymorphism. Since the basic principle for T cell alertness is the presence of an unfamiliar change on the MHC/peptide surface, the chance for detecting such a change on the entire surface (foreign MHC) is much higher than on only half of it (self MHC plus peptide). In addition, the available repertoire for self MHC plus peptide is grossly diminished by negative selection.[27]

Above considerations are confirmed (and, of course, inspired) by the multitude of possibilities found for the antigen specificity of alloreactive T cells (Fig. 5.1).[53] It is not known whether alloreactive T cells exist that recognize 'empty' MHC molecules, that is, heavy chain/β2m complexes without peptide. Recognition of TAP-deficient cells by alloreactive T cells is frequently seen; however, since TAP negative cells present TAP-independent peptides,[53,58] this cannot be taken as proof for recognition of empty molecules.[53] Thus, alloreactive T cells recognizing TAP-deficient cells belong either to a category 'without peptide' or to one of the 'peptide-dependent' categories. Among the peptide-dependent alloreactive T cells, several subclasses have been observed:[53] peptide-dependent, but without specificity, so that any peptide will suffice for recognition; peptide selective, which means that out of a collection of peptides, only a fraction will be recognized; and peptide-specific, so that only one peptide is recognized[59,53,51] (or at least so few peptides that the crossreactivity is comparable to that seen for self-restricted T cells); and perhaps an unlikely subclass that is specific for a peptide only and does not care about its MHC context. An illustration of these categories is in Fig. 5.1. Most of the alloreactive T cells commonly seen in mixed lymphocyte cultures and, by analogue, probably also those involved in graft rejection belong to the categories showing no or low peptide specificity. On the other hand, the peptide specific ones might be of special importance, e.g., by recognizing tissue-specific peptides, and thus might be responsible for organ-specific destruction. In clinical transplantation, alloreactivity has to be avoided or suppressed. Dependent on the organ transplanted, HLA matching between donor and recipient is sought.[60] This is logistically difficult, as seen for kidney transplantation, but improves the outcome.[60-62] For bone marrow transplantation, at least partial identity is a prerequisite for success (here also due to matching MHC restriction of the developing T cells).[60,63,64] For transplantation of other organs, e.g., liver, HLA matching is not an advantage.[65] Regardless of HLA matching, immunosuppression is obligatory for all organ transplantation and usually has to be applied indefinitely to suppress alloreactivity.

An interesting aspect arises from the subclass of alloreactive T cells specifically recognizing individual peptides.[53] Such T cells might be involved in the positive effects of the so-called graft-versus-leukemia (GvL) reaction.[66] If bone marrow is transplanted as a therapeutic measure for leukemia, especially for chronic myelogenic leukemia (CML), it is observed that these recipients suffering from GvH have a lower incidence of leukemia relapse.[66] It is believed that either a fraction of the GvH T cells or a separate set of GvL T cells mediate leukemia cell destruction; indeed, additional transfusion of donor T cells after engraftment of the transplanted bone marrow or stem cells is used as a therapeutic measure against relapse.[67] At least in haploidentical donor-recipient combinations, the possibility exists that some of the GvL T cells recognize leukemia-specific peptides on recipient MHC molecules allogeneic to the T cells. Along these lines, it has been speculated that 'allorestricted' T cells, that is, those recognizing a specific peptide on foreign MHC molecules, might be useful to generate T cells against all sorts of peptides including those not seen by self-MHC restricted T cells due to self tolerance.[68] This would be especially interesting for antigen being expressed predominantly in certain tumor cells but only marginally in normal cells, such as the tumor suppressor molecule p53. Indeed, allorestricted T cells specific for a tumor-associated antigen, MDM2, have been described recently.[69] These CTL are able to recognize tumor cells and even show some in vivo effects. Although associated with several problems, allorestricted T cells might have a future for certain applications in tumor therapy. I use this possibility to attach a paper on allorestricted T cells that was written in 1984, but was never published, maybe because it was premature at that time. The manuscript, stemming from the 'pre-peptide' era of MHC–immunology, discusses aspects that might still be interesting, especially when applied with our modern tools and knowledge on MHC and peptides.

Historical manuscript written naively in 1984 but never published since. Reprinted here without alterations.

TISSUE SPECIFIC CYTOTOXIC T-CELLS PRODUCED BY SUBTRACTIVE IMMUNIZATION IN VITRO

Hans-Georg Rammensee

Cytotoxic T lymphocytes (CTL) specific for polymorphic tissue specific antigens coded for by genes outside of the major histocompatibility complex (MHC) can be readily obtained (1,2) after in vivo immunization between pairs of congenic strains of mice, which differ in genes coding for the tissue specific antigens, but have identical sets of major histocompatibility complex genes (due to the MHC-restricted recognition of antigen by CTL (3). These requirements preclude the production of CTL specific for monomorphic antigens with conventional methods, and make it almost impossible to demonstrate tissue specific CTL in outbred populations, such as humans. Here I show in an example, that a new technology of subtractive immunization entirely in vitro allows the production of tissue specific CTL lines, potentially in outbred populations, regardless of whether or not the antigen recognized is polymorphic. Such tissue specific CTL might be useful for removing unwanted tissue, like tumors, in vivo. Due to the requirement of self tolerance, there is a blind spot in the T cell repertoire of any individual. Self aggressive T cells which recognize self antigens in context of self MHC are not allowed in a healthy immune system. In contrast, T cells recognizing self antigens in context of foreign MHC are allowed (4,7) and can be detected in spleens of normal animals after the excess of T cells reacting against the foreign MHC alone had been removed .These findings implicate that the allorestricted repertoire of T cells is potentially unlimited, or does not need to have a blind spot, in contrast to the self restricted repertoire (8). Potentially, the entire genomic T cell repertoire can be tapped by using the allorestricted repertoire of several MHC-different strains. We have proposed, based on such considerations, that the use of the allorestricted T cell repertoire would make it possible to produce tissue specific CTL, regardless of whether the tissue specific antigen is monomorphic (i.e., it is identical to a self antigen for the responding T cell) or not (4).

In the experiments described below, I show in an example that tissue specific CTL can be obtained by subtractive immunization entirely in vitro, following the schedule: A minus B1 anti B2. A stands here for T cells from mouse A, B1 stands for tissue 1 from a mouse B (which differs from A in the MHC genes), B2 stands for tissue 2 from mouse B. CTL recognizing B2, but not B1, are then considered as tissue specific CTL. In addition to allorestricted, tissue-specific CTL, this system would potentially also reveal any MHC Class I antigen expressed on B2, but not on B1 or in the mouse A; this underlines the potency of this system,

Splenic T cells of B10.BR (H-2^k) mice were depleted of reactivity against C57BL/6 (B6, H-2^b) spleen cells with the Bromodeoxyuridine and light method. The surviving cells were primed in limiting dilution against B6-lymphoma cells (EL4). The priming in limiting dilution rather than in bulk culture was necessary because the depletion of alloreactive cells is incomplete with this method; the screening of many single clones enhances the chance to detect the allorestricted CTL among the remaining alloreactive ones, [In the meantime, we have developed a better method for removing alloreactive CTL using antibodies against the transferrin receptor (H.-G.R., J. Lesley, I. Trowbridge and M.J. Bevan, manuscript in preparation). After restimulation, all the EL4 reactive clones and lines obtained were tested for killing of EL4 tumor cells and Concanavalin A induced blasts of B6 origin (Fig. 1). Clones or lines killing virtually only EL4 cells, but not B6 blasts, were expanded and tested again on both targets with titrated effector:target ratios. Some CTL lines turned out to kill EL4 strongly but at high effector: target cell ratios, they lysed also B6 blasts to some extent. These lines were discarded. A few CTL lines, however, were truly specific for EL4 and did not kill B6 blasts at all, as can be seen

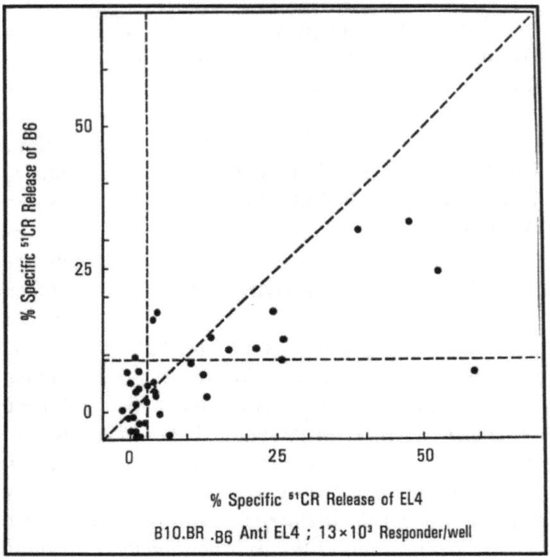

Fig. 1. B10.BR(H-2^k) spleen cells were depleted of reactivity against C57BL/6 (B6, H-2^b) stimulator cells as described. Briefly, responder cells were cultured with irradiated (3000 R) stimulators for 7 days. 6 x 10^{-5} M 5-bromo-2'-deoxyundine (Sigma) was added one day after initiation of the culture (day 1), and on days 3, 4, 5, 6 and 7, the cultures were exposed to light for 90 min. Fresh Bromodeoxyuridine (10^{-4} M), 5% rat Concanavalin A Sup and 50 mM-methyl--D-mannoside was added on day 4. The surviving cells were primed in vitro under limiting dilution conditions in round bottomed 96-well microtiter plates (Costar 3799) with 7 x 10^3 irradiated (6000 R) EL4 thymoma cells (H-2^b, of B6 origin) per well as source of antigen and 7 x 10^5 irradiated (3000 R) B6 spleen cells per well as fillers in the presence of rat Concanavalin A supernatant and methyl mannoside for 7 days, in a total volume of 0.2 ml . Then each plate was split by transferring half of the cell suspension of each well to a new plate. New medium, stimulators and fillers were added to each well to reconstitute the culture volume. After additional 6 days of culture, the contents of each individual well were split and tested in a ^{51}Cr release assay for the killing of B6 blasts of EL4 tumor targets, Each point in the figure represents the effector cells from a single well seeded at 1.3 x 10^4 responder cells/well on day 7 in 38 replicates, Spontaneous release in presence of stimulators alone was 5,3% for EL4 and 9,4% for B6 blasts. The dotted parallels to the axis represent % specific ^{51}Cr release in the absence of responders plus 3 standard deviations for each target.

for one of the CTL lines, called 1304-1E5 in Fig. 2. This line was tested, after further expansion, on a panel of target cells, which is shown in Fig. 2b-d; these data and the characteristics of the target cells are summarized in Table 1. No lysis of Concanavalin A induced blasts of B6 female, B10 male, or BALB.B origin excludes H-2^b alone or H-2^b plus the male specific H-Y antigen as being recognized by 1E5. EL4, as well as its subline 2F6, which has been separated from EL4 several years ago, are killed. An H-2^b expressing T lymphoma is not killed, indicating the antigen in question is not common to all tumors of T lineage. Two lymphomas of the mouse strain AKR (H-2^k) are not lysed, excluding unrestricted recognition of TL determinants (which so far has not been reported for CTL anyway). B6 and B10.BR thymocytes are not lysed, excluding an antigen common on all thymus-derived cells. H-2^d or (H-2^b x H-2^d) tumors of the B-cell lineage and an H-2^b tumor of the fibroblast lineage are not killed, illustrating the tissue specificity of this antigen. Surprisingly, of five H-2^b CTL clones tested as target cells, one, of BALB.B origin and specific for H-$2D^d$, was lysed well; another one, also of BALB.B origin, but specific for H-$2L^d$ was not lysed. The three others were killed intermediately. This might suggest that a determinant on the T cell receptor for antigen, or on a molecule physically associated to the latter, is recognized, The killing efficiency of two of these targets (G4 and CTLL; both are CTL clones) was considerably variable between different experiments; compare for example the lysis of G4 in Fig. 2B and- 2D. In another experiment (not shown), CTLL target cells were killed as efficiently as EL4 targets, in contrast to the experiment in Figure 2D, where CTLL targets were lysed only intermediately. This could be due to different levels of antigen expression during the culture cycles of these CTL clones. G4 is restimulated every seven days with antigen plus IL-2; CTLL

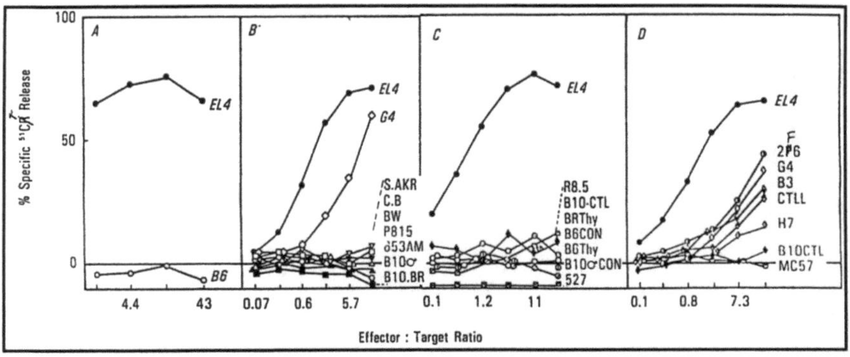

Fig. 2. The contents of the well shown in Fig. 1 to kill 55% of EL4 targets but no significant portion of B6 blasts were expanded for one week in one well of a 24-well plate (Costar 3424) in a total of 2 ml of the same medium used in limiting dilution cultures with 5×10^4 EL4 stimulators and 5×10^6 B6 fillers. Thereafter, this CTL line, called 1304-1E5, was maintained in 50 ml culture flasks (Falcon 3013) in upright position with 2×10^5 EL4 stimulators and 2×10^7 B10.BR fillers in a total volume of 10ml. Four to 6 days after restimulation, samples of the cells were tested in 3-fold titration in 51Cr release assays on the targets indicated in the figure. The characteristics of these target cells are given in Table 1. Spontaneous release of the individual targets was between 4.9% and 23.5%, except for H-7 (43.6%) and the hybridoma 527 (58.9%)o A, B, C, and D represent four independent assays.

is grown in IL-2 containing medium and is split when a high density is reached.

The reactivity pattern of another EL4-specific CTL line obtained in the same experiment is shown in Figure 3 and Table 1. The specificity of this line is very similar to that of 1E5, in that it kills EL4 tumor cells, but no cells of other tissues tested, except some CTL clones of H-2^b origin. In contrast to 1E5, however, the CTL line 3A8 does not kill G4, indicating that the two CTL lines recognize different epitopes. Both CTL lines lyse in vivo passaged EL4 cells suggesting that the antigen recognized is not due to a culture-induced artifact (data not shown).

Although these reactivity patterns do not reveal the identity of the antigens being recognized by both CTL lines, they indicate one thing: Highly tissue specific, or cell-line specific, cell surface antigens are involved, present on at least one, but not all, tumors of the T lineage, and on some, but not all, CTL clones. It is possible that these antigens are encoded not by cellular but by viral genes expressed only in certain cells, which again underlines the potency of the method of subtractive immunization. Both tissue specific antigens are probably recognized in context of H-2K^b products because monoclonal antibodies against K^b completely block the killing of EL4 target cells by both CTL lines (data not shown), There are, however, alternative possibilities, what these CTL defined antigens on EL4 and some H-2^b CTL clones could be. (I) It is not a distinct antigen at all, but just a difference in density of the K^b molecule on EL4 cells as compared to Con A blasts, fibroblasts or thymocytes; this tissue-specific difference in antigen density could then be detected by CTL(9). (II) A somatic mutation in a class I molecule during the 40 years or so EL4 cells have been maintained created a new antigenic determinant. However, this is unlikely because the same mutation should have occurred then independently in the four CTL clones killed by 1304-1E5. Moreover, the EL4 cells used in these experiments kill B6 mice, when injected i.p. (data not shown), suggesting that they do not express strong transplantation antigens different from B6 antigens. (III) The antigen is a tissue specific Ia-like antigen crossreacting with K^b such as Qam208, which has been described recently. (10) Whichever of these four possibilities is the correct one will be difficult to prove. The point of this paper, however, is not to demonstrate and to identify on lymphoma cells a CTL-defined antigen, which may or may not be identical with cell surface

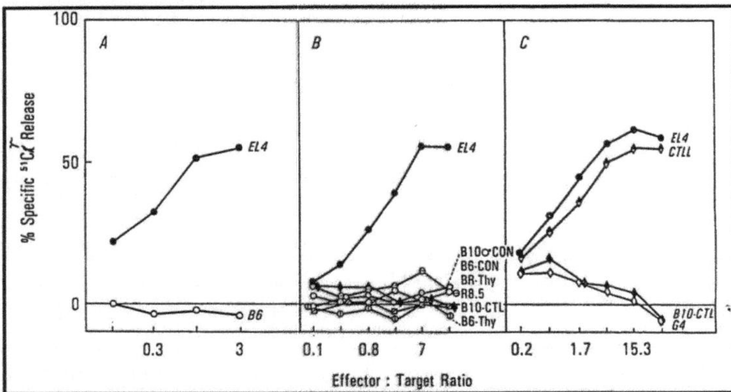

Fig. 3. Reactivity pattern of another EL-4 specific CTL line, 1304-3A8, derived from the experiment in Fig. 1. This line was propagated as described in Fig. 2 for 1304-1E5, and tested on the targets indicated in the figure. The characteristics of these targets and additional ones not included in this figure are shown in Table 1. Spontaneous release was between 4.9% and 37.6%. A, B, and C represent three independent assays.

antigens already described by use of other immunological methods. The significance of this paper lies in the demonstration of a method which allows potentially the production of tissue specific CTL, regardless whether or not the genes encoding the recognized antigens display allelic variation within the species, and regardless of whether or not inbred strains are available in that species.

The availability of a method to produce such allogeneic, allorestricted, tissue specific CTL could be useful for the now somewhat ailing field of tumor immunology. Namely, the dilemma of this field is the uncertainty whether tumor specific antigens exist on spontaneous tumors, i.e., antigens expressed only on the tumor cells. but not at all on any of the other cells of the host. The recent revelations on the relation between oncogenes and genes involved in the normal growth of cells suggest that tumor cells do not need to express new antigens absent from normal cells. A more promising strategy for the immunotherapy of tumors would be to look for such tissue specific antigens which are for sure expressed on the tumor cells, are not expressed on cells of vital function in the host and may or may not be expressed on normal host cells without vital function. If such antigens can be found on a given tumor, immunological reagents can be engineered to remove from the host the tumor cells together with the innocent bystander cells (with non-vital function) expressing the target antigen. Candidates for such tissue specific tumor antigens limited to cells of non-vital function include especially such differentiation antigens which are expressed only in certain tissues and only during certain stages of the cell cycle.

This strategy of immune therapy is now widely explored with antibodies directed against tissue specific antigens. For one example, E. Vitetta and colleagues treated mice from an IgD-expressing B cell lymphoma by injecting toxin-conjugated antibodies anti-IgD. IgD is expressed on all immature B cells during a certain stage of differentiation; the transient removal of the IgD-positive cells during the therapy had no intolerable side effects to the mice. This example shows that it is possible to remove tumor cells from a body together with some other cells of non-vital function without killing the host altogether. However, the use of antibodies for the elimination of tumor cells in vivo has limitations: naked antibodies may frequently not be sufficiently cytotoxic in vivo, and treatment with toxin conjugated antibodies bears the risk of side effects on the host by the toxin itself, especially when antibody and toxin fall apart, or are degradated in vivo.

Target Cells	H-2	Lysis by 1304-1E5	Lysis by 1304-3A8
B6 (♀) Con A Blasts	b	-	-
B10 (♂) Con A Blasts	b	-	-
BALB.B Con A Blasts	b	-	N.D.
B10.BR Con A Blasts	b	-	-
EL4; B6 Lymphoma	b	+++	+++
2F6; Subline of EL4	b	++	N.D.
R8.5; (B6xBALB/c)F_1 T Lymphoma	b/d	-	-
BW5147; AKR Lymphoma	k	-	-
S.AKR; AKR Lymphoma	k	-	N.D.
B6 Thymocytes	b	-	-
B10.BR Thymocytes	k	-	-
P815; DBA/2 Mastocytoma	d	-	-
653AM; BALB/c Myeloma	d	-	-
527; (B6xSP2) B Hybridoma	b/d	-	-
MC57; B6 Fibroblast Line	b	-	N.D.
G4; BALB.B CTL CLone Anti H-2D^d	b	++	-
B10; BALB.B CTL Clone Anti H-2L^d	b	-	-
B3; B6 CTL Clone Anti BALB.B	b	++	+
H7; B6 CTL CLone Anti BALB.B	b	+	N.D.
CTLL; B6 CTL Clone	b	++	+++

Table 1. Specificity of CTL lines 1304-1E5 and 1304-3A8

Tissue specific CTL could be used for immunotherapy in vivo instead of toxin conjugated tissue-specific antibodies, Established tumors, as well as allografts, can be destroyed with participation of CTL by adoptive transfer of in vivo primed T cells. However, the use of in vitro propagated T cells, especially CTL, turned out to be problematic. Cloned IL-2 dependent CTL were shown to destroy tissue in vivo when applied locally. However, when IL-2 dependent CTL were applied systemically, they did migrate only poorly to lymphoid tissues (16). This could be due to the lack of specific homing receptors which are needed by T cells for orientation within the lymphoid system. Another reason, however, could be the IL-2 dependency of most in vitro propagated CTL. IL-2 levels in body fluids, like serum, are kept down by inhibitors and are too low to be detected, so that IL-2 dependent CTL would die soon after in vivo inoculation (17). Indeed, administration of IL-2 in vivo, together with in vitro grown tumor-specific CTL and cyclophosphamide, which is believed to inhibit IL-2 inhibition in vivo (18), cured a significant portion of mice from leukemia. In other studies, the migration of IL-2-dependent tumor-specific CTL to the tumor was improved by the in vivo administration of IL-2 (19,20). Finally, IL-2 independent CTL clones could mediate tumor rejection after application, suggesting that the requirements for the in vivo performance of cloned CTL are not yet sufficiently explored. Taken together, it is possible that tumor therapy with in vivo propagated CTL will become feasible, and if so, the method of subtractive immunization described in this paper will enable the production of CTL with the desired specificities also in outbred populations, like humans.

Such allorestricted, tissue specific CTL produced by the described subtractive immunization, however, cause an additional problem. They are, by design, MHC-incompatible to the individual whose tissue they recognize. Inoculation of these allogeneic cells into that individual will lead to their rejection unless the host has been made tolerant to the MHC products on the tissue-specific CTL or is at least transiently immunosuppressed. Alternatively, the CTL must be applied in such a way that they act fast enough to have finished their job of eliminating their target cells before they are killed themselves (15).

In addition to all these eventually manageable problems, there is a principal limitation to the application of CTL in general, which lies in their manner to recognize antigen always in context of MHC products. For cells lacking MHC expression, no CTL can be produced.

Taken together, the use of allogeneic, allorestricted, tissue specific CTL produced by subtractive immunization in vitro may lead to progress in tumor immunology, although limited to such tumors expressing (1) MHC products, and (2) a tissue specific antigen not shared with cells of vital function in the host.

I would like to thank L. Sherman, J. Shiel, B. Froscher, R. Ahmed and L. Lefrancois for providing cell lines, L. Sherman and M. Bevan for helpful discussions, and M. Bevan for giving me the opportunity to work in his laboratory. This work was supported by Grant RA 369/1-1 of the Deutsche Forschungsgemeinschaft.

REFERENCES

1. *Forman, J. Ciavarra, R, and Vitetta, E.J. J. Exp. Med. 154:1357 (1981).*
2. *Steinmuller, D., Tyler, J.D., and David, C.S. J. Immunol. 126:1747 (1981).*
3. *Bevan, M.J. Nature 256:419 (1975).*
4. *Rammensee, H.-G. and Bevan, M.J. Nature 308:741 (1984).*
5. *Dos Reis, G.A. and Shevach, E.M, J. Exp. Med. 157:1287 (1983).*
6. *Groves, E.S. and Singer, A.J. Exp, Med, 158:1483 (1983).*
7. *Matzinger, P., Zamoyska, R. and Waldmann, H. Nature 308:738 (1984).*
8. *Ishii, N., Nagy, Z.A, and Klein, J. Nature 295:531 (1982).*
9. *Bevan, M.J . Immunol. Today, in press (1984).*
10. *Oudshoorn-Snoek, M., Mellor, A.L., Flavell, R.A., and Demant, P. Immunogenetics 19:461 (1984).*
11. *Weiss, D.W. Transpl. Proceed. 16:545 (1984).*
12. *Doolittle, R. et al. Science 221:275 (1983).*
13. *Vitetta, E.S., Krulick, K.A., Miyama-Inaba, M., Cashley, W. and Uhr, J.W. Science 219:644 (1983).*
14. *Mills, C.D. and North, R.J. J. Exp. Med, 157:1448 (1983).*
15. *Tyler, J.D., Gralli, S.J., Snider, M.E., Dvorak, A.M. and Steinmuller, D. J. Exp. Med. 159:234 (1984).*
16. *Caroll, A.M., Palladino, M.A., Oettgen, H., and Defonsa, M. Cell. Immunol. 76:69 (1983).*
17. *Gallatin, W.M., Weissman, I.L., and Butcher, E.C. Nature 304:30 (1983).*
18. *Hardt, C., Rollinghoff, M., Pfizenmaier, K., Mosmann, H. and Wagner, H. J. Exp. Med. 154:262 (1981).*
19. *Cheever, M.A., Greenberg, P.O., Fefer, A., and Gillis, S. J. Exp. Med. 155:968 (1982).*
20. *Palladino, M.A., Welte, K., Caroll, A.M, and Oettgen, H.F. Cell. Immunol. 86:299 (1984).*
21. *Engers, H.D., Glasebrook, A.L. and Sorensorl, G.D, J. Exp. Med. 156:1280 (1982).*
22. *Engers, H.D., Lahaye, T., Sorenson, G.D., Glasebrook, A.L. Horvath, C., and Brunner, K.T.J. Immunol. 133:1664 (1984).*
23. *Rammensee, H.-G., Bevan, M.J. and Fink, P.J. Immunol. Today, in press (1984).*

A special situation of alloreactivity occurs when organs are grafted between HLA identical individuals, or between MHC identical animal strains that differ at non-MHC loci.[70-73] In these cases, recipient T cells can react against MHC-presented peptides derived from polymorphic gene products differing between donor and recipient.[74,75] This reaction is usually weaker as compared to alloreactivity against MHC incompatibility; the antigens recognized here are therefore called 'minor histocompatibility antigens'.[71,73,76] The molecular identification of these peptides started only recently;[74,77-82] a list of the few peptides known to date is in Table 5.2. It is assumed that each of the normal MHC ligands, such as those listed in Table 5.2, can behave as a minor histocompatibility antigen if donor and recipient happen to differ in their peptide sequences, or in their expression altogether, as is the case with the male-specific peptides upon transplantation of male cells into female recipients.[83-85] In addition to polymorphic MHC-presented peptides, allelic forms of β2-microglobulin can behave as minor histocompatibility antigens.[86]

IMMUNITY AGAINST INFECTION

The first line of defense against viral and bacterial infections are the different non-adaptive branches of the immune system, such as the complement system and antigen-nonspecific effector cells activated by disturbances of their normal surroundings. The specific, adaptive immune response against infections by virus, bacteria, and eukaryotic parasites is strictly controlled by MHC-restricted antigen presentation. Antibody responses upstream of IgM are regulated by T-B interaction. This holds true for the initiation of the response, for its magnitude, and the antibody isotype eventually produced. Helper T cells recognize MHC II-presented fragments of the same antigen as seen by the B cell's surface immunoglobulin. Thus, MHC restricted antigen presentation mediates cell-to-cell contact of helper T cells with the matching B cell.

For cell-mediated immunity, as well as the initiation of T helper cells, the antigens on the infectious agent have to be internalized by antigen-presenting cells before T cells can take action. Bacteria or other particles are engulfed by the professional antigen presenting cells, macrophages and dendritic cells, their antigens processed, and peptides thereby presented on MHC II, sometimes also MHC I, molecules to be seen by T cells. For cell-mediated immunity against viral infections, the infected cell presents fragments of the newly produced viral antigens on their MHC I molecule to be recognized by $CD8^+$ cytotoxic T cells.[93] All MHC I expressing cells can present viral peptides after infection and are then prone to recognition and destruction by cytotoxic T cells. For the initiation of CTL to occur, however, antigen has to be presented on dendritic cells or macrophages.[94] The viral antigen can reach MHC I molecules of antigen-presenting cells either upon direct infection of these cells or upon engulfment of viral particles, or upon uptake of debris of infected cells.[95] An interesting hypothesis here is that priming of $CD8^+$ T cells against cellular antigens in general, including those of viral origin, is mediated by APC that have taken up a peptide loaded chaperone, gp96, released from the infected or affected cells.[96]

In addition to antigens regularly presented by MHC molecules, T cells can be activated by superantigens that bridge MHC molecules and T cell receptor α or β chains (see Fig. 5.1) independent of the MHC-bound peptide.[97,98,99] Such responses are potentially associated with septic shock, food poisoning, and other diseases. Superantigens also influence the available T cell repertoire, since the responding T cells can undergo anergy or deletion.[100,101]

Peptide antigens derived from viruses or bacteria and recognized by specific $CD4^+$ or $CD8^+$ T cells have been studied for a long time. The identification of naturally MHC processed peptides of viral origin was first reported for influenza and vesicular stomatitis virus in 1990.[102,103] Since then, a large number of natural ligands or T cell epitopes from all kinds of infectious agents have been reported. Tables 5.3, 5.4, and 5.5 show collections of MHC-restricted peptides from viral and other sources.

A comment on the distinction between natural MHC ligand and T cell epitope seems appropriate here. A peptide is classified as a natural MHC ligand only if it has been eluted from MHC molecules and either directly sequenced, or identified by biochemical comparison with synthetic peptides. If there are T cells for it, the ligand is of course also a T cell epitope. If a peptide, however, is only known to be recognized by MHC-restricted T cells, it cannot be classified as a ligand at the same time, even if it fits well to an MHC motif, and its nature as a ligand is very likely. Only peptides recognized by T cells that also recognize the relevant infected or otherwise antigen-expressing cell are classified as T cell epitopes. If a peptide is recognized by T cells after priming and stimulation with that peptide, and the T cells do not recognize the relevant natural target (e.g., virus-infected cell), the peptide is irrelevant and not treated differently from peptides that merely bind to MHC molecules: such peptides are only occasionally considered in this book. Two reasons could account for the frequently observed situation that a peptide-specific T cell is not relevant for the natural target:

1) The peptide-stimulated T cell is of low affinity, e.g., needs 20 000 or so peptide copies on the target cell,[361] whereas the natural target may have only a few hundred or less.[223]
2) The peptide-stimulated T cell, if of high affinity, does not find its peptide on the natural target cell since it is not processed.[362]

This situation can happen, e.g., if a motif selected peptide is used for stimulation. Thus, for T cell epitopes to determine, or for evaluating the relevance of peptide stimulated T cells, the 'acid test'[95] of testing recognition of the natural target is unavoidable.

AUTOIMMUNITY AND SELF TOLERANCE

Most of the peptides presented by MHC I or II molecules on the cells of a healthy individual are self peptides derived from all kinds of physiological proteins (Tables 5.6 to 5.7). T cells specific for such self peptides underly the various mechanisms of self tolerance, e.g., central clonal deletion in the thymus for all peptides presented with sufficient abundance on thymic antigen-presenting cells,[27] or peripheral mechanisms such as clonal anergy and deletion following continuous presentation of self antigen to T cells in the absence of costimulatory signals.[363,364] However, self antigen reactive T cells still exist among the mature T cell population,[30] and activation of these may occur, e.g., upon crossreactivity with foreign antigens.[365,366] The result of such self-reactive T cells can be autoimmune disease.

The involvement of MHC molecules in autoimmune diseases is indicated by the HLA association shown by most if not all autoimmune diseases (Table 5.8). In most cases, neither the autoantigen involved nor the mechanism responsible for the HLA-association are known. Presentation of the disease-inducing peptides by the associated HLA-molecule is only one of the possible explanations. Another explanation is that a fragment of the associated HLA-molecule itself is crossreactive to the disease-inducing antigen, and therefore, affects the T cell repertoire directly or indirectly.

Comparing the peptide specificity of disease-associated and of closely-related non-associated HLA molecules may give some insight into the mechanism underlying the disease, and may help to identify the disease in many peptides.[374, 382,462] An example for such a consideration is rheumatoid arthritis. At least for certain populations, this disease is associated with HLA-DR4 subtypes DRB1*0401 and DRB1*0404, and not at all with DRB1*0402. Other alleles are associated intermediately. A comparison of the peptide motifs of associated and non-associated allelic products indicate disease-associated characteristics of the motifs, e.g., preference of a negative charge and disfavoring of a positive charge at P4 of the associated DRB1*0401 and DRB1*0404 motifs, whereas the opposite is true for the non-associated DRB1*0402.[463,447] These features can be satisfactorily explained by the structure of the respective pockets. Thus, one may postulate that the RA-inducing peptide must have a negative charge at P4 (and otherwise be conform to the rest of the respective DR4 motifs). Similar considerations can be drawn for other autoimmune diseases, when associated and non-associated MHC molecules are closely related. An especially interesting HLA polymorphism is at residue 57 of the HLA class II beta chain, β57, which is frequently an Asp, whereas a number of autoimmune diseases are associated with HLA DR or DQ molecules with a non-Asp β57, e.g., β57Ser.[464,465] Table 5.8 shows a list of autoimmune diseases together with their associated HLA alleles.

TUMOR IMMUNOLOGY

Tumor immunology came of age with the identification of structurally defined tumor antigens.[466] Antibodies specific for tumor-associated antigen have been beneficial for diagnosis and therapy.[467-470] For an impressive example, antibodies against an epithelial antigen (that is, a tissue rather than a tumor-specific antigen) have been used successfully for treatment of minimal residue disease in breast cancer patients.[470] Definition of tumor antigens recognized by T cells, pioneered by Thierry Boon and colleagues,[471,472] has revolutionized the possibilities for development of vaccine and therapeutic measures.[466,473-475]

Tumor-expressed antigens recognized by patient T cells are not necessarily tumor-specific. The first human T cell-recognized tumor antigen, MAGE1, for example, is not only expressed on melanoma cells but also in testis;[472] another CTL-recognized tumor antigen, tyrosinase, is even a tissue-specific antigen expressed on melanocytes.[425,423,427] These antigens, recognized by tumor-destroying T cells from a patient, teach us that a number of additional antigens highly expressed in the tumor but with low or restricted expression otherwise might be suitable candidates for T cell mediated tumor immunity, in addition to the really tumor-specific but rare antigens, e.g., mutated gene products. The sorts of antigen that may be considered here include oncogene and tumor-suppressor gene products, viral antigens, differentiation antigens, aberrantly expressed frameshift mutations, or fusion proteins.[476] For many of these antigens, T cell response will not spontaneously arise in patients. Thus, there are two problems. First, the antigens actually presented by MHC molecules on tumor cells have to be identified. For this task, the knowledge of MHC motifs allows prediction of expected T cell epitopes from candidate proteins. Second, ways have to be found to use tumor-associated epitopes for activating patient T cells. The second task is formidable. The easiest would be to immunize patients with synthetic peptides representing the tumor antigens.[477] This has the disadvantage that the peptides to be used have to be selected individually for each patient, depending on tumor type and HLA expression. Initial attempts in this direction are encouraging.[477] However, depending on the immune status of the patient and the state of the disease, more efficient measures might be necessary, such as immunization together with an adjuvant or with lipopeptides; the extreme being in vitro stimulation and expansion of T cells followed by adoptive transfer back to the patient.[475] For such in vitro stimulation, as well as for more efficient in vivo T cell activation, antigen presentation on dendritic cells might be the most promising approach.[478] Choices for the delivery of the antigens range from transfection of antigen-presenting cells to the use of recombinant viral vesicles, protein preparations, or synthetic peptides. No matter which of the forms of delivery are used, monitoring of the success of such treatment requires information on the T cell epitopes involved. The MHC motifs collected in this book should be of help in identifying such T cell epitopes. Table 5.9 shows a list of MHC class I-restricted tumor-associated peptides already known. The identification of class II restricted tumor-associated epitopes has only recently begun;[479] such epitopes might be important to initiate and sustain a $CD8^+$ T cell response.[480]

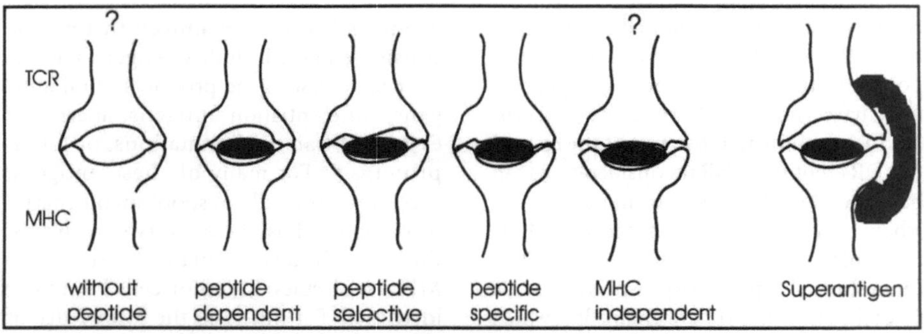

Fig. 5.1. Possibilities for the antigen specificity of alloreactive and superantigen reactive T cells.

*Table 5.1. Natural killer inhibitory receptors and MHC counterparts**

Receptor	Type	Inhibitory MHC molecules
Mouse		
Ly-49A	C-type lectin	H2-D^d, H2-D^k
Ly-49C	C-type lectin	H2-K^b, $H2^d$, $H2^k$, $H2^s$
Ly-49G2	C-type lectin	H2-D^d, H2-L^d
Human		
NKAT1	Two Ig-SF domains (p58.1)	HLA-Cw2, Cw4, Cw5, Cw6
NKAT2	Two Ig-SF domains (p58.2)	HLA-Cw1, Cw3, Cw7, Cw8, Cw9
NKAT3	Three Ig-SF domains (p70)	HLA-B*5101, B*5801, B*2705, HLA-G
NKAT4	Three Ig-SF domains (p140)	HLA-A*0301
CD94/NKG2A	C-type lectin heterodimer	HLA-A, Bw6, C

*See references 6-12; SF, Superfamily.

Table 5.2. Minor histocompatibility peptides

Protein/Gene	AA position	T cell epitope/MHC ligand	MHC molecule	References
B6 (dom)	-	AAPDNRETF	H2-D^b	87
Human SMCY	-	SPSVDKARAEL	HLA-B7	88
Murine SMCY	-	TENSGKDI	H2-K^k	89
Myosin family	-	YIGEVLVSV	HLA-A*0201	90
ND1α	1-17	fMFFINILTLLVPILIAM	H2-M3	91
ND1α	1-12	fMFFINILTLLVP	H2-M3	92
ND1β	1-17	fMFFINALTLLVPILIAM	H2-M3	91
ND1β	1-12	fMFFINALTLLVP	H2-M3	92
UTY protein (mouse)		WMHHNMDLI	H2-D^b	78

Table 5.3. Viral epitopes on MHC class I molecules

Virus	Protein	AA position	T cell epitope/ MHC ligand	MHC molecule	Ref.
Adenovirus 3	E3 9Kd	30-38	LIVIGILIL	HLA-A*0201	104
Adenovirus 5	E1A	234-243	SGPSNTPPEI	H2-D^b	105
Adenovirus 5	E1B	192-200	VNIRNCCYI	H2-D^b	106
Adenovirus 5	E1A	234-243	SGPSNIPPEI (T>I)	H2-D^b	106
CSFV	NS polyprotein	2276-2284	ENALLVALF	SLA, haplotype d/d	107
Dengue virus 4	NS3	500-508	TPEGIIPTL	HLA-B*3501	108, 109
EBV	LMP-2	426-434	CLGGLLTMV	HLA-A*0201	110
EBV	EBNA-1	480-484	NIAEGLRAL	HLA-A*0201	111
EBV	EBNA-1	519-527	NLRRGTALA	HLA-A*0201	111
EBV	EBNA-1	525-533	ALAIPQCRL	HLA-A*0201	111
EBV	EBNA-1	575-582	VLKDAIKDL	HLA-A*0201	111
EBV	EBNA-1	562-570	FMVFLQTHI	HLA-A*0201	111
EBV	EBNA-2	15-23	HLIVDTDSL	HLA-A*0201	111
EBV	EBNA-2	22-30	SLGNPSLSV	HLA-A*0201	111
EBV	EBNA-2	126-134	PLASAMRML	HLA-A*0201	111
EBV	EBNA-2	132-140	RMLWMANYI	HLA-A*0201	111
EBV	EBNA-2	133-141	MLWMANYIV	HLA-A*0201	111
EBV	EBNA-2	151-159	ILPQGPQTA	HLA-A*0201	111
EBV	EBNA-2	171-179	PLRPTAPTI	HLA-A*0201	111
EBV	EBNA-2	205-213	PLPPATLTV	HLA-A*0201	111
EBV	EBNA-2	246-254	RMHLPVLHV	HLA-A*0201	111
EBV	EBNA-2	287-295	PMPLPPSQL	HLA-A*0201	111
EBV	EBNA-2	294-302	QLPPPAAPA	HLA-A*0201	111
EBV	EBNA-2	381-389	SMPELSPVL	HLA-A*0201	111
EBV	EBNA-2	453-461	DLDESWDYI	HLA-A*0201	111
EBV	BZLF1	43-51	PLPCVLWPV	HLA-A*0201	111
EBV	BZLF1	167-175	SLEECDSEL	HLA-A*0201	111
EBV	BZLF1	176-184	EIKRYKNRV	HLA-A*0201	111
EBV	BZLF1	195-203	QLLQHYREV	HLA-A*0201	111
EBV	BZLF1	196-204	LLQHYREVA	HLA-A*0201	111
EBV	BZLF1	217-225	LLKQMCPSL	HLA-A*0201	111
EBV	BZLF1	229-237	SIIPRTPDV	HLA-A*0201	111
EBV	EBNA-6	284-293	LLDFVRFMGV	HLA-A*0201	112
EBV	EBNA-3	464-472	SVRDRLARL	HLA-A*0203	113
EBV	EBNA-4	416-424	IVTDFSVIK	HLA-A*1101	114, 115
EBV	EBNA-4	399-408	AVFDRKSDAK	HLA-A*0201	116
EBV	EBNA-3	246-253	RYSIFFDY	HLA-A24	113
EBV	EBNA-6	881-889	QPRAPIRPI	HLA-B7	117
EBV	EBNA-3	379-387	RPPIFIRRL	HLA-B7	117
EBV	EBNA-1	426-434	EPDVPPGAI	HLA-B7	111
EBV	EBNA-1	228-236	IPQCRLTPL	HLA-B7	111
EBV	EBNA-1	546-554	GPGPQPGPL	HLA-B7	111
EBV	EBNA-1	550-558	QPGPLRESI	HLA-B7	111
EBV	EBNA-1	72-80	RPQKRPSCI	HLA-B7	111
EBV	EBNA-2	224-232	PPTPLLTVL	HLA-B7	111
EBV	EBNA-2	241-249	TPSPPRMHL	HLA-B7	111
EBV	EBNA-2	244-252	PPRMHLPVL	HLA-B7	111
EBV	EBNA-2	254-262	VPDQSMHPL	HLA-B7	111
EBV	EBNA-2	446-454	PPSIDPADL	HLA-B7	111
EBV	BZLF1	44-52	LPCVLWPVL	HLA-B7	111
EBV	BZLF1	222-231	CPSLDVDSII	HLA-B7	111
EBV	BZLF1	234-242	TPDVLHEDL	HLA-B7	111
EBV	EBNA-3	339-347	FLRGRAYGL	HLA-B8	118
EBV	EBNA-3	26-34	QAKWRLQTL	HLA-B8	113
EBV	EBNA-3	325-333	AYPLHEQHG	HLA-B8	116
EBV	EBNA-3	158-166	YIKSFVSDA	HLA-B8	116
EBV	LMP-2	236-244	RRRWRRLTV	HLA-B*2704	119
EBV	EBNA-6	258-266	RRIYDLIEL	HLA-B*2705	119
EBV	EBNA-3	458-466	YPLHEQHGM	HLA-B*3501	120
EBV	EBNA-3	458-466	YPLHEQHGM	HLA-B*3503	113

Table 5.3. (con't)

Virus	Protein	AA position	T cell epitope/ MHC ligand	MHC molecule	Ref.
EBV	EBNA-6	335-343	KEHVIQNAF	HLA-B44	121
EBV	EBNA-6	130-139	EENLLDFVRF	HLA-B*4403	122
EBV	EBNA-2	42-51	DTPLIPLTIF	HLA-B51	121
EBV	EBNA-6	213-222	QNGALAINTF	HLA-B62	112
EBV	EBNA-3	603-611	RLRAEAGVK	HLA-A3	123
HBV	sAg	348-357	GLSPTVWLSV	HLA-A*0201	124
HBV	sAg	335-343	WLSLLVPFV	HLA-A*0201	124
HBV	cAg	18-27	FLPSDFFPSV	HLA-A*0201	125,126,127
HBV	cAg	18-27	FLPSDFFPSV	HLA-A*0202	127
HBV	cAg	18-27	FLPSDFFPSV	HLA-A*0205	127
HBV	cAg	18-27	FLPSDFFPSV	HLA-A*0206	127
HBV	pol	575-583	FLLSLGIHL	HLA-A*0201	128
HBV	pol	816-824	SLYADSPSV	HLA-A*0201	128
HBV	pol	455-463	GLSRYVARL	HLA-A*0201	128
HBV	env	338-347	LLVPFVQWFV	HLA-A*0201	129
HBV	pol	642-650	ALMPLYACI	HLA-A*0201	129
HBV	env	378-387	LLPIFFCLWV	HLA-A*0201	129
HBV	pol	538-546	YMDDVVLGA	HLA-A*0201	129
HBV	env	250-258	LLLCLIFLL	HLA-A*0201	130
HBV	env	260-269	LLDYQGMLPV	HLA-A*0201	130
HBV	env	370-379	SIVSPFIPLL	HLA-A*0201	130
HBV	env	183-191	FLLTRILTI	HLA-A*0201	130
HBV	cAg	88-96	YVNVNMGLK	HLA-A*1101	131
HBV	cAg	141-151	STLPETTVVRR	HLA-A*3101	132
HBV	cAg	141-151	STLPETTVVRR	HLA-A*6801	132
HBV	cAg	18-27	FLPSDFFPSV	HLA-A*6801	127
HBV	sAg	28-39	IPQSLDSWWTSL	H2-L^d	133
HBV	cAg	93-100	MGLKFRQL	H2-K^b	134
HBV	preS	141-149	STBXQSGXQ	HLA-A*0201	135
HCMV	gp B	618-628	FIAGNSAYEYV	HLA-A*0201	124
HCMV	E1	978-989	SDEEEAIVAYTL	HLA-B18	136
HCMV	pp65	397-411	DDVWTSGSDSDEELV	HLA-B35	137
HCMV	pp65	123-131	IPSINVHHY	HLA-B*3501	136
HCMV	pp65	495-504	NLVPMVATVQ	HLA-A*0201	137
HCMV	pp65	415-429	RKTPRVTGGGAMAGA	HLA-B7	137
HCV	MP	17-25	DLMGYIPLV	HLA-A*0201	138
HCV	MP	63-72	LLALLSCLTV	HLA-A*0201	139
HCV	MP	105-112	ILHTPGCV	HLA-A*0201	139
HCV	env E	66-75	QLRRHIDLLV	HLA-A*0201	139
HCV	env E	88-96	DLCGSVFLV	HLA-A*0201	139
HCV	env E	172-180	SMVGNWAKV	HLA-A*0201	139
HCV	NS1	308-316	HLHQNIVDV	HLA-A*0201	139
HCV	NS1	340-348	FLLLADARV	HLA-A*0201	139
HCV	NS2	234-246	GLRDLAVAVEPVV	HLA-A*0201	139
HCV	NS1	18-28	SLLAPGAKQNV	HLA-A*0201	139
HCV	NS1	19-28	LLAPGAKQNV	HLA-A*0201	139
HCV	NS4	192-201	LLFNILGGWV	HLA-A*0201	129
HCV	NS3	579-587	YLVAYQATV	HLA-A*0201	129
HCV	core protein	34-43	YLLPRRGPRL	HLA-A*0201	129
HCV	MP	63-72	LLALLSCLTI	HLA-A*0201	129
HCV	NS4	174-182	SLMAFTAAV	HLA-A*0201	140
HCV	NS3	67-75	CINGVCWTV	HLA-A*0201	140
HCV	NS3	163-171	LLCPAGHAV	HLA-A*0201	141
HCV	NS5	239-247	ILDSFDPLV	HLA-A*0201	141
HCV	NS4A	236-244	ILAGYGAGV	HLA-A*0201	142
HCV	NS5	714-722	GLQDCTMLV	HLA-A*0201	142
HCV	NS3	281-290	TGAPVTYSTY	HLA-A*0201	143
HCV	NS4A	149-157	HMWNFISGI	HLA-A*0201	144
HCV	NS5	575-583	RVCEKMALY	HLA-A3	145
HCV	NS1	238-246	TINYTIFK	HLA-A*1101	145
HCV	NS2	109-116	YISWCLWW	HLA-A23	145
HCV	core protein	40-48	GPRLGVRAT	HLA-B7	145

Table 5.3. (con't)

Virus	Protein	AA position	T cell epitope/ MHC ligand	MHC molecule	Ref.
HCV	NS3	389-397	HSKKKCDEL	HLA-B8	145
HCV	env E	44-51	ASRCWVAM	HLA-B*3501	146
HCV	core protein	27-35	GQIVGGVYL	HLA-B*40012	147
HCV	NS1	77-85	RPLTDFDQGW	HLA-B*5301	145
HCV	core protein	18-27	LMGYIPLVGA	H2-D^d	138
HCV	core protein	16-25	ADLMGYIPLV	H2-D^d	148
HCV	NS5	409-424	MSYSWTGALVTPCAEE	H2-D^d	149
HCV	NS1	205-213	KHPDATYSR	Papa-A06	150
HCV-1	NS3	400-409	KLVALGINAV	HLA-A*0201	141
HCV-1	NS3	440-448	GDFDSVIDC	Patr-B16	151
HCV-1	env E	118-126	GNASRCWVA	Patr-B16	151
HCV-1	NS1	159-167	TRPPLGNWF	Patr-B13	151
HCV-1	NS3	351-359	VPHPNIEEV	Patr-B13	151
HCV-1	NS3	438-446	YTGDFDSVI	Patr-B01	151
HCV-1	NS1	328-335	SWAIKWEY	Patr-A11	151
HCV-1	NS1	205-213	KHPDATYSR	Patr-A04	150
HCV-1	NS3	440-448	GDFDSVIDC	Patr-A04	150
HIV	gp41	583-591	RYLKDQQLL	HLA-A24	152
HIV	gag p24	267-275	IVGLNKIVR	HLA-A*3302	153, 154
HIV	gag p24	262-270	EIYKRWIIL	HLA-B8	155, 156
HIV	gag p24	261-269	GEIYKRWII	HLA-B8	155, 156
HIV	gag p17	93-101	EIKDTKEAL	HLA-B8	155, 157
HIV	gp41	586-593	YLKDQQLL	HLA-B8	158
HIV	gag p24	267-277	ILGLNKIVRMY	HLA-B*1501	153
HIV	gp41	584-592	ERYLKDQQL	HLA-B14	158
HIV	nef	115-125	YHTQGYFPQWQ	HLA-B17	159
HIV	nef	117-128	TQGYFPQWQNYT	HLA-B17	159
HIV	gp120	314-322	GRAFVTIGK	HLA-B*2705	160, 184
HIV	gag p24	263-271	KRWIILGLN	HLA-B*2702	161
HIV	nef	72-82	QVPLRPMTYK	HLA-B*3501	159
HIV	nef	117-125	TQGYFPQWQ	HLA-B*3701	159
HIV	gag p24	143-151	HQAISPRTL	HLA-Cw*0301	162
HIV	gag p24	140-151	QMVHQAISPRTL	HLA-Cw*0301	162
HIV	gp120	431-440	MYAPPIGGQI	H2-K^d	163
HIV	gp160	318-327	RGPGRAFVTI	H2-D^d	164, 165
HIV	gp120	17-29	MPGRAFVTI	H2-L^d	166, 167
HIV-1	RT	476-484	ILKEPVHGV	HLA-A*0201	168, 169
HIV-1	nef	190-198	AFHHVAREL	HLA-A*0201	170
HIV-1	gp160	120-128	KLTPLCVTL	HLA-A*0201	171
HIV-1	gp160	814-823	SLLNATDIAV	HLA-A*0201	171
HIV-1	RT	179-187	VIYQYMDDL	HLA-A*0201	172
HIV-1	gag p17	77-85	SLYNTVATL	HLA-A*0201	173
HIV-1	gp160	315-329	RGPGRAFVTI	HLA-A*0201	174
HIV-1	gp41	768-778	RLRDLLLIVTR	HLA-A3	175, 178
HIV-1	nef	73-82	QVPLRPMTYK	HLA-A3	176
HIV-1	gp120	36-45	TVYYGVPVWK	HLA-A3	177
HIV-1	gag p17	20-29	RLRPGGKKK	HLA-A3	177
HIV-1	gp120	38-46	VYYGVPVWK	HLA-A3	179
HIV-1	nef	74-82	VPLRPMTYK	HLA-A*1101	114
HIV-1	gag p24	325-333	AIFQSSMTK	HLA-A*1101	114
HIV-1	nef	73-82	QVPLRPMTYK	HLA-A*1101	180
HIV-1	nef	83-94	AAVDLSHFLKEK	HLA-A*1101	159
HIV-1	gag p24	349-359	ACQGVGGPGGHK	HLA-A*1101	181
HIV-1	gag p24	203-212	ETINEEAAEW	HLA-A25	182
HIV-1	nef	128-137	TPGPGVRYPL	HLA-B7	159
HIV-1	gag p17	24-31	GGKKKYKL	HLA-B8	183
HIV-1	gp120	2-10	RVKEKYQHL	HLA-B8	181
HIV-1	gag p24	298-306	DRFYKTLRA	HLA-B14	173
HIV-1	nef	132-147	GVRYPLTFGWCYKLVP	HLA-B18	159
HIV-1	gag p24	265-24	KRWIILGLNK	HLA-B*2705	184, 153
HIV-1	nef	190-198	AFHHVAREL	HLA-B*5201	170

Table 5.3. (con't)

Virus	Protein	AA position	T cell epitope/ MHC ligand	MHC molecule	Ref.
HIV-1	gp120	380-388	SFNCGGEFF	HLA-Cw*0401	185
HIV-1	RT	206-214	TEMEKEGKI	H2-K^k	186
HIV-1	p17	18-26	KIRLRPGGK	HLA-A*0301	187
HIV-1	p17	20-29	RLRPGGKKKY	HLA-A*0301	188
HIV-1	RT	325-333	AIFQSSMTK	HLA-A*0301	188
HIV-1	p17	84-92	TLYCVHQRI	HLA-A11	188
HIV-1	RT	508-517	IYQEPFKNLK	HLA-A11	188
HIV-1	p17	28-36	KYKLKHIVW	HLA-A24	188
HIV-1	gp120	53-62	LFCASDAKAY	HLA-A24	189
HIV-1	gag p24	145-155	QAISPRTLNAW	HLA-A25	188
HIV-1	gag p24	167-175	EVIPMFSAL	HLA-A26	188
HIV-1	RT	593-603	ETFYVDGAANR	HLA-A26	188
HIV-1	gp41	775-785	RLRDLLLIVTR	HLA-A31	190
HIV-1	RT	559-568	PIQKETWETW	HLA-A32	187
HIV-1	gp120	419-427	RIKQIINMW	HLA-A32	187
HIV-1	RT	71-79	ITLWQRPLV	HLA-A*6802	188
HIV-1	RT	85-93	DTVLEEMNL	HLA-A*6802	188
HIV-1	RT	71-79	ITLWQRPLV	HLA-A*7401	188
HIV-1	gag p24	148-156	SPRTLNAWV	HLA-B7	188
HIV-1	gag p24	179-187	ATPQDLNTM	HLA-B7	188
HIV-1	gp120	303-312	RPNNNTRKSI	HLA-B7	188
HIV-1	gp41	843-851	IPRRIRQGL	HLA-B7	188
HIV-1	p17	74-82	ELRSLYNTV	HLA-B8	188
HIV-1	nef	13-20	WPTVRERM	HLA-B8	188
HIV-1	nef	90-97	FLKEKGGL	HLA-B8	188
HIV-1	gag p24	183-191	DLNTMLNTV	HLA-B14	191
HIV-1	p17	18-27	KIRLRPGGKK	HLA-B27	188
HIV-1	p17	19-27	IRLRPGGKK	HLA-B27	188
HIV-1	gp41	791-799	GRRGWEALKY	HLA-B27	188
HIV-1	nef	73-82	QVPLRPMTYK	HLA-B27	188
HIV-1	gp41	590-597	RYLKDQQL	HLA-B27	192
HIV-1	nef	105-114	RRQDILDLWI	HLA-B*2705	188
HIV-1	nef	134-141	RYPLTFGW	HLA-B*2705	188
HIV-1	p17	36-44	WASRELERF	HLA-B35	188
HIV-1	gag p24	262-270	TVLDVGDAY	HLA-B35	188
HIV-1	gp120	42-52	VPVWKEATTTL	HLA-B35	188
HIV-1	p17	36-44	NSSKVSQNY	HLA-B35	193
HIV-1	gag p24	254-262	PPIPVGDIY	HLA-B35	193
HIV-1	RT	342-350	HPDIVIYQY	HLA-B35	193
HIV-1	gp41	611-619	TAVPWNASW	HLA-B35	194
HIV-1	gag	245-253	NPVPVGNIY	HLA-B35	193
HIV-1	nef	120-128	YFPDWQNYT	HLA-B37	188
HIV-1	gag p24	193-201	GHQAAMQML	HLA-B39	188
HIV-1	p17	20-29	RLRPGGKKKY	HLA-B42	188
HIV-1	RT	438-446	YPGIKVRQL	HLA-B42	188
HIV-1	RT	591-600	GAETFYVDGA	HLA-B45	188
HIV-1	gag p24	325-333	NANPDCKTI	HLA-B51	188
HIV-1	gag p24	275-282	RMYSPTSI	HLA-B52	188
HIV-1	gp120	42-51	VPVWKEATTT	HLA-B*5501	192
HIV-1	gag p24	147-155	ISPRTLNAW	HLA-B57	188
HIV-1	gag p24	240-249	TSTLQEQIGW	HLA-B57	188
HIV-1	gag p24	162-172	KAFSPEVIPMF	HLA-B57	188
HIV-1	gag p24	311-319	QASQEVKNW	HLA-B57	188
HIV-1	gag p24	311-319	QASQDVKNW	HLA-B57	188
HIV-1	nef	116-125	HTQGYFPDWQ	HLA-B57	188
HIV-1	nef	120-128	YFPDWQNYT	HLA-B57	188
HIV-1	gag p24	240-249	TSTLQEQIGW	HLA-B58	188
HIV-1	p17	20-29	RLRPGGKKKY	HLA-B62	188
HIV-1	p24	268-277	LGLNKIVRMY	HLA-B62	188
HIV-1	RT	415-426	LVGKLNWASQIY	HLA-B62	188
HIV-1	RT	476-485	ILKEPVHGVY	HLA-B62	188
HIV-1	nef	117-127	TQGYFPDWQNY	HLA-B62	188
HIV-1	nef	84-91	AVDLSHFL	HLA-B62	195

Table 5.3. (con't)

Virus	Protein	AA position	T cell epitope/ MHC ligand	MHC molecule	Ref.
HIV-1	gag p24	168-175	VIPMFSAL	HLA-Cw*0102	188
HIV-1	gp120	376-384	FNCGGEFFY	HLA-A29	196
HIV-1	gp120	375-383	SFNCGGEFF	HLA-B15	196
HIV-1	nef	136-145	PLTFGWCYKL	HLA-A*0201	197
HIV-1	nef	180-189	VLEWRFDSRL	HLA-A*0201	197
HIV-1	nef	68-77	FPVTPQVPLR	HLA-B7	197
HIV-1	nef	128-137	TPGPGVRYPL	HLA-B7	197
HIV-1	gag p24	308-316	QASQEVKNW	HLA-Cw*0401	521
HIV-1 IIIB	RT	273-282	VPLDEDFRKY	HLA-B35	181
HIV-1 IIIB	RT	25-33	NPDIVIYQY	HLA-B35	181
HIV-1 IIIB	gp41	557-565	RAIEAQAHL	HLA-B51	181
HIV-1 IIIB	RT	231-238	TAFTIPSI	HLA-B51	181
HIV-1 IIIB	p24	215-223	VHPVHAGPIA	HLA-B*5501	181
HIV-1 IIIB	gp120	156-165	NCSFNISTSI	HLA-Cw8	181
HIV-1 IIIB	gp120	241-249	CTNVSTVQC	HLA-Cw8	181
HIV-1_{SF2}	gp120	312-320	IGPGRAFHT	H2-D^d	198
HIV-1_{SF2}	pol	25-33	NPDIVIYQY	HLA-B*3501	199
HIV-1_{SF2}	pol	432-441	EPIVGAETFY	HLA-B*3501	199
HIV-1_{SF2}	pol	432-440	EPIVGAETF	HLA-B*3501	199
HIV-1_{SF2}	pol	6-14	SPAIFQSSM	HLA-B*3501	199
HIV-1_{SF2}	pol	59-68	VPLDKDFRKY	HLA-B*3501	199
HIV-1_{SF2}	pol	6-14	IPLTEEAEL	HLA-B*3501	199
HIV-1_{SF2}	nef	69-79	RPQVPLRPMTY	HLA-B*3501	199
HIV-1_{SF2}	nef	66-74	FPVRPQVPL	HLA-B*3501	199
HIV-1_{SF2}	env	10-18	DPNPQEVVL	HLA-B*3501	199
HIV-1_{SF2}	env	7-15	RPIVSTQLL	HLA-B*3501	199
HIV-1_{SF2}	pol	6-14	IPLTEEAEL	HLA-B51	199
HIV-1_{SF2}	env	10-18	DPNPQEVVL	HLA-B51	199
HIV-1_{SF2}	gag p24	199-207	AMQMLKETI	H2-K^d	198
HIV-2	gag p24	182-190	TPYDINQML	HLA-B*5301	200
HIV-2	gag	260-269	RRWIQLGLQK	HLA-B*2703	188
HIV_{SF2}	gp41	593-607	GIWGCSGKLICTTAV	HLA-B17	201
HIV_{SF2}	gp41	753-767	ALIWEDLRSLCLFSY	HLA-B22	201
HPV 6b	E7	21-30	GLHCYEQLV	HLA-A*0201	202
HPV 6b	E7	47-55	PLKQHFQIV	HLA-A*0201	202
HPV11	E7	4-12	RLVTLKDIV	HLA-A*0201	202
HPV16	E7	86-94	TLGIVCPIC	HLA-A*0201	129
HPV16	E7	85-93	GTLGIVCPI	HLA-A*0201	129
HPV16	E7	12-20	MLDLQPETT	HLA-A*0201	129
HPV16	E7	11-20	YMLDLQPETT	HLA-A*0201	203
HPV16	E6	15-22	RPRKLPQL	HLA-B7	204
HPV16	E7	49-57	RAHYNIVTF	H2-D^b	205
HSV	gp B	498-505	SSIEFARL	H2-K^b	206
HSV-1	gp C	480-488	GIGIGVLAA	HLA-A*0201	104
HSV-1	ICP27	448-456	DYATLGVGV	H2-K^d	207
HSV-1	ICP27	322-332	LYRTFAGNPRA	H2-K^d	207
HSV-1	UL39	822-829	QTFDFGRL	H2-K^b	208
HSV-2	gp C	446-454	GAGIGVAVL	HLA-A*0201	104
HTLV-1	TAX	11-19	LLFGYPVYV	HLA-A*0201	209
Influenza	MP	58-66	GILGFVFTL	HLA-A*0201	68,169,209, 210, 211
Influenza	MP	59-68	ILGFVFTLTV	HLA-A*0201	168, 212, 213
Influenza	NP	265-273	ILRGSVAHK	HLA-A3	214
Influenza	NP	91-99	KTGGPIYKR	HLA-A*6801	215, 216
Influenza	NP	380-388	ELRSRYWAI	HLA-B8	217
Influenza	NP	381-388	LRSRYWAI	HLA-B*2702	218
Influenza	NP	339-347	EDLRVLSFI	HLA-B*3701	219
Influenza	NS1	158-166	GEISPLPSL	HLA-B44	220
Influenza	NP	338-346	FEDLRVLSF	HLA-B44	220
Influenza	NS1	158-166	GEISPLPSL	HLA-B*4402	220
Influenza	NP	338-346	FEDLRVLSF	HLA-B*4402	220
Influenza A	PB1	591-599	VSDGGPNLY	HLA-A1	214, 29

Table 5.3. (con't)

Virus	Protein	AA position	T cell epitope/ MHC ligand	MHC molecule	Ref.
Influenza A	NP	44-52	CTELKLSDY	HLA-A1	29
Influenza A	NS1	122-130	AIMDKNIIL	HLA-A*0201	221
Influenza A	NS1	123-132	IMDKNIILKA	HLA-A*0201	221
Influenza A	NP	383-391	SRYWAIRTR	HLA-B*2705	160,184
Influenza A	NP	147-155	TYQRTRALV	H2-K^{d}	222, 223
Influenza A	HA	210-219	TYVSVSTSTL	H2-K^{d}	224, 225
Influenza A	HA	518-526	IYSTVASSL	H2-K^{d}	224
Influenza A	HA	259-266	FEANGNLI	H2-K^{k}	226, 227, 228
Influenza A	HA	10-18	IEGGWTGMI	H2-K^{k}	226, 227, 228
Influenza A	NP	50-57	SDYEGRLI	H2-K^{k}	229, 230
Influenza A	NS1	152-160	EEGAIVGEI	H2-K^{k}	231
Influenza A34	NP	366-374	ASNENMETM	H2-D^{b}	168, 222, 219
Influenza A68	NP	366-374	ASNENMDAM	H2-D^{b}	232
Influenza B	NP	85-94	KLGEFYNQMM	HLA-A*0201	233
Influenza B	NP	85-94	KAGEFYNQMM	HLA-A*0201	234
Influenza JAP	HA	204-212	LYQNVGTYV	H2-K^{d}	235
Influenza JAP	HA	210-219	TYVSVGTSTL	H2-K^{d}	225
Influenza JAP	HA	523-531	VYQILAIYA	H2-K^{d}	235
Influenza JAP	HA	529-537	IYATVAGSL	H2-K^{d}	235
Influenza JAP	HA	210-219	TYVSVGTSTI (L>I)	H2-K^{d}	236
Influenza JAP	HA	255-262	FESTGNLI	H2-K^{k}	237
JHMV	cAg	318-326	APTAGAFFF	H2-L^{d}	238
LCMV	NP	118-126	RPQASGVYM	H2-L^{d}	239, 240
LCMV	NP	396-404	FQPQNGQFI	H2-D^{b}	241
LCMV	GP	276-286	SGVENPGGYCL	H2-D^{b}	242
LCMV	GP	33-42	KAVYNFATCG	H2-D^{b}	243, 244
MCMV	pp89	168-176	YPHFMPTNL	H2-L^{d}	245
MHV	spike protein	510-518	CLSWNGPHL	H2-D^{b}	248
MMTV	env gp36	474-482	SFAVATTAL	H2-K^{d}	246
MMTV	gag p27	425-433	SYETFISRL	H2-K^{d}	246
MMTV	env gp73	544-551	ANYDFICV	H2-K^{b}	247
MuLV	env p15E	574-581	KSPWFTTL	H2-K^{b}	249, 250
MuLV	env gp70	189-196	SSWDFITV	H2-K^{b}	251, Sijts et al. submitted
MuLV	gag 75K	75-83	CCLCLTVFL	H2-D^{b}	252
MuLV	env gp70	423-431	SPSYVYHQF	H2-L^{d}	253
MV	F protein	437-447	SRRYPDAVYLH	HLA-B*27	254
MV	F protein	438-446	RRYPDAVYL	HLA-B*2705	255
MV	NP	281-289	YPALGLHEF	H2-L^{d}	256
MV	HA	343-351	DPVIDRLYL	H2-L^{d}	257
MV	HA	544-552	SPGRSFSYF	H2-L^{d}	257
Poliovirus	VP1	111-118	TYKDTVQL	H2-K^{d}	258
Poliovirus	VP1	208-217	FYDGFSKVPL	H2-K^{d}	258
Pseudorabiesvirus	gp GIII	455-463	IAGIGILAI	HLA-A*0201	104
Rabiesvirus	NS	197-205	VEAEIAHQI	H2-K^{k}	227, 228
Rotavirus	VP7	33-40	IIYRFLLI	H2-K^{b}	259
Rotavirus	VP6	376-384	VGPVFPPGM	H2-K^{b}	260
Rotavirus	VP3	585-593	YSGYIFRDL	H2-K^{b}	260
RSV	M2	82-90	SYIGSINNI	H2-K^{d}	261
SIV	gag p11C	179-190	EGCTPYDINQML	Mamu-A*01	266
SV	NP	324-332	FAPGNYPAL	H2-D^{b}	262
SV	NP	324-332	FAPGNYPAL	H2-K^{b}	263, 264, 265
SV40	T	404-411	VVYDFLKC	H2-K^{b}	267
SV40	T	206-215	SAINNYAQKL	H2-D^{b}	268, 269
SV40	T	223-231	CKGVNKEYL	H2-D^{b}	268, 269
SV40	T	489-497	QGINNLDNL	H2-D^{b}	268, 269
SV40	T	492-500 (501)	NNLDNLRDY(L)	H2-D^{b}	270
SV40	T	560-568	SEFLLEKRI	H2-K^{k}	271
VSV	NP	52-59	RGYVYQGL	H2-K^{b}	272

Table 5.4 Other T cell epitopes on MHC class I molecules

Source/Organism	Protein	AA position	T cell epitope/MHC ligand	MHC molecule	Ref.
B. polymyxa	β-endoxylanase	149-157	GAGIGVLTA	HLA-A*0201	104
Chicken	Ovalbumin	257-264	SIINFEKL	H2-K^b	168, 273, 274
E. coli	Methionine synthase	590-598	AAGIGIIQI	HLA-A*0201	104
E. coli	hypothetical protein	4-12	QAGIGILLA	HLA-A*0201	104
E. coli	β-gal	876-884	TPHPARIGL	H2-L^d	136
Human	CDK4-R24C	22-32	KACDPHSGHFV	HLA-A*0201	275
Human	CDK4-R24C	23-32	ACDPHSGHFV	HLA-A*0201	275
Human	HLA-A24	170-179	RYLENGKETL	H2-K^d	168, 276
Human	HLA-Cw3	170-179	RYLKNGKETL	H2-K^d	168, 276
L. monocytogenes	p60	217-225	KYGVSVQDI	H2-K^d	277
L. monocytogenes	p60	449-457	IYVGNGQMI	H2-K^d	278
L. monocytogenes	Fr38		fMIVIL	H2-M3	279
L. monocytogenes	Lem A	1-6	fMIGWII	H2-M3	280
L. monocytogenes	Lem A	1-7	fMIGWIIA	H2-M3	280
L. monocytogenes	Lysteriolysin O	91-99	GYKDGNEYI	H2-K^d	281
P. aeruginosa	Leu-Val-Ile binding prot.	123-131	GYKLIFRTI	H2-K^d	282
P. aeruginosa	Leu-Val-Ile binding prot.	162-171	QYGEGIATEV	H2-K^d	282
P. berghei	CSP	252-260	SYIPSAEKI	H2-K^d	283
P. falciparum	CSP	334-342	YLNKIQNSL	HLA-A*0201	285
P. falciparum	CSP	1-10	MMRKLAILSV	HLA-A*0201	285
P. falciparum	TRAP	3-11	HLGNVKYLV	HLA-A*0201	286
P. falciparum	TRAP	500-508	GIAGGLALL	HLA-A*0201	286
P. falciparum	STARP	523-531	MINAYLDKL	HLA-A*0202	286
P. falciparum	CSP	300-308	MPNDPNRNV	HLA-B7	286
P. falciparum	SSP2	107-115	ASKNKEKAL	HLA-B8	287
P. falciparum	CSP	105-113	LRKPKHKKL	HLA-B8	286
P. falciparum	LSA-1	1854-1861	KSLYDEHI	HLA-B17	286
P. falciparum	CSP	368-375	KPKDELDY	HLA-B*3501	288
P. falciparum	CSP	368-375	KSKDELDY	HLA-B*3501	288
P. falciparum	LSA-1	1850-1857	KPNDKSLY	HLA-B*3501	288
P. falciparum	LSA-1	1786-1794	KPIVQYDNF	HLA-B*53	288
P. falciparum	CSP	39-47	NYDNAGTNL	H2-K^d	289
P. falciparum	CSP	333-342	KYLKKIKNSL	H2-K^d	289
P. falciparum	CSP	375-383	YENDIEKKI	H2-K^k	290

Table 5.4. (con't)

Source/Organism	Protein	AA position	T cell epitope/MHC ligand	MHC molecule	Ref.
P. falciparum	CSP	371-379	DELDYENDI	$H2\text{-}K^k$	290
P. yoelii	CSP	281-289	SYVPSAEQI	$H2\text{-}K^d$	284
S. lincolnensis	lmrA		LAGIGLIAA	HLA-A*0201	104
Yeast	ysa-1	77-85	VDGIGILTI	HLA-A*0201	104
Yeast	PRAI-SCS	95-102	EPKYKTQL	HLA-B8	155
Yersinia	HSP60	35-43	GRNVVLDKS	HLA-B*27	291
Yersinia	HSP60	117-125	DRGIDKAVI	HLA-B*27	291
Yersinia	HSP60	420-428	IRAASAITA	HLA-B*27	291
Yersinia	YOP 51	249-257	IQVGNTRTI	$H2\text{-}K^b$	292

Table 5.5 MHC class II T cell epitopes

Protein	AA position	Sequence	MHC molecule	Ref.
Acetyl-Choline-receptor (torpedo fish)	97-112	DGDFAIVHMTKLLLDY	$RT1.B^L$	293
Avian infectious bronchitis virus	67-83	QHGYWRRQARFKPGKGG	$RT1.B^L$	293
β_2-microglobulin	46-55	YVTQFHPPHI	$H2\text{-}E^d$	355
Bacillus Calmette-Guérin protein BCGap	84-100	EEYLILSAR	HLA-DRB1*1405	294
bcr-abl p210, b3a2		ATGFKQSSKALQRPVAS	HLA-DRB1*0401 (DR4Dw4)	295
Bovine type II collagen	276-288	AGFKGEQGPKGEP	HLA-DRB1*0401 (DR4Dw4)	296
Carboxypeptidase H	362-382	KNSLINYLEQIHRGVKGFVR	$H2\text{-}A^{g7}$	297
Carboxypeptidase H	440-464	FSPAVGVDFELESFSERKEEEKEEL	$H2\text{-}A^{g7}$	297
Cardiac myosin a (rat)	1539-1555	KLELQSALEEAEASLEH	$RT1.B^L$	298
Chlamydial histone-like protein hc-1	13-28	LLESIQQNLLKAEKGN	HLA-DRB1*0401 (DR4Dw4)	299
Chlamydial histone-like protein hc-1	19-34	QNLLKAEKGNKAAAQR	HLA-DRB1*0401 (DR4Dw4)	299
Cholera toxin B subunit	89-100	NNKTPHAIAAIS	$H2\text{-}A^b$	300
Der pI	113-127	ISNYCQIYPPNANKI	$H2\text{-}A^b$	301
Der pI	15-29	DLRQMRTVTPIRMQG	$H2\text{-}A^b$	301
Der pII	28-40	IIHRGKPFQLEAV	HLA-DRB1*1101	302
Der pII	58-73	IDGLEVDVPGIDPNA	HLA-DRB1*0405 (DR4Dw14)	303
Der pII	33-47	KPFQLEAVFEANQNT	HLA-DRB1*1502	303
Desmoglein 3	190-204	LNSKIAFKIVSQEPA	HLA-DRB1*0402 (DR4Dw10)	304
DRB1*0101-chain	22-35	ERVRLLERCIYNQE	HLA-DRB1*0101	305
EBV lytic Ag BHRF1	171-189	AGLTLSLLVICSYLFISRG	HLA-DR2	306
EqMb	69-77	LTALGGILK	$H2\text{-}E^k$	307
Flavivirus NS3 prot.	146-154	VIGLYGNGV	HLA-DRB1*1501 (DR2b)	308

GAD65	524-543	SRLSKVAPVIKARMMEYGTT	H2-A^{g7}	310
GAD65	509-528	IPPSLRYLLDNEERMSRLSK	H2-A^{g7}	311
GAD65	247-266	NMYAMMIARFKMFPEVKEKG	H2-A^{g7}	311
GBP	73-84	QKSQRSQDENPV	RT1.B^{L}	312
HBV core	145-155	ETTVVRRRGRS	HLA-DRB1*1302	313
HBV core	93-103	VGLKIRQLLW	HLA-DRB1*1302	313
HBV core	52-62	HTALRQAILCW	HLA-DRB1*1302	313
HBV pre-S1 protein	10-24	PLGFFPDHQLDPAFG	RT1.B^{L}	293
HCMV-IE1	162-175	DKREMWMACIKELH	HLA-DRB1*0801	314
HCV NP	111-130	DPRRRSRNLGKVIDTFTCGL	HLA-DRB1*08032	147
HCV NP	161-180	SVNYATGNLPGCSFSIFLLA	HLA-DRB1*08032	147
HEL	1-18	KVFGRCELAAAMKRHGLD	H2-E^{k}	315, 316
HEL	81-96	SALLSSDITASVNCAK	H2-E^{k}	309
HEL	108-119	WVAWRNRCKGTD	H2-E^{k}	309
HEL	108-119	WVAWRNRCKGTD	H2-E^{d}	309, 317
HEL	46-61	NTDGSTOYGILQINSR	RT1.B^{L}	293
HEL	9-29	AAAMKRHGLDNYRGYSLGNW	H2-A^{g7}	318
HEL	90-104	SVNCAKKIVSDGNGM	H2-A^{g7}	319
HIV-1 gag p17	17-28	EKIRLRPGGKKK	H2-E^{d}	320
HSP65	180-188	TFGLQLELT	RT1.B^{L}	293
HSP65	418-427	LQAAPALDKL	HLA-DRB5*0101 (DR2a)	321, 322
HSP65 (p277)	437-460	VLGGGCALLRCIPALDSLTPANED	H2-A^{g7}	297
Human GAD65	115-127	MNILLQYVVKSFD	HLA-DRB1*0401 (DR4Dw4)	323
Human GAD65	274-286	IAFTSEHSHFSLK	HLA-DRB1*0401 (DR4Dw4)	323
Ig l chain	91-108	ALWFRNHFVFGGGTKVTV	H2-E^{d}	324
Influenza HA	306-318	PKYVKQNTLKLAT	HLA-DRB5*0101 (DR2a)	325
Influenza HA	130-142	HNTNGVTAASSHE	RT1.B^{L}	293
Influenza HA	307-316	KYVKQNTLKL	H2-E^{d}	326
Influenza PR8 HA	109-119	SSFERFEIFPK	H2-E^{d}	309
Influenza PR8 NP	260-283	ARSALILRGSVAHKSCLPACVYGP	H-2A^{k}	327
Influenza PR8 NP	260-283	ARSALILRGSVAHKSCLPACVYGP	H-2A^{b}	327
Influenza PR8 NP	413-435	SVQRNLPFDRTTVMAAFTGNTEG	H-2A^{b}	327
Influenza PR8 NP	260-283	ARSALILRGSVAHKSCLPACVYGP	H-2A^{s}	327
Influenza PR8 NP	206-229	FWRGENGRKTRIAYERMCNILKGK	H-2A^{d}	327
Influenza PR8 NP	45-60	TELKLSDYEGRLIQNS	H-2A^{d}	327
Insulin B chain	9-23	SHLVEALYLVCGERG	H2-A^{g7}	328
IRBP (bovine)	1181-1191	SWEGVGVVPD	RT1.B^{L}	293
Japanese cedar pollen Ag, CRY J I	356-367	TPQLTKNAGVLT	HLA-DRB3*0301 (DR52Dw26)	329
λ repressor	12-26	LEDARRLKAIYEKKK	H2-A^{g7}	330
Link	61-73	AKFYRDPTAFGSG	HLA-DRB1*0401 (DR4Dw4)	331

Table 5.5. (con't)

Protein	AA position	Sequence	MHC molecule	Ref.
LLO	218-226	IAKFGTAFK	H2-E^k	307
Lol pol	171-190	GDVVAVVDIKEKGKDKWIELK	HLA-DRB1*0301(DR17)	332
Lol p1	121-132	EQNVRSAGELEL	RT1.B^L	293
Lol p9	105-116	AKYDAFVTALTE	HLA-DRB4	333
Lol p9	193-207	ETYKFIPSLEAA	HLA-DRB4	333
L-plastin	581-595	NNAKYAISMARKIGA	HLA-DRB4*0101	334
M. leprae HSP70	468-487	TGKENTIKIQEGSGLSKEEI	HLA-DRB1*0101	335
M. leprae HSP70	71-90	RHMGSDWSIEIDGKKYTAQE	HLA-DR3	335
M. leprae HSP70	261-280	DSDKNPLFLDEQLIRAEFQR	HLA-DR3	335
M. leprae HSP70	408-427	QPSVQIQVYQGEREIASHNK	HLA-DR3	335
M. leprae HSP70	241-260	AKIELSSSQSTSVNLPYITV	HLA-DR7	335
M. leprae 28 kD protein	121-140	VTGSPICTAPDLNLGGTCPS	H2-A^b	336
M. leprae HSP70	298-317	KDAGISVESEIDHVVLVGGST	HLA-DRw52	335
M. leprae HSP70	388-407	ERNTTIPTKRSETFTTADDN	HLA-DRw52 or HLA-DQ2	335
M. tuberculosis	248-254	FQDAYNAAGGHNAVF	H2-A^b	337
M. tuberculosis 19kD protein	61-80	VTGSVVCTTAAGNVNIAIGG	H2-A^b	336
M. bovis HSP65	3-13	KTIAYDEEARR	HLA-DRB1*0301(DR17)	343
M. leprae HSP18	38-50	EFVVEFDLPGIKA	HLA-DRB1*0401 (DR4Dw4)	344
M. tuberculosis HSP65	180-188	TFGLQLELT	RT1.B^L	345
M. tuberculosis HSP65	396-410	DAVRNAKAAVEEGIV	RT1.B^L	345
M. tuberculosis HSP65	446-460	ALPKQIAFNSGLEPG	RT1.B^L	345
MBP	1-11	ASQKRPSQRHG	H2-A^u	346
MBP	85-95	PVVHFFKNIVT	HLA-DRB1*1501 (DR2b)	338
MBP	87-99	VHFFKNIVTPRTP	HLA-DRB5*0101 (DR2a)	339
MBP	131-145	ASDYKSAHKGFKGVD	HLA-DRB5*0101 (DR2a)	321
MBP	139-153	KGFKGVDAQGTLSKI	HLA-DRB5*0101 (DR2a)	321
MBP	72-85	QKSQRSQDENPV	RT1.B^L	293
MBP	12-35	YLATASTMDHARHGFLPRHRDTGI	H2-A^{g7}	340
MBP (rat)	72-85	QKSQRTQDENPV	RT1.B^L	293
MBP	87-99	VHFFKNIVTPRTP	RT1.B^L	293
MCC	91-103	RADLIAYLKQATK	H2-E^k	307
MCC	93-103	DLIAYLKQATK	H2-E^s	315,307
MCC	93-103	DLIAYLKQATK	H2-E^b	315,307
MOG	8-22	PGYPIRALVGDEQED	H2-A^{g7}	340
MOG	35-55	MEVGWYRSPFSRVVHLVRNGK	H2-A^{g7}	342
MOG	35-55	MEVGWYRSPFSRVVHLYRNGK	H2-A^b	347

MoHb	68-76	ITAFNEGLK	H2-E^{k}	307
MoMb	69-77	LTALGTILK	H2-E^{k}	307
MV fusion protein	51-65	HQSLVIKLMPNITLL	HLA-DRB1*0101	341
Myelin P2 (bovine)	53-78	TESPFKNTEISFKLGQEFEETTADNR	RT1.B^{L}	293
Myoglobin	110-121	IIIEVLKKRHSG	H2-A^{g7}	348
Myoglobulin	69-78	LTALGTILKK	H2-A^{g7}	348
Myosin (rat)	1539-1555	KLELQSALEEAEASLEH	RT1.B^{L}	293
OVA	323-339	ISQAVHAAHAEINEAGR	RT1.B^{L}	293
OVA	323-339	ISQAVHAAHAEINEAGR	H2-A^{g7}	330
PCC	91-104	RADLIAYLKQATAK	H2-E^{k}	307
PLP	56-70	DYEYLINVIHAFQYV	H2-A^{g7}	340
PLP (rat)	217-240	KVCGSNLLSICKTAEFQMTFHLFI	RT1.B^{L}	293
PLP	30-49	WTTCQSIAFPSKTSASIGSL	HLA-DRB1*1501 (DR2b)	349
PLP	180-199	LFCGCGHEALTGTEKLIETY	HLA-DRB1*1501 (DR2b)	349
PLP	30-49	WTTCQSIAFPSKTSASIGSL	HLA-DRB5*0101 (DR2a)	349
PLP	180-199	LFCGCGHEALTGTEKLIETY	HLA-DRB5*0101 (DR2a)	349
rep	12-26	LEDARRLKAIYEKKK	H2-E^{k}	315
rep	12-26	LEDARRLKAIYEKKK	H2-E^{d}	309
Ribosomal protein S30	1-22	KVHGSLARAGKVRGQTPKVAKQ	H2-A^{g7}	348
Rotavirus major capsid protein VP6	289-302	RLSFQLVRPPNMTP	H2-E^{d}	350
Rubella virus peptid E1	273-284	EVWVTPVIGSQA	HLA-DRB1*0403 (DR4Dw13)	351
S100β (rat)	76-91	FVSMVTTACHEFFEHE	RT1.B^{L}	352, 293
SNase	51-70	VEKYGPEASAFTKKMVENAK	H2-E^{k}	315
SNase	81-100	RTDKYGRGLAYIYADGKMVN	H2-E^{k}	315
SNase	121-140	HEHQLRKSEAQAKKEKLNIW	H2-E^{k}	320
SNase	112-129	AYVYKPNNTHEQHLRKSE	H2-E^{d}	354
Snase	81-100	RTDKYGRGLAYIYADGKMVN	H2-E^{b}	315,307
Staphylococcal enteroxin B	121-136	HNGNQLDKYRSITVRV	H2-A^{b}	356
SV M protein	146-161	IFNANKVALAPQCLPV	H2-A^{b}	353
SV M protein	331-346	FRYYPNVVAKNIGRIR	H2-A^{b}	353
SWMb	102-118	KYLEFISEAIIHVLHSR	H2-E^{d}	309
SWMb	132-146	NKALELFRKDIAAKY	H2-E^{d}	325
SWMb	26-40	QDILIRLFKSHPETL	H2-E^{k}	315
SWMb	66-78	VTVLTALGAILKK	H2-E^{k}	309
TCR	77-86	TLTVNNARPE	RT1.B^{L}	357
TCR Vβ6	38-60	DSGKGLRLIYYSITENDLQKGDL	H2-A^{g7}	348
TCR Vβ8.2	38-60	DTGHGLRLIHYSYGAGSTEKGDI	H2-A^{g7}	348
Tetanus toxin	830-843	QYIKANSKFIGITE	HLA-DRB1*1302	358
Tyrosinase	56-70	QNILLSNAPLGPQFP	HLA-DRB1*0401 (DR4Dw4)	359

Table 5.5. (con't)

Protein	AA position	Sequence	MHC molecule	Ref.
Tyrosinase	448-462	DYSYLQDSDPDSFQD	HLA-DRB1*0401 (DR4Dw4)	359
Y. enterocolitica 60 kD HSP	214-225	ELESPFILLADK	H2-A^b	360
Y. enterocolitica 60 kD HSP	74-86	VKEVAAKANDAAG	H2-A^b	360

Table 5.6 Normal self ligands of MHC class I molecules

Protein/Gene	AA position	MHC ligand	MHC molecule	Ref.
[GLCNac]-P-transferase	371-379	KVFGPIHER	HLA-A*3101	367
3-PGAL-dehydrogenase (hamster)	172-186	LMTTVHAITATQKTV	HCMV class I homolog UL18	368
40 kD peptide	89-96	GAYEFTTL	H2-K^b	369
40 kD peptide E92 R	89-96	GAYRFTTL	H2-K^b	369
40S ribosomal protein S11	70-79	GRILSGVVTK	HLA-B*2705	370
40S ribosomal protein S15	114-122	YLGEFSITY	HLA-B*1501	371
40S ribosomal protein S15	116-123	GEFSITYK	HLA-B*4006	371
40S ribosomal protein S16	40-48	MIEPRTLQY	HLA-A1	367, 214
40S ribosomal protein S17	95-105	IEVDPDTKEML	HLA-B*40012	371
40S ribosomal protein S17	77-84	RERRDNYV	HLA-B*4006	371
40S ribosomal protein S17	49-57	KIAGYVTHL	HLA-G	372
40S ribosomal protein S17 homolog		DGPVRGISI	H2-D^d	373
40S ribosomal protein S19	93-101	GVMPSHFSR	HLA-A*1101	367
40S ribosomal protein S21	6-13	GEFVDLYV	HLA-B*4006	371
40S ribosomal protein S21	37-46	AEVDKVTGRF	HLA-B44	220
40S ribosomal protein S21	60-67	GQFKTYAI	HLA-B*5201	374
40S ribosomal protein S24	53-60	DDHRAGKI	H2-K^k	375
40S ribosomal protein S25	103-111	HRAQVIYTR	HLA-B*2705	370
40S ribosomal protein S26	107-115	APAPPPKPM	HLA-B7	376
40S ribosomal protein S26	63-71	VLPKLYVKL	HLA-G	372
40S ribosomal protein S29 (rat)	3-11	QQLYWSHPR	HLA-A*3101	367
40S ribosomal protein S3	54-62	RTQNVLGEK	HLA-A*1101	377
40S ribosomal protein S30	114-125	RRFVNVVPTFGK	HLA-B*2705	370
40S ribosomal protein S30	113-121	NRRFVNVVP	HLA-B*7301	378
40S ribosomal protein S6	107-115	SVLNLVIVK	HLA-A*1101	377
40S ribosomal protein S7/S8	137-144	SEIVGKRI	H2-K^k	375
40S ribosomal protein S7/S8A	135-144	FPSEIVGKRI	HLA-B*5102	374
60S ribosomal protein L18 (rat)	94-102	VPKLKVXAL	HLA-B8	155

60S ribosomal protein L19	137-145	ILMEHIHKL	HLA-A*0201	379
60S ribosomal protein L19	137-145	ILMEHIHKL	HLA-A*0214	380
60S ribosomal protein L19	137-145	ILMEHIHKL	Qa-2	381
60S ribosomal protein L27	98-106	DVFRDPALK	HLA-A*6801	215
60S ribosomal protein L27	66-74	KIKSFVKVY	HLA-B*1501	371
60S ribosomal protein L28	68-76	GQRKPATSY	HLA-B*1501	371
60S ribosomal protein L28	37-45	FRYNGLIHR	HLA-B*2705	160
60S ribosomal protein L30	23-31	RTDGKVFQF	HLA-B*5801	371
60S ribosomal protein L35	18-27	FQLDDLKVEL	HLA-A*0214	380
60S ribosomal protein L36	36-44	GRLTKHTKF	HLA-B*2705	382
60S ribosomal protein L36 (rat)	36-44	GRLTKHTKF	HLA-B*2702	382
60S ribosomal protein L36 (rat)	3-11	LRYPMAVGL	HLA-B*2709	370
60S ribosomal protein L4 (rat)		NMNTDLSRILKSPEIQR	HCMV class I homolog UL18	368
60S ribosomal protein L44	39-48	RRYDRKQSGY	HLA-B*2705	370
60S ribosomal protein L7A	25-33	KVVNPLFEK	HLA-A*1101	377
60S ribosomal protein L8	173-181	GRIDKPILK	HLA-B*2705	160
60S ribosomal protein L8	162-170	NRAVVGVVA	HLA-B*7301	378
60S ribosomal protein L8 (human)	7-16	GQRKGAGSVY	HLA-B*1501	151
60S ribosomal protein L8 (rat)	7-15	GQRKGAGSV	HLA-B*1501	371
α actin	39-47	RPRHQGVMV	HLA-B*3501	383
Actin	364-372	ESGPSIVHR	HLA-A*3302	367
Actin	63-71	KRGILTLKY	HLA-B*2702	382
Adenosine phosphoribosyl transferase (mouse)		SLVELTSL	$H2\text{-}K^b$	384
Aldehyde dehydrogenase	5572-5595	XQYTSRMI	HLA-A*0201	135
Amidophosphoribosyltansferase precursor	354-362	GRTFIQPNM	HLA-B*2705	370
Amidophosphoribosyltransferase precursor	354-362	GRTFIQPNM	HLA-B*2709	370
APC frameshift		KYLKIKHLL	$H2\text{-}K^d$	385
associated microfibril. protein	72-80	EEFQFIKKA	HLA-B*4006	371
ATPase	653-660	IPVMGLMMV	$H2\text{-}K^k$	386
ATP-dependent RNA helicase	148-156	YLLPAIVHI	HLA-A*0201	387
ATP-dependent RNA helicase	77-85	RRSKEITVR	HLA-B*2705	160
β-5 GTP binding protein	320-329	ILFGHENRV	HLA-A*0201	379
β-actin	275-282	HETTFNSI	$H2\text{-}K^k$	375
β-actin	170-179	ALPHAILRLD	HCMV class I homolog UL18	368
β-actin	170-178	ALPHAILRL	HCMV class I homolog UL18	368
β-actin	364-373	ESGPSIVHRK	HLA-A*6801	389
β-actin	37-45	RPRHQGVMV	HLA-B*0702	391
β-actin	37-45	RPRHQGVMV	HLA-B*5502	391
β-catenin (mutated)	29-37	SYLDSGIHF	HLA-A24	418
β-galactosidase (rat)		ILPDGTXKF	HCMV class I homolog UL18	368

Table 5.6. (con't)

Protein/Gene	AA position	MHC ligand	MHC molecule	Ref.
B cell transl. Gene 1 protein	103-111	TLWVDPYEV	HLA-A*0201	388
BIP	158-165	EAYLGKKV	H2-K^k	375
Bovine hemoglobin	112-121	HLPSDFTPAV	HLA-A*0214	380
Bovine metalloproteinase	19-27	GQYGNPLNK	HLA-A*1101	367
Butyryl cholinesterase	256-264	NAPWAVTSL	HLA-Cw*0102	81
Ca^{2+} dependent protease	172-181	KRWQAIYKQF	HLA-B*2705	370
Calreticulin signal sequence	1-10	MLLSVPLLLG	HLA-A*0201	387
Carboxypeptidase M	91-99	HLIDYLVTS	HLA-A*0201	389
CArG binding factor A	209-216	EEDPVKKV	H2-K^k	375
Cathepsin B (rat)		VMGGHAIRI	HCMV class I homolog UL18	368
Cathepsin D	255-262	GELSYLNV	H2-K^k	386
CCAAT-binding transcription factor	240-248	RGYRPRFRR	HLA-A*3101	367
CD20	222-230	RPKSNIVLL	HLA-B7	390
CD20	222-230	RPKSNIVLL	HLA-B*0702	391
CDC25 homol.	560-567	LPFTVILV	HLA-B*5102	374
$CDK4^{wt}$	22-32	KARDPHSGHFV	HLA-A*0201	275
Cholera toxin B subunit	89-100	NNKTPHAIAAIS	H2-A^b	300
CKS-2	11-19	KYFDEHYEY	HLA-Cw*0702	392
CKShs1 protein		EPEPHILLF	HLA-B*3501	393
c-myc	241-249	HEETPPTTS	HLA-B40*	389
Cofilin	127-135	KLTGIKHEL	Qa-2	381
COI	1-6	fMFINRW	H2-M3	80
Collagen 1α2	4-12	SFVDTRTLL	H2-K^d	394
Collagen α1	1106-1112	VQGPVGL	HLA-B*1501	371
Collagen Type IV	51-59	GSPATWTTR	HLA-A*1101	395
Complement C3b	776-783	QEKINLNV	H2-K^k	386
Core histone (rat)	188-196	ARLQTALL	HLA-B*2705	382
Cyclin	152-159	SHIGDAVV	HLA-B*3801	396
Cyclin	152-159	SHIGDAVV	HLA-B*39011	396
Cyclin (mouse)	67-75	AMGVNLTSM	H2-D^b	T. Dumrese et al, unpubl.
Cyclin A	178-186	YHEDIHTYL	HLA-B*3801	396
Cyclin B	313-321	GEVDVEQHT	HLA-B40*	389
Cyclin B	269-277	FAFVTDNTY	HLA-B*4601	81
Cyclin D1 (mouse)	20-28	TNLLNDRVL	H2-D^b	397
Cyclin-like protein	135-143	ATDFKFAMY	HLA-A1	367, 377
Cytochrome C	38-47	GRKTGQAPGY	HLA-B*2705	370
Cytochrome C oxidase	42-50	KRKKAYADF	HLA-B*2702	382

Cytochrome C oxidase	154-163	ITSQDVLHSW	HLA-B*5801	371
Cytochrome C oxidase II	110-121	YTDYGGLIFNSY	HLA-A1	367, 377
Cytochrome P450	20-28	TRYPILAGH	HLA-B*2705	382
Cytokine receptor		KGPPAALTL	HLA-G	372
Cytosine methyl transferase	238-246	YLDDPDLKY	HLA-A1	377
DEAD box protein p68 RNA helicase	547-554	SNFVFAGI	H2-K^b	398
DP signal sequence	9-17	APRTVALTA	HLA-B*3501	383
Elongation factor (hamster)	429-444	IMGPNYTPGKKEDLYLKPIQ	HCMV class I homolog UL18	368
Elongation factor 1-α 1	431-441	ETVAVGVIKAV	HLA-A*6901	380
Elongation factor 1α	271-280	VLKPGMVVTF	HLA-B*1501	371
Elongation factor 1α	208-216	MPWFKGwKV	HLA-B*5102	374
Elongation factor 2	265-275	YFDPANGKFSK	HLA-A*1101	367
Elongation factor 2	341-349	RRWLPAGda	HLA-B*2705	160
Elongation factor 2	265-273	YPDPANGKF	HLA-B*3801	396
Elongation factor 2	48-57	AEMGKGSFKY	HLA-B*4403	399
Elongation factor 2	265-273	YPDPANGKF	HLA-B*5201	374
Epithelial cell mucin MUC-1	9-17	STAPPAHGV	HLA-A*1101	400
ERP72	1-9	MRPRKAFLL	HLA-G	372
Ets-1	154-162	YTSDYFISY	HLA-A1	367, 377
Expressed sequence tag		IMEETGKXF	HCMV class I homolog UL18	368
Expressed sequence tag		LMPNGPMRL	HCMV class I homolog UL18	368
Fatty acid synthase	751-759	HVPEHAVVL	HLA-G	372
Feline leukemia virus envelope polyprotein homolog		FGPYKLNRL	H2-D^d	373
Fibrillarin	177-188	VSDIVGPDGLVY	HLA-A1	367, 238
Fibrinogen α-chain	261-269	LERPEGNEI	HLA-A*0201	379
Fibrinogen β-chain	51-59	KKREEAPSL	HLA-A*0201	379
Fructose-6-amino transferase	217-225	STDHIPILY	HLA-A1	377
γ actin	126-135	ETFNTPAHYV	HLA-A*6901	380
GBLP	35-42	SRDKTIIM	HLA-B*39011	396
GBLP	192-200	TGYLNTVTV	HLA-B*5101	374
GBLP	192-200	TGYLNTVTV	HLA-B*5102	374
GBLP	192-200	TGYLNTVTV	HLA-B*5103	374
GBLP	192-200	TGYLNTVTV	HLA-B*5201	374
Glucose transporter 5	322-330	gAVNVVMTf	HLA-B*5801	371
Glutamic acid decarboxylase	114-123	VMNILLQYVV	HLA-A*0201	401
Glutamyl-tRNA synthetase	343-351	IRKPYIwEY	HLA-Cw*0702	392
Glutathion peroxidase	38-46	LLIENVASL	HLA-A*0201	379
GPIX	8-10	FLL	HLA-A*0201	379
GPIX	11-16	WATAEA	HLA-A*0201	379
GPIX	8-15	FLLWATAE	HLA-A*0201	379
GPIX	8-16	FLLWATAEA	HLA-A*0201	379

Table 5.6. (con't)

Protein/Gene	AA position	MHC ligand	MHC molecule	Ref.
Granulin	162-170	ITPTGHSL	HLA-Cw*0102	81
HBBCP	190-198	ARLFGIRAK	HLA-B*2705	160, 382
H2-D^k	112-119	SEGGSHTI	H2-K^k	375
HFPS	191-199	KRYKSIVKY	HLA-B*2702	382
HGNBP β-subunit	35-43	SRDKTIIMW	HLA-B*2702	382
Histone 3.1/3.3	118-129	TIMPKDIQLARR	HLA-A*3302	367
Histone H1	40-50	AASKERSGVSL	HLA-B*0702	391
Histone H2a	23-32	LQFPVGRVHR	HLA-A*3101	367
Histone H4	65-73	NVIRDAVTY	HLA-A3	383
Histone	83-91	LRFQSSAVM	HLA-B*2705	370
Histone 2a Z	25-32	KQFPVGRI	HLA-B*5201	374
Histone binding protein	627-635	QDEAVAQF	HLA-B*3801	396
Histone H1	49-59	AASKERSGVSL	HLA-B7	390
Histone H2A	77-85	RIIPRHLQL	HLA-G	402,372
Histone H3.3	52-60	RRYQKSTEL	HLA-B*2705	160
Histone H3.3	40-48	RYRPGTVAL	HLA-Cw*0702	392
HLA class I α chain	161-169	DMAAQITQR	HLA-A*3302	367
HLA class I α chain	111-123	QSEDGSHTIQIMY	HLA-A1	367
HLA class III gene		GVPKTHLEL	HLA-G	372
HLA-A2.1 signal sequence	5-13	APRTLVLLL	HLA-B7	390
HLA-A α3 domain		YPAEITLTW	HLA-B*3501	393
HLA-B7 signal sequence	2-10	LVMAPRTVL	HLA-B7	390
HLA-DP signal sequence	9-17	APRTVALTA	HLA-B7	390
HLA-DP signal sequence	9-18	APRTVALTAL	HLA-B7	390
HLA-DP signal sequence	9-17	APRTVALTA	HLA-B*0702	391
HLA-DP signal sequence	9-17	APRTVALTA	HLA-B*5501	391
HLA-DP signal sequence	9-17	APRTVALTA	HLA-B*5502	391
HLA-DP signal sequence	9-17	APRTVALTA	HLA-B*5601	391
HLA-DQα	33-41	EEFYVDLER	HLA-B*40*	389
HLA-E	116-126	FAYDGKDYLTL	HLA-Cw*0304	403
HLA-E precursor	137-145	FAYDGKDYL	HLA-A*0214	380
HLA-E signal sequence	1-9	MVDGTLLLL	HLA-A*0201	388
hnRNP K	159-167	SLAGGIIGV	HLA-A*0201	379
hnRNA-binding protein M4	360-368	GRFGSGMNM	HLA-B*2705	370
hnRNP A1	257-265	GSYNDFGNY	RT1.A^l	404
hnRNP A2	281-290	GGYGGGYDNY	RT1.A^l	404

hnRNP A2 or B1 homolog	277-288	NYGGGNYGSGSY	HLA-Cw*0702	392
hnRNP C protein	84-91	EEEPVKKI	H2-K^k	375
hnRNP complex K homolog		SGPERLLSXY	H2-D^d	373
hnRNP F	238-246	AGYGGYEEY	RT1.A^l	404
HS1 protein	160-168	MQPTHPIRL	HLA-G	372
HSB 66EST	18-29	AVILPPLSPYFK	HLA-A*1101	367
HSHM02C05		YEIHDGMNL	HLA-B*40012	371
HSP27	69-77	AAPAYSRAL	HLA-Cw*0102	81
HSP60	284-292	RRKAMFEDI	HLA-B*2705	405
HSP60 (mouse)	499-508	SALQNAASIA	H2-D^b	406
HSP60 (mouse)	162-170	KDIGNIISDA	H2-D^b	406
HSP70/HSP70	126-134	KMKEIAEAY	HLA-B*4601	81
HSP70B/HSC70	66-76	TVFDAKRLIGR	HLA-A*6801	215
HSP86	200-209	RRIKEIVKKH	HLA-B*2705	382
HSP89α	200-208	RRIKEIVKK	HLA-B*2705	160
HSP89β	195-203	RRVKEVVKK	HLA-B*2705	160
HSP90	703-711	AVPDEIPPL	HLA-A*0205	380
HSP90	427-436	AEDKENYKKF	HLA-B*4403	399
HSP90α	481-490	XEKYIDQEEL	HLA-A*2902	137
HSP90β	24-32	MSLIINTEFY	RT1.A^l	404
HSrn	234-242	DAYRrIHSL	HLA-B14	155
Human autoantigen LA (SS-B)	51-58	IMIKFNRL	H2-K^b	407
Human autoantigen LA (SS-B)	51-58	IMIKFXRL	H2-K^b	407
Human CD9		AVGIGIAVV	HLA-A*0201	104
Human G protein coupled receptor	164-172	ALGLGLLPV	HLA-A*0201	104
Human glutamyltransferase		LVVLGLLAV	HLA-A*0201	104
Human HSP60	140-148	IRRGVMLAV	HLA-B*27	291
Human HSP60	369-377	KRIQEIIEQ	HLA-B*27	291
Human HSP60	469-477	KRTLKIPAM	HLA-B*27	291
Human MHC Iα	140-148	FAYDGKDYI	HLA-A*0205	380
Human protein translation factor-sui	65-74	DYIHIRIQQR	HLA-A*3302	367
Human vinculin	358-366	GLDVLTAKV	HLA-A*0201	408
Human vinculin	823-831	RILGAVAKV	HLA-A*0201	408
Human vinculin	983-991	QVCERIPTI	HLA-A*0201	408
Hypoxanthine phosphoribosyltransferase homolog		IGPERGHNL	H2-D^d	373
IEF 9306	127-135	GEFGGFGSV	HLA-B*4006	371
IFN-induced 15kD protein	45-54	LAVHPSGVAL	HLA-Cw*0304	403
Ig gamma-4 C region	279-287	DSDGSFFLY	HLA-A1	377
Ig VH	49-58	AYISSGSSTL	H2-K^d	225
IL-1 receptor antagonist homolog		GRVFIIKE	HLA-B*2705	382

Table 5.6. (con't)

Protein/Gene	AA position	MHC ligand	MHC molecule	Ref.
IL-6 precursor	161-169	ILKQKIAdI	HLA-B8	155
IL-7 receptor α-chain	289-296	KPKTSLNV	H2-K^k	386
Immediate early response gene	87-95	RRFGDKLNF	HLA-B*2705	382
Immediate early response gene	87-95	RRFGDKLNF	HLA-B*2709	370
Insulin B chain	7-15	CGSHLVEAL	H2-K^b	409
Insulin receptor precursor homolog		SXPKTDXQTL	H2-D^d	373
Int-6	24-32	KRTTVVAQL	HLA-B*2709	370
Interferon binding protein	339-347	RLPDGRVVL	HLA-G	372
IP-30 signal sequence	27-35	LLDVPTAAV	HLA-A*0201	388
IP-30 signal sequence	26-35	LLLDVPTAAV	HLA-A*0201	388
IP-30 signal sequence	26-37	LLLDVPTAAVQA	HLA-A*0201	388
IP-30 signal sequence	26-36	LLLDVPTAAVQ	HLA-A*0201	388
IRE-BP	695-703	GEILDVFDA	HLA-B40*	389
JAK1 (tyrosine kinase)	355-363	SYFPEITHI	H2-K^d	168, 410
J-chain	102-110	YTAVVPLVY	HLA-A1	377
Lamin B receptor	14-23	GRWPGSSLYY	HLA-B*2705	370
Lamin B2		RYMDAWNTYSR	HLA-A*3101	367
Lamin C	490-498	KAGQVVTIW	HLA-B*5801	371
LDH M chain	115-122	NIFKFIIP	RT1.A^l	404
Lipopolysaccharide binding protein (mouse)		EQYKFYSV	H2-K^b	411
LMP-2		APTGDLPRA	HLA-B*5502	391
LMP-2		APTGDLPRA	HLA-B*5601	391
MARCKS homolog (cattle)	155-163	KRFSFKKSF	HLA-B*2705	382
mdm2 (mouse)	100-107	YAMIYRNL	H2-K^b	69, 397
mdm2 (mouse)	441-449	GRPKNGCIV	H2-D^b	397
Met Adenosyltransferase	312-320	RRVLVQVSY	HLA-B*2705	370
Metalloproteinase 2 inhibitor homolog		KGPDKGNEF	H2-D^d	373
MHC α chain	140-148	YAYDGKDYI	HLA-B*5102	374
MHC α chain	140-148	FAYDGKDYI	HLA-B*5102	374
MHC class I	221-230	HEATLRCWAL	HLA-B*40012	371
MHC class I	260-268	AGDRTFQKW	HLA-B*5801	371
MHC class IIβ	209-217	VTSPLTVEW	HLA-B*5801	371
MHC I α chain	140-148	FAYDGKDYI	HLA-A*0214	380
MHC II β chain	150-158	GFYPGSIEV	HLA-B*5201	374
mRNA CD40 homolog (mouse)		SGPRKXIXL	H2-D^d	373
N-acetylglucosaminyltransferase V Gnt-V	intron	VLPDVFIRCV	HLA-A*0201	412
N-acetylglucosaminyltransferase V Gnt-V	intron	VLPDVFIRC	HLA-A*0201	412

NADH-Dehydrogenase	98-105	MEVFLICV	H2-K[k]	386
NADH-Dehydrogenase	1-9	fMYFINILTL	H2-M3	413
Nascent polypeptide complex α chain		KSPASDTYIV	HLA-G	372
Neuronal acetylcholine receptor	141-149	GRFEGTSTK	HLA-B*2705	370
NK/T cell activation protein	107-115	YYEEQHPEL	HLA-A24	377
Nuclear protein (TTP)	130-138	RHPKYKTEL	HLA-G	372
Nucleic acid binding protein	53-61	NXPERIITL	HLA-Cw*0102	81
OGDH	104-112	QLSPYPFDL	H2-L[d]	414
OGDH	105-112	LSPFPFDL	H2-L[d]	415, 59
OGDH	97-112	VAITRIEQLSPFPFDL	H2-L[d]	415, 59
OGDH	105-112	LSPFPFDL	H2-K[b]	416
OGDH	105-112	LSPYPFDL	H2-L[d]	416
Ornithin decarboxylase	23-31	ILDQKINEV	HLA-A*0201	379
Ornithin decarboxylase	309-317	SSEQTFMYY	HLA-A1	214
P1-CDC21	259-266	HSTIMPRL	HLA-B*5201	374
Phosphatidyl-inositol-3-kinase	373-382	RKGGNNKLIK	HLA-B*2705	370
Phosphoglycerate kinase	180-189	XPQKAGGFLM	H2-L[d]	417
Phospholipase A 2-activating protein (mouse)	102-111	ILPEQGLMLT	HCMV class I homolog UL18	368
Phosphoribosyltransferase	15-22	QELGVGCV	H2-K[k]	386
Pm5 protein	270-278	TFDVAPSRL	HLA-B*3801	396
Prohibitin (rat)	229-240	ATAGDGLIELRK	HLA-A*1101	367, 377
Proliferating cell nucleolar antigen P40 homologue		SGPERGEKL	H2-D[d]	373
Proliferation cell nuclear antigen	241-249	IADMGHLKY	HLA-A1	367, 214, 377
Proteasome C3		DPSGAYFAW	HLA-B*3501	393
Proteasome subunit homologue C5	127-135	RRFMQYYVY	HLA-B*2705	382
Proteasome SVC8	150-159	YMIDPSGVSY	HLA-B*4601	81
Protein phosphatase 1	113-121	KYPENFFLL	HLA-A24	377
Protein phosphatase 2A	389-397	SLLPAIVEL	HLA-A*0201	388
Protein synthesis factor eIFC	87-95	NKADVILKY	HLA-Cw*0702	392
Pyrimidine binding protein	168-176	AAVDAGMAM	HLA-Cw*0304	403
RBAP-2	266-273	VQIFGNKM	HLA-B*5201	374
Restin	1273-1281	ELKVKNLEL	HLA-B8	155
Ribonucl Reductase	290-297	REIIINAV	HLA-B*4006	371
Ribonucleoprotein L	312-322	RRMGPPVGGHR	HLA-B*2705	382
Ribosomal protein (Human fau)	114-123	RRFVNVVPTF	HLA-B*2702	382
Signal peptidase	45-54	SESPIVVVL	HLA-B*40012	371
SKShs1 protein	59-66	IHEPEPHI	HLA-B*39011	396
Splicing factor	3-11	RVYIGRLSY	HLA-A3	383
SSR α signal sequence	12-25	VLFRGGPRGLLAVA	HLA-A*0201	419, 387
Synthetic peptide		DIKVGIEF	H2-K[b]	420

Table 5.6. (con't)

Protein/Gene	AA position	MHC ligand	MHC molecule	Ref.
Synthetic peptide		SIYRYYGL	$H2\text{-}K^b$	421
T cell transcript. Factor 1 homolog		KEMKAKVI	$H2\text{-}K^k$	375
Talin	777-785	ALNELLQHV	HLA-A*0201	379
TF II B	116-124	NAFKEITTM	$RT1.A^l$	404
TF NF-E2	35-42	TELQGLNV	$H2\text{-}K^k$	386
Thymidilate synthase	253-261	DAHIYLNHI	HLA-B*5103	374
Thymidylate synthase	253-261	DAHIYLNHI	HLA-B*5101	374
Thymosin β-10	11-20	ASFDKAKLKK	HLA-A*1101	367
Thymosin β-10	11-19	ASFDKAKLK	HLA-A*1101	377
TIS 11B protein	325-333	RRXPIFSRL (X=L)	HLA-B*2705	382
TIS 11B protein	325-333	RRLPIFSRL	HLA-B*2709	370
Tissue inhibitor of metalloproteinase	125-133	VAPWNSLSL	HLA-Cw*0102	81
Topoisomerase II	801-809	SPRYIFTML	HLA-B7	390
Transforming protein spi-1 homolog (human)		SXHKEQPAT	$H2\text{-}D^d$	373
Tristetraproline	148-155	HPKYKTEL	HLA-B8	155
TRP-2	181-188	VYDFFVWL	$H2\text{-}K^b$	422
Tyrosin protein kinase	557-562	LLPPPP	HLA-A*0201	379
Tyrosinase	369-377	YMNGTMSQV	HLA-A*0201	423-426
Tyrosinase	369-377	YMDGTMSQV	HLA-A*0201	427
Tyrosinase	1-9	MLLAVLYCL	HLA-A*0201	423, 424
Tyrosinase	206-215	AFLPWHRLFL	HLA-A24	428
Tyrosinase	206-214	AFLPWHRLF	HLA-A24	428
Tyrosinase	192-200	SEIWRDIDF	HLA-B*4402	429
Tyrosinase	192-200	SEIWRDIDF	HLA-B*4403	429
UBC5 (yeast)	61-68	YPFKPPKV	HLA-B*5101	374
UBC5 (yeast)	61-68	YPFKPPKV	HLA-B*5102	374
Ubiquitin	65-73	STLHLVRL	HLA-A*0214	380
Ubiquitin	53-61	GRTLSDYNI	HLA-B*2709	370
Ubiquitin	63-71	KESTLHLVL	HLA-B40	389
Ubiquitin	63-71	KESTLHLVL	HLA-B*40012	371
Ubiquitin	64-72	KESTLHLVL	HLA-A*2902	137
Ubiquitin carrier protein E2		NLPPHIIRL	HCMV class I homolog UL18	368
Urease canavalia ensiformis homolog		DGPVREHNL	$H2\text{-}D^d$	373
Vector artefact		SVVEFSSL	$H2\text{-}K^b$	384
Vimentin	51-61	SLYASSPGGVY	HLA-A3	383

Table 5.7. Normal ligands of MHC class II molecules

Protein	AA position	Sequence	MHC molecule	Ref.
α1-antitrypsin	397-410	YDRNTKSPLFVGKV	$H2\text{-}E^k$	430
α1-antitrypsin	149-164	VDTFLEDVKNLYHSEA	HLA-DRB1*0301(DR17)	431
α-enolase	23-?	AEVYHDVAASEFF...	HLA-DRB1*0801	435
β_2-microglobulin	83-96	YLLYYTEFTPTEKD	HLA-DRB1*0405 (DR4Dw15)	432
β_2-microglobulin	84-98	LLYYTEFTPTEKDEY	HLA-DRB1*0405 (DR4Dw15)	439
β_2-microglobulin	85-96	LYYTEFTPTEKD	HLA-DRB1*0405 (DR4Dw15)	439
β_2-microglobulin	4-21	TPKIQVYSRHPAENGKSN	HLA-DRB1*1104	437
β_2-microglobulin	21-38	TPKIQVYSRHPAENGKSN	HLA-DRB1*1301	437
β_2-microglobulin	21-37	TPKIQVYSRHPAENGKS	HLA-DRB1*1301	441
β_2-microglobulin	21-36	TPKIQVYSRHPAENGK	HLA-DRB1*1301	441
β_2-microglobulin	21-35	TPKIQVYSRHPAENG	HLA-DRB1*1301	441
β_2-microglobulin	21-34	TPKIQVYSRHPAEN	HLA-DRB1*1301	441
β_2-microglobulin	21-38	TPKIQVYSRHPAENGKSN	HLA-DRB1*1302	437
β_2-microglobulin	42-56	HPPHIEIQMLKNGKK	$H2\text{-}E^k$	433
β_2-microglobulin	84-98	LLYYTEFTPTEKDEY	HLA-DRB1*0405 (DR4Dw15)	432
β_2-microglobulin	42-56	HPPHIEIQMLKNGKK	$H2\text{-}E^s$	433
β-actin	286-303	MQKEITALAPSTMKIKII	$H2\text{-}E^s$	433
40S ribosomal protein S30	1-22	KVHGSLARAGKVRGQTPKVAKQ	$H2\text{-}A^k$	434
4F2	318-338	VTQYLNATGNRWCSWSLSQAR	HLA-DRB1*0701	435
4F2	318-334	VTQYLNATGNRWCSWSL	HLA-DRB1*0701	435
ACh receptor	289-304	VFLLLLADKVPETSLS	HLA-DRB1*0301(DR17)	435
Actin	195-210	ERGYSFTTTAEREIVR	$RT1.B^l$	436
Actin B	8-21	LVVDNGSGMCKAGF	$H2\text{-}E^d$	430
Alkaline phosphatase	479-496	YIPHVMAYAACIGANRDH	HLA-DRB1*0102	437
Apolipoprotein	196-213	SPLALIKGMTRPLSTLIS	HLA-DRB1*1104	437
Apolipoprotein	3344-3361	KSSVITLNTNAELFNQSD	HLA-DRB3*0202 (DR52Dw25)	437
Apolipoprotein	3345-3360	SXVITLNTNVGLYXQS	HLA-DR11 or Dw52	451
Apolipoprotein	3345-3360	SSVITLNTNVGLYXQT	HLA-DRB1*1201	450
Apolipoprotein B	2646-2663	STPEFTILNTFHIPSFTI	HLA-DRB1*0101	437
Apolipoprotein B	2877-2894	ISNQLTLDSNTKYFHKLN	HLA-DRB1*0301(DR17)	431
Apolipoprotein B	2877-2893	ISNQLTLDSNTKYFHKL	HLA-DRB1*0301(DR17)	431
Apolipoprotein B	2877-2892	ISNQLTLDSNTKYFHK	HLA-DRB1*0301(DR17)	431
Apolipoprotein B	1207-1224	YANILLDRRVPQTDMTF	HLA-DRB1*0301(DR17)	435
Apolipoprotein B	1276-1295	NLFLKSDGRIKYTLNKNSLK	HLA-DRB1*0301(DR17)	435
Apolipoprotein B	1273-1292	IPDNLFLKSDGRIKYTLNKN	HLA-DRB1*0301(DR17)	435

Table 5.7. (con't)

Protein	AA position	Sequence	MHC molecule	Ref.
Apolipoprotein B	1273-1291	IPDNLFLKSDGRIKYTLNK	HLA-DRB1*0301(DR17)	435
Apolipoprotein B	1273-1290	IPDNLFLKSDGRIKYTLN	HLA-DRB1*0301(DR17)	431, 435
Apolipoprotein B	1273-1289	IPDNLFLKSDGRIKYTL	HLA-DRB1*0301(DR17)	435
Apolipoprotein B	1276-1291	NLFLKSDGRIKYTLNK	HLA-DRB1*0301(DR17)	435
Apolipoprotein B	1276-1290	NLFLKSDGRIKYTLN	HLA-DRB1*0301(DR17)	435
Apolipoprotein B	1294-1310	VTTLNSDLKYNALDLTN	HLA-DRB1*0301(DR17)	435
Apolipoprotein B	2211-2224	SLDEHYHIRVHLVK	$H2-E^d$	430
Apolipoprotein B	2614-2628	TPDFIVPLTDLRIPS	HLA-DRB1*0404 (DR4Dw14)	438
Apolipoprotein B	2614-2627	TPDFIVPLTDLRIP	HLA-DRB1*0404 (DR4Dw14)	438
Apolipoprotein B	2615-2627	PDFIVPLTDLRIP	HLA-DRB1*0404 (DR4Dw14)	438
Apolipoprotein B	2615-2630	PDFIVPLTDLRIPSVQ	HLA-DRB1*0404 (DR4Dw14)	438
Apolipoprotein B	2617-2628	FIVPLTDLRIPS	HLA-DRB1*0404 (DR4Dw14)	438
Apolipoprotein B	2612-2631	FQTPDFIVPLTDLRIPSVQI	HLA-DRB1*0404 (DR4Dw14)	438
Apolipoprotein B-100	2804-2816	LNFDFQAKQLSDP	HLA-DQA1*0301/DQB1*0301 (DQ3.1)	Friede et al. (unpubl.)
Apolipoprotein B-100	2647-2662	TPEFTILNTLHIPSFT	HLA-DRB1*0801	435
Apolipoprotein B-100	3218-3230	KPYNEAKTXFDKY	HLA-DRB1*0405 (DR4Dw15)	439
Apolipoprotein B-100	1585-1598	NKVDLTFSKQHALL	HLA-DRB1*0901	440
Apolipoprotein B-100	43-58	APRFKHLRKYTYNYEA	HLA-DRB1*1302	441
Apolipoprotein B-100	3342-3361	SSVITLNVGLYDQSDIAK	HLA-DRB1*1302	441
Apolipoprotein B-100	3342-3358	SSVITLNVGLYDQSD	HLA-DRB1*1302	441
Apolipoprotein B-100	1724-1743	KNIFHFKVNQEGLKLSNDMM	HLA-DRB1*0801	435
Apolipoprotein B-100	1724-1739	KNIFHFKVNQEGLKLS	HLA-DRB1*0801	435
Apolipoprotein B-100	1780-1799	YKQTVSLDIQPYSLVTTLNS	HLA-DRB1*0801	435
Apolipoprotein B-100	2646-1662	STPEFTILNTLHIPSFT	HLA-DRB1*0801	435
Apolipoprotein B-100	2647-2664	TPEFTILNTLHIPSFTID	HLA-DRB1*0801	435
Apolipoprotein B-100	2885-2900	SNTKYFHKLNIPQLDF	HLA-DRB1*0801	435
Apolipoprotein B-100	2072-2088	LPFFKFLPKYFEKKRNT	HLA-DRB1*0801	435
Apolipoprotein B-100	2072-2086	LPFFKFLPKYFEKKR	HLA-DRB1*0801	435
Apolipoprotein B-100	4022-4036	WNFYYSPQSSPDKKL	HLA-DRB1*0801	435
Apolipoprotein B-100	1586-1608	KVDLTFSKQHALLCSDYQADYES	HLA-DRB1*0701	435
Apolipoprotein B-100	1586-1600	KVDLTFSKQHALLCS	HLA-DRB1*0701	435
Apolipoprotein B-100	1942-1954	FSHDYRGSTSHRL	HLA-DRB1*0701	435
Apolipoprotein B-100	2077-2089	LPKYFEKKRNTII	HLA-DRB1*0701	435
Apolipoprotein B-100	1200-1220	FPKSLHTYANILLDRRVPQTD	HLA-DR2	435
Apolipoprotein B-100	1200-1218	FPKSLHTYANILLDRRVPQ	HLA-DR2	435
Apolipoprotein E	268-284	WANLMEKIQASVATNPI	$H2-A^d$	442

Apolipoprotein E	268-283	WANLMEKIQASVATNP	H2-A^d	442
Apolipoprotein E	236-252	EEQTQQIRLQAEIFQAR	H2-A^d	442
Apolipoprotein E	237-252	EQTQQIRLQAEIFQAR	H2-A^d	442
Apolipoprotein-E prec.	222-236	ERAEAWRQKLHGRL	H2-E^d	430
Apolipoprotein-E prec.	223-236	RAEAWRQKLHGRL	H2-E^d	430
BLAST-1	62-78	FDQKIVEWDSRKSKYFE	HLA-DRB1*0402 (DR4Dw10)	432
BLAST-1	63-77	DQKIVEWDSRKSKYF	HLA-DRB1*0402 (DR4Dw10)	432
Bovine fetuin	342-355	IPGGPVRLCPGRIR	H2-E^k	430
BSA	152-170	ADEKKFWGKYLYEIARRHP	HLA-DPA1*0102/DPB1*0201	445
BSA	141-155	GKYLYEIARRHPYFY	H2-E^b	446
BST-2	128-142	HKLQDASAEVERLRR	HLA-DQA1*0301/DQB1*0301 (DQ3.1)	Friede et al., (unpubl.)
C. elegans cDNA homol.	74-87	GQFYFLIRKRIHLR	H2-E^d	430
Ca^{2+} release channel	2614-1623	RPSMLQHLLR	HLA-DRB1*0801	435
Calcitonin receptor	38-53	EPFLYILGKSRVLEAQ	HLA-DRB1*0801	435
Carboxypeptidase A	44-54	LYVLKIGKKDG	H2-E^s	433
Cathepsin C	170-185	YDHNFVKAINAIQKSW	HLA-DRB1*0401 (DR4Dw4)	432
Cathepsin C	58-73	XXXXKKVVVYLQKLDT	HLA-DRB1*0405 (DR4Dw15)	439
Cathepsin C	62-76	KKVVVYLQKLDTAYD	HLA-DRB1*0405 (DR4Dw15)	439
Cathepsin C	63-76	KVVVYLQKLDTAYD	HLA-DRB1*0405 (DR4Dw15)	439
Cathepsin C (rat) homol.	170-184	YDHNFVKAINAIQKS	HLA-DRB1*0407 (DR4Dw13)	447
Cathepsin D	221-238	IGRYYTVFDRDNNRVGFA	HLA-DRB1*1101	437
Cathepsin D	134-151	GPVDEVRELQKAIGAVPL	HLA-DRB1*1104	437
Cathepsin E	89-112	QNFTVIFDTGSSNLWVPSVYCTSP	HLA-DRB1*0801	435
Cathepsin E	89-104	QNFTVIFDTGSSNLWV	HLA-DRB1*0801	435
Cathepsin H	185-198	LPSQAFEYILYNKG	HLA-DPA1*0102/DPB1*0201	445
Cathepsin H	77-92	YILYNKGIMGEDSYPY	H2-A^k	443
Cathepsin H	72-92	YILYNKGIMGEDSYPY	H2-A^k	433
Cathepsin L-like	237-247	ESFLXYKKGIY	HLA-DRB1*1302	437
Cathepsin S	21-42	DPTLDHHWHLWKKTYGKQYKE	HLA-DRB1*1302	441
Cathepsin S	21-41	DPTLDHHWHLWKKTYGKQYK	HLA-DRB1*1302	441
Cathepsin S	189-205	TAFQYIIDNKGIDSDAS	HLA-DRB1*0801	435
Cattle fetuin	45-62	IDSVKVWPRRPTGEVYDI	HLA-DRB1*1301	437
Cattle hemoglobin	26-41	AEALERMFLSFPTTKT	HLA-DRB1*0401 (DR4Dw4)	435
Cattle serum albumin	419-436	TPTLVEVSRSLGKVGTRC	HLA-DRB1*1101	437
Cattle serum albumin	419-436	TPTLVEVSRSLGKVGTRC	HLA-DRB1*1104	437
Cattle transferrin	68-82	DVAFVKDQTVIQNTD	HLA-DRB1*0401 (DR4Dw4)	432
Cattle transferrin	261-281	DVIWELLNHAQEHFGKDKSKE	HLA-DRB1*0801	435
Cattle transferrin	261-275	DVIWELLNHAQEHFG	HLA-DRB1*0801	435
Cattle transferrin	261-273	DVIWELLNHAQEH	HLA-DRB1*0801	435

Table 5.7. (con't)

Protein	AA position	Sequence	MHC molecule	Ref.
CD20	260-270	EDIEIIPIGEE	HLA-DQA1*0501/DQB1*0201 (DQ2)	448
CD20	261-270	DIEIIPIGEE	HLA-DQA1*0501/DQB1*0201 (DQ2)	448
CD23	163-180	CPEKWINFQRKCYYFGKG	HLA-DRB1*1301	437
CD35	359-380	DDFMGQLLNGRVLFPVNLQLGA	HLA-DRB1*0801	435
CD45	1071-1084	GQVKKNNHQEDKIE	HLA-DR17 or DRw52	435
CD48	62-77	FDQKIVEWDSRKSKYF	HLA-DRB1*0402 (DR4Dw10)	438
CD48	62-78	FDQKIVEWDSRKSKYFE	HLA-DRB1*0402 (DR4Dw10)	438
CD48	62-79	FDQKIVEWDSRKSKYFES	HLA-DRB1*0402 (DR4Dw10)	438
CD48	62-75	FDQKIVEWDSRKSK	HLA-DRB1*0402 (DR4Dw10)	438
CD75	106-122	IPRLQKIWKNYLSMNKY	HLA-DRB1*0801	435
Clusterin	41-55	VNKEIQNAVQGVKHI	H2-E^k	433
c-myc	371-385	KRSFFALRDQIPDL	HLA-DRB1*0801	435
Coagulation factor V	39-56	TTYKKVVFRKYLDSTFTK	HLA-DRB1*1101	437
Complement C9	465-483	APVLISQKLSPIYNLVPVK	HLA-DRB1*0701	435
Cys-C	40-55	DAYHSRAIQVVRARKQ	H2-A^d	442
Cystatin SN	41-58	DEYYRRLLRVLRAREQIV	HLA-DRB1*0801	435
Cyt-b5	155-172	GFKAIRPDKKSNPIIRTV	HLA-DRB1*0301(DR17)	435
Cytoplasmic actin	47-62	MGQKDSYVGDEAQSKR	HLA-DRB1*0404 (DR4Dw14)	438
Cytoplasmic actin	66-81	TLKYPIEHGIVTNWDD	HLA-DRB1*0404 (DR4Dw14)	438
Cytoplasmic actin	69-82	YPIEHGIVTNWDDM	HLA-DRB1*0404 (DR4Dw14)	438
Cytoplasmic actin	96-114	VAPEEHPVLLTEAPLNPKA	HLA-DRB1*0404 (DR4Dw14)	438
Cytoplasmic actin	28-48	AVFPSIVGRPRHQGVMV	HLA-DRB1*0404 (DR4Dw14)	438
DEAD box protein		LHLGYLPNQLFR	H2-E^k	430
Dihydrolipoamide dehydrogenase (unpubl.)	138-152	AHLFKQNKVVHVNG	HLA-DRB1*1201	Falk et al,
DNA-B	92-108	DPFKGDDYNEENPTEPS	H2-A^k	443
EBV gp220	592-606	TGHGARTSTEPTTDY	HLA-DR17 or DRw52	435
EBV MCP	1264-1282	VPGLYSPCRAFFNKEELL	HLA-DRB1*0701	435
EBV MCP	1264-1277	VPGLYSPCRAFFNK	HLA-DRB1*0701	435
EBV tegument p140	1395-1407	KELKRQYEKKLRQ	HLA-DR17 or DRw52	435
Elongation factor Tu	342-359	AQVIILNHPGQISAGYAP	HLA-DRB3*0301 (DR52Dw26)	437
ER60	448-461	GFPTIYFSPANKKL	H2-E^k	430
Factor VIII	1775-1790	LWDYGMSSSPHVLRNR	HLA-DR2	435
Fcε Receptor II	298-310	SFLDAWVCEQLAT	H2-A^k	443
Fetuin (cattle)	56-74	YKHTLNQIDSVKVWPRRPT	HLA-DRB1*0101	354
Fibronectin receptor α	586-616	LSPIHIALNFSLDPQAPVDSHGLRPALHYQ	HLA-DR2	435

GAPDH	9-24	FGRIGRLVTRAAFNSG	HLA-DRB1*0402 (DR4Dw10)	432
GAPDH	9-22	FGRIGRLVTRAAFN	HLA-DRB1*0402 (DR4Dw10)	432
GAPDH	9-24	GFGRIGRLVTRAAFNSG	HLA-DRB1*0402 (DR4Dw10)	432
GAPDH	9-23	FGRIGRLVTRAAFNS	HLA-DRB1*0402 (DR4Dw10)	444
GAPDH	8-22	GFGRIGRLVTRAAFN	HLA-DRB1*0402 (DR4Dw10)	444
GAPDH	139-154	YDNSLKIISNASCTTN	HLA-DRB1*0404 (DR4Dw14)	432
GAPDH	292-305	STFDAGAGIALNDH	HLA-DQA1*0301/DQB1*0301 (DQ3.1)	Friede et al, unpubl
Glucose transporter	459-474	TFDEIASGFRQGGASQ	HLA-DR17 or DRw52	435
Granulin D	41-56	CPAGYTCNVKARSCEK	HLA-DRB1*1101	451
Granulin D	41-58	CPAGYTCNVKARSCEKEV	HLA-DRB1*1101	437
Guanylate binding protein 2	434-450	QELKNKYYQVPRKGIQA	HLA-DR2	435
H2-Aβ^k	37-53	VRFDSDVGEFRAVTEL	H2-A^k	443
H2-Aβ^k	165-179	TPRRGEVYTCHVEHP	H2-A^k	434
H2-Aβ^k	37-53	FVRFDSDVGEFRAVTEL	H2-A^k	433
H2-Aβ^k	3-17	XXXFVHQFQPFCYF	H2-A^k	433
H2-Aβ^k	10-20	QFQPFXYFTNT	H2-A^k	433
H2-Aβ	55-66	RPDAEYWNSQPE	H2-A^b	446
H2-Eα	52-68	ASFEAQGALANIAVDKA	H2-A^b	446
H2-Eα^d	52-67	ASFEAQGALANIAVDK	H2-A^d	442
H2-Eα^d	52-68	ASFEAQGALANIAVDKA	H2-A^d	442
H2-Eβ^k	33-47	XNLRFDSDVGEFRAV	H2-A^k	433
H2-L^d	160-174	EGECVEWLHRYLKNG	H2-E^s	433
Hemoglobin-like	124-141	SLDKFLANVSTVLTGKYR	HLA-DRB3*0202 (DR52Dw25)	437
HEL	48-61	DGSTDYGILQINSR	H2-A^k	434
HEL	48-60	DGSTDYGILQINS	H2-A^k	434
HEL	48-62	DGSTDYGILQINSRW	H2-A^k	434
HEL	52-63 (64)	DYGILQINSRWW(C)	H2-A^k	434
Histone H3	110-?	CAIHAKRVTIMPKDIQLA...	HLA-DRB1*0405 (DR4Dw15)	432
HLA-C	52-?	VDDTQFVRFDSDAASPRGEP...	HLA-DRB1*0401 (DR4Dw4)	432
HLA-class I	104-119	GPDGRLLRGHNQYAYD	HLA-DRB1*1201	450
HLA-class Iα	46-60	EPRAPWIEQEGPEYW	HLA-DQA1*0501/DQB1*0201 (DQ2)	448
HLA-class Iα	47-59	PRAPWIEQEGPEY	HLA-DQA1*0501/DQB1*0201 (DQ2)	448
HLA-class Iα	46-59	EPRAPWIEQEGPEY	HLA-DQA1*0501/DQB1*0201 (DQ2)	448
HLA-class Iα	46-58	EPRAPWIEQEGPE	HLA-DQA1*0501/DQB1*0201 (DQ2)	448
HLA-class Iα	52-60	IEQEGPEYW	HLA-DQA1*0501/DQB1*0201 (DQ2)	448
HLA-A	145-156	KDYIALNEDLRS	HLA-DRB1*0404 (DR4Dw14)	438
HLA-A	145-158	KDYIALNEDLRSWT	HLA-DRB1*0404 (DR4Dw14)	438
HLA-A	145-159	KDYIALNEDLRSWTA	HLA-DRB1*0404 (DR4Dw14)	438
HLA-A	146-161	DYIALNEDLRSWTAAD	HLA-DRB1*0404 (DR4Dw14)	438

Table 5.7. (con't)

Protein	AA position	Sequence	MHC molecule	Ref.
HLA-A	146-160	DYIALNEDLRSWTAA	HLA-DRB1*0404 (DR4Dw14)	438
HLA-A	146-158	DYIALNEDLRSWT	HLA-DRB1*0404 (DR4Dw14)	438
HLA-A1	119-136	KDYIALNEDLRSWTAADT	HLA-DRB3*0202 (DR52Dw25)	437
HLA-A11	143-156	KRKWEAAHAAEQQR	HLA-DRB1*0901	440
HLA-A2	103-117	VGSDWRFLRGYHQYA	HLA-DRB1*0101	354
HLA-A2	103-120	VGSDWRFLRGYHQYQYDG	HLA-DRB1*0101	354
HLA-A2	103-116	VGSDWRFLRGYHQY	HLA-DRB1*0101	354
HLA-A2	104-117	GSDWRFLRGYHQYA	HLA-DRB1*0101	354
HLA-A2	103-117	VGSDWRFLRGYHQYA	HLA-DRB1*0301(DR17)	435
HLA-A2	33-47	FVRFDSDAASQRMEP	HLA-DRB1*0401 (DR4Dw4)	432
HLA-A2	52-69	VDDTQFVRFDSDAASQRM	HLA-DRB1*0401 (DR4Dw4)	432
HLA-A2	33-45	FVRFDSDAASQRM	HLA-DRB1*0401 (DR4Dw4)	432
HLA-A2	103-120	VGSDWRFLRGYHQYAYDG	HLA-DRB1*1101	437
HLA-A2	103-120	VGSDWRFLRGYHQYAYDG	HLA-DRB1*0701	435
HLA-A29	234-253	RPAGDGTFQKWASVVVPSGQ	HLA-DRB1*0701	435
HLA-A29	234-249	RPAGDGTFQKWASVVV	HLA-DRB1*0701	435
HLA-A29	237-258	GDGTFQKWASVVVPSGQEQRYT	HLA-DRB1*0701	435
HLA-A29	237-254	GDGTFQKWASVVVPSGQE	HLA-DRB1*0701	435
HLA-A29	239-252	GTFQKWASVVVPSG	HLA-DRB1*0701	435
HLA-A29	239-253	GTFQKWASVVVPSGQ	HLA-DRB1*0701	435
HLA-A29	239-261	GTFQKWASVVVPSGQEQRYTCHV	HLA-DRB1*0701	435
HLA-A3	152-166	EAEQLRAYLDGTGVE	HLA-DRB1*1501 (DR2b)	321
HLA-A3	135-151	AADMAAQITKRKWEAAH	HLA-DRB5*0101 (DR2a)	321
HLA-A3	134-149	TAADMAAQITKRKWEA	HLA-DRB5*0101 (DR2a)	321
HLA-A30	52-67	VDDTQFVRFDSDAASQ	HLA-DRB1*0301(DR17)	435
HLA-A33	323-340	AGAVVAAVRWRRKSSDRK	HLA-DRB1*1302	437
HLA-B38	128-?	GPDGRLLRGHNQFAYDGKDY...	HLA-DRB1*0402 (DR4Dw10)	432
HLA-B38	128-146	GPDGRLLRGHNQFAYDGKD	HLA-DRB1*0402 (DR4Dw10)	432
HLA-B38	128-145	GPDGRLLRGHNQFAYDGK	HLA-DRB1*0402 (DR4Dw10)	432
HLA-B38	128-144	GPDGRLLRGHNQFAYDG	HLA-DRB1*0402 (DR4Dw10)	432
HLA-B38	131-145	GRLLRGHNQFAYDGK	HLA-DRB1*0402 (DR4Dw10)	432
HLA-B38	104-121	GPDGRLLRGYDQFAYDGK	HLA-DRB1*1201	450
HLA-B39	128-145	GPDGRLLRGHNQFAYDGK	HLA-DRB1*0402 (DR4Dw10)	444
HLA-B39	128-143	GPDGRLLRGHNQFAYD	HLA-DRB1*0402 (DR4Dw10)	444
HLA-B39	128-147	GPDGRLLRGHNQFAYDGKDY	HLA-DRB1*0402 (DR4Dw10)	444
HLA-B39	127-143	VGPDGRLLRGHNQFAYD	HLA-DRB1*0402 (DR4Dw10)	444

HLA-B*4001	27-40	SHSMRYFHTAMSRP	HLA-DRB1*0404 (DR4Dw14)	444
HLA-B*4001	26-41	GSHSMRYFHTAMSRPG	HLA-DRB1*0404 (DR4Dw14)	444
HLA-B*4001	27- 41	SHSMRYFHTAMSRPG	HLA-DRB1*0404 (DR4Dw14)	444
HLA-B*4001	26-43	GSHSMRYFHTAMSRPGRG	HLA-DRB1*0404 (DR4Dw14)	444
HLA-B44	143-156	DGKDYIALNEDLSS	HLA-DRB1*0401 (DR4Dw4)	432
HLA-B44	154-168	LSSWTAADTAAQITQ	HLA-DRB1*0401 (DR4Dw4)	432
HLA-B44	154-167	LSSWTAADTAAQIT	HLA-DRB1*0401 (DR4Dw4)	432
HLA-B44	6-23	RYFYTAMSRPGRGEPRFI	HLA-DRB1*1302	437
HLA-B44	158-169	TAADTAAQITQR	HLA-DQA1*0301/DQB1*0301 (DQ3.1)	Friede et al, unpubl.
HLA-B44	83-99	RETQISKTNTQTYRENL	HLA-DRB1*0701	435
HLA-B44	83-98	RETQISKTNTQTYREN	HLA-DRB1*0701	435
HLA-B44	83-97	RETQISKTNTQTYRE	HLA-DRB1*0701	435
HLA-B60	1-13	GSHSMRYFHTAMSRPGRGE	HLA-DRB1*0404 (DR4Dw14)	432
HLA-B60	2-13	SHSMRYFHTAMSRPGRGE	HLA-DRB1*0404 (DR4Dw14)	432
HLA-B61	5-20	MRYFHTSVSRPGRGEP	HLA-DRB1*1101	451
HLA-B62	130-144	LSSWTAADTAAQITQ	HLA-DRB1*0401 (DR4Dw4)	452
HLA-B62	129-150	DLSSWTAADTAAQITQRKWEAA	HLA-DRB1*0401 (DR4Dw4)	435
HLA-B7	104-123	GPDGRLLRGHDQYAYDGKDY	HLA-DRB1*1301	441
HLA-B7	104-122	GPDGRLLRGHDQYAYDGKD	HLA-DRB1*1301	441
HLA-C	56-72	GPEYWDRETQKYKRQAQ	HLA-DRB1*1302	441
HLA-C	56-71	GPEYWDRETQKYKRQA	HLA-DRB1*1302	441
HLA-C	56-70	GPEYWDRETQKYKRQ	HLA-DRB1*1302	441
HLA-Class I	153-166	DLRSWTAADTAAQI	HLA-DRB1*0407 (DR4Dw13)	447
HLA-Class I	153-168	DLRSWTAADTAAQITQ	HLA-DRB1*0407 (DR4Dw13)	447
HLA-Class I	154-167	LRSWTAADTAAQIT	HLA-DRB1*0407 (DR4Dw13)	447
HLA-Class I	29-40	MRYFYTAVSRPG	HLA-DRB1*0407 (DR4Dw13)	447
HLA-Class I	28-41	VDDTQFVRFDSDAA	HLA-DRB1*0407 (DR4Dw13)	447
HLA-Cw*03	27-40	SHSMRYFYTAVSRP	HLA-DRB1*0404 (DR4Dw14)	444
HLA-Cw*03	27-41	SHSMRYFYTAVSRPG	HLA-DRB1*0404 (DR4Dw14)	444
HLA-Cw*03	26-41	GSHSMRYFYTAVSRPG	HLA-DRB1*0404 (DR4Dw14)	444
HLA-Cw*03	26-42	GSHSMRYFYTAVSRPGR	HLA-DRB1*0404 (DR4Dw14)	444
HLA-Cw*03	27-43	SHSMRYFYTAVSRPGRG	HLA-DRB1*0404 (DR4Dw14)	444
HLA-Cw9	130-150	LRSWTAADTAAQITQRKWEAA	HLA-DRB1*0401 (DR4Dw4)	435
HLA-DPβ	80-92	RHNYELDEAVTLQ	HLA-DRB1*0801	435
HLA-DPw4β	25-44	LERYIYNREEFVRFDSDVGE	HLA-DRB3*0202 (DR52Dw25)	437
HLA-DQ 3.2	24-38	SPEDFVYQFKGMCYF	HLA-DRB1*0401 (DR4Dw4)	435
HLA-DQα	97-119	NIVIKRSNSTAATNEVPEVTVFS	HLA-DR2	435
HLA-DQα	97-112	NIVIKRSNSTAATNEV	HLA-DR2	435
HLA-DQα	179-?	SLQSPITVEWRAQSESAQSKMLSGIGGFVL	HLA-DRB1*0701	435
HLA-DQα*0501	1-15	EDIVADHVASYGVNL	HLA-DQA1*0501/DQB1*0201 (DQ2)	448
HLA-DQα*0501	1-11	EDIVADHVASY	HLA-DQA1*0501/DQB1*0201 (DQ2)	448

Table 5.7. (con't)

Protein	AA position	Sequence	MHC molecule	References
HLA-DQα*0501	16-30	YQSYGPSGQYTHEFD	HLA-DQA1*0501/DQB1*0201 (DQ2)	448
HLA-DQα*0301	153-168	YLTFLPSADEIYDCKV	HLA-DQA1*0501/DQB1*0201 (DQ2)	448
HLA-DQα*0501	16-30	YQSYGPSGQYTHEFD	HLA-DQA1*0501/DQB1*0201 (DQ2)	448
HLA-DQB1*06	53-70	TERVRLVTRHIYNREEYV	HLA-DRB1*1301	437
HLA-DQB1*06	53-68	TERVRLVTRHIYNREE	HLA-DRB1*1301	441
HLA-DQB1*06	53-67	TERVRLVTRHIYNRE	HLA-DRB1*1301	441
HLA-DQB1*06	53-66	TERVRLVTRHIYNR	HLA-DRB1*1301	441
HLA-DQB1*06	53-70	TERVRLVTRHIYNREEYV	HLA-DRB1*1302	437
HLA-DQB1*0604	123-140	FYPGQIKVRWFRNDQEET	HLA-DRB1*1301	437
HLA-DQβ	42-59	SDVGVYRAVTPQGRPDAE	HLA-DR2	435
HLA-DQβ	43-59	DVGVYRAVTPQGRPDAE	HLA-DR2	435
HLA-DQβ	43-57	DVGVYRAVTPQGRPD	HLA-DR2	435
HLA-DQβ	43-55	DVEVYRAVTPLGPEVAGQF	HLA-DQA1*0501/DQB1*0301 (DQ7)	450
HLA-DQw6	43-58	DVGVYRAVTPQGRPDA	HLA-DRB1*1501 (DR2b)	321
HLA-DQw6	43-56	DVGVYRAVTPQGRP	HLA-DRB5*0101 (DR2a)	321
HLA-DQw6	43-58	DVGVYRAVTPQGRPDA	HLA-DRB5*0101 (DR2a)	321
HLA-DQw6	41-57	DSDVGVYRAVTPQGRPD	HLA-DRB5*0101 (DR2a)	321
HLA-DQw6	41-58	DSDVGVYRAVTPQGRPDA	HLA-DRB5*0101 (DR2a)	321
HLA-DQw6	41-60	DSDVGVYRAVTPQGRPDAEY	HLA-DRB5*0101 (DR2a)	321
HLA-DR	238-252	IIKGVRKSNAAERRG	HLA-DRB1*0402 (DR4Dw10)	432
HLA-DR	45-58	LEEFGRFASFEAQG	HLA-DRB1*1501 (DR2b)	321
HLA-DR13β	43-60	DVGEFRAVTELGRPDEEY	HLA-DRB1*1302	437
HLA-DR2b	43-61	DVGEFAAVTEKRRPDAEYW	HLA-DRB5*0101 (DR2a)	321
HLA-DR4	248-266	IYFRNQKGHSGLQPTGFLS	HLA-DRB1*0402 (DR4Dw10)	432
HLA-DR4	248-261	IYFRNQKGHSGLQP	HLA-DRB1*0402 (DR4Dw10)	432
HLA-DR4	250-261	FRNQKGHSGLQP	HLA-DRB1*0402 (DR4Dw10)	432
HLA-DR4	249-266	FIYFRNQKGHSGLQPTGFLS	HLA-DRB1*0402 (DR4Dw10)	432
HLA-DR4	252-270	IYFRNQKGSHSGLQPTGFL	HLA-DRB1*0401 (DR4Dw4)	432
HLA-DR4β*0401	124-135	VYPEVTVYPAKT	HLA-DRB1*0401 (DR4Dw4)	438
HLA-DR4β*0401	124-134	VYPEVTVYPAK	HLA-DRB1*0401 (DR4Dw4)	438
HLA-DR52β	43-60	DVGEYRAVTELGRPDEEY	HLA-DRB1*1302	437
HLA-DRα	110-127	VPPEVTVLTNSPVELREP	HLA-DRB3*0301 (DR52Dw26)	437
HLA-DRα	33-50	IQAEFYLNPDQSGEFMFD	HLA-DRB3*0202 (DR52Dw25)	437
HLA-DRα	101-126	RSNYTPITNPPEVTVLTNSPVELREP	HLA-DRB1*0701	435
HLA-DRα	58-78	GALANIAVDKANLEIMTKRSN	HLA-DRB1*0701	435
HLA-DRα	182-200	APSPLPETTENVVCALGLTV	HLA-DRB1*0701	435

HLA-DRα	182-198	APSPLPETTENVVCALG	HLA-DRB1*0801	435
HLA-DRα	158-180	SETVFLPREDHLFRKFHYLPFLP	HLA-DRB1*0801	435
HLA-DRα chain	86-101	ANIAVDKANLEIMTKR	HLA-DRB1*0404 (DR4Dw14)	438
HLA-DRα chain	85-101	LANIAVDKANLEIMTKR	HLA-DRB1*0404 (DR4Dw14)	438
HLA-DRα chain	82-96	QGALANIAVDKANLE	HLA-DRB1*0404 (DR4Dw14)	438
HLA-DRα chain	82-98	QGALANIAVDKANLEIM	HLA-DRB1*0404 (DR4Dw14)	438
HLA-DRα chain	81-99	AQGALANIAVDKANLEIMT	HLA-DRB1*0404 (DR4Dw14)	438
HLA-DRB1*0101	22-35	ERVRLLERCIYNQE	HLA-DRB1*0101	305,449
HLA-DRB1*1501	94-111	RVQPKVTVYPSKTQPLQH	HLA-DR2	435
HLA-DRB1*1501	94-108	RVQPKVTVYPSKTQP	HLA-DR2	435
HSC70 Homol.	238-252	VNHFIAEFKRKHKKD	HLA-DRB1*1101	451
HSC70 Homol.	238-250	VNHFIAEFKRKHK	HLA-DRB1*1101	451
HSC70	445-?	GERAMTKDNNLLG...	HLA-DRB1*0401 (DR4Dw4)	432
HSC70	574-585	CNEIINWLDKNQ	HLA-DRB1*0402 (DR4Dw10)	432
HSC70	291-305	IDFYTSITRARFEE	HLA-DRB1*1101	451
HSC70	62-79	NPTNTVFDAKRLIGRRFD	HLA-DRB1*1104	437
HSC70	234-248	DNRMVHFIAEFKRK	H2-E^k	433
Hsp90-β	68-81	KELKIDIIPNPQER	HLA-DRB1*0405 (DR4Dw15)	432
HSP60	478-492	EGSLIVEKIMQSSSE	H2-E^s	433
HSP70	420-437	TIPTKQTQTFTTYSDNQP	RT1.B^l	436
HSP70	38-54	TPSYVAFTDTERLIGDA	HLA-DRB1*0701	435
HSP70	38-52	TPSYVAFTDTERLIG	HLA-DRB1*0701	435
HSP70	28-41	IIANDQGNRTTPSY	H2-A^k	434
ICAM-2	64-76	LNKILLDEQAQWK	HLA-DRB1*0301(DR17)	435
IFN α receptor	271-287	GNHLYKWKQIPDCENVK	HLA-DRB1*0801	435
IFN γ receptor	128-147	GPPKLDIRKEEKQIMIDIFH	HLA-DRB1*0301(DR17)	435
IFN γ receptor	128-148	GPPKLDIRKEEKQIMIDIFHP	HLA-DRB1*0301(DR17)	435
Igλ chain	11-28	FPPSSEELQANKATLVCL	HLA-DRB3*0301 (DR52Dw26)	437
Igλ chain C region	80-?	KHKVYACEVTHQG...	HLA-DRB1*0401 (DR4Dw4)	432
Igλ chain C region	81-?	HKVYACEVTHQGL...	HLA-DRB1*0401 (DR4Dw4)	432
Ig heavy chain	121-?	GVYFYLQWGRSTLVSVS	HLA-DRB1*0401 (DR4Dw4)	435
Igκ chain	63-80	FTFTISRLEPEDFAVYYC	HLA-DRB1*0801	435
Igκ chain	63-77	FTFTISRLEPEDFAV	HLA-DRB1*0801	435
Igκ chain	188-201	KHKVYACEVTHQGL	HLA-DRB1*0701	435
Igκ chain Homol.	190-204	KHKVYACEVTHQGLS	HLA-DRB1*1101	451
Igκ chain	39-?	KPGKAPKLLIYAASSL...	HLA-DRB1*0404 (DR4Dw14)	438
Igκ chain	43-?	APKLLIYAASSL...	HLA-DRB1*0404 (DR4Dw14)	438
Igκ chain	111-126	AAPSVFIFPPSDEQLK	HLA-DQA1*0501/DQB1*0201 (DQ2)	448
Igκ chain V region A	30 63-74	PGKAPKRLIYAA	HLA-DRB1*0404 (DR4Dw14)	444
Igκ chain V region	60-80	PGQPPRLLIYDASNRATGIPA	HLA-DRB1*0401 (DR4Dw4)	438

Table 5.7. (con't)

Protein	AA position	Sequence	MHC molecule	Ref.
Igκ chain V region	59-80	KPGQPPRLLIYDASNRATGIPA	HLA-DRB1*0401 (DR4Dw4)	438
Igκ chain V region	61-80	**pEPPRLLIYDASNRATGIPA	HLA-DRB1*0401 (DR4Dw4)	438
Igκ chain V region	71-77	pEPPRLLIYDASNRATG	HLA-DRB1*0401 (DR4Dw4)	438
Igκ chain precursor	88-102	SGTDFTLTISRLEPE	HLA-DRB1*0407 (DR4Dw13)	447
IgE Fc receptor	203-222	SPEEQDFLTKHASHTGSWIG	HLA-DRB1*0402 (DR4Dw10)	438
IgE Fc receptor	206-222	EQDFLTKHASHTGSWIG	HLA-DRB1*0402 (DR4Dw10)	438
IgE Fc receptor	207-222	QDFLTKHASHTGSWIG	HLA-DRB1*0402 (DR4Dw10)	438
IgG Vμ	59-74	XNADFKTPATLTVDKP	$H2\text{-}A^b$	446
IgG2a	194-210	WQSQSITCNVAHPASST	$H2\text{-}A^s$	454
IgG2a	281-296	NVEVHTAQTQTHREDY	$H2\text{-}A^s$	454
IgG2a, membrane domain	384-395	KQTISPDYRNMI	HLA-DRB1*0301(DR17)	431
IgM μ chain homol.	173-187	GPTTYKVTSSLQIKE	HLA-DRB1*0407 (DR4Dw13)	447
IL-2 receptor chain	168-182	SQLELRWKSRHIKER	$H2\text{-}E^d$	430
IL-2 receptor chain	170-182	LELRWKSRHIKER	$H2\text{-}E^d$	430
IL-3 receptor α-chain	127-146	GPGAPADVQYDLYLNVANRR	HLA-DPA1*0201/DPB1*0401 (DPw4)	450
IL-8 receptor	169-188	LPFFLFRQAYHPNNSSPVCY	HLA-DRB1*0801	435
Influenza HA	306-318	PKYVKQNTLKLAT	HLA-DRB1*0101	455
Influenza NP	265-279	IASNENMDAMESSTLY	HLA-DQA1*0501/DQB1*0201 (DQ2)	448
Invariant chain	97-118	LPKPPKPVSKMRMATPLLMQAL	HLA-DRB1*0101	449
Invariant chain	97-120	LPKPPKPVSKMRMATPLLMQALPM	HLA-DRB1*0101	354
Invariant chain	97-118	LPKPPKPVSKMRMATPLLMQAL	HLA-DRB1*0102	437
Invariant chain	97-113	LPKPPKPVSKMRMATPL	HLA-DRB1*0301(DR17)	456, 435, 457
Invariant chain	97-119	LPKPPKPVSKMRMATPLLMQALP	HLA-DRB1*0301(DR17)	456, 435, 457
Invariant chain	97-120	LPKPPKPVSKMRMATPLLMQALPM	HLA-DRB1*0301(DR17)	456, 435, 457
Invariant chain	98-113	PKPPKPVSKMRMATPL	HLA-DRB1*0301(DR17)	456, 435, 457
Invariant chain	98-117	PKPPKPVSKMRMATPLLMQA	HLA-DRB1*0301(DR17)	456, 435, 457
Invariant chain	99-116	KPPKPVSKMRMATPLLMQ	HLA-DRB1*0301(DR17)	456, 435, 457
Invariant chain	99-119	KPPKPVSKMRMATPLLMQALPM	HLA-DRB1*0301(DR17)	456, 435, 457
Invariant chain	131-149	ATKYGNMTEDHVMHLLQNA	HLA-DRB1*0301(DR17)	435
Invariant chain	97-114	LPKPPKPVSKMRMATPLLQ	HLA-DRB1*0402 (DR4Dw10)	432
Invariant chain	185-199	MHHWLLFEMSRHSLE	HLA-DRB1*0402 (DR4Dw10)	438
Invariant chain	186-199	HHWLLFEMSRHSLE	HLA-DRB1*0402 (DR4Dw10)	438
Invariant chain	188-202	WLLFEMSRHSLEQKP	HLA-DRB1*0402 (DR4Dw10)	438
Invariant chain	97-120	LPKPPKPVSKMRMATPLLMQALPM	HLA-DRB1*1301	441
Invariant chain	97-119	LPKPPKPVSKMRMATPLLMQALP	HLA-DRB1*1301	441
Invariant chain	66-83	TTAYFLYQQQGRLDKLTV	HLA-DRB1*1302	437
Invariant chain	66-80	TTAYFLYQQQGRLDK	HLA-DRB1*1302	441

Invariant chain	97-120	LPKPPKPVSKMRMATPLLMQALPM	HLA-DRB1*1302	441
Invariant chain	111-126	TPLLMQALPMGALPQG	HLA-DQA1*0501/DQB1*0301 (DQ7)	450
Invariant chain	111-125	TPLLMQALPMGALPQ	HLA-DQA1*0501/DQB1*0301 (DQ7)	450
Invariant chain	99-117	KPPKPVSKMRMATPLLMQA	HLA-DQA1*0501/DQB1*0301 (DQ7)	450
Invariant chain	97-115	LPKPPKPVSKMRMATPLLM	HLA-DQA1*0501/DQB1*0301 (DQ7)	450
Invariant chain	99-112	KPPKPVSKMRMATP	HLA-DQA1*0501/DQB1*0201 (DQ2)	448
Invariant chain	108-123	RMATPLLMQALPMGAL	HLA-DQA1*0501/DQB1*0201 (DQ2)	448
Invariant chain	108-118	RMATPLLMQAL	HLA-DQA1*0501/DQB1*0201 (DQ2)	448
Invariant chain	109-123	MATPLLMQALPMGAL	HLA-DQA1*0501/DQB1*0201 (DQ2)	448
Invariant chain	98-119	PKPPKPVSKMRMATPLLMQALP	HLA-DRB1*0701	435
Invariant chain	86-100	KPVSQMRMATPLLMR	H2-A^b	446
Invariant chain	85-101	KPVSQMRMATPLLMRPM	H2-A^d	442
IP30	38-59	SPLQALDFFGNGPPVNYKTGNL	HLA-DR17 or DRw52	435
K^+ channel protein	492-516	GDMYPKTWSGMLVGALCALAGVLTI	HLA-DRB1*0701	435
K^+ channel protein	173-190	DGILYYYQSGGRLRRPVN	HLA-DR2	435
K-ras	164-180	RQYRLKKISKEEKTPGC	HLA-DRB1*0801	435
L plastin	581-595	NNAKYAISMARKIGA	HLA-DRB1*0901	440
λ repressor	12-26	LEDARRLKAIYEKKK	H2-A^d	442
LAM Blast-1	88-108	DPQSGALYISKVQKEDNSTYI	HLA-DRB1*0801	435
LAM Blast-1	92-108	GALYISKVQKEDNSTYI	HLA-DRB1*0801	435
LAM Blast-1	129-146	DPVPKPVIKIEKIEDMDD	HLA-DRB1*0801	435
LAM Blast-1	129-143	DPVPKPVIKIEKIED	HLA-DRB1*0801	435
LAR	1302-1316	DPVEMRRLNYQTPG	HLA-DRB1*0801	435
LDL-Receptor	518-532	KPRAIVVDPVHGFMY	HLA-DRB1*0301(DR17)	431
Leucine-rich 2-glycoprotein	200-211	QPDLRYLFLNGN	HLA-DRB1*0402 (DR4Dw10)	432
LIF receptor	854-866	TSILCYRKREWIK	HLA-DRB1*0701	435
LIF receptor	709-726	YQLLRSMIGYIEELAPIV	HLA-DRB1*0801	435
Lymphocyte activ. antigen	414-431	DPGSLLSLFRRLSDQRSK	HLA-DRB1*1104	437
Macrophage inflam. prot.	47-64	KPGVIFLTKRSRQVCADP	HLA-DRB1*1104	437
Mannose binding protein	174-193	IQNLIKEEAFLGITDEKTEG	HLA-DR2	435
Mannose-6-phosphate receptor	185-202	DLNPLIKLSGAYLVDDSD	HLA-DRB1*0102	437
MBI	177-193	EDENLYEGLNLDDCSMY	H2-A^k	443
MBI	177-194	EDENLYEGLNLDDCSMYY	H2-A^k	433
Membrane cofactor prot.	315-332	VPYRYLQRRKKKGKADGG	HLA-DRB1*1101	437
MET protooncogene	59-81	EHHIFLGATNYIYVLNEEDLQKV	HLA-DR2	435
MIF	32-45	KPPQYIAVHVVPDQ	HLA-DRB1*0405 (DR4Dw15)	432
MIF	32-47	KPPQYIAVHVVPDQLM	HLA-DRB1*0405 (DR4Dw15)	439
MIF	32-46	KPPQYIAVHVVPDQL	HLA-DRB1*0405 (DR4Dw15)	439
MIF	32-45	KPPQYIAVHVVPDQ	HLA-DRB1*0405 (DR4Dw15)	439

Table 5.7. (con't)

Protein	AA position	Sequence	MHC molecule	Ref.
MIF Homol.	32-46	XXXQYIAVHVVPDQT	HLA-DRB1*0405 (DR4Dw15)	453
MIL-1 Receptor	185-199	AILLDKGNKEFLSAG	H2-A^k	443
MuLV env	255-269	IRLKITDSGPRVPIGPN	H2-A^s	454
MuLV env	255-267	IRLKITDSGPRVPIG	H2-A^s	458
MuLV env	145-158	HNEGFYVCPGPHRP	H2-A^b	446
MuLV env	454-469	SPSYVYHQFERRAKYK	H2-E^b	446
MuLV env	454-475	SPSYVYHQFERRAKYKREPVSL	H2-E^b	446
MuLV env	454-467	SPSYVYHQFERRAK	H2-E^b	446
M. bovis 65 kD Ag	243-255	KPLLIIAEDVEGEY	HLA-DQA1*0501/DQB1*0201 (DQ2)	448
M. leprae 18 kD Ag	31-43	DAWREGEEFVVEF/DQB1*0201 (DQ2)	HLA-DQA1*0501/DQB1*0201 (DQ2)	448
Myosin β heavy chain	1027-1047	HELEKIKKQVEQEKCEIQAAL	HLA-DRB1*0801	435
Na+ channel protein	384-397	YGYTSYDTFSWAFL	HLA-DR17 or DRw52	435
Na^+-K^+-ATPase	199-216	IPADLRIISANGCK	HLA-DRB1*0101	354
Neuropeptide Y-like receptor	306-317	GAKFKTSAQHAL	HLA-DRB1*0901	440
Nidogen	429-446	DLHSYVVMNHGRSYTAIS	HLA-DRB1*1101	437
Nucleobindin	140-153	LDPQNQHTFEARDL	RT1.B^l	436
Ovalbumin	267-276	WTSSNVMEERY	HLA-DQA1*0501/DQB1*0201 (DQ2)	448
Ovalbumin	323-336	ISQAVHAAHAEINE	H2-A^d	442
PAI-1	261-281	AAPYEKEVPLSALTNILSAQL	HLA-DRB1*0401 (DR4Dw4)	435
PAI-1	378-396	DRPFLFVVRHNPTGTVLFM	HLA-DRB1*0801	435
PAI-1	133-148	MPHFFRLFRSTVKQVD	HLA-DRB1*0801	435
PGSG	1-19	YPTQRARYQWVRCNPDSNS	HLA-DRB1*0405 (DR4Dw15)	432
PGSG	4-19	QRARYQWVRCNPDSNS	HLA-DRB1*0405 (DR4Dw15)	432
PGSG	5-19	RARYQWVRCNPDSNS	HLA-DRB1*0405 (DR4Dw15)	432
PGSG	28-46	YPTQRARYQWVRCNPDSNS	HLA-DRB1*0407 (DR4Dw13)	447
Phosphoglycerate kinase	216-228	VADKIQLINNMLD	HLA-DRB1*0405 (DR4Dw15)	432
PKM2	99-112	SDPILYRPVAVALD	HLA-DRB1*0405 (DR4Dw15)	453
PKM2	101-118	DPILYRPVAVALDTKGPE	HLA-DRB1*0405 (DR4Dw15)	439
PKM2	101-117	DPILYRPVAVALDTKGP	HLA-DRB1*0405 (DR4Dw15)	439
Pleckstrin	161-178	VIDWLVSNQSVRNRQEGL	HLA-DRB3*0202 (DR52Dw25)	437
Pyruvate kinase	264-278	IKIISKIENHEGVRR	HLA-DRB1*0402 (DR4Dw10)	432
Pyruvate kinase	264-277	IKIISKIENHEGVR	HLA-DRB1*0402 (DR4Dw10)	432
Rabies virus NP	11-25	NNQVVSLKPEIIVDQY	HLA-DQA1*0501/DQB1*0201 (DQ2)	448
ras-related protein RAB-5A	123-140	SPNIVIALSGNKADLANK	HLA-DRB1*0102	437
ras-related protein RAB-7 (rat)	86-98	APNTFKTLDSWRD	HLA-DRB1*0405 (DR4Dw15)	432
Ribophorin I	86-103	SGRFFTVKLPVALDPGAK	HLA-DRB1*1101	437

Ribophorin I	203-218	DIPAYSQDTFKVHYEN	RT1.B[l]	436
Ryudocan	84-100	EPLVPLDNHIPENAQPG	H2-A[k]	434
Serotonin receptor	359-376	LPFFIVALVLPFCESSCH	HLA-DRB1*1101	437
Serum albumin	347-361	TPTLVEAARNLGRVG	H2-E[k]	433
Sialyltransferase	206-223	DAVLRFNGAPTANFQQDV	HLA-DRB1*1301	437
Sialyltransferase	288-305	HPNQPFYILKPQMPWELW	HLA-DRB1*0101	437,449
Sphingolipid activator protein 3	165-176	TGNYRIESVLSS	HLA-DRB1*0401 (DR4Dw4)	432
Substance P receptor	255-269	CTFAICWLPFHVFFL	H2-E[s]	433
Tf receptor	442-459	VPQLNQMVRTAAEVAGQX	H2-A[d]	442
Thromboxane-A synthase	406-420	PAFRFTREAAQDCEV	HLA-DRB1*0701	435
Thyroid peroxidase	632-645	IDVWLGGLAENFLPY	HLA-DQA1*0501/DQB1*0201 (DQ2)	448
TIMP-1	101-118	NRSEEFLIAGKLQDGLLH	HLA-DRB1*0801	435
TIMP-1	102-117	RSEEFLIAGKLQDGLL	HLA-DRB1*0801	435
TIMP-1	103-117	SEEFLIAGKLQDGLL	HLA-DRB1*0801	435
TIMP-1	101-112	NRSEEFLIAGKL	HLA-DRB1*0801	435
TIMP-2	187-214	QAKFFACIKRSDGSCAWYRGAAPPKQEF	HLA-DRB1*0801	435
TIMP-2	187-205	QAKFFACIKRSDGSCAWYR	HLA-DRB1*0801	435
Transferrin	92-107	THYYAVAVVKKDTDFK	HLA-DRB1*0405 (DR4Dw15)	432
Transferrin	88-108	DNPQTHYYAVAVVKKDTDFKL	HLA-DRB1*0405 (DR4Dw15)	439
Transferrin	88-107	DNPQTHYYAVAVVKKDTDFK	HLA-DRB1*0405 (DR4Dw15)	439
Transferrin	89-108	NPQTHYYAVAVVKKDTDFKL	HLA-DRB1*0405 (DR4Dw15)	439
Transferrin	89-107	NPQTHYYAVAVVKKDTDFK	HLA-DRB1*0405 (DR4Dw15)	439
Transferrin	88-103	DNPQTHYYAVAVVKKD	HLA-DRB1*0405 (DR4Dw15)	439
Transferrin	92-106	THYYAVAVVKKDTDF	HLA-DRB1*0405 (DR4Dw15)	439
Transferrin	100-113	XXKKGTDFQLNQLE	H2-A[k]	433
Transferrin	103-117	KGTDFQLNQLEGKKG	H2-A[k]	433
Transferrin receptor	680-696	RVEYHFLSPYVSPKESP	HLA-DRB1*0101	354
Transferrin receptor	737-754	LATWTIQGAANALSGDVW	HLA-DRB1*0101	437,449
Transferrin receptor	332-349	LPNIPVQTISRAAAEKLF	HLA-DRB1*0102	437
Transferrin receptor	618-632	LLSFVRDLNQYRADI	HLA-DRB1*0301(DR17)	431
Transferrin receptor	383-399	EIKILNIFGVIKGFVEP	HLA-DRB1*0404 (DR4Dw14)	438
Transferrin receptor	383-398	EIKILNIFGVIKGFVE	HLA-DRB1*0404 (DR4Dw14)	438
Transferrin receptor	384-400	IKILNIFGVIKGFVEPD	HLA-DRB1*0404 (DR4Dw14)	438
Transferrin receptor	384-399	IKILNIFGVIKGFVEP	HLA-DRB1*0404 (DR4Dw14)	438
Transferrin receptor	384-398	IKILNIFGVIKGFVE	HLA-DRB1*0404 (DR4Dw14)	438
Transferrin receptor	173-186	FREFKLSKVWRDQH	HLA-DRB1*0405 (DR4Dw15)	432
Transferrin receptor	173-185	FREFKLSKVWRDQ	HLA-DRB1*0405 (DR4Dw15)	432
Transferrin receptor	174-186	REFKLSKVWRDQH	HLA-DRB1*0405 (DR4Dw15)	432

Table 5.7. (con't)

Protein	AA position	Sequence	MHC molecule	Ref.
Transferrin receptor	174-185	REFKLSKVWRDQ	HLA-DRB1*0405 (DR4Dw15)	432
Transferrin receptor	397-411	VEPDHYVVVGAQRDA	HLA-DRB1*0405 (DR4Dw15)	432
Transferrin receptor	398-411	EPDHYVVVGAQRDA	HLA-DRB1*0405 (DR4Dw15)	432
Transferrin receptor	215-230	NPGGYVAYSKAATVTG	HLA-DRB1*0901	440
Transferrin receptor	580-597	IPELNKVARAAAEVAGQF	HLA-DRB1*1104	437
Transferrin receptor	142-155	TGTIKLLNENSYVP	HLA-DRB1*1201	450
Transferrin receptor	144-156	TIKLLNENSYVPR	HLA-DRB1*1201	450
Transferrin receptor	141-156	FTGTIKLLNENSYVPR	HLA-DRB1*1201	450
Transferrin receptor	140-156	DFTGTIKLLNENSYVPR	HLA-DRB1*1201	450
Transferrin receptor	215-232	NPGGYVAYSKAATVTGKL	HLA-DRB1*1302	441
Transferrin receptor	215-230	NPGGYVAYSKAATVTG	HLA-DRB1*1302	441
Transferrin receptor	579-597	IPELNKVARAAA	HLA-DQA1*0501/DQB1*0301 (DQ7)	450
Transferrin receptor	15-31	GEPLSYTRFSLARQVDG	HLA-DPA1*0102/DPB1*0201	445
Transferrin receptor	203-218	KPTEVSGKLVHANFGT	$H2\text{-}A^s$	454
Transferrin receptor Homol.	580-595	XPELNKVARAAAEVAG	HLA-DR11 or Dw52	451
Tubulin α-1 chain	207-223	EAIYDICRRNLDIERPT	HLA-DRB1*0801	435
Tubulin α-1 chain	207-219	EAIYDICRRNLDI	HLA-DRB1*0801	435
Tubulin α-1 chain	391-408	LDHKFDLMYAKRAFVHWY	HLA-DRB1*0101	437,449
Tubulin α-chain	220-237	ERPTYTNLNRLIGQIVSS	HLA-DRB1*1101	437
Ubiquitin	3-20	IFVKTLTGKTITLEVEPS	HLA-DRB1*0102	437
Valosin-cont. protein p97	78-93	SDEKIRMNRVVRNNLR	HLA-DRB1*1201	450
VLA-4	229-247	GSLFVYNITTNKYKAFLKQ	HLA-DRB1*0401 (DR4Dw4)	435
von Willebrand factor	617-636	IALLLMASQEPQRMSRNFVR	HLA-DRB1*0801	435
von Willebrand factor	617-630	IALLLMASQEPQRM	HLA-DRB1*0801	435

Table 5.8. Associations between HLA expression and autoimmune diseases

Disease	Associated molecules	Relative risk
Birdshot Chorioretinopathy	A29	224.3
Idiopathic haemochromatosis	A3; B14; B7; HLA-H[459]	8.2; 4.5; -; -
Psoriasis vulgaris	Cw6	34.9
Adrenogenital syndrome		
- salt-losing form	B47	54.0
- viril. form	B51	3.8
- late-onset form	B14	48.5
Ankylosing spondylitis	B27	91.0
Reiter's disease	B27	37.0
Post-salmonella arthritis	B27	29.7
Post-shigella arthritis	B27	20.7
Post-yersinia arthritis	B27	17.6
Post-gonococcal arthritis	B27	14.0
Uveitis	B27	10.5
Amyloidosis in rheumatid arthritis	B27	8.2
Subacute thyroiditis	B35	18.9
Behcet's disease	B51	8.1
Narcolepsy	DR2; DRB1*1501-DRB5*0101-DQA*0102-DQB1*0602; B7	231.0; -; -
Goodpasture's syndrome	DR2	17.1
Multiple sclerosis	DR2; DRB1*1501-DQA1*0102-DQB1*0602; B7	4.1; -; -
Tuberculoid leprosy	DR2	8.1
Systemic lupus erythematodes	DR3; DRB*1501-DRB5*0101-DQB1*0602	5.8; -
Coeliac disease	DR3; DQA1*0501 (DR3+5); DQB1 *0201 (DR3+7)	19.8; -;-
Dermatitis herpetiformis	DR3; A1; B8	56.4; 4; 9
Myasthenia gravis	DR3; B8; B46; DR9	4.0; 4.4; -; -
Insulin-dependent diabetes mellitus (IDDM)	DR3; DR4; DR3/4; DR2; DQ8 (DQA1 *0301+DQB1*0302); DQ2 (DQA1*0501 +DQB1*0201); DQA1*0102+DQB1*06	4.9;9.5;14.3;0.2;-;-;-
Grave's disease (Thyrotoxicosis)	DR3; DR5	3.7; -
Sjögren/Sicca syndrome	DR3	9.7
Addison's disease	DR3; B8	9.3; 4
Hereditary IgA deficiency	DR3	17.0
Idiopathic membraneous glomerulonephritis	DR3	12.0
Neonatal alloimmune thrombopeny	DR3	9.2
Chronic active hepatitis (autoimmune)	DR3	13.9
IgA nephropathy (type Berger)	DR4	4.0; -
Hydralazin induced lupus erythematodes	DR4	5.6
Pernicious anemia	DR5	5.3
Pemphigus vulgaris	DR4	14.4
Vitiligo	DR4	-
Rheumatoid arthritis	DR4;DRB1*0401;DRB1*0404:DRB1*0405	4.0
Felty syndrome	DR4	76.0
Hashimoto's disease	DR5	3.2
Juvenile rheumatoid arthritis	DR5;DRB1*08/DQA1*0501/DQB1*0301; DRB1*08DQA1*0401/DQB1*0402	5.2; -; -
Idiopathic nephrotic syndrome	DR7; DR2; DQA1*0201; DQA1*0102-DQB1*0602	-
Hodgin's disease	DPB1*0301; DPB1*0401; DPB1*0901	-

The data are mainly taken from Roitt, 1994[460] and Wegener, 1994.[461]
-: unknown

Table 5.9. Tumor associated epitopes on MHC class I molecules

Protein/Gene	Examples for tumor expression	AA position	T cell epitope/MHC ligand	MHC molecule	Ref.
BAGE	Melanoma	2-10	AARAVFLAL	HLA-Cw*1601	481
c-abl	many	793-800	AADDXFKD	HLA-B13	135
c-abl	many	793-800	AADDXFKD	HLA-B44	135
Connexin 32		135-143	YVISVVFRL	HLA-A*0214	380
Draft-1	many	1-16	XXLNSQDQQCDSSLVE	HLA-B*2705	482
GAGE-1	Melanoma	9-16	YRPRPRRY	HLA-Cw*0601	483
GAGE-2	Melanoma	9-16	YRPRPRRY	HLA-Cw*0601	483
gp100	Melanoma	457-466	LLDGTATLRL	HLA-A*0201	484
gp100	Melanoma	209-217	ITDQVPFSV	HLA-A*0201	484
gp100	Melanoma	154-162	KTWGQYWQV	HLA-A*0201	484
gp100	Melanoma	208-217	TITDQVPFSV	HLA-A*0201	484
gp100	Melanoma	476-485	VLYRYGSFSV	HLA-A*0201	484
gp75	Melanoma	294-321	MSLQRQFLR	HLA-A*3101	485
HER-2	Mamma carcinoma	369-377	KIFGSLAFL	HLA-A*0201	486
HER-2	Mamma carcinoma	971-979	ELVSEFSRM	HLA-A*0201	486
HER-2	Mamma carcinoma	971-979	ELVSEFSRV	HLA-A*0201	487
MAGE-1	Melanoma	161-169	EADPTGHSY	HLA-A1	488, 489
MAGE-1	Melanoma	230-238	SAYGEPRKL	HLA-Cw*1601	376
MAGE-3	Melanoma	168-176	EVDPIGHLY	HLA-A1	490, 491
MAGE-3	Melanoma	271-279	FLWGPRALV	HLA-A*0201	492
MAGE-3	Melanoma	167-176	MEVDPIGHLY	HLA-B*4402	493
MAGE-3	Melanoma	167-176	MEVDPIGHLY	HLA-B*4403	493,
Melan A/MART-1	Melanoma	27-35	AAGIGILTV	HLA-A*0201	494, 495, 496, 497
Melan A/MART-1	Melanoma	32-40	ILTVILGVL	HLA-A*0201	498
Melan A/MART-1	Melanoma	27-35	AAGIGILTV	HLA-A*0202	499
Melan A/MART-1	Melanoma	27-35	AAGIGILTV	HLA-A*0204	499
Melan A/MART-1	Melanoma	27-35	AAGIGILTV	HLA-A*0205	499
Melan A/MART-1	Melanoma	27-35	AAGIGILTV	HLA-A*0206	499
Melan A/MART-1	Melanoma	27-35	AAGIGILTV	HLA-A*0209	499
Melan A/MART-1	Melanoma	27-35	AAGIGILTV	HLA-A*6901	499
Melan-A/MART-1	Melanoma	24-34	AEEAAGIGILT	HLA-B*4501	Schneider et al., pers. communication
Melan-A/MART-1	Melanoma	24-33	AEEAAGIGIL	HLA-B*4501	Schneider et al., pers.

					communication
mimic epitope of a natural tumor AG			AHYLFRNL	H2-K^{b}	500
mimic epitope of a natural tumor AG			THYLFRNL	H2-K^{b}	500
mimic epitope of a natural tumor AG			AQHPNAELL	H2-D^{b}	500
MUM-1	Melanoma		EEKLIVVLF	HLA-B*4402	493, 501
MUM-1	Melanoma		EEKLIVVAF	HLA-B*4402	493, 501
MUM-1	Melanoma		EEKLIVVAF	HLA-B*4403	493, 501
MUM-1	Melanoma		EEKLIVVLF	HLA-B*4403	493, 501
MUT1			FEQNTAQP	H2-K^{b}	502
MUT2			FEQNTAQA	H2-K^{b}	502
p15	Melanoma	10-18	AYGLDFYIL	HLA-A24	503
p53	many	343-351	ELNEALELK	HLA-A*1101	114
p53	many	321-330	KPLDGEYFTL	HLA-B7	504
p53	many	26-35	LPENNVLSPL	HLA-B7	504
p53	many	249-257	RPILTIITL	HLA-B7	504
p53	many	266-274	GRNSFEVRV	HLA-B*2709	370
p53 (mouse)	many	227-234	TTIHYKYM	H2-L^{d}	397
p53 mutant	many	126-145	FYQLAKTCPV	H2-K^{d}	505
p53 mutant		122-130	TYSPPLNEL	H2-K^{d}	506
p53^{wt} (mouse)	many	232-240	KYMCNSSCM	H2-D^{b}	507
P815	Tum-p 198	14-22	KYQAVTTTL	H2-K^{d}	168, 508, 509
P91A tum^{-}	Melanoma	15-22	QNHRALDL	H2-L^{d}	510
pmel17/gp100	Melanoma	280-288	YLEPGPVTA	HLA-A*0201	511
pmel17/gp100	Melanoma	456-466	ILDGTATLRL	HLA-A*0201	512
pmel17/gp100	Melanoma	17-25	ALLAVGATK	HLA-A3	513
Rage-1 from ORF2	Melanoma	11-20	SPSSNRIRNT	HLA-B7	514
ras P21 oncogene mutant	Melanoma	4-12	YKLVVVGAV	H2-K^{d}	515
TRP-2	Melanoma	197-205	LLPGGRPYR	HLA-A*3101	516
Tumor antigen P815	P91A	12-20	ISTQNHRAL	H2-L^{d}	517
Tumor antigen P815	P1A	35-43	LPYLGWLVF	H2-L^{d}	518, 519
Tum-P35B		4-13	GPPHSNNFGY	H2-D^{d}	520
Tyrosinase	Melanoma	369-377	YMNGTMSQV	HLA-A*0201	423, 424, 425,426
Tyrosinase	Melanoma	369-377	YMDGTMSQV	HLA-A*0201	427
Tyrosinase	Melanoma	1-9	MLLAVLYCL	HLA-A*0201	423, 424
Tyrosinase	Melanoma	206-215	AFLPWHRLFL	HLA-A24	428
Tyrosinase	Melanoma	206-214	AFLPWHRLF	HLA-A24	428
Tyrosinase (MZ-2C)	Melanoma	192-200	SEIWRDIDF	HLA-B*4402	429
Tyrosinase (MZ-2C)	Melanoma	192-200	SEIWRDIDF	HLA-B*4403	429

REFERENCES

1. Kärre K. Natural killer cells and the MHC class I pathway of peptide presentation. Semin Immunol 1993; 5:127-45.
2. Ljunggren HG, Karre K. In search of the 'missing self': MHC molecules and NK cell recognition. Immunol Today 1990; 11:237-44.
3. Ohlen C, Bastin J, Ljunggren HG et al. Resistance to H-2-restricted but not to allo-H2-specific graft and cytotoxic T lymphocyte responses in lymphoma mutant. J Immunol 1990; 145:52-8.
4. Ljunggren HG, Karre K. Host resistance directed selectively against H-2-deficient lymphoma variants. Analysis of the mechanism. J Exp Med 1985; 162: 174 5-59.
5. Kärre K. Express yourself or die: peptides, MHC molecules, and NK cells. Science 1995; 267:978-9.
6. Colonna M. Natural killer cell receptors specific for MHC class I molecules. Curr Opin Immunol 1996; 8:101-7.
7. Long EO, Colonna M, Lanier LL. Inhibitory MHC class I receptors on NK and T cells: a standard nomenclature. Immunol Today 1996; 17:100.
8. Lanier LL. Natural killer cell receptors and MHC class I interactions. Curr Opin Immunol 1997; 9:126-31.
9. Phillips JH, Chang C, Mattson J et al. CD94 and a novel associated protein (94AP) form a NK cell receptor involved in the recognition of HLA-A, HLA-B, and HLA-C allotypes. Immunity 1996; 5:163-72.
10. Carretero M, Cantoni C, Bellon T et al. The CD94 and NKG2-A C-type lectins covalently assemble to form a natural killer cell inhibitory receptor for HLA class I molecules. Eur J Immunol 1997; 27:563-7.
11. Brooks AG, Posch PE, Scorzelli CJ et al. NKG2 complexed with CD94 defines a novel inhibitory natural killer cell receptor. J Exp Med 1997; 185:795-800.
12. Münz C, Holmes N, King A et al. HLA-G molecules inhibit NKAT3 expressing natural killer cells. J Exp Med 1997; 185:385-91.
13. Cella M, Longo A, Ferrara GB et al. NK3-specific natural killer cells are selectively inhibited by Bw4-positive HLA alleles with isoleucine 80. J Exp Med 1994; 180:1235-42.
14. Colonna M, Borsellino G, Falco M et al. HLA-C is the inhibitory ligand that determines dominant resistance to lysis by NK1- and NK2-specific natural killer cells. Proc Natl Acad Sci U S A 1993; 90:12000-4.
15. Raulet DH, Correa I, Corral L et al. Inhibitory effects of class I molecules on murine NK cells: speculations on function, specificity and self-tolerance. Semin Immunol 1995; 7:103-7.
16. Raulet DH, Held W. Natural killer cell receptors: the offs and ons of NK cell recognition. Cell 1995; 82:697-700.
17. Held W, Roland J, Raulet DH. Allelic exclusion of Ly49-family genes encoding class I MHC-specific receptors on NK cells. Nature 1995; 376:355-8.
18. Dorfman JR, Raulet DH. Major histocompatibility complex genes determine natural killer cell tolerance. Eur J Immunol 1996; 26:151-5.
19. Gumperz JE, Valiante NM, Parham P et al. Heterogenous phenotypes of expression of the NKB1 natural killer cell class I receptor among individuals of different human histocompatibility leukocyte antigen types appear genetically regulated, but not linked to major histocompatibility complex haplotype. J Exp Med 1996; 183:1817-27.
20. Correa I, Raulet DH. Binding of diverse peptides to MHC class I molecules inhibits target cell lysis by activated natural killer cells. Immunity 1995; 2:61-71.
21. Malnati MS, Peruzzi M, Parker KC et al. Peptide specificity in the recognition of MHC class I by natural killer cell clones. Science 1995; 267:1016-8.
22. Orange JS, Wang B, Terhorst C et al. Requirement for natural killer cell-produced interferon gamma in defense against murine cytomegalovirus infection and enhancement of this defense pathway by interleukin 12 administration. J Exp Med 1995; 182:1045-56.
23. Germann T, Rude E. Interleukin-12. Int Arch Allergy Immunol 1995; 108:103-12.
24. Chien YH, Davis MM. How alpha beta T-cell receptors 'see' peptide/MHC com-

plexes. Immunol Today 1993; 14:597-602.
25. Schild H, Chien YH. The recognition of MHC molecules by gamma delta T cells. Behring Inst Mitt 1994; 113-23.
26. Schild H, Mavaddat N, Litzenberger C et al. The nature of major histocompatibility complex recognition by gamma delta T cells. Cell 1994; 76:29-37.
27. Sprent J. Central tolerance of T cells. Int Rev Immunol 1995; 13:95-105.
28. Kisielow P, von Boehmer H. Development and selection of T cells: facts and puzzles. Adv Immunol 1995; 58:87-209.
29. DiBrino M, Parker KC, Shiloach J et al. Endogenous peptides with distinct amino acid anchor residue motifs bind to HLA-A1 and HLA-B8. J Immunol 1994; 152: 620-31.
30. Matzinger P. Tolerance, danger, and the extended family. Annu Rev Immunol 1994; 12:991-1045.
31. Garboczi DN, Ghosh P, Utz U et al. Structure of the complex between human T cell receptor, viral peptide and HLA A2. Nature 1996; 384:134-141.
32. Garcia KC, Degano M, Stanfield RL et al. An alphabeta T cell receptor structure at 2.5 Å and its orientation in the TCR-MHC complex. Science 1996; 274:209-19.
33. Schwartz RH. Costimulation of T lymphocytes: the role of CD28, CTLA-4, and B7/BB1 in interleukin-2 production and immunotherapy. Cell 1992; 71:1065-8.
34. Romagnani S. Th1 and Th2 in human diseases. Clin Immunol Immunopathol 1996; 80:225-35.
35. Cantrell D. T cell antigen receptor signal transduction pathways. Annu Rev Immunol 1996; 14:259-74.
36. Mosmann TR, Sad S, Krishnan L et al. Differentiation of subsets of $CD4^+$ and $CD8^+$ T cells. Ciba Found Symp 1995; 195-1/97.
37. Erard F, Dunbar PR, Le Gros G. The IL4- induced switch of $CD8^+$ T cells to a TH2 phenotype and its possible relationship to the onset of AIDS. Res Immunol 1994; 145:643-5.
38. Sun J, Leahy DJ, Kavathas PB. Interaction between CD8 and major histocompatibility complex (MHC) class I mediated by multiple contact surfaces that include the alpha 2 and alpha 3 domains of MHC class I. J Exp Med 1995; 182: 1275-80.
39. von Boehmer H. Thymic selection: a matter of life and death. Immunol Today 1992; 13:454-8.
40. Bluethmann H, Kisielow P, Uematsu Y et al. T-cell-specific deletion of T-cell receptor transgenes allows functional rearrangement of endogenous alpha- and beta-genes. Nature 1988; 334:156-9.
41. Kisielow P, Bluethmann H, Staerz UD et al. Tolerance in T-cell-receptor transgenic mice involves deletion of nonmature $CD4^+8^+$ thymocytes. Nature 1988; 333:742-6.
42. Kisielow P, Teh HS, Bluethmann H et al. Positive selection of antigen-specific T cells in thymus by restricting MHC molecules. Nature 1988; 335:730-3.
43. Kagi D, Ledermann B, Burki K et al. Lymphocyte-mediated cytotoxicity in vitro and in vivo: mechanisms and significance. Immunol Rev 1995; 146: 95-115.
44. Kagi D, Vignaux F, Ledermann B et al. Fas and perforin pathways as major mechanisms of T cell-mediated cytotoxicity. Science 1994; 265:528-30.
45. Mosmann TR. Cytokines, differentiation and functions of subsets of CD4 and CD8 T cells. Behring Inst Mitt 1995; 1-6.
46. Trinchieri G. The two faces of interleukin 12: a pro-inflammatory cytokine and a key immunoregulatory molecule produced by antigen-presenting cells. Ciba Found Symp 1995; 195:203-20.
47. Magram J, Connaughton SE, Warrier RR et al. IL-12-deficient mice are defective in IFN gamma production and type 1 cytokine responses. Immunity 1996; 4:471-81.
48. Doherty TM. T-cell regulation of macrophage function. Curr Opin Immunol 1995; 7:400-4.
49. Foy TM, Aruffo A, Bajorath J et al. Immune regulation by CD40 and its ligand GP39. Annu Rev Immunol 1996; 14: 591-617.
50. Banchereau J, Bazan F, Blanchard D et al. The CD40 antigen and its ligand. Annu Rev Immunol 1994; 12:881-922.
51. Sherman LA, Chattopadhyay S. The mo-

lecular basis of allorecognition. Annu Rev Immunol 1993; 11:385-402.
52. Rammensee HG, Falk K, Rötzschke O. Peptides naturally presented by MHC class I molecules. Annu Rev Immunol 1993; 11:213-44.
53. Rötzschke O, Falk K, Faath S et al. On the nature of peptides involved in T cell alloreactivity. J Exp Med 1991; 174: 1059-71.
54. Klein J. Natural History of the Major Histocompatibility Complex. New York: J. Wiley & Sons; 1986.
55. Gorer PA. The genetic and antigenic basis of tumor transplantation. J Pathol Bacteriol. 1937; 44:691-7.
56. von Boehmer H, Teh HS, Kisielow P. The thymus selects the useful, neglects the useless and destroys the harmful. Immunol Today 1989; 10:57-61.
57. Jameson SC, Hogquist KA, Bevan MJ. Positive selection of thymocytes. Annu Rev Immunol 1995; 13:93-126.
58. Hosken NA, Bevan MJ. An endogenous antigenic peptide bypasses the class I antigen presentation defect in RMA-S. J Exp Med 1992; 175:719-29.
59. Udaka K, Tsomides TJ, Walden P et al. A ubiquitous protein is the source of naturally occurring peptides that are recognized by a CD8+ T-cell clone. Proc Natl Acad Sci U S A 1993; 90:11272-6.
60. van Rood JJ. The impact of the HLA-system in clinical medicine. Schweiz Med Wochenschr 1993; 123:85-92.
61. van Rood JJ, Claas FH, Doxiadis II et al. The role of HLA typing in clinical kidney transplants: 30 years later HLA matching is prime importance in bone marrow transplantation. Clin Transpl 1993; 434-5.
62. Opelz G, Wujciak T. Cadaveric kidneys should be allocated according to the HLA match. Transplant Proc 1995; 27:93-9.
63. Gale RP, Opelz G. Immunologic and clinical perspectives in human bone marrow transplantation. Transplant Proc 1978; 10:265-8.
64. Opelz G, Gale RP, Feig SA et al. Significance of HLA and non-HLA antigens in bone marrow transplantation. Transplant Proc 1978; 10:43-6.
65. Wong T, Donaldson P, Devlin J et al. Repeat HLA-B and -DR loci mismatching at second liver transplantation improves patient survival. Transplantation 1996; 61:440-4.
66. Kolb HJ, Schattenberg A, Goldman JM et al. Graft-versus-leukemia effect of donor lymphocyte transfusions in marrow grafted patients. European Group for Blood and Marrow Transplantation Working Party Chronic Leukemia. Blood 1995; 86:2041-50.
67. Stachel D, Schmid I, Straka C et al. Allogenic peripheral blood stem cell (PBSC) transplantation in two patients with graft failure. Bone Marrow Transplant 1995; 16:839-42.
68. Rammensee HG, Bevan MJ. Evidence from in vitro studies that tolerance to self antigens is MHC-restricted. Nature 1984; 308:741-4.
69. Sadovnikova E, Stauss HJ. Peptide-specific cytotoxic T lymphocytes restricted by nonself major histocompatibility complex class I molecules: Reagents for tumor immunotherapy. Proc Natl Acad Sci U S A 1996; 93:13114-8.
70. Roopenian DC, Christianson GJ, Davis AP et al. The genetic origin of minor histocompatibility antigens. Immunogenetics 1993; 38:131-40.
71. Counce S, Smith P, Barth R et al. Strong and weak histocompatibility gene differences in mice an their role in the rejection of homografts of tumors and skin. Ann Surg 1956; 144:198-204.
72. Goulmy E. Human minor histocompatibility antigens. Curr Opin Immunol 1996; 8:75-81.
73. Fischer-Lindahl K. Minor histocompatibility antigens. Trends Genet 1991; 7:219-24.
74. Rötzschke O, Falk K, Wallny HJ et al. Characterization of naturally occurring minor histocompatibility peptides including H-4 and H-Y. Science 1990; 249:283-7.
75. Wallny HJ, Rammensee HG. Identification of classical minor histocompatibility antigen as cell-derived peptide. Nature 1990; 343:275-8.
76. Simpson E. Mechanisms of transplantation immunity. Springer Semin Immunopathol 1992; 14:17-32.

77. Rodgers JR, Mehta V, Cook RG. Surface expression of beta 2-microglobulin-associated thymus-leukemia antigen is independent of TAP2. Eur J Immunol 1995; 25:1001-7.
78. Greenfield A, Scott D, Pennisi D et al. An H-YD^b epitope is encoded by a novel mouse Y chromosome gene. Nature Genetics 1996; 14:474-8.
79. Scott DM, Ehrmann IE, Ellis PS et al. Identification of a mouse male-specific transplantation antigen, H-Y. Nature 1995; 376:695-8.
80. Morse MC, Bleau G, Dabhi VM et al. The COI mitochondrial gene encodes a minor histocompatibility antigen presented by H2-M3. J Immunol 1996; 156:3301-7.
81. Barber LD, Percival L, Valiante NM et al. The inter-locus recombinant HLA-B*4601 has high selectivity in peptide binding and functions characteristic of HLA-C. J Exp Med 1996; 184:735-40.
82. Wang CR, Loveland BE, Lindahl KF. H-2M3 encodes the MHC class I molecule presenting the maternally transmitted antigen of the mouse. Cell 1991; 66: 335-45.
83. Eichwald EJ, Silmser CS. Communication. Transpl Bull 1955; 2:148
84. Hurme M, Hetherington CM, Chandler PR et al. Cytotoxic T-cell responses to H-Y: mapping of the Ir genes. J Exp Med 1978; 147:758-67.
85. Gordon RD, Samelson LE, Simpson E. Selective response to H-Y antigen by F1 female mice sensitized to F1 male cells. J Exp Med 1977; 146:606-10.
86. Rammensee HG, Robinson PJ, Crisanti A et al. Restricted recognition of beta 2-microglobulin by cytotoxic T lymphocytes. Nature 1986; 319:502-4.
87. Perreault C, Jutras J, Roy DC et al. Identification of an immunodominant mouse minor histocompatibility antigen (MiHA). T cell response to a single dominant MiHA causes graft-versus-host disease. J Clin Invest 1996; 98:622-8.
88. Wang W, Meadows LR, den Haan JM et al. Human H-Y: a male-specific histocompatibility antigen derived from the SMCY protein. Science 1995; 269:1588-90.
89. Scott DM, Ehrmann IE, Ellis PS et al. Identification of a mouse male-specific transplantation antigen, H-Y. Nature 1995; 376:695-8.
90. den Haan JM, Sherman NE, Blokland E et al. Identification of a graft versus host disease-associated human minor histocompatibility antigen. Science 1995; 268:1476-80.
91. Loveland B, Wang CR, Yonekawa H et al. Maternally transmitted histocompatibility antigen of mice: a hydrophobic peptide of a mitochondrially encoded protein. Cell 1990; 60:971-80.
92. Fischer-Lindahl K, Hermel E, Loveland BE et al. Maternally transmitted antigen of mice: a model transplantation antigen. Annu Rev Immunol 1991; 9:351-72.
93. Oldstone MB. The role of cytotoxic T lymphocytes in infectious disease: history, criteria, and state of the art. Curr Top Microbiol Immunol 1994; 189:1-8.
94. Paglia P, Girolomoni G, Robbiati F et al. Immortalized dendritic cell line fully competent in antigen presentation initiates primary T cell responses in vivo. J Exp Med 1993; 178:1893-901.
95. Bevan MJ. Immunology. Stimulating killer cells. Nature 1989; 342:478-9.
96. Srivastava PK, Udono H, Blachere NE et al. Heat shock proteins transfer peptides during antigen processing and CTL priming. Immunogenetics 1994; 39:93-8.
97. Kotzin BL, Leung DY, Kappler J et al. Superantigens and their potential role in human disease. Adv Immunol 1993; 54:99-166.
98. Marrack P, Winslow GM, Choi Y et al. The bacterial and mouse mammary tumor virus superantigens; two different families of proteins with the same functions. Immunol Rev 1993; 131:79-92.
99. Jardetzky TS, Brown JH, Gorga JC et al. Three-dimensional structure of a human class II histocompatibility molecule complexed with superantigen. Nature 1994; 368:711-8.
100. Renno T, Hahne M, Tschopp J et al. Peripheral T cells undergoing superantigen-induced apoptosis in vivo express B220 and upregulate Fas and Fas ligand. J Exp Med 1996; 183:431-7.
101. Rammensee HG, Kroschewski R, Fran-

goulis B. Clonal anergy induced in mature V beta 6+ T lymphocytes on immunizing Mls-1b mice with Mls-1a expressing cells. Nature 1989; 339:541-4.
102. Rötzschke O, Falk K, Deres K et al. Isolation and analysis of naturally processed viral peptides as recognized by cytotoxic T cells. Nature 1990; 348:252-4.
103. van Bleek GM, Nathenson SG. Isolation of an immunodominant viral peptide from the class I H-2K^b molecule. Nature 1990; 348:213-6.
104. Loftus DJ, Castelli C, Clay TM et al. Identification of epitope mimics recognized by CTL reactive to the melanoma/melanocyte-derived peptide MART-1. J Exp Med 1996; 184:647-57.
105. Kast WM, Offringa R, Peters PJ et al. Eradication of adenovirus E1-induced tumors by E1A-specific cytotoxic T lymphocytes. Cell 1989; 59:603-14.
106. Toes RE, Offringa R, Blom RJ et al. An adenovirus type 5 early region 1B-encoded CTL epitope-mediating tumor eradication by CTL clones is down-modulated by an activated ras oncogene. J Immunol 1995; 154:3396-405.
107. Pauly T, Elbers K, König M et al. Classical swine fever virus-specific cytotoxic T lymphocytes and identification of a T cell epitope. J Gen Virol 1995; 76:3039-49.
108. Livingston PG, Kurane I, Dai LC et al. Dengue virus-specific, HLA-B35-restricted, human CD8$^+$ cytotoxic T lymphocyte (CTL) clones. Recognition of NS3 amino acids 500 to 508 by CTL clones of two different serotype specificities. J Immunol 1995; 154:1287-95.
109. Zivny J, Kurane I, Leporati AM et al. A single nine-amino acid peptide induces virus-specific, CD8$^+$ human cytotoxic T lymphocyte clones of heterogeneous serotype specificities. J Exp Med 1995; 182:853-63.
110. Lee SP, Thomas WA, Murray RJ et al. HLA A2.1-restricted cytotoxic T cells recognizing a range of Epstein-Barr virus isolates through a defined epitope in latent membrane protein LMP2. J Virol 1993; 67:7428-35.
111. Stuber G, Dillner J, Modrow S et al. HLA-A0201 and HLA-B7 binding peptides in the EBV-encoded EBNA-1, EBNA-2 and BZLF-1 proteins detected in the MHC class I stabilization assay. Low proportion of binding motifs for several HLA class I alleles in EBNA-1. Int Immunol 1995; 7:653-63.
112. Kerr BM, Kienzle N, Burrows JM et al. Identification of type B-specific and cross-reactive cytotoxic T-lymphocyte responses to Epstein-Barr virus. J Virol 1996; 70:8858-64.
113. Burrows SR, Gardner J, Khanna R et al. Five new cytotoxic T cell epitopes identified within Epstein-Barr virus nuclear antigen 3. J Gen Virol 1994; 75:2489-93.
114. Zhang QJ, Gavioli R, Klein G et al. An HLA-A11-specific motif in nonamer peptides derived from viral and cellular proteins. Proc Natl Acad Sci U S A 1993; 90:2217-21.
115. Gavioli R, Kurilla MG, de Campos Lima PO et al. Multiple HLA A11-restricted cytotoxic T-lymphocyte epitopes of different immunogenicities in the Epstein-Barr virus-encoded nuclear antigen 4. J Virol 1993; 67:1572-8.
116. Steven NM, Leese AM, Annels NE et al. Epitope focusing in the primary cytotoxic T cell response to Epstein-Barr virus and its relationship to T cell memory. J Exp Med 1996; 184:1801-13.
117. Hill A, Worth A, Elliott T et al. Characterization of two Epstein-Barr virus epitopes restricted by HLA-B7. Eur J Immunol 1995; 25:18-24.
118. Burrows SR, Sculley TB, Misko IS et al. An Epstein-Barr virus-specific cytotoxic T cell epitope in EBV nuclear antigen 3 (EBNA 3). J Exp Med 1990; 171:345-9.
119. Brooks JM, Murray RJ, Thomas WA et al. Different HLA-B27 subtypes present the same immunodominant Epstein-Barr virus peptide. J Exp Med 1993; 178: 879-87.
120. Lee SP, Morgan S, Skinner J et al. Epstein-Barr virus isolates with the major HLA B35.01-restricted cytotoxic T lymphocyte epitope are prevalent in a highly B35.01-positive African population. Eur J Immunol 1995; 25:102-10.
121. Moss DJ, Burrows SR, Khanna R et al. Immune surveillance against Epstein-Barr virus. Semin Immunol 1992; 4: 97-104.

122. Khanna R, Burrows SR, Kurilla MG et al. Localization of Epstein-Barr virus cytotoxic T cell epitopes using recombinant vaccinia: implications for vaccine development. J Exp Med 1992; 176:169-76.
123. Hill AB, Lee SP, Haurum JS et al. Class I major histocompatibility complex-restricted cytotoxic T lymphocytes specific for Epstein-Barr virus (EBV)-transformed B lymphoblastoid cell lines against which they were raised. J Exp Med 1995; 181:2221-8.
124. Nayersina R, Fowler P, Guilhot S et al. HLA A2 restricted cytotoxic T lymphocyte responses to multiple hepatitis B surface antigen epitopes during hepatitis B virus infection. J Immunol 1993; 150:4659-71.
125. Bertoletti A, Costanzo A, Chisari FV et al. Cytotoxic T lymphocyte response to a wild type hepatitis B virus epitope in patients chronically infected by variant viruses carrying substitutions within the epitope. J Exp Med 1994; 180:933-43.
126. Bertoletti A, Chisari FV, Penna A et al. Definition of a minimal optimal cytotoxic T-cell epitope within the hepatitis B virus nucleocapsid protein. J Virol 1993; 67:2376-80.
127. del Guercio MF, Sidney J, Hermanson G et al. Binding of a peptide antigen to multiple HLA alleles allows definition of an A2-like supertype. J Immunol 1995; 154:685-93.
128. Rehermann B, Fowler P, Sidney J et al. The cytotoxic T lymphocyte response to multiple hepatitis B virus polymerase epitopes during and after acute viral hepatitis. J Exp Med 1995; 181:1047-58.
129. Wentworth PA, Vitiello A, Sidney J et al. Differences and similarities in the A2.1-restricted cytotoxic T cell repertoire in humans and human leukocyte antigen-transgenic mice. Eur J Immunol 1996; 26:97-101.
130. Rehermann B, Pasquinelli C, Mosier SM et al. Hepatitis B virus (HBV) sequence variation of cytotoxic T lymphocyte epitopes is not common in patients with chronic HBV infection. J Clin Invest 1995; 96:1527-34.
131. Tsai SL, Chen MH, Yeh CT et al. Purification and characterization of a naturally processed hepatitis B virus peptide recognized by CD8+ cytotoxic T lymphocytes. J Clin Invest 1996; 97:577-84.
132. Missale G, Redeker A, Person J et al. HLA-A31- and HLA-Aw68-restricted cytotoxic T cell responses to a single hepatitis B virus nucleocapsid epitope during acute viral hepatitis. J Exp Med 1993; 177:751-62.
133. Schirmbeck R, Melber K, Kuhrober A et al. Immunization with soluble hepatitis B virus surface protein elicits murine H-2 class I-restricted CD8+ cytotoxic T lymphocyte responses in vivo. J Immunol 1994; 152:1110-9.
134. Kuhöber A, Pudollek HP, Reifenberg K et al. DNA immunization induces antibody and cytotoxic T cell responses to hepatitis B core antigen in H-2b mice. J Immunol 1996; 156:3687-95.
135. Kobayashi H, Sato K, Miyokawa N et al. Analysis of naturally processed human histocompatibility leukocyte antigen class I-bound peptides from hepatocellular carcinoma tissues in vivo. Jpn J Cancer Res 1995; 86:962-8.
136. Gavin MA, Gilbert MJ, Riddell SR et al. Alkali hydrolysis of recombinant proteins allows for the rapid identification of class I MHC-restricted CTL epitopes. J Immunol 1993; 151:3971-80.
137. Wills MR, Carmichael AJ, Mynard K et al. The human cytotoxic T-lymphocyte (CTL) response to cytomegalovirus is dominated by structural protein pp65: frequency, specifity, and T-cell receptor usage of pp65-specific CTL. J Virol 1996; 70:7569-79.
138. Shirai M, Okada H, Nishioka M et al. An epitope in hepatitis C virus core region recognized by cytotoxic T cells in mice and humans. J Virol 1994; 68: 3334-42.
139. Shirai M, Arichi T, Nishioka M et al. CTL responses of HLA-A2.1-transgenic mice specific for hepatitis C viral peptides predict epitopes for CTL of humans carrying HLA-A2.1. J Immunol 1995; 154:2733-42.
140. Cerny A, Fowler P, Brothers MA et al. Induction in vitro of a primary human antiviral cytotoxic T cell response. Eur J Immunol 1995; 25:627-30.
141. Cerny A, McHutchison JG, Pasquinelli C

et al. Cytotoxic T lymphocyte response to hepatitis C virus-derived peptides containing the HLA A2.1 binding motif. J Clin Invest 1995; 95:521-30.
142. Battegay M, Fikes J, Di Bisceglie AM et al. Patients with chronic hepatitis C have circulating cytotoxic T cells which recognize hepatitis C virus-encoded peptides binding to HLA-A2.1 molecules. J Virol 1995; 69:2462-70.
143. Kurokohchi K, Akatsuka T, Pendleton CD et al. Use of recombinant protein to identify a motif-negative human cytotoxic T-cell epitope presented by HLA-A2 in the hepatitis C virus NS3 region. J Virol 1996; 70:232-40.
144. Wentworth PA, Sette A, Celis E et al. Identification of A2-restricted hepatitis C virus-specific cytotoxic T lymphocyte epitopes from conserved regions of the viral genome. Int Immunol 1996; 8: 651-9.
145. Koziel MJ, Dudley D, Afdhal N et al. HLA class I-restricted cytotoxic T lymphocytes specific for hepatitis C virus. Identification of multiple epitopes and characterization of patterns of cytokine release. J Clin Invest 1995; 96:2311-21.
146. Koziel MJ, Dudley D, Wong JT et al. Intrahepatic cytotoxic T lymphocytes specific for hepatitis C virus in persons with chronic hepatitis [published erratum appears in J Immunol 1993; 150:2563]. J Immunol 1992; 149: 3339-44.
147. Kaneko T, Nakamura I, Kita H et al. Three new cytotoxic T cell epitopes identified within the hepatitis C virus nucleoprotein. J Gen Virol 1996; 77:1305-9.
148. Rehermann B, Chang K, McHutchison JG et al. Quantitative analysis of the peripheral blood cytotoxic T lymphocyte response in patients with chronic hepatitis C virus infection. J Clin Invest 1996; 98:1432-40.
149. Shirai M, Chen M, Arichi T et al. Use of intrinsic and extrinsic helper epitopes for in vivo induction of anti-hepatitis C virus cytotoxic T lymphocytes (CTL) with CTL epitope peptide vaccines. J Infect Dis 1996; 173:24-31.
150. Cooper S, Kowalski H, Erickson AL et al. The presentation of a hepatitis C viral peptide by distinct major histocompatibility complex class I allotypes from two chimpanzee species. J Exp Med 1996; 183:663-8.
151. Kowalski H, Erickson AL, Cooper S et al. Patr-A and B, the orthologues of HLA-A and B, present hepatitis C virus epitopes to CD8+ cytotoxic T cells from two chronically infected chimpanzees. J Exp Med 1996; 183:1761-75.
152. Dai LC, West K, Littaua R et al. Mutation of human immunodeficiency virus type 1 at amino acid 585 on gp41 results in loss of killing by $CD8^+$ A24-restricted cytotoxic T lymphocytes. J Virol 1992; 66:3151-4.
153. Buseyne F, McChesney M, Porrot F et al. Gag-specific cytotoxic T lymphocytes from human immunodeficiency virus type 1-infected individuals: Gag epitopes are clustered in three regions of the p24gag protein. J Virol 1993; 67:694-702.
154. Buseyne F, Riviere Y. HIV-specific $CD8^+$ T-cell immune responses and viral replication. AIDS 1993; 7 Suppl 2:s81-5.
155. DiBrino M, Parker KC, Margulies DH et al. The HLA-B14 peptide binding site can accommodate peptides with different combinations of anchor residues. J Biol Chem 1994; 269:32426-34.
156. Phillips RE, Rowland Jones S, Nixon DF et al. Human immunodeficiency virus genetic variation that can escape cytotoxic T cell recognition. Nature 1991; 354:453-9.
157. Achour A, Picard O, Zagury D et al. HGP-30, a synthetic analogue of human immunodeficiency virus (HIV) p17, is a target for cytotoxic lymphocytes in HIV-infected individuals. Proc Natl Acad Sci U S A 1990; 87:7045-9.
158. Johnson RP, Trocha A, Buchanan TM et al. Identification of overlapping HLA class I-restricted cytotoxic T cell epitopes in a conserved region of the human immunodeficiency virus type 1 envelope glycoprotein: definition of minimum epitopes and analysis of the effects of sequence variation. J Exp Med 1992; 175:961-71.
159. Culmann B, Gomard E, Kieny MP et al. Six epitopes reacting with human cytotoxic $CD8^+$ T cells in the central region

of the HIV-1 NEF protein. J Immunol 1991; 146:1560-5.
160. Jardetzky TS, Lane WS, Robinson RA et al. Identification of self peptides bound to purified HLA-B27. Nature 1991; 353: 326-9.
161. Nietfield W, Bauer M, Fevrier M et al. Sequence constraints and recognition by CTL of an HLA-B27-restricted HIV-1 gag epitope. J Immunol 1995; 154: 2189-97.
162. Littaua RA, Oldstone MB, Takeda A et al. An HLA-C-restricted CD8+ cytotoxic T-lymphocyte clone recognizes a highly conserved epitope on human immunodeficiency virus type 1 gag. J Virol 1991; 65:4051-6.
163. Renggli J, Valmori D, Romero JF et al. $CD8^+$ T-cell protective immunity induced by immunization with Plasmodium berghei CS protein-derived synthetic peptides: evidence that localization of peptide-specific CTLs is crucial for protection against malaria. Immunol Lett 1995; 46:199-205.
164. Takahashi H, Cohen J, Hosmalin A et al. An immunodominant epitope of the human immunodeficiency virus envelope glycoprotein gp160 recognized by class I major histocompatibility complex molecule-restricted murine cytotoxic T lymphocytes. Proc Natl Acad Sci U S A 1988; 85:3105-9.
165. Bergmann C, Stohlmann SA, McMillan M. An endogenously synthesized decamer peptide efficiently primes cytotoxic T cells specific for the HIV-1 envelope glycoprotein. Eur J Immunol 1993; 23:2777-81.
166. Bergmann CC, Stohlman SA. Specificity of the H-2 L(d)-restricted cytotoxic T-lymphocyte response to the mouse hepatitis virus nucleocapsid protein. J Virol 1996; 70:3252-7.
167. Bergmann CC, Tong L, Cua RV et al. Cytotoxic T cell repertoire selection - A single amino acid determines alternative class I restriction. J Immunol 1994; 152:5603-12.
168. Falk K, Rötzschke O, Stevanović S et al. Allele-specific motifs revealed by sequencing of self-peptides eluted from MHC molecules. Nature 1991; 351:290-6.
169. Gotch F, McMichael A, Rothbard J. Recognition of influenza A matrix protein by HLA-A2-restricted cytotoxic T lymphocytes. Use of analogues to orientate the matrix peptide in the HLA-A2 binding site. J Exp Med 1988; 168:2045-57.
170. Hadida F, Haas G, Zimmermann N et al. CTLs from lymphoid organs recognize an optimal HLA-A2-restricted and HLA-B52-restricted nonapeptide and several epitopes in the C-terminal region of HIV-1 Nef. J Immunol 1995; 154: 4174-86.
171. Dupuis M, Kundu SK, Merigan TC. Characterization of HLA-A*0201-restricted cytotoxic T cell epitopes in conserved regions of the HIV type 1 gp160 protein. J Immunol 1995; 155:2232-9.
172. Harrer E, Harrer T, Barbosa P et al. Recognition of the highly conserved YMDD region in the human immunodeficiency virus type 1 reverse transcriptase by HLA-A2-restricted cytotoxic T lymphocytes from an asymptomatic long-term nonprogressor. J Infect Dis 1996; 173:476-9.
173. Yang OO, Kalams SA, Rosenzweig M et al. Efficient lysis of human immunodeficiency virus type 1-infected cells by cytotoxic T lymphocytes. J Virol 1996; 70:5799-806.
174. Alexander-Miller MA, Parker KC, Tsukui T et al. Molecular analysis of presentation by HLA-A2.1 of a promiscuously binding V3 loop peptide from the HIV-1 envelope protein to human cytotoxic T lymphocytes. Int Immunol 1996; 8:641-9.
175. Takahashi K, Dai LC, Fuerst TR et al. Specific lysis of human immunodeficiency virus type 1-infected cells by a HLA-A3.1-restricted $CD8^+$ cytotoxic T-lymphocyte clone that recognizes a conserved peptide sequence within the gp41 subunit of the envelope protein. Proc Natl Acad Sci U S A 1991; 88:10277-81.
176. Koenig S, Fuerst TR, Wood LV et al. Mapping the fine specificity of a cytolytic T cell response to HIV-1 nef protein. J Immunol 1990; 145:127-35.
177. Venet A, Walker BD. Cytotoxic T-cell epitopes in HIV/SIV infection. AIDS 1993; 7 Suppl 1:S117-26.

178. Safrit JT, Andrews CA, Zhu T et al. Characterization of human immunodeficiency virus type 1-specific cytotoxic T lymphocyte clones isolated during acute seroconversion: recognition of autologous virus sequences within a conserved immunodominant epitope. J Exp Med 1994; 179:463-72.
179. Johnson RP, Hammond SA, Trocha A et al. Induction of a major histocompatibility complex class I-restricted cytotoxic T-lymphocyte response to a highly conserved region of human immunodeficiency virus type 1 (HIV-1) gp120 in seronegative humans immunized with a candidate HIV-1 vaccine. J Virol 1994; 68:3145-53.
180. Couillin I, Connan F, Culmann Penciolelli B et al. HLA-dependent variations in human immunodeficiency virus Nef protein alter peptide/HLA binding. Eur J Immunol 1995; 25:728-32.
181. Sipsas NV, Kalams SA, Trocha A et al. Identification of type-specific cytotoxic T lymphocyte responses to homologous viral proteins in laboratory workers accidentally infected with HIV-1. J Clin Invest 1997; 99:752-62.
182. van Baalen CA, Klein MR, Huisman RC et al. Fine-specificity of cytotoxic T lymphocytes which recognized conserved epitopes of the GAG protein of human immunodeficiency virus type 1. J Gen Virol 1996; 77:1659-65.
183. Phillips RE, Rowland-Jones S, Nixon DF et al. Human immunodeficiency virus genetic variation that can escape cytotoxic T cell recognition. Nature 1991; 354:453-559.
184. Huet S, Nixon DF, Rothbard JB et al. Structural homologies between two HLA B27-restricted peptides suggest residues important for interaction with HLA B27. Int Immunol 1990; 2:311-6.
185. Johnson RP, Trocha A, Buchanan TM et al. Recognition of a highly conserved region of human immunodeficiency virus type 1 gp120 by an HLA-Cw4-restricted cytotoxic T-lymphocyte clone. J Virol 1993; 67:438-45.
186. Hosmalin A, Clerici M, Houghten R et al. An epitope in human immunodeficiency virus 1 reverse transcriptase recognized by both mouse and human cytotoxic T lymphocytes. Proc Natl Acad Sci U S A 1990; 87:2344-8.
187. Harrer T, Harrer E, Kalams SA et al. Cytotoxic T lymphocytes in asymptomatic long-term nonprogressing HIV-1 infection. Breadth and specificity of the response and relation to in vivo viral quasispecies in a person with prolonged infection and low viral load. J Immunol 1996; 156:2616-23.
188. Brander C, Walker B. The HLA-class I restricted CTL response in HIV-1 infection: Identification of optimal epitopes. In: Korber B, Brander C, Walker B et al, eds. HIV Molecular Immunology Database 1996. Los Alamos: Los Alamos National Laboratory, Theoretical Biology and Biophysics, 1996.
189. Lieberman J, Fabry JA, Kuo MC et al. Cytotoxic T lymphocytes from HIV-1 seropositive individuals recognize immunodominant epitopes in gp160 and reverse transcriptase. J Immunol 1992; 148:2738-47.
190. Safrit JT, Andrews CA, Zhu T et al. Characterization of human immunodeficiency virus type 1-specific cytotoxic T lymphocyte clones isolated during acute seroconversion: recognition of autologous virus sequences within a conserved immunodominant epitope. J Exp Med 1994; 179:463-72.
191. Johnson RP, Trocha A, Buchanan TM et al. Identification of overlapping HLA class I-restricted cytotoxic T cell epitopes in a conserved region of the human immundeficiency virus type 1 envelope glycoprotein: definition of minimum epitopes and analysis of the effects of sequence variation. J Exp Med 1992; 175:961-71.
192. Shankar P, Fabry JA, Fong D et al. Three regions of gp160 contain overlapping CTL epitopes restricted by multiple HLA class I alleles. J Cellular Biochem 1995; S21B:D4-345.
193. Rowland-Jones S, Sutton J, Ariyoshi K et al. HIV-specific cytotoxic T-cells in HIV-exposed but uninfected Gambian women. Nature Med 1995; 1:59-64.
194. Johnson RP, Hammond SA, Trocha A et al. Induction of a major histocompatibil-

ity complex class I-restricted cytotoxic T lymphocyte response to a highly conserved region of human immunodeficiency virus type 1 (HIV-1) gp120 in seronegative humans immunized with a candidate HIC-1 vaccine. J Virol 1994; 68:3145-53.
195. Culmann-Penciolelli B, Lamhamedi-Cherradi S, Couillin I et al. Identification of multirestricted immunodominant regions recognized by cytolytic T lymphocytes in the human immunodeficiency virus type 1 nef protein. J Virol 1994; 68:7336-43.
196. Wilson CC, Kalams SA, Wilkes BM et al. Overlapping epitopes in human immunodeficiency virus type 1 gp120 presented by HLA A, B, and C molecules: effects of viral variation on cytotoxic T lymphocyte recognition. J Virol 1997; 71:1256-64.
197. Haas G, Plikat U, Debre P et al. Dynamics of viral variants in HIV-1 Nef and specific cytotoxic T lymphocytes in vivo. J Immunol 1996; 157:4212-21.
198. Doe B, Selby M, Barnett S et al. Induction of cytotoxic T lymphocytes by intramuscular immunization with plasmid DNA is facilitated by bone marrow-derived cells. Proc Natl Acad Sci U S A 1996; 93:8578-83.
199. Shiga H, Shioda T, Tomiyama H et al. Identification of multiple HIV-1 cytotoxic T-cell epitopes presented by human leukocyte antigen B35 molecules. AIDS 1996; 10:1075-83.
200. Gotch F, McAdam SN, Allsopp CE et al. Cytotoxic T cells in HIV2 seropositive Gambians. Identification of a virus-specific MHC-restricted peptide epitope. J Immunol 1993; 151:3361-9.
201. Carmichael A, Jin Y, Sissons P. Analysis of the human env-specific cytotoxic T-lymphocyte (CTL) response in natural human immunodeficiency virus Type 1 infection: Low prevalence of broadly cross-reactive env-specific CTL. J Virol 1996; 70:8468-76.
202. Tarpey I, Stacey S, Hickling J et al. Human cytotoxic T lymphocytes stimulated by endogenously processed human papillomavirus type 11 E7 recognize a peptide containing a HLA-A2 (A*0201) motif. Immunology 1994; 81:222-7.
203. Ressing ME, Sette A, Brandt RM et al. Human CTL epitopes encoded by human papillomavirus type 16 E6 and E7 identified through in vivo and in vitro immunogenicity studies of HLA-A*0201-binding peptides. J Immunol 1995; 154: 5934-43.
204. Ellis JR, Keating PJ, Baird J et al. The association of an HPV16 oncogene variant with HLA-B7 has implications for vaccine design in cervical cancer. Nature Med 1995; 1:464-70.
205. Feltkamp MC, Smits HL, Vierboom MP et al. Vaccination with cytotoxic T lymphocyte epitope-containing peptide protects against a tumor induced by human papillomavirus type 16-transformed cells. Eur J Immunol 1993; 23:2242-9.
206. Bonneau RH, Salvucci LA, Johnson DC et al. Epitope specificity of H-2Kb-restricted, HSV-1-, and HSV-2-cross-reactive cytotoxic T lymphocyte clones. Virology 1993; 195:62-70.
207. Banks TA, Nair S, Rouse BT. Recognition by and in vitro induction of cytotoxic T lymphocytes against predicted epitopes of the immediate-early protein ICP27 of herpes simplex virus. J Virol 1993; 67:613-6.
208. Salvucci LA, Bonneau RH, Tevethia SS. Polymorphism within the herpes simplex virus (HSV) ribonucleotide reductase large subunit (ICP6) confers type specificity for recognition by HSV type 1-specific cytotoxic T lymphocytes. J Virol 1995; 69:1122-31.
209. Utz U, Koenig S, Coligan JE et al. Presentation of three different viral peptides, HTLV-1 Tax, HCMV gB, and influenza virus M1, is determined by common structural features of the HLA-A2.1 molecule. J Immunol 1992; 149:214-21.
210. Falk K, Rötzschke O, Stevanović S et al. Analysis of a naturally occurring HLA class I-restricted viral epitope. Immunology 1994; 82:337-42.
211. Bednarek MA, Sauma SY, Gammon MC et al. The minimum peptide epitope from the influenza virus matrix protein. Extra and intracellular loading of HLA-A2. J Immunol 1991; 147:4047-53.
212. Henderson RA, Cox AL, Sakaguchi K et al. Direct identification of an endogenous

peptide recognized by multiple HLA-A2.1-specific cytotoxic T cells. Proc Natl Acad Sci U S A 1993; 90:10275-9.
213. Walker BD, Flexner C, Birch Limberger K et al. Long-term culture and fine specificity of human cytotoxic T-lymphocyte clones reactive with human immunodeficiency virus type. Proc Natl Acad Sci U S A 1989; 86:9514-8.
214. DiBrino M, Tsuchida T, Turner RV et al. HLA-A1 and HLA-A3 T cell epitopes derived from influenza virus proteins predicted from peptide binding motifs. J Immunol 1993; 151:5930-5.
215. Guo HC, Jardetzky TS, Garrett TP et al. Different length peptides bind to HLA-Aw68 similarly at their ends but bulge out in the middle. Nature 1992; 360: 364-6.
216. Silver ML, Guo HC, Strominger JL et al. Atomic structure of a human MHC molecule presenting an influenza virus peptide. Nature 1992; 360:367-9.
217. Sutton J, Rowland Jones S, Rosenberg W et al. A sequence pattern for peptides presented to cytotoxic T lymphocytes by HLA B8 revealed by analysis of epitopes and eluted peptides. Eur J Immunol 1993; 23:447-53.
218. Tussey LG, Rowland Jones S, Zheng TS et al. Different MHC class I alleles compete for presentation of overlapping viral epitopes. Immunity 1995; 3:65-77.
219. Townsend AR, Rothbard J, Gotch FM et al. The epitopes of influenza nucleoprotein recognized by cytotoxic T lymphocytes can be defined with short synthetic peptides. Cell 1986; 44:959-68.
220. DiBrino M, Parker KC, Margulies DH et al. Identification of the peptide binding motif for HLA-B44, one of the most common HLA-B alleles in the Caucasian population. Biochemistry 1995; 34: 10130-8.
221. Man S, Newberg MH, Crotzer VL et al. Definition of a human T cell epitope from influenza A non-structural protein 1 using HLA-A2.1 transgenic mice. Int Immunol 1995; 7:597-605.
222. Rötzschke O, Falk K, Deres K et al. Isolation and analysis of naturally processed viral peptides as recognized by cytotoxic T cells. Nature 1990; 348:252-4.
223. Falk K, Rötzschke O, Deres K et al. Identification of naturally processed viral nonapeptides allows their quantification in infected cells and suggests an allele-specific T cell epitope forecast. J Exp Med 1991; 174:425-34.
224. Kuwano K, Braciale TJ, Ennis FA. Localization of a cross-reactive CTL epitope to the transmembrane region on the hemaglutinin of influenza H1 and H2 viruses. FASEB J 1988; 2:2221.
225. Cao W, Myers Powell BA, Braciale TJ. Recognition of an immunoglobulin VH epitope by influenza virus-specific class I major histocompatibility complex-restricted cytolytic T lymphocytes. J Exp Med 1994; 179:195-202.
226. Gould KG, Scotney H, Brownlee GG. Characterization of two distinct major histocompatibility complex class I Kk-restricted T-cell epitopes within the influenza A/PR/8/34 virus hemagglutinin. J Virol 1991; 65:5401-9.
227. Larson JK, Wunner WH, Otvos L, Jr. et al. Identification of an immunodominant epitope within the phosphoprotein of rabies virus that is recognized by both class I-and class II-restricted T cells. J Virol 1991; 65:5673-9.
228. Gould KG, Scotney H, Townsend AR et al. Mouse H-2k-restricted cytotoxic T cells recognize antigenic determinants in both the HA1 and HA2 subunits of the influenza A/PR/8/34 hemagglutinin. J Exp Med 1987; 166:693-701.
229. Bastin J, Rothbard J, Davey J et al. Use of synthetic peptides of influenza nucleoprotein to define epitopes recognized by class I-restricted cytotoxic T lymphocytes. J Exp Med 1987; 165:1508-23.
230. Gould K, Cossins J, Bastin J et al. A 15 amino acid fragment of influenza nucleoprotein synthesized in the cytoplasm is presented to class I-restricted cytotoxic T lymphocytes. J Exp Med 1989; 170: 1051-6.
231. Cossins J, Gould KG, Smith M et al. Precise prediction of a Kk-restricted cytotoxic T cell epitope in the NS1 protein of influenza virus using an MHC allele-specific motif. Virology 1993; 193:289-95.
232. Cerundolo V, Elliott T, Elvin J et al. The binding affinity and dissociation rates of

peptides for class I major histocompatibility complex molecules. Eur J Immunol 1991; 21:2069-75.
233. Robbins PA, Lettice LA, Rota P et al. Comparison between two peptide epitopes presented to cytotoxic T lymphocytes by HLA-A2. Evidence for discrete locations within HLA-A2. J Immunol 1989; 143:4098-103.
234. Robbins PA, Garboczi DN, Strominger JL. HLA-A*0201 complexes with two 10-mer peptides differing at the P2 anchor residue have distinct refolding kinetics. J Immunol 1995; 154:703-9.
235. Braciale TJ, Braciale VL, Winkler M et al. On the role of the transmembrane anchor sequence of influenza hemagglutinin in target cell recognition by class I MHC-restricted, hemagglutinin-specific cytolytic T lymphocytes. J Exp Med 1987; 166:678-92.
236. Cao W, Tykodi SS, Esser MT et al. Partial activation of $CD8^+$ T cells by a self-derived peptide. Nature 1995; 378:295-8.
237. Sweetser MT, Morrison LA, Braciale VL et al. Recognition of pre-processed endogenous antigen by class I but not class II MHC-restricted T cells. Nature 1989; 342:180-2.
238. Bergmann C, McMillan M, Stohlman S. Characterization of the L^d-restricted cytotoxic T-lymphocyte epitope in the mouse hepatitis virus nucleocapsid protein. J Virol 1993; 67:7041-9.
239. Whitton JL, Tishon A, Lewicki H et al. Molecular analyses of a five-amino-acid cytotoxic T-lymphocyte (CTL) epitope: an immunodominant region which induces nonreciprocal CTL cross-reactivity. J Virol 1989; 63:4303-10.
240. Schulz M, Aichele P, Schneider R et al. Major histocompatibility complex binding and T cell recognition of a viral nonapeptide containing a minimal tetrapeptide. Eur J Immunol 1991; 21:1181-5.
241. Yanagi Y, Tishon A, Lewicki H et al. Diversity of T-cell receptors in virus-specific cytotoxic T lymphocytes recognizing three distinct viral epitopes restricted by a single major histocompatibility complex molecule. J Virol 1992; 66: 2527-31.
242. Oldstone MB, Whitton JL, Lewicki H et al. Fine dissection of a nine amino acid glycoprotein epitope, a major determinant recognized by lymphocytic choriomeningitis virus-specific class I-restricted H-$2D^b$ cytotoxic T lymphocytes. J Exp Med 1988; 168:559-70.
243. Oldstone MB, Tishon A, Eddleston M et al. Vaccination to prevent persistent viral infection. J Virol 1993; 67:4372-8.
244. Klavinskis LS, Whitton JL, Joly E et al. Vaccination and protection from a lethal viral infection: identification, incorporation, and use of a cytotoxic T lymphocyte glycoprotein epitope. Virology 1990; 178:393-400.
245. Reddehase MJ, Rothbard JB, Koszinowski UH. A pentapeptide as minimal antigenic determinant for MHC class I-restricted T lymphocytes. Nature 1989; 337:651-3.
246. Wei WZ, Gill RF, Jones RF et al. Induction of cytotoxic T lymphocytes to murine mammary tumor cells with a K^d-restricted immunogenic peptide. Int J Cancer 1996; 66:659-63.
247. Malarkannan S, Serwold T, Nguyen V et al. The mouse mammary tumor virus *env* gene is the source of a $CD8^+$ T-cell-stimulating peptide presented by a major histocompatibility complex class I molecule in a murine thymoma. Proc Natl Acad Sci USA 1996; 93:13991-6.
248. Bergmann CC, Yao Q, Lin M et al. The JHM strain of mouse hepatitis virus induces a spike protein-specific D^b-restricted cytotoxic T cell response. J Gen Virol 1996; 77:315-25.
249. Sijts AJ, Ossendorp F, Mengede EA et al. Immunodominant mink cell focus-inducing murine leukemia virus (MuLV)-encoded CTL epitope, identified by its MHC class I-binding motif, explains MuLV-type specificity of MCF-directed cytotoxic T lymphocytes. J Immunol 1994; 152:106-16.
250. White HD, Roeder DA, Green WR. An immunodominant K^b-restricted peptide from the p15E transmembrane protein of endogenous ecotropic murine leukemia virus (MuLV) AKR623 that restores susceptibility of a tumor line to anti-AKR/gross MuLV cytotoxic T lymphocytes [published erratum appears in J Virol 1994; 68:3452]. J Virol 1994; 68:897-904.

251. Neisig A, Roelse J, Sijts AJ et al. Major differences in transporter associated with antigen presentation (TAP)-dependent translocation of MHC class I-presentable peptides and the effect of flanking sequences. J Immunol 1995; 154:1273-9.
252. Chen W, Qin H, Chesebro B et al. Identification of a *gag*-encoded cytotoxic T-lymphocyte epitope from FBL-3 leukemia shared by Friend, Moloney, and Rauscher murine leukemia virus-induced tumors. J Virol 1996; 70:7773-82.
253. Huang AYC, Gulden PH, Woods AS et al. The immunodominant major histocompatibility complex class I-restricted antigen of a murine colon tumor derives from an endogenous retroviral gene product. Proc Natl Acad Sci U S A 1996; 93:9730-5.
254. Verjans GM, Janssen R, UytdeHaag FG et al. Intracellular processing and presentation of T cell epitopes, expressed by recombinant Escherichia coli and Salmonella typhimurium, to human T cells. Eur J Immunol 1995; 25:405-10.
255. van Binnendijk RS, Versteeg van Oosten JP, Poelen MC et al. Human HLA class I- and HLA class II-restricted cloned cytotoxic T lymphocytes identify a cluster of epitopes on the measles virus fusion protein. J Virol 1993; 67:2276-84.
256. Beauverger P, Buckland R, Wild TF. Measles virus antigens induce both type-specific and canine distemper virus cross-reactive cytotoxic T lymphocytes in mice: localization of a common L^d-restricted nucleoprotein epitope. J Gen Virol 1993; 74:2357-63.
257. Beauverger P, Buckland R, Wild F. Measles virus hemagglutinin induces an L^d-restricted $CD8^+$ cytotoxic T lymphocyte response to two specific epitopes. Virology 1994; 200:281-3.
258. Kutubuddin M, Simons J, Chow M. Poliovirus-specific major histocompatibility complex class I-restricted cytolytic T-cell epitopes in mice localize to neutralizing antigenic regions. J Virol 1992; 66: 5967-74.
259. Franco MA, Prieto I, Labbe M et al. An immunodominant cytotoxic T cell epitope on the VP7 rotavirus protein overlaps the H2 signal peptide. J Gen Virol 1993; 74:2579-86.
260. Franco MA, Lefevre P, Willems P et al. Identification of cytotoxic T cell epitopes on the VP3 and VP6 rotavirus proteins. J Gen Virol 1994; 75:589-96.
261. Kulkarni AB, Morse HC, Bennink JR et al. Immunization of mice with vaccinia virus-M2 recombinant induces epitope-specific and cross-reactive Kd-restricted $CD8^+$ cytotoxic T cells. J Virol 1993; 67:4086-92.
262. Haurum JS, Tan L, Arsequell G et al. Peptide anchor residue glycosylation: effect on class I major histocompatibility complex binding and cytotoxic T lymphocyte recognition. Eur J Immunol 1995; 25:3270-6.
263. Kast WM, Roux L, Curren J et al. Protection against lethal Sendai virus infection by in vivo priming of virus-specific cytotoxic T lymphocytes with a free synthetic peptide. Proc Natl Acad Sci U S A 1991; 88:2283-7.
264. Schumacher TN, De Bruijn ML, Vernie LN et al. Peptide selection by MHC class I molecules. Nature 1991; 350:703-6.
265. Liu T, Zhou X, Orvell C et al. Heat-inactivated Sendai virus can enter multiple MHC class I processing pathways and generate cytotoxic T lymphocyte responses in vivo. J Immunol 1995; 154: 3147-55.
266. Yasutomi Y, Koenig S, Woods RM et al. A vaccine-elicited, single viral epitope-specific cytotoxic T lymphocyte response does not protect against intravenous, cell-free simian immunodeficiency virus challenge. J Virol 1995; 69:2279-84.
267. Mylin LM, Deckhut AM, Bonneau RH et al. Cytotoxic T lymphocyte escape variants, induced mutations, and synthetic peptides define a dominant $H\text{-}2K^b$-restricted deteriminant in simian virus 40 tumor antigen. Virology 1995; 159-72.
268. Deckhut AM, Lippolis JD, Tevethia SS. Comparative analysis of core amino acid residues of H-2D(b)-restricted cytotoxic T-lymphocyte recognition epitopes in simian virus 40 T antigen. J Virol 1992; 66:440-7.
269. Tevethia SS, Lewis M, Tanaka Y et al. Dissection of $H\text{-}2D^b$-restricted cytotoxic T-lymphocyte epitopes on simian virus 40 T antigen by the use of synthetic pep-

tides and H-2D^{bm} mutants. J Virol 1990; 64:1192-200.
270. Alsheikhly AR. Interaction of in vitro- and in vivo-generated cytotoxic T cells with SV40 T antigen: analysis with synthetic peptides. Scand J Immunol 1994; 39:467-79.
271. Rawle FC, O'Connell KA, Geib RW et al. Fine mapping of an H-2K^{k} restricted cytotoxic T lymphocyte epitope in SV40 T antigen by using in-frame deletion mutants and a synthetic peptide. J Immunol 1988; 141:2734-9.
272. van Bleek GM, Nathenson SG. Isolation of an endogenously processed immunodominant viral peptide from the class I H-2K^{b} molecule. Nature 1990; 348: 213-6.
273. Rötzschke O, Falk K, Stevanović S et al. Exact prediction of a natural T cell epitope. Eur J Immunol 1991; 21:2891-4.
274. Carbone FR, Moore MW, Sheil JM et al. Induction of cytotoxic T lymphocytes by primary in vitro stimulation with peptides. J Exp Med 1988; 167:1767-79.
275. Wölfel T, Hauer M, Schneider J et al. A p16INK4a-insensitive CDK4 mutant targeted by cytolytic T lymphocytes in a human melanoma. Science 1995; 269: 1281-4.
276. Maryanski JL, Pala P, Corradin G et al. H-2-restricted cytolytic T cells specific for HLA can recognize a synthetic HLA peptide. Nature 1986; 324:578-9.
277. Pamer EG. Direct sequence identification and kinetic analysis of an MHC class I-restricted Listeria monocytogenes CTL epitope. J Immunol 1994; 152:686-94.
278. Sijts AJ, Neisig A, Neefjes J et al. Two Listeria monocytogenes CTL epitopes are processed from the same antigen with different efficiencies. J Immunol 1996; 156:683-92.
279. Gulden PH, Fischer P III, Sherman NE et al. A Listeria monocytogenes pentapeptide is presented to cytolytic T lymphocytes by the H2-M3 MHC class Ib molecule. Immunity 1996; 5:73-9.
280. Lenz LL, Dere B, Bevan MJ. Identification of an H2-M3-restricted Listeria epitope: Implications for antigen presentation by M3. Immunity 1996; 5:63-72.
281. Pamer EG, Harty JT, Bevan MJ. Precise prediction of a dominant class I MHC-restricted epitope of Listeria monocytogenes. Nature 1991; 353:852-5.
282. Yamazaki H, Tanaka M, Nagoya M et al. Epitope selection in major histocompatibility complex class I-mediated pathway is affected by the intracellular localization of an antigen. Eur J Immunol 1997; 27:347-53.
283. Romero P, Maryanski JL, Corradin G et al. Cloned cytotoxic T cells recognize an epitope in the circumsporozoite protein and protect against malaria. Nature 1989; 341:323-6.
284. Weiss WR, Mellouk S, Houghten RA et al. Cytotoxic T cells recognize a peptide from the circumsporozoite protein on malaria-infected hepatocytes. J Exp Med 1990; 171:763-73.
285. Blum-Tirouvanziam U, Servis C, Habluetzel A et al. Localization of HLA-A2.1-restricted T cell epitopes in the circumsporozoite protein of Plasmodium falciparum. J Immunol 1995; 154: 3922-31.
286. Aidoo M, Lalvani A, Allsopp CE et al. Identification of conserved antigenic components for a cytotoxic T lymphocyte-inducing vaccine against malaria. Lancet 1995; 345:1003-7.
287. Wizel B, Houghten RA, Parker KC et al. Irradiated sporozoite vaccine induces HLA-B8-restricted cytotoxic T lymphocyte responses against two overlapping epitopes of the Plasmodium falciparum sporozoite surface protein 2. J Exp Med 1995; 182:1435-45.
288. Hill AV, Elvin J, Willis AC et al. Molecular analysis of the association of HLA-B53 and resistance to severe malaria. Nature 1992; 360:434-9.
289. Blum-Tirouvanziam U, Beghdadi-Rais C, Roggero MA et al. Elicitation of specific cytotoxic T cells by immunization with malaria soluble synthetic polypeptides. J Immunol 1994; 153:4134-41.
290. Kumar S, Miller LH, Quakyi IA et al. Cytotoxic T cells specific for the circumsporozoite protein of Plasmodium falciparum. Nature 1988; 334:258-60.
291. Huang F, Hermann E, Wang J et al. A patient-derived cytotoxic T-lymphocyte clone and two peptide-dependent mono-

clonal antibodies recognize HLA-B27-peptide complexes with low stringency for peptide sequences. Infect Immun 1996; 64:120-7.
292. Starnbach MN, Bevan MJ. Cells infected with Yersinia present an epitope to class I MHC-restricted CTL. J Immunol 1994; 153:1603-12.
293. Wauben MHM, van der Kraan M, Grosfeld-Stulemeyer MC et al. Definition of an extended MHC class II-peptide binding motif for the autoimmune disease-associated Lewis rat RT1.B^{L} molecule. Int Immunol 1997; 9:281-90.
294. Matsushita S, Yokomizo H, Kohsaka H et al. Diversity of a human CD4+ T cell repertoire recognizing one TCR ligand. Immunol Letters 1996; 51:191-4.
295. ten Bosch GJA, Joosten AM, Kessler JH et al. Recognition of BCR-ABL Positive leukemic blasts by human CD4^{+} T cells elicited by primary in vitro immunization with a BCR-ABL breakpoint peptide. Blood 1996; 88:3522-7.
296. Fugger L, Rothbard JB, Sonderstrup McDevitt G. Specificity of an HLA-DRB1*0401-restricted T cell response to type II collagen. Eur J Immunol 1996; 26:928-33.
297. Carrasco-Marin E, Shimizu J, Kanagawa O et al. The class II MHC I-A^{g7} molecules from non-obese diabetic mice are poor peptide binders. J Immunol 1996; 156:450-8.
298. Wegmann KW, Zhao W, Griffin AC et al. Identification of myocarditogenic peptides derived from cardiac myosin capable of inducing experimental allergic myocarditis in the Lewis rat. The utility of a class II binding motif in selecting self-reactive peptides. J Immunol 1994; 153:892-900.
299. Gaston JSH, Deane KHO, Jecock RM et al. Identification of 2 *Chlamydia trachomatis* antigens recognized by synovial fluid T cells from patients with Chlamydia induced reactive arthritis. J Rheumatol 1996; 23:130-6.
300. Cong Y, Bowdon HR, Elson CO. Identification of an immunodominant T cell epitope on cholera toxin. Eur J Immunol 1996; 26:2587-95.
301. Kristensen NM, Hoyne GF, Hayball JD et al. Induction of T cell responses to the invariant chain derived peptide CLIP in mice immunized with the group 1 allergen of house dust mite. Int Immunol 1996; 8:1091-8.
302. Tsitoura DC, Holter W, Cerwenka A et al. Induction of anergy in human T helper 0 cells by stimulation with altered T cell antigen receptor ligands. J Immunol 1996; 156:2801-8.
303. Okano M, Nagano T, Nakada M et al. Epitope analysis of HLA-DR-restricted helper T-cell responses to DER P II, a major allergen molecule of dermatophagoides pteronyssinus. Allergy 1996; 51: 29-35.
304. Wucherpfennig KW, Yu B, Bhol K et al. Structural basis for major histocompatibility complex (MHC)-linked susceptibility to autoimmunity: charged residues of a single MHC binding pocket confer selective presentation of self-peptides in pemphigus vulgaris. Proc Natl Acad Sci USA 1995; 92:11935-9.
305. Colovai AI, Liu Z, Harris PE et al. Allopeptide-specific T cell reactivity altered by peptide analogs. J Immunol 1997; 158:48-54.
306. White CA, Cross SM, Kurilla MG et al. Recruitment during infectious mononucleosis of CD3^{+}CD4^{+}CD8^{+} virus-specific cytotoxic T cells which recognise Epstein-Barr virus lytic antigen BHRF1. Virology 1996; 219:489-92.
307. Reay PA, Kantor RM, Davis MM. Use of global amino acid replacements to define the requirements for MHC binding and T cell recognition of moth cytochrome c (93-103). J Immunol 1994; 152:3946-57.
308. Kurane I, Okamoto Y, Dai LC et al. Flavivirus-cross-reactive, HLA-DR15-restricted epitope on NS3 recognized by human CD4^{+} CD8^{-} cytotoxic T lymphocyte clones. J Gen Virol 1995; 76:2243-9.
309. Spouge JL, Guy HR, Cornette JL et al. Strong conformational propensities enhance T cell antigenicity. J Immunol 1987; 138:204-12.
310. Chen S, Whiteley PJ, Freed DC et al. Responses of NOD congenic mice to a glutamic acid decarboxylase-derived peptide. J Autoimmunity 1994; 7:635-41.
311. Kaufman DL, Clare Salzler M, Tian J et al. Spontaneous loss of T-cell tolerance

to glutamic acid decarboxylase in murine insulin-dependent diabetes. Nature 1993; 366:69-72.

312. Mannie MD, Paterson PY, U'Prichard DC et al. The N- and C-terminal boundaries of myelin basic protein determinants required for encephalitogenic and proliferative responses of Lewis rat T cells. J Neuroimmunol 1990; 26:201-11.
313. Diepolder HM, Jung M, Wierenga E et al. Anergic TH1 clones specific for hepatitis B virus (HBV) core peptides are inhibitory to other HBV core-specific CD4+ T cells in vitro. J Virol 1996; 70:7540-8.
314. Gautier N, Chavant E, Prieur E et al. Characterization of an epitope of the human cytomegalovirus protein IE1 recognized by a CD4+ T cell clone. Eur J Immunol 1996; 26:1110-7.
315. Altuvia Y, Berzofsky JA, Rosenfeld R et al. Sequence features that correlate with MHC restriction [published erratum appears in Mol Immunol 1994; 31: 703]. Mol Immunol 1994; 31:1-19.
316. Adorini L, Appella E, Doria G et al. Mechanisms influencing the immunodominance of T cell determinants. J Exp Med 1988; 168:2091-104.
317. Adorini L, Sette A, Buus S et al. Interaction of an immunodominant epitope with Ia molecules in T-cell activation. Proc Natl Acad Sci U S A 1988; 85: 5181-5.
318. Hurtenbach U, Lier E, Adorini L et al. Prevention of autoimmune diabetes in non-obese diabetic mice by treatment with a class II major histocompatibility complex-blocking peptide. J Exp Med 1993; 177:1499-594.
319. Deng H, Apple M, Clare-Salzler M et al. Determinant capture as a possible mechanism of protection afforded by major histocompatibility complex class II molecules in autoimmune disease. J Exp Med 1993; 178:1675-80.
320. Sette A, Buus S, Appella E et al. Prediction of major histocompatibility complex binding regions of protein antigens by sequence pattern analysis. Proc Natl Acad Sci USA 1989; 86:3296-300.
321. Vogt AB, Kropshofer H, Kalbacher H et al. Ligand motifs of HLA-DRB5*0101 and DRB1*1501 molecules delineated from self-peptides. J Immunol 1994; 153:1665-73.
322. Anderson DC, van Schooten WC, Barry ME et al. A Mycobacterium leprae-specific human T cell epitope cross-reactive with an HLA-DR2 peptide. Science 1988; 242:259-61.
323. Wicker LS, Chen S, Nepom GT et al. Naturally processed T cell epitopes from human glutamic acid decarboxylase identified using mice transgenic for the Type 1 diabetes-associated human MHC Class II allele, DRB1*0401. J Clin Invest 1996; 98:2597-603.
324. Bogen B, Snodgrass R, Briand JP et al. Synthetic peptides and beta-chain gene rearrangements reveal a diversified T cell repertoire for a lambda light chain third hypervariable region. Eur J Immunol 1986; 16:1379-84.
325. O'Sullivan D, Arrhenius T, Sidney J et al. On the interaction of promiscuous antigenic peptides with different DR alleles. Identification of common structural motifs. J Immunol 1991; 147:2663-9.
326. Fahrer AM, Geysen HM, White DO et al. Analysis of the requirements for class II-restricted T cell recognition of a single determinant reveals considerable diversity in the T cell response and degeneracy of peptide binding to I-E^d. J Immunol 1995; 155:2849-57.
327. Brett SJ, Tite JP. Both H-2- and non-H-2-linked genes influence influenza nucleoprotein epitope recognition by CD4+ T cells. Immunology 1996; 87:42-8.
328. Daniel D, Wegmann DR. Protection of nonobese diabetic mice from diabetes by intranasal or subcutaneous administration of insulin peptide B-(9-23). Proc Natl Acad Sci U S A 1996; 93:956-60.
329. Ikagawa S, Matsushita S, Chen YZ et al. Single amino acid substitutions on a Japanese cedar pollen allergen (Cry j 1)-derived peptide induced alterations in human T cell responses and T cell receptor antagonism. J Allergy Clin Immunol 1996; 97:53-64.
330. Smilek DE, Lock CB, McDevitt HO. Antigen recognition and peptide-mediated immunotherapy in autoimmune disease. Immunol Rev 1990; 118:37-71.
331. Hammer J, Gallazzi F, Bono E et al. Peptide binding specificity of HLA-DR4

molecules: correlation with rheumatoid arthritis association. J Exp Med 1995; 181:1847-55.
332. Geluk A, van Meijgaarden KE, Southwood S et al. HLA-DR3 molecules can bind peptides carrying two alternative specific submotifs. J Immunol 1994; 152:5742-8.
333. Blaher B, Suphioglu C, Knox RB et al. Identification of T-cell epitopes of Lol p 9, a major allergen of ryegrass (*Lolium perenne*) pollen. J Allergy Clin Immunol 1996; 98:124-32.
334. Kobayashi H, Kokubo T, Abe Y et al. Analysis of anchor residues in a naturally processed HLA-DR53 ligand. Immunogenetics 1996; 44:366-71.
335. Adams E, Basten A, Rodda S et al. Human T-cell clones to the 70-kilodalton heat shock protein of Mycobacterium leprae define mycobacterium-specific epitopes rather than shared epitopes. Infection and Immunity 1997; 65:1061-70.
336. Harris DP, Vordermeier HM, Singh M et al. Cross-recognition by T cells of an epitope shared by two unrelated mycobacterial antigens. Eur J Immunol 1995; 25:3173-9.
337. Yanagisawa S, Koike M, Kariyone A et al. Mapping of Mβ11$^+$ helper T cell epitopes on mycobacterial antigen in mouse primed with *Mycobacterium tuberculosis.* Int Immunol 1997; 9:227-37.
338. Wucherpfennig KW, Sette A, Southwood S et al. Structural requirements for binding of an immunodominant myelin basic protein peptide to DR2 isotypes and for its recognition by human T cell clones. J Exp Med 1994; 179:279-90.
339. Martin R, Howell MD, Jaraquemada D et al. A myelin basic protein peptide is recognized by cytotoxic T cells in the context of four HLA-DR types associated with multiple sclerosis. J Exp Med 1991; 173:19-24.
340. Amor S, O'Neill JK, Morris MM et al. Encephalitogenic epitopes of myelin basic protein, proteolipid protein, myelin oligodendrocyte glycoprotein for experimental allergic encephalomyelitis induction in Biozzi ABH (H-2A^{g7}) mice share an amino acid motif. J Immunol 1996; 156:3000-8.
341. Muller CP, Ammerlaan W, Fleckenstein B et al. Activation of T cells by the ragged tail of MHC class II-presented peptides of the measles virus fusion protein. Int Immunol 1996; 8:445-56.
342. Bernard CCA, Johns TG, Slavin A et al. Myelin oligodendrocyte glycoprotein: a novel candidate autoantigen in multiple sclerosis. J Mol Med 1997; 75:77-88.
343. Hawes GE, Struyk L, Godthelp BC et al. Limited restriction in the TCR-alpha beta V region usage of antigen-specific clones. Recognition of myelin basic protein (amino acids 84-102) and Mycobacterium bovis 65-kDa heat shock protein (amino acids 3-13) by T cell clones established from peripheral blood mononuclear cells of monozygotic twins and HLA-identical individuals. J Immunol 1995; 154:555-66.
344. McNicholl JM, Whitworth WC, Oftung F et al. Structural requirements of peptide and MHC for DR(alpha, beta 1*0401)-restricted T cell antigen recognition. J Immunol 1995; 155:1951-63.
345. Anderton SM, van der Zee R, Noordzij A et al. Differential mycobacterial 65-kDa heat shock protein T cell epitope recognition after adjuvant arthritis-inducing or protective immunization protocols. J Immunol 1994; 152:3656-64.
346. Samson MF, Smilek DE. Reversal of acute experimental autoimmune encephalomyelitis and prevention of relapses by treatment with a myelin basic protein peptide analogue modified to form long-lived peptide-MHC complexes. J Immun 1995; 155:2737-46.
347. Mendel I, Kerlero de Rosbo N, Ben-Nun A. Delineation of the minimal encephalitogenic epitope within the immunodominant region of myelin oligodendrocyte glycoprotein: diverse Vβ gene usage by T cells recognizing the core epitope encephalitogenic for T cell receptor Vβ^b and T cell receptor Vβ^a H-2^b mice. Eur J Immunol 1996; 26:2470-9.
348. Ridgway WM, Fasso M, Lanctot A et al. Breaking self-tolerance in nonobese diabetic mice. J Exp Med 1996; 183:1657-62.
349. Markovic Plese S, Fukaura H, Zhang J et al. T cell recognition of immunodominant and cryptic proteolipid protein

epitopes in humans. J Immunol 1995; 155:982-92.
350. Baños DM, Lopez S, Arias CF et al. Identification of a T-helper cell epitope on the rotavirus VP6 protein. J Virol 1996; 71:419-26.
351. Ou D, Mitchell LA, Domeier ME et al. Characterization of the HLA-restrictive elements of a rubella virus-specific cytotoxic T cell clone: influence of HLA-DR4β chain residue 74 polymorphism on antigenic peptide-T cell interaction. Int Immunol 1996; 8:1577-86.
352. Kojima K, Berger T, Lassmann H et al. Experimental autoimmune panencephalitis and uveoretinitis transferred to the Lewis rat by T lymphocytes specific for the S100 beta molecule, a calcium binding protein of astroglia. J Exp Med 1994; 180:817-29.
353. Cole GA, Tao T, Hogg TL et al. Binding motifs predict major histocompatibility class II-restricted epitopes in the Sendai virus M protein. J Virol 1995; 69:8057-60.
354. Chicz RM, Urban RG, Lane WS et al. Predominant naturally processed peptides bound to HLA-DR1 are derived from MHC-related molecules and are heterogeneous in size. Nature 1992; 358:764-8.
355. Guery JC, Sette A, Appella E et al. Constitutive presentation of dominant epitopes from endogenous naturally processed self-beta 2-microglobulin to class II-restricted T cells leads to self-tolerance. J Immunol 1995; 154:545-54.
356. Wen R, Broussard DR, Surman S et al. Carboxy-terminal residues of major histocompatibility complex class II-associated peptides control the presentation of the bacterial superantigen toxic shock syndrome toxin-1 to T cells. Eur J Immunol 1997; 27:772-81.
357. Broeren CP, Lucassen MA, van Stipdonk MJ et al. CDR1 T-cell receptor beta-chain peptide induces major histocompatibility complex class II-restricted T-T cell interactions. Proc Natl Acad Sci U S A 1994; 91:5997-6001.
358. Boitel B, Blank U, Mege D et al. Strong similarities in antigen fine specificity among DRB1* 1302-restricted tetanus toxin tt830-843-specific TCRs in spite of highly heterogeneous CDR3. J Immunol 1995; 154:3245-55.
359. Topalian SL, Gonzales MI, Parkhurst M et al. Melanoma-specific CD4+ T cells recognize nonmutated HLA-DR-restricted tyrosinase epitopes. J Exp Med 1996; 183:1965-71.
360. Noll A, Autenrieth IB. Yersinia-hsp60-reactive T cells are efficiently stimulated by peptides of 12 and 13 amino acid residues in a MHC class II (I-A^b)-restricted manner. Clin Exp Immunol 1996; 105: 231-7.
361. Schild H, Deres K, Wiesmüller KH et al. Efficiency of peptides and lipopeptides for in vivo priming of virus-specific cytotoxic T cells. Eur J Immunol 1991; 21:2649-54.
362. Schild H, Rötzschke O, Kalbacher H et al. Limit of T cell tolerance to self proteins by peptide presentation. Science 1990; 247:1587-9.
363. Miller JF. Autoantigen-induced deletion of peripheral self-reactive T cells. Int Rev Immunol 1995; 13:107-14.
364. Miller JF, Morahan G. Peripheral T cell tolerance. Annu Rev Immunol 1992; 10:197.
365. von Herrath MG, Oldstone MB. Role of viruses in the loss of tolerance to self-antigens and in autoimmune diseases. Trends Microbiol 1995; 3:424-30.
366. von Herrath MG, Dockter J, Oldstone MB. How virus induces a rapid or slow onset insulin-dependent diabetes mellitus in a transgenic model. Immunity 1994; 1:231-42.
367. Falk K, Rötzschke O, Takiguchi M et al. Peptide motifs of HLA-A1, -A11, -A31, and -A33 molecules. Immunogenetics 1994; 40:238-41.
368. Fahnestock ML, Johnson JL, Feldman RM et al. The MHC class I homolog encoded by human cytomegalovirus binds endogenous peptides. Immunity 1995; 3:583-90.
369. Brossart P, Bevan MJ. Selective activation of Fas/Fas ligand-mediated cytotoxicity by a self peptide. J Exp Med 1996; 183:2449-58.
370. Fiorillo MT, Meadows L, D'Amato M et al. Susceptibility to ankylosing spondylitis

correlates with the C-terminal residue of peptides presented by various HLA-B27 subtypes. Eur J Immunol 1997; 27: 368-73.

371. Falk K, Rötzschke O, Takiguchi M et al. Peptide motifs of HLA-B58, B60, B61, and B62 molecules. Immunogenetics 1995; 41:165-8.

372. Lee N, Malacko AR, Ishitani A et al. The membrane-bound and soluble forms of HLA-G bind identical sets of endogenous peptides but differ with respect to TAP association. Immunity 1995; 3:591-600.

373. Corr M, Boyd LF, Padlan EA et al. H-2D^{d} exploits a four residue peptide binding motif. J Exp Med 1993; 178:1877-92.

374. Falk K, Rötzschke O, Takiguchi M et al. Peptide motifs of HLA-B51, -B52 and -B78 molecules, and implications for Behcet's disease. Int Immunol 1995; 7:223-8.

375. Brown EL, Wooters JL, Ferenz CR et al. Characterization of peptide binding to the murine MHC class I H-2Kk molecule. Sequencing of the bound peptides and direct binding of synthetic peptides to isolated class I molecules.J Immunol 1994; 153:3079-92.

376. Engelhard VH. Structure of peptides associated with MHC class I molecules. Curr Opin Immunol 1994; 6:13-23.

377. Kubo RT, Sette A, Grey HM et al. Definition of specific peptide motifs for four major HLA-A alleles. J Immunol 1994; 152:3913-24.

378. Barber LD, Percival L, Parham P. Characterization of the peptide-binding specificity of HLA-B*7301. Tissue Antigens 1996; 47:472-7.

379. Diehl, M. Untersuchungen zur Peptidpräsentation gewebsspezifischer HLA-Moleküle 1995; Phillips-Universität Marburg.

380. Barouch D, Friede T, Stevanović S et al. HLA-A2 subtypes are functionally distinct in peptide binding and presentation. J Exp Med 1995; 182:1847-56.

381. Joyce S, Tabaczewski P, Angeletti RH et al. A nonpolymorphic major histocompatibility complex class Ib molecule binds a large array of diverse self-peptides. J Exp Med 1994; 179:579-88.

382. Rötzschke O, Falk K, Stevanović S et al. Dominant aromatic/aliphatic C-terminal anchor in HLA-B*2702 and B*2705 peptide motifs. Immunogenetics 1994; 39: 74-7.

383. Stevanović S, Pomer S, Rammensee H-G. Oberflächenantigene im Nierenzellkarzinom - Präsentation von MHC I-gebundenen Selbstpeptiden. Akt Urol 1995; Sonderheft:45-6.

384. Malarkannan S, Gonzalez F, Nguyen V et al. Alloreactive CD8^{+} T cell can recognize unusual, rare, and unique processed peptide/MHC complexes. J Immunol 1996; 157:4464-73.

385. Townsend A, Ohlen C, Rogers M et al. Source of unique tumour antigens. Nature 1994; 371:662

386. Burrows GG, Ariail K, Celnik B et al. Variation in H-2K^{k} peptide motif revealed by sequencing naturally processed peptides from T-cell hybridoma class I molecules. J Neurosci Res 1996; 45:803-11.

387. Henderson RA, Michel H, Sakaguchi K et al. HLA-A2.1-associated peptides from a mutant cell line: a second pathway of antigen presentation. Science 1992; 255:1264-6.

388. Hunt DF, Henderson RA, Shabanowitz J et al. Characterization of peptides bound to the class I MHC molecule HLA-A2.1 by mass spectrometry. Science 1992; 255:1261-3.

389. Harris PE, Colovai A, Liu Z et al. Naturally processed HLA class I bound peptides from c-myc-transfected cells reveal allele-specific motifs. J Immunol 1993; 151:5966-74.

390. Huczko EL, Bodnar WM, Benjamin D et al. Characteristics of endogenous peptides eluted from the class I MHC molecule HLA-B7 determined by mass spectrometry and computer modeling. J Immunol 1993; 151:2572-87.

391. Barber LD, Gillece Castro B, Percival L et al. Overlap in the repertoires of peptides bound in vivo by a group of related class I HLA-B allotypes. Curr Biol 1995; 5:179-90.

392. Falk K, Rötzschke O, Grahovać B et al. Allele-specific peptide ligand motifs of HLA-C molecules. Proc Natl Acad Sci U S A 1993; 90:12005-9.

393. Davenport MP, Smith KJ, Barouch D et al. HLA class I binding motifs derived from random peptide libraries differ at the COOH terminus from those of eluted peptides. J Exp Med 1997; 185:367-71.
394. Reich EP, von Grafenstein H, Barlow A et al. Self peptides isolated from MHC glycoproteins of non-obese diabetic mice. J Immunol 1994; 152:2279-88.
395. Merkel F, Kalluri R, Marx M et al. Autoreactive T-cells in Goodpasture's syndrome recognize the N-terminal NC1 domain on alpha 3 type IV collagen. Kidney Int 1996; 49:1127-33.
396. Falk K, Rötzschke O, Takiguchi M et al. Peptide motifs of HLA-B38 and B39 molecules. Immunogenetics 1995; 41:162-4.
397. Dahl AM, Beverley PC, Stauss HJ. A synthetic peptide derived from the tumor-associated protein mdm2 can stimulate autoreactive, high avidity cytotoxic T lymphocytes that recognize naturally processed protein. J Immunol 1996; 157:239-46.
398. Dubey P, Hendrickson RC, Meredith SC et al. The immunodominant antigen of an ultraviolet-induced regressor tumor is generated by a somatic point mutation in the DEAD box helicase p68. J Exp Med 1997; 185:695-706.
399. Fleischhauer K, Avila D, Vilbois F et al. Characterization of natural peptide ligands for HLA-B*4402 and -B*4403: implications for peptide involvement in allorecognition of a single amino acid change in the HLA-B44 heavy chain. Tissue Antigens 1994; 44:311-7.
400. Doménech N, Henderson RA, Finn OJ. Identification of an HLA-A11-restricted epitope from the tandem repeat domain of the epithelial tumor antigen mucin. J Immunol 1995; 155:4766-74.
401. Panina-Bordignon P, Lang R, van Endert PM et al. Cytotoxic T cells specific for glutamic acid decarboxylase in autoimmune diabetes. J Exp Med 1995; 181:1923-7.
402. Diehl M, Münz C, Keilholz W et al. Nonclassical HLA-G molecules are classical peptide presenters. Curr Biol 1996; 6:305-14.
403. Tzeng C, Adams EJ, Gumperz JE et al. Peptides bound endogenously by HLA-Cw*0304 expressed in LCL 721.221 cells include a peptide derived from HLA-E. Tissue Antigens 1996; 48:325-8.
404. Reizis B, Schild H, Stevanović S et al. Peptide binding motifs of the MHC class I molecules ($RT1.A^l$) of the Lewis rat. Immunogenetics 1997; 45:278-9.
405. Cerrone MC, Ma JJ, Stephens RS. Cloning and sequence of the gene for heat shock protein 60 from Chlamydia trachomatis and immunological reactivity of the protein. Infect Immun 1991; 59:79-90.
406. Zügel U, Schoel B, Yamamoto S et al. Crossrecognition by CD8 T cell receptor alpha beta cytotoxic T lymphocytes of peptides in the self and the mycobacterial hsp60 which share intermediate sequence homology. Eur J Immunol 1995; 25:451-8.
407. Chen W, Ede JN, Jackson DC et al. CTL recognition of an altered peptide associated with asparagine bond rearrangement—implications for immunity and vaccine design. J Immunol 1996; 157:1000-5.
408. di Marzo Veronese F, Arnott D, Barnaba V et al. Autoreactive cytotoxic T lymphocytes in human immunodeficiency virus type 1-infected subjects. J Exp Med 1996; 183:2509-16.
409. Sheil JM, Shepherd SE, Klimo GF et al. Identification of an autologous insulin B chain peptide as a target antigen for H-$2K^b$-restricted cytotoxic T lymphocytes. J Exp Med 1992; 175:545-52.
410. Harpur AG, Zimiecki A, Wilks AF et al. A prominent natural H-2 K^d ligand is derived from protein tyrosine kinase JAK1. Immunol Lett 1993; 35:235-7.
411. Tallquist MD, Yun TJ, Pease LR. A single T cell receptor recognizes structurally distinct MHC/peptide complexes with high specificity. J Exp Med 1996; 184:1017-26.
412. Guilloux Y, Lucas S, Brichard VG et al. A peptide recognized by human cytolytic T lymphocytes on HLA-A2 melanomas is encoded by an intron sequence of the N-acetylglucosaminyltransferase V gene. J Exp Med 1996; 183:1173-83.
413. Wang C, Castano AR, Peterson PA et al. Nonclassical binding of formylated pep-

tide in crystal structure of the MHC class Ib molecule H2-M3. Cell 1995; 82: 655-64.
414.Sykulev Y, Joo M, Vturina I et al. Evidence that a single peptide-MHC complex on a target cell can elicit a cytolytic T cell response. Immunity 1996; 4: 565-71.
415.Udaka K, Tsomides TJ, Eisen HN. A naturally occurring peptide recognized by alloreactive CD8+ cytotoxic T lymphocytes in association with a class I MHC protein. Cell 1992; 69:989-98.
416.Wu MX, Tsomides TJ, Eisen HN. Tissue distribution of natural peptides derived from a ubiquitous dehydrogenase, including a novel liver-specific peptide that demonstrates the pronounced specificity of low affinity T cell reactions. J Immunol 1995; 154:4495-502.
417.Corr M, Boyd LF, Frankel SR et al. Endogenous peptides of a soluble major histocompatibility complex class I molecule, H-2Lds: sequence motif, quantitative binding, and molecular modeling of the complex. J Exp Med 1992; 176: 1681-92.
418.Robbins PF, el Gamil M, Li YF et al. A mutated beta-catenin gene encodes a melanoma-specific antigen recognized by tumor infiltrating lymphocytes. J Exp Med 1996; 183:1185-92.
419.Wei ML, Cresswell P. HLA-A2 molecules in an antigen-processing mutant cell contain signal sequence-derived peptides. Nature 1992; 356:443-6.
420.Walden P, Wiesmüller KH, Jung G. Elucidation of T-cell epitopes: a synthetic approach with random peptide libraries. Biochem Soc Trans 1995; 23:678-81.
421.Udaka K, Wiesmüller K, Kienle S et al. Self-MHC restricted peptides recognized by an alloreactive T lymphocyte clone. Journal of Immunology 1996; 157:670-8.
422.Bloom M., Perry-Lalley D, Robbins PF et al. Identification of tyrosinase-related protein 2 as a tumor rejection antigen for the B16 melanoma. J Exp Med 1997; 185:453-9.
423.Wölfel T, Van Pel A, Brichard V et al. Two tyrosinase nonapeptides recognized on HLA-A2 melanomas by autologous cytolytic T lymphocytes. Eur J Immunol 1994; 24:759-64.
424.Robbins PF, el Gamil M, Kawakami Y et al. Recognition of tyrosinase by tumor-infiltrating lymphocytes from a patient responding to immunotherapy [published erratum appears in Cancer Res 1994; 54:3952]. Cancer Res 1994; 54:3124-6.
425.Brichard V, Van Pel A, Wölfel T et al. The tyrosinase gene codes for an antigen recognized by autologous cytolytic T lymphocytes on HLA-A2 melanomas. J Exp Med 1993; 178:489-95.
426.Engelhard VH, Appella E, Benjamin DC et al. Mass spectrometric analysis of peptides associated with the human class I MHC molecules HLA-A2.1 and HLA-B7 and identification of structural features that determine binding. Chem Immunol 1993; 57:39-62.
427.Skipper JC, Hendrickson RC, Gulden PH et al. An HLA-A2-restricted tyrosinase antigen on melanoma cells results from posttranslational modification and suggests a novel pathway for processing of membrane proteins. J Exp Med 1996; 183:527-34.
428.Kang X, Kawakami Y, el Gamil M et al. Identification of a tyrosinase epitope recognized by HLA-A24-restricted, tumor-infiltrating lymphocytes. J Immunol 1995; 155:1343-8.
429.Brichard VG, Herman J, Van Pel A et al. A tyrosinase nonapeptide presented by HLA-B44 is recognized on a human melanoma by autologous cytolytic T lymphocytes. Eur J Immunol 1996; 26: 224-30.
430.Schild H, Grüneberg U, Pougialis G et al. Natural ligand motifs of H-2E molecules are allele specific and illustrate homology to HLA-DR molecules. Int Immunol 1996; 7:1957-65.
431.Malcherek G, Falk K, Rötzschke O et al. Natural peptide ligand motifs of two HLA molecules associated with myasthenia gravis. Int Immunol 1993; 5: 1229-37.
432.Friede T, Gnau V, Jung G et al. Natural ligand motifs of closely related HLA-DR4 molecules predict features of rheumatoid arthritis associated peptides. Biochim Biophys Acta 1996; 1316:85-101.
433.Marrack P, Ignatowicz L, Kappler JW et al. Comparison of peptides bound to

spleen and thymus class II. J Exp Med 1993; 178:2173-83.
434.Nelson CA, Roof RW, McCourt DW et al. Identification of the naturally processed form of hen egg white lysozyme bound to the murine major histocompatibility complex class II molecule I-A^k. Proc Natl Acad Sci U S A 1992; 89: 7380-3.
435.Chicz RM, Urban RG, Gorga JC et al. Specificity and promiscuity among naturally processed peptides bound to HLA-DR alleles. J Exp Med 1993; 178:27-47.
436.Reizis B, Mor F, Eisenstein M et al. The peptide binding specificity of the MHC class II I-A molecule of the Lewis rat, RT1B^l. Int Immunol 1996; 8:1825-32.
437.Verreck FA, van de Poel A, Drijfhout JW et al. Natural peptides isolated from Gly86/Val86-containing variants of HLA-DR1, -DR11, -DR13, and -DR52. Immunogenetics 1996; 43:392-7.
438.Kirschmann DA, Duffin KL, Smith CE et al. Naturally processed peptides from rheumatoid arthritis associated and non-associated HLA-DR alleles. J Immunol 1995; 155:5655-62.
439.Kinouchi R, Kobayasi H, Sato K et al. Peptide motifs of HLA-DR4/DR53 (DRB1*0405/DRB4*0101) molecules. Immunogenetics 1994; 40:376-8.
440.Futaki G, Kobayashi H, Sato K et al. Naturally processed HLA-DR9/DR53 (DRB1*0901/DRB4*0101)-bound peptides. Immunogenetics 1995; 42:299-301.
441.Davenport MP, Quinn CL, Chicz RM et al. Naturally processed peptides from two disease-resistance-associated HLA-DR13 alleles show related sequence motifs and the effects of the dimorphism at position 86 of the HLA-DR beta chain. Proc Natl Acad Sci U S A 1995; 92:6567-71.
442.Hunt DF, Michel H, Dickinson TA et al. Peptides presented to the immune system by the murine class II major histocompatibility complex molecule I-A^d. Science 1992; 256:1817-20.
443.Nelson CA, Viner NJ, Young SP et al. A negatively charged anchor residue promotes high affinity binding to the MHC class II molecule I-A^k. J Immunol 1996; 157:755-62.
444.Hayden JB, McCormack AL, Yates III JR et al. Analysis of naturally processed peptides eluted from HLA DRB1*0402 and *0404. J Neurosci Res 1996; 45:795-802.
445.Rötzschke O, Falk K. Origin, structure and motifs of naturally processed MHC class II ligands. Curr Opin Immunol 1994; 6:45-51.
446.Rudensky AY, Preston Hurlburt P, Hong SC et al. Sequence analysis of peptides bound to MHC class II molecules. Nature 1991; 353:622-7.
447.Davenport MP, Godkin A, Friede T et al. A distinctive peptide binding motif for HLA-DRB1*0407, an HLA-DR4 subtype not associated with rheumatoid arthritis. Immunogenetics 1997; 45:229-32.
448.Vartdal F, Johannsen BH, Friede T et al. The peptide binding motif for the disease associated HLA-DQ (α1*0501, β1*0201) molecule. Eur J Immunol 1996; 26:2764-72.
449.Verreck FAW, Vermeulen C, v.d.Poel A et al. The generation of SDS-stable HLA DR dimers is independent of efficient peptide binding. Int Immunol 1996; 8:397-404.
450.Falk K, Rötzschke O, Stevanović S et al. Pool sequencing of natural HLA-DR, DQ, and DP ligands reveals detailed peptide motifs, constraints of processing, and general rules. Immunogenetics 1994; 39:230-42.
451.Newcomb JR, Cresswell P. Characterization of endogenous peptides bound to purified HLA-DR molecules and their absence from invariant chain-associated alpha beta dimers. J Immunol 1993; 150:499-507.
452.Adibzadeh M, Friccius H, Bornhak S et al. Role of three quantitatively dominant endogenous peptides from HLA-DRB1*0401 molecules in class II specific allreactivity. Transplant Immunol 1994; 2:293-9.
453.Matsushita S, Takahashi K, Motoki M et al. Allele specificity of structural requirement for peptides bound to HLA-DRB1*0405 and -DRB1*0406 complexes: implication for the HLA-associated susceptibility to methimazole-induced insulin autoimmune syndrome. J Exp Med 1994; 180:873-83.
454.Rudensky AY, Preston Hurlburt P, al Ramadi BK et al. Truncation variants of

peptides isolated from MHC class II molecules suggest sequence motifs. Nature 1992; 359:429-31.
455.Stern LJ, Brown JH, Jardetzky TS et al. Crystal structure of the human class II MHC protein HLA-DR1 complexed with an influenza virus peptide. Nature 1994; 368:215-21.
456.Riberdy JM, Newcomb JR, Surman MJ et al. HLA-DR molecules from an antigen-processing mutant cell line are associated with invariant chain peptides. Nature 1992; 360:474-7.
457.Sette A, Ceman S, Kubo RT et al. Invariant chain peptides in most HLA-DR molecules of an antigen-processing mutant. Science 1992; 258:1801-4.
458.Schmidt CM, Orr HT. Maternal/fetal interactions: the role of the MHC class I molecule HLA-G. Crit Rev Immunol 1993; 13:207-24.
459.Feder JN, Gnirke A, Thomas W et al. A novel MHC class I-like gene is mutated in patients with hereditary haemochromatosis. Nat Genet 1996; 13:399-408.
460.Roitt IM. Essential Immunology. 8th ed. Oxford: Blackwell Scientific Publications; 1994.
461.Wegener S. HLA und Krankheitsassoziationen. Infusionsther Transfusionsmed 1994; 21:213-9.
462.Hammer J, Gallazzi F, Bono E et al. Peptide binding specificity of HLA-DR4 molecules: correlation with rheumatoid arthritis association. J Exp Med 1995; 181:1847-55.
463.Friede T, Gnau V, Jung G et al. Natural ligand motifs of closely related HLA-DR4 molecules predict features of rheumatoid arthritis associated peptides. Biochim Biophys Acta 1996; 1316:85-101.
464.Todd JA, Bell JI, McDevitt HO. HLA-DQ beta gene contributes to susceptibility and resistance to insulin-dependent diabetes mellitus. Nature 1987; 329:599-604.
465.Morel PA, Dorman JS, Todd JA et al. Aspartic acid at position 57 of the HLA-DQ beta chain protects against type I diabetes: a family study [published erratum appears in Proc Natl Acad Sci U S A 1989; 86:1317]. Proc Natl Acad Sci U S A 1988; 85:8111-5.
466.Boon T, Cerottini JC, van den Eynde B et al. Tumor antigens recognized by T lymphocytes. Annu Rev Immunol 1994; 12:337-65.
467.Reisfeld RA, Gillies SD. Recombinant antibody fusion proteins for cancer immunotherapy. Curr Top Microbiol Immunol 1996; 213:27-53.
468.Handgretinger R, Anderson K, Lang P et al. A phase I study of human/mouse chimeric antiganglioside GD2 antibody ch14.18 in patients with neuroblastoma. Eur J Cancer 1995; 31A:261-7.
469.Reisfeld RA, Greene ML, Yachi A. Fifth Annual Sapporo Cancer Seminar. Monoclonal antibodies—progress in cancer immunobiology and clinical application. Cancer Res 1986; 46:2193-6.
470. Pantel K, Riethmuller G. Micrometastasis detection and treatment with monoclonal antibodies. Curr Top Microbiol Immunol 1996; 213:1-18.
471.De Plaen E, Lurquin C, Van Pel A et al. Immunogenic (tum-) variants of mouse tumor P815: cloning of the gene of tum-antigen P91A and identification of the tum- mutation. Proc Natl Acad Sci U S A 1988; 85:2274-8.
472.van der Bruggen P, Traversari C, Chomez P et al. A gene encoding an antigen recognized by cytolytic T lymphocytes on a human melanoma. Science 1991; 254:1643-7.
473.Rosenberg SA. The immunotherapy of solid cancers based on cloning the genes encoding tumor-rejection antigens. Annu Rev Med 1996; 47:481-91.
474.Pardoll DM. Tumour antigens. A new look for the 1990s. Nature 1994; 369: 357.
475.Riddell SR, Greenberg PD. Principles for adoptive T cell therapy of human viral diseases. Annu Rev Immunol 1995; 13: 545-86.
476.Toes RE, Offringa R, Feltkamp MC et al. Tumor rejection antigens and tumor specific cytotoxic T lymphocytes. Behring Inst Mitt 1994; 94:72-86.
477.Marchand M, Weynants P, Rankin E et al. Tumor regression responses in melanoma patients treated with a peptide encoded by gene MAGE-3. Int J Cancer 1995; 63:883-5.
478.Young JW, Inaba K. Dendritic cells as adjuvants for class I major histocompat-

ibility complex-restricted antitumor immunity. J Exp Med 1996; 183:7-11.
479.Topalian SL, Gonzales MI, Parkhurst M et al. Melanoma-specific CD4+T cells recognize nonmutated HLA-DR-restricted tyrosinase epitopes. J Exp Med 1996; 183:1965-71.
480.Topalian SL. MHC class II restricted tumor antigens and the role of CD4+ T cells in cancer immunotherapy. Curr Opin Immunol 1994; 6:741-5.
481.Boel P, Wildmann C, Sensi ML et al. BAGE: a new gene encoding an antigen recognized on human melanomas by cytolytic T lymphocytes. Immunity 1995; 2:167-75.
482.Frumento G, Harris PE, Gawinowicz MA et al. Sequence of a prominent 16-residue self-peptide bound to HLA-B27 in a lymphoblastoid cell line. Cell Immunol 1993; 152:623-6.
483. van den Eynde B, Peeters O, De Backer O et al. A new family of genes coding for an antigen recognized by autologous cytolytic T lymphocytes on a human melanoma. J Exp Med 1995; 182:689-98.
484.Kawakami Y, Eliyahu S, Jennings C et al. Recognition of multiple epitopes in the human melanoma antigen gp100 by tumor-infiltrating T lymphocytes associated with in vivo tumor regression. J Immunol 1995; 154:3961-8.
485.Wang RF, Parkhurst MR, Kawakami Y et al. Utilization of an alternative open reading frame of a normal gene in generating a novel human cancer antigen. J Exp Med 1996; 183:1131-40.
486.Fisk B, Blevins TL, Wharton JT et al. Identification of an immunodominant peptide of HER-2/neu protooncogene recognized by ovarian tumor-specific cytotoxic T lymphocyte lines. J Exp Med 1995; 181:2109-17.
487.Fisk B, Savary C, Hudson JM et al. Changes in an HER-2 peptide upregulating HLA-A2 expression affect both conformational epitopes and CTL recognition: implications for optimization of antigen presentation and tumor-specific CTL induction. J Immunother Emphasis Tumor Immunol 1995; 18:197-209.
488.Traversari C, van der Bruggen P, Luescher IF et al. A nonapeptide encoded by human gene MAGE-1 is recognized on HLA-A1 by cytolytic T lymphocytes directed against tumor antigen MZ2-E. J Exp Med 1992; 176:1453-7.
489.van der Bruggen P, Traversari C, Chomez P et al. A gene encoding an antigen recognized by cytolytic T lymphocytes on a human melanoma. Science 1991; 254:1643-7.
490.Gaugler B, van den Eynde B, van der Bruggen P et al. Human gene MAGE-3 codes for an antigen recognized on a melanoma by autologous cytolytic T lymphocytes. J Exp Med 1994; 179: 921-30.
491.Celis E, Tsai V, Crimi C et al. Induction of anti-tumor cytotoxic T lymphocytes in normal humans using primary cultures and synthetic peptide epitopes. Proc Natl Acad Sci U S A 1994; 91: 2105-9.
492.van der Bruggen P, Bastin J, Gajewski T et al. A peptide encoded by human gene MAGE-3 and presented by HLA-A2 induces cytolytic T lymphocytes that recognize tumor cells expressing MAGE-3. Eur J Immunol 1994; 24:3038-43.
493.Herman J, van der Bruggen P, Luescher IF et al. A peptide encoded by the human MAGE3 gene and presented by HLA-B44 induces cytolytic T lymphocytes that recognize tumor cells expressing MAGE3. Immunogenetics 1996; 43: 377-83.
494.Coulie PG, Brichard V, Van Pel A et al. A new gene coding for a differentiation antigen recognized by autologous cytolytic T lymphocytes on HLA-A2 melanomas. J Exp Med 1994; 180:35-42.
495.Kawakami Y, Eliyahu S, Delgado CH et al. Cloning of the gene coding for a shared human melanoma antigen recognized by autologous T cells infiltrating into tumor. Proc Natl Acad Sci U S A 1994; 91:3515-9.
496.Kawakami Y, Eliyahu S, Sakaguchi K et al. Identification of the immunodominant peptides of the MART-1 human melanoma antigen recognized by the majority of HLA-A2-restricted tumor infiltrating lymphocytes. J Exp Med 1994; 180:347-52.
497.Rivoltini L, Kawakami Y, Sakaguchi K et al. Induction of tumor-reactive CTL

from peripheral blood and tumor-infiltrating lymphocytes of melanoma patients by in vitro stimulation with an immunodominant peptide of the human melanoma antigen MART-1. J Immunol 1995; 154:2257-65.
498.Castelli C, Storkus WJ, Maeurer MJ et al. Mass spectrometric identification of a naturally processed melanoma peptide recognized by CD8+ cytotoxic T lymphocytes. J Exp Med 1995; 181:363-8.
499.Fleischhauer K, Tanzarella S, Wallny H et al. Multiple HLA-A alleles can present an immunodominant peptide of the human melanoma antigen Melan-A/MART-1 to a peptide-specific HLA-A*0201+ cytotoxic T cell line. J Immunol 1996; 157:787-97.
500.Blake J, Johnston JV, Hellstrom KE et al. Use of combinatorial peptide libraries to construct functional mimics of tumor epitopes recognized by MHC class I-restricted cytolytic T lymphocytes. J Exp Med 1996; 184:121-30.
501.Coulie PG, Lehmann F, Lethe B et al. A mutated intron sequence codes for an antigenic peptide recognized by cytolytic T lymphocytes on a human melanoma. Proc Natl Acad Sci U S A 1995; 92: 7976-80.
502.Mandelboim O, Berke G, Fridkin M et al. CTL induction by a tumour-associated antigen octapeptide derived from a murine lung carcinoma. Nature 1994; 369:67-71.
503.Robbins PF, el Gamil M, Li YF et al. Cloning of a new gene encoding an antigen recognized by melanoma-specific HLA-A24-restricted tumor-infiltrating lymphocytes. J Immunol 1995; 154: 5944-50.
504.Gnjatić S, Bressac de Paillerets B, Guillet JG et al. Mapping and ranking of potential cytotoxic T epitopes in the p53 protein: effect of mutations and polymorphism on peptide binding to purified and refolded HLA molecules. Eur J Immunol 1995; 25:1638-42.
505.Ciernik F, Berzofsky JA, Carbone DP. Induction of cytotoxic T lymphocytes and antitumor immunity with DNA vaccines expressing single T cell epitopes. J Immunol 1996; 156:2369-75.
506.Bertholet S, Iggo R, Corradin G. Cytotoxic T lymphocyte responses to wild-type and mutant mouse p53 peptides. Eur J Immunol 1997; 27:798-801.
507.Lacabanne V, Viguier M, Guillet J et al. A wild-type p53 cytotoxic T cell epitope is presented by mouse hepatocarcinoma cells. Eur J Immunol 1996; 26:2635-9.
508.Sibille C, Chomez P, Wildmann C et al. Structure of the gene of tum- transplantation antigen P198: a point mutation generates a new antigenic peptide. J Exp Med 1990; 172:35-45.
509.Wallny HJ, Deres K, Faath S et al. Identification and quantification of a naturally presented peptide as recognized by cytotoxic T lymphocytes specific for an immunogenic tumor variant. Int Immunol 1992; 4:1085-90
510. McCormick D, Stauss HJ, Thorpe C et al. Major histocompatibility complex and T cell receptor interaction of the P91 tum- peptide. Eur J Immunol 1996; 26:2895-902.
511.Cox AL, Skipper J, Chen Y et al. Identification of a peptide recognized by five melanoma-specific human cytotoxic T cell lines. Science 1994; 264:716-9.
512.Kawakami Y, Eliyahu S, Delgado CH et al. Identification of a human melanoma antigen recognized by tumor-infiltrating lymphocytes associated with in vivo tumor rejection. Proc Natl Acad Sci U S A 1994; 91:6458-62.
513.Skipper JCA, Kittlesen DJ, Hendrickson RC et al. Shared epitopes for HLA-A3-restricted melanoma-reactive human CTL include a naturally processed epitope from Pmel-17/gp100. J Immunol 1996; 157:5027-33.
514.Gaugler B, Brouwenstijn N, Vantomme V et al. A new gene coding for an antigen recognized by autologous cytolytic T lymphocytes on a human renal carcinoma. Immunogenetics 1996; 44:323-30.
515.Abrams SI, Stanziale SF, Lunin SD et al. Identification of overlapping epitopes in mutant ras oncogene peptides that activate CD4+ and CD8+ T cell responses. Eur J Immunol 1996; 26:435-43.
516.Wang R, Appella E, Kawakami Y et al. Identification of TRP-2 as a human tu-

mor antigen recognized by cytotoxic T lymphocytes. J Exp Med 1996; 184: 2207-16.

517.Lurquin C, Van Pel A, Mariame B et al. Structure of the gene of tum- transplantation antigen P91A: the mutated exon encodes a peptide recognized with Ld by cytolytic T cells. Cell 1989; 58:293-303.

518.van den Eynde B, Mazarguil H, Lethe B et al. Localization of two cytotoxic T lymphocyte epitopes and three anchoring residues on a single nonameric peptide that binds to H-2L_d and is recognized by cytotoxic T lymphocytes against mouse tumor P815. Eur J Immunol 1994; 24:2740-5.

519.Lethé B, van den Eynde B, Van Pel A et al. Mouse tumor rejection antigens P815A and P815B: two epitopes carried by a single peptide. Eur J Immunol 1992; 22:2283-8.

520.Szikora JP, Van Pel A, Boon T. Tum- mutation P35B generates the MHC-binding site of a new antigenic peptide. Immunogenetics 1993; 37:135-8.

521.Buseyne F, Stevanović, Rammensee HG et al. Characterizaton of an HIV-1 $p24^{gag}$ epitope recognized by a $CD8^+$ cytotoxic T cell clone. Immunol Letters 1997; 55:145-149.

522.von Boehmer H. Thymic selection: a matter of life and death. Immunol Today 1992; 13:454-8.

APPENDIX A

USEFUL INTERNET ADDRESSES

Six years ago, Walter Gilbert urged that scientists "hook our individual computers into the worldwide network that gives us access to daily changes in the databases and also makes immediate our communications with each other."[1] The Internet expands constantly and with it the wealth of information; today's scientists can hardly do without it. New and additional data come up every day—not to speak of the daily communication processes over the net. Many data found in the present book were retrieved from various www addresses (see below) and subsequently collected in order to offer a specific and comprehensive compilation of data relating to the structure and function of MHC molecules. As the present data will continuously be updated, we have listed below some helpful addresses which we think may serve the molecular biologist's and immunologist's interests.

WWW Entrez: http://www.ncbi.nlm.nih.gov

This network browser is provided by the National Center for Biotechnology Information and allows searching and browsing of protein and nucleic acid databases, as well as related references from MEDLINE.

DBGET: http://www.genome.ad.jp/dbget/:

This is a database retrieval system and allows retrieval of related entries in different databases such as GenBank, EMBL, SWISS-PROT, PIR etc.

Pedro's Biomolecular Research Tools:

http: //www.public.iastate. edu/~pedro/research_tools.html. This is an outstanding collection of WWW links to services useful for molecular biologists. It comprises a list of molecular biology database search and analysis facilities, and bibliographies.

Sequence databases

EMBL: http://www.ebi.ac.uk/ebi_docs/embl_db/ebi/topembl.html
GENBANK: http://www.ncbi.nlm.nih.gov/Genbank/index.html
GSDB:http://www.ncgr.org/gsdb/gsdb.html
PIR:http://www.gdb.org/Dan/proteins/pir.html
SWISS-PROT: http://www.ebi.ac.uk/ebi_docs/swiss-prot_db/swisshome.html

MHC Resources

http://www.uni-tuebingen.de/uni/kxi/:

Our own homepage provides access to MHC ligands and peptide motifs.

http://www.icnet.uk/axp/tia/index.html:

This page provides links to resources available from the Tissue Antigen Laboratory at the Imperial Cancer Research Fund. Included are HLA sequence data, HLA nomenclature including monthly updates.

http://histo.cryst.bbk.ac.uk:

Histo is dedicated to the investigation of the relationship between sequence, structure and function of the proteins of the MHC. There are also collections of mouse class II sequences and non human and non mouse sequences.

http://www.hgmp.mrc.ac.uk:

This is a database of the human MHC and contains cDNA sequences of all current alleles as well as physical maps.[2]

http://wehi.wehi.edu.au/mhcpep/:

Database of Major Histocompatibility Complex binding peptides at the Walter and Eliza Hall Institute-Melbourne, Australia.

http://www3.ncbi.nlm.nih.gov:

This access is provided by the National Center for Biotechnology Information and offers gene maps of the human genome as well as human/mouse homology map.

http://www.swmed.edu/home_pages/ASHI/ashi.htm:

This is organized by the American Society for Histocompatibility and Immunogenetics and offers access to HLA sequence alignments.

http://hiv-web.lanl.gov/immuno:

HIV Molecular Immunology Database. Offers T cell epitope maps on HIV proteins, alignments, and annotation, as well as a summary and map of linear B cell epitopes and monoclonal antibodies.

References

1. Gilbert W. Towards a paradigm shift in biology. Nature 1991; 349:99.
2. Newell WR, Trowsdale J, Beck S. MHCDB: database of the human MHC (release 2). Immunogenetics 1996; 45:6-8.

APPENDIX B

COMPUTER PROGRAMS ARE AVAILABLE FROM THE FOLLOWING SOURCES:

Joe D'Amaro
Department of Immunohematology and Blood Bank
University Hospital Leiden
PO Box 9600
2300 RD Leiden
The Netherlands

Miles Davenport
Molecular Immunology Group
Institute of Molecular Medicine
Nuffield Department of Medicine
University of Oxford
John Radcliffe Hospital
Headington, OX3 9DU
United Kingdom

Burkhard Fleckenstein
NMI (Naturwissenschaftliches und Medizinisches Institut an der Universität Tübingen in Reutlingen)
Eberhardstr. 29
72762 Reutlingen
Germany

Jürgen Hammer
Roche Milano Ricerche
Via Olgettina 58
20132 Milano
Italy

APPENDIX C

ABBREVIATIONS

4F2	lymphocyte activation antigen 4F2
AA	amino acids
ACh	acetylcholine
Ag	antigen
APC	adenomatous polyposis coli protein
B. polymyxa	*Bacillus polymyxa*
β_2m	β2-microglobulin
BAGE	tumor antigen
Bf	factor B
β-gal	β-galactosidase
BHRF	Epstein-Barr virus bcl-2 homologue
BIP	bone inducing protein
BLAST-1	B-lymphocyte activation marker
BSA	bovine serum albumin
BST-2	bone marrow stromal cell membrane protein
BZLF1	Epstein-Barr virus trans-activator protein
C.	*Caenorhabditis* spec.
cAg	core antigen
CArG	mouse CArG-binding factor A
CD	cluster of differentiation
CDK4wt	cycline dependent kinase
CKS-2	cylcine dependent kinase subunit 2
CKShs1	cycline-dependent kinases regulatory subunit 1
CLIP	class II associated invariant chain peptide
cM	centiMorgans
c-myc	proto-oncogene
COI	cytochrome c oxidase polypeptide I
CRE	cAMP response element
CRY	*Cryptomeria japonica* major allergen
CSFV	classical swine fever virus
CSP	circumsporozoite protein
CYP21	steroid 21-hydroxylase
Derp	*Dermatophagoides pteronyssinus*
E. coli	*Escherichia coli*
E1-E7	immediate early protein
EBNA	Epstein-Barr virus nuclear antigen
EBV	Epstein-Barr-virus

elFC	protein translation factor
env	envelope
EqMb	equine myoglobin
ER	endoplasmic reticulum
ER60	endoplasmic reticulum resident protein
ERP72	endoplasmic reticulum resident protein
Fc	fragment cystallizable
FLU	Influenza
Fr	fraction
GAD	glutamic acid decarboxylase
gag	group-specific antigen
GAGE	tumor antigen
GBLP	guanine nucleotide binding protein β subunit-like protein
gp	gylcoprotein
gp100	—›pmel
GPIX	platelet glycoprotein IX (syn.: CD42A)
HA	hemagglutimin
HBBCP	human cytomegalovirus
HCV	Hepatitis B virus
HEL	hen egg lysozyme
HER-2	proto-oncogene
HER-2/neu	—›HER-2
HFPS	human fasyl pyrophosphate synthetase
HGNBP	human nucleotide binding protein
HIV	human immunodeficiency virus
HLA	human lymphocyte antigen
hn RNP	heterogenous ribonucleoprotein
HPV	human papilloma virus
HS1	hematopoietic lineage cell specific protein
HSC	heat shock protein constitutive
HSHM	human expressed sequence tag
HSP	heat shock protein
HSrn	human C6.1A protein (proto-oncogene)
HSV	Herpes simplex virus
HTLV	Human T-lymphotrophic virus
ICAM	intercellular adhesion molecule
ICP-27	HSV infected cell protein (transciptional regulator IE63)
ICS	IFN consensus sequence
IDDM	insulin dependent diabetes mellitus
IE	immediate early
IEF	human retinoblastoma binding protein P48
IFN	interferon
Ig	immunoglobulin
Ig VH	immunoglobulin variable region of heavy chain
Ig-SF	immunoglobulin super family
Ii	invariant chain
IL	interleukin
Int-6	a highly conserved, widely expressed gene, which is mutated by mouse mammary tumor virus in mammary preneoplasia
IP	prostacyclin receptor gene
IRBP	interphotoreceptor retinoid-binding protein

IRS	IFN response sequence
JAK1	Janus kinase
JHMV	JHM strain of mouse hepatitus virus
kb	kilobase pairs
kD	kilo-Dalton
K-ras	Kirsten-ras
L.	*Listeria* spec.
LAR	leucocyte antigen related
LCMV	lymphocytic choriomeningitis virus
LDH	lactate dehydrogenase
LDL	low density lipoprotein
lem A	putative regulator protein in L.monocytogenes
LIF	leukemia inhibitory factor
LLO	listeriolysin O
lmp-1	latent membrane protein 1
lmp-2	latent membrane protein 2
lmrA	lincomycin resistance protein from *S. lincolnensis*
Lol P	*Lolium perenne*
LSA-1	liver-stage antigen-1
Ly	lymphocyte antigen
M.	*Mycobacterium* spec.
MAGE	melanoma associated antigen
MART-1	melanoma antigen
MBP	myelin basic protein
Mbp	megabase pairs
MCC	moth cytochrome c
MCMV	murine cytomegalovirus
mdm	tumor antigen
Melan/MART-1	—›Mart-1
MET	oncogene
MHV	mouse hepatitis virus
MIF	migration inhibitory factor
miHAg	minor histocompatibility antigen
MMTV	murine mammory tumor virus
MOG	myelin oligodendrocyte glycoprotein
MoHb	mouse hemoglobin
MoMb	mouse myoglobin
MP	matrix protein
MuLV	murine leukemia virus
MUM-1	tumor antigen
MUT	tumor antigen
MV	measles virus
nef	negative factor
NK	natural killer
NKAT	natural killer associated transcript
NP	nucleoprotein
NRE	negative response element
NS	nonstructural proteins
OGDH	oxoglutarate dehydrogenase
ORF	open reading frame
OVA	ovalbumin

P.	*Plasmodium* spec.
P1-CDC21	human CDC21 homolog (chromatin binding protein)
p2CA	murine alpha-ketoglutarate dehydrogenase homologue
PA28	20S proteasome regulator (syn.: 11S regulator)
PAI-1	plasminogen activator inhibitor-1
PB1	RNA-directed RNA polymerase subunit P1
PCC	pigeon cytochrome c
PGAL	phosphoglyceraldehyde
PGSG	platelet proteolycan core protein
PKM-2	pyruvate kinase M1 (muscle) isoenzyme
PLP	proteolipid protein
pmel	melanoma antigen (syn.: gp 100)
pol	polymerase
pp	phosphoprotein
PR	Puerto Rico
PRAI-SCS	yeast phosphoribosyl aminomidazole succinocarboxamide cynthase
prec.	precursor
preS	Hepatitis B virus S antigen precursos
RAGE	tumor antigen
ras	proto-oncogene
RBAP-2	retinoblastoma associated protein 2
rep	regulator of replication and gene expression
RSV	respiratory syncytial virus
RT	reverse transcriptase
S. lincolnensis	*Streptomyces lincolnensis*
sAg	soluble antigen
SEC61	endoplasmic reticulum peptide exporter
SFV	Semliki Forest virus
SIV	simian immunodeficiency virus
SLE	systemic lupus erythematosus
SMCY	male-specific transplantation antigen (ubiquitously transcribed teratricopeptide repeat gene on the Y chromosome)
SNase	Staphylococcal nuclease
SSP2	sporozoite S protein 2
SSR	signal sequence receptor
STARP	sporozoite threonine and asparagine rich protein
Substance P	neuropeptide
SV	Sendai virus
SWM	→SWMb
SWMb	sperm whale myoglobin
T	T-antigen
TAP	transporter associated with antigen processing
tax	HTLV-1 derived trans-activator
TCR	T cell receptor
TCR V	T cell-receptor variable segment
TF	transcription factor
Tf	transferrin
TIMP-1	tissue inhibitor of metalloproteinase 1
TIMP-2	tissue inhibitor of metalloproteinase 2
TIS	EGF-response factor 1

TNF	tumor necrosis factor
TRAP	thrombospondin related anonymous protein
TRP-2	tyrosinase related protein
UBC	ubiquitin conjugating enzyme
UC	unrelated chromatin
UL-18	HCMV gene encoding a class I heavy chain homologue
VLA	adhesion receptor
YOP	*Yersinia* outer membrane protein
ysa-1	yeast protein (*Saccharomyces cerevisiae*)
miHAg	minor histocompatibility antigen
UL	viral gene locus

INDEX

MIX
Papier aus verantwortungsvollen Quellen
Paper from responsible sources
FSC® C105338

If you have any concerns about our products, you can contact us on
ProductSafety@springernature.com

In case Publisher is established outside the EU, the EU authorized representative is:
Springer Nature Customer Service Center GmbH
Europaplatz 3, 69115 Heidelberg, Germany

Printed by Libri Plureos GmbH
in Hamburg, Germany